Powwowing in Pennsylvania
Braucherei & the Ritual of Everyday Life

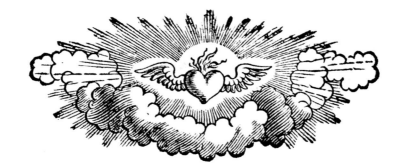

Powwowing in Pennsylvania

Braucherei & the Ritual of Everyday Life

Featuring Dr. Helfenstein's

Secrets of Sympathy

A New & Improved Translation

Patrick J. Donmoyer

Pennsylvania German Cultural Heritage Center
Kutztown University of Pennsylvania

2017

Powwowing in Pennsylvania: Braucherei & the Ritual of Everyday Life

By Patrick J. Donmoyer

Volume VI of the Annual Publication Series
The Pennsylvania German Cultural Heritage Center
Kutztown University of Pennsylvania

Printed in the United States on acid-free paper by Masthof Press, Morgantown, PA

Text, layout, and cover art by Patrick J. Donmoyer
Photography by the author, unless otherwise stated.

Copyright © 2018 Patrick J. Donmoyer

All rights reserved. No part of this book may be reprinted or reproduced or utilized in any form or by any electronic, mechanical or other means, now known or hereafter invented, including photocopying and recording or in any information storage or retrieval system, without permission in writing from the author and the publisher.

ISBN: 978-0-9987074-3-3 (Paperback)
ISBN: 978-0-9987074-8-8 (Hardback)
Library of Congress Control Number: 2017961881

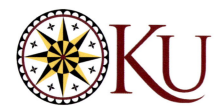

22 Luckenbill Road
Kutztown, Pennsylvania 19530
(610) 683-1589
heritage@kutztown.edu
www.kutztown.edu/pgchc

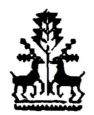

Masthof Press
219 Mill Road
Morgantown, PA 19543
(610) 286-0258
www.masthof.com

Dedicated
to
Ada Fox
&
Tom Nissley

In Memory
of
Don Yoder
(1921-2015)

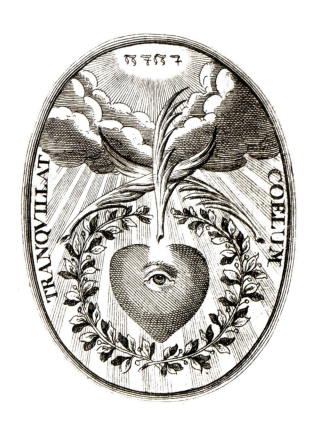

Contents

Preface: 13

Chapter I. Ritual Traditions of the Pennsylvania Dutch: 23

Chapter II. Faces of Powwowing: 33
Healers, Practitioners, and Facilitators

Chapter III. European Origins: 59
Benediction, Blessing, Brauchen

Chapter IV. Healing, Cosmology, & Faith: 99
Ritual Space & Performance

Chapter V. Ritual Literature: 127
Manuscripts, Books, Broadsides

Chapter VI. Hexerei & Ritual Harm: 175
Cursing, Hexing, Sorcery

Chapter VII. Herbal Rituals: 197
Trees, Shrubs, and Botanicals

Chapter VIII. Ritual Objects of Power: 215
Canes, Knives, Stones, Carvings

Chapter IX. Powwow & The Authorities: 231
Medical, Legal, Educational, Media

Chapter X. Rituals of Everyday Life: 257
Domestic, Agricultural, Sacred

Conclusion: 283

Appendix. Dr. Helfenstein's *Secrets of Sympathy*: 285

Endnotes: 307

Bibliography: 331

Index: 337

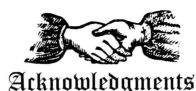

Acknowledgments

I am deeply grateful for the assistance, encouragement, and support of so many people, without whom this work would not have been possible. Because this book is the result of work in the community for over a decade, there is insufficient space here to thank every person who has had an impact on this project. Nevertheless, I would like to express my gratitude to all those who have directly contributed to the development of this work in no particular order and regretting in advance any unintended omission:

To Tom Nissley, for his support, encouragement, and friendship throughout the duration of this important project. To William Woys Weaver, for his friendship, insights, and assistance in assembling the materials featured throughout this work. To Reg Good, for his invaluable contributions to expanding the scope of the folk-religious materials featured in this work, especially those representative of the European experience. To Clarke Hess and Lee Stolzfus, for welcoming me on so many visits to document Clarke's early American powwowing materials.

To the staff at Glencairn Museum, Brian Henderson, Ed Gyllenhaal, and Bret Bostock for hosting the exhibition that not only showcased the collections featured in this book, but also provided a venue for the material culture of powwowing to inspire thoughtful dialogue about the role of spiritual traditions in fostering empathy and building understanding among all people. To the Schwenkfelder Library and Heritage Center, especially David Luz and Candace Perry for their role in hosting the first exhibition and conference. To Lisa Randolph and Michael Emery for graciously allowing the powwowing collection of the late Lester Breininger to play such a significant role in this project. To Willard Martin, for entrusting the carved powwowing Bible-board to this project. To Anna Mae Grubb for the powwowing papers of her grandfather, Nathan Fernsler Krall.

To Russell Earnest and Patricia Suter for the use of materials from The Earnest Archive and Library. To Ned and Linda Heindel for their hospitality and access to Hexenkopf and the Raubsville powwowing materials. To Thomas Gable and family, for allowing me to feature the family photographs of Reading healer Joseph H. Hageman. To the Rev. Brian Haas and Lee Haas and family for the extensive materials on Dennis Rex of Slatedale. To Gregory Wonders and family for allowing me to feature the manuscript of Levi Laydom in this work, and to Mark Hagenbuch for introducing and facilitating the exchange. To Jim and Maria Houston for permission to feature materials in this book and in the exhibition. To Sharon O'Neal-Lehner for sharing her family history. To Carl and Minerva Arner for generously sharing their Good Friday eggs and rain water with the Heritage Center.

To Dr. Bill Donner, chair of the Publications Committee, and Dr. Jennifer Schlegel of the Advisory Committee, as readers of the text and for their encouragement and thoughtful assistance in preparing this project for publication. To Daniel Harms for his camaraderie, and helpful suggestions in preparing the work, as a reader of the text. To Edward E. Quinter for his thorough attention to language, and his assistance and shared enthusiasm over many years in transcribing and translating early German manuscripts. To Natacha Klein Käfer, for her important contributions in the field, and for expanding my horizons beyond North America and Europe, to include South American Brazilian experience. To Jack Montgomery, for his friendship and encouragement throughout this project and in the years leading up to it's publication. To Joyce Munro for her stellar editorial assistance and helpful suggestions. To Mark Louden for his friendship, sound advice, and encouragement, as well as his editorial support in this project and in the creation of the Powwowing in Pennsylvania exhibition booklet.

To all of the institutions that lent or provided permission for materials to appear in this book and the exhibition at Glencairn Museum, especially The Mercer Museum and Bucks County Historical Society, The Library Company of Philadelphia, The Landis Valley Museum, Kutztown Historical Society, The Pennsylvania Folklife Society Collection at Ursinus College, Historic Schaefferstown Inc., The Evangelical & Reformed Historical Society, Lancaster, The Lehigh Valley Heritage Museum, Special Collections at the Franklin & Marshall College Library, The First United Church of Christ Easton, Williams Township Historical and Genealogical Society, Lower Macungie Township Historical Society, and Albany Township Historical Society.

To all those who shared their talents, energies, stories, memories, experiences, and those who provided materials essential to this project, especially, Mark Alwein and Annabel Karnes, Terry Berger, Dennis Boyer, Donald Breininger, Josh Brown, Keith Brintzenhof, Eric Claypoole, Robert Cook, David DelNegro, Cody Dickerson, Dave Dietrich, Marlin Dietrich and Family, Robert Ensminger, Fred Fritch, Peter V. Fritsch, Rev. John Heffner, Susan Hess, Richard Hummel, Alan Keyser, Julie Kresge, Annabel Knorr, John Messner, Tammy Mitgang, Scott and Leslie Mertz, Kevin Nelson, Anna Mae Peterson, Harry Quinter, John Rausch, Marylynn Rathman, Richard Savidge, Bernard Schuman, Richard Shaner, Michael Showalter, Matthew Sicher and Jesse Tobin, Milton Sonday, Brendan and Meredith Strasser, Bill Unger, David Valuska, Elaine Vardjan, Sarajane Williams, Chris Witmer, Michael Yarnall, and especially all those who remain anonymous, out of respect for their contributions in continuing the tradition.

To all of my colleagues at the Pennsylvania German Cultural Heritage Center at Kutztown University, especially Naomi Pauley and Lucy Kern for their helpful support throughout this project. To the staff at Masthof Press for their helpful assistance and patience as I prepared this project for print.

To my family, my parents Daniel and Susan Donmoyer, my grandmother J. LaRue Baeshore Galbraith, my inlaws John and Joyce Munro, and especially my wife Becca Munro and our daughter Ada Fox, for their unwavering support, assistance, patience, and love throughout the long year that this project was brought to life.

DISCLAIMER

A Caution to the Reader:

This book gives no medical or legal advice.

This work explores the cultural significance of ritual traditions, including remedies, and is intended for reference and folk-cultural study only. The author is not a physician, and does not advocate for use or experimentation with any of the rituals, procedures, or recipes described in this book that might be ineffective or harmful to your health.

This work is not indended to be used, nor should it be used, to diagnose, treat, or advise anyone in matters of health. Consult your doctor before any attempt to make use of the contents of this book. The reader assumes full responsibility for their own actions, and the author and the publisher are not liable for any consequences or negative outcomes arising from attempts to use or adopt any of the ideas contained herein.

CAVEAT LECTOR.

Preface

A Personal Journey

Under the light of the full moon, my great-great-grandfather took his knife and cut a potato in half. The cross-section shone in the moonlight, as he whispered a prayer in Pennsylvania Dutch, and began to rub a wart on my grandmother's hand with the potato. He repeated this three times, before putting the halves back together, and burying them under the downspout at the eaves of farm house. My grandmother was just a little girl, but she recalled that within a few days, her wart had vanished.

This was the very first powwow story that I heard as a child growing up in south central Pennsylvania. At the time that my grandmother told me about her experience, I hadn't the slightest notion that I would later feel compelled as a young adult to collect stories of ritual healing experiences from across the state and beyond.

Although many years have passed since my first exposure to the tradition, I can still remember that the most compelling part about the story was not the ritual procedure itself – but the nonchalance with which scores of people in Pennsylvania relate this very same experience, as though it were as commonplace as eating pie.

Although at present, my work among the Pennsylvania Dutch community of southeastern and central Pennsylvania has been in a professional capacity, my connection to the community in which I live, work, and study has also been a deeply personal reflection of my upbringing and cultural values.

Born in Pennsylvania, my roots extend across Lebanon, Berks, and Schuylkill counties, and like most others in that region, I am descended from diverse ancestry. My Pennsylvania Dutch roots are Alsatian, Swiss, and German, but generously mixed with Scotch-Irish, Welsh, English, and a touch of Shawnee. I grew up in an average American household, attended a Lutheran Church, and spent summers in the mountains of Northern Pennsylvania. Some of my grandparents remembered a time when there were still family farms, but many of my relatives worked for Bethlehem Steel in Lebanon City where I was born. At the same time, I was distinctly aware that my family was Pennsylvania Dutch. One of my grandfathers spoke Pennsylvania Dutch language to me when I was a child, and dressed plain for a significant portion of his life. All of my grandparents and two of my great-grandmothers spoke English with noticeably Dutchified accents, we all ate pork, sauerkraut, and potato filling on New Year's Day.

As the son of a Lutheran minister, my family moved a few times, first from Lebanon to Gettysburg, and then to southern York County. I later relocated to Berks and Montgomery counties, and everywhere I go, powwow stories seem to follow me.

My last remaining paternal great-grandmother died in 2004, and not long after that the stories began to come out that both she and her mother had powwowed. As with many families, such stories are rarely told unless someone has the forethought to ask. One relative remembered being powwowed for childhood illnesses with salt, which was disposed of in the griddle of the wood-fired cook-stove. I had been very close with my great-grandmother. She had adopted and raised my father, and our family had lived with her for a short while before moving to Gettysburg. She was an intelligent and spirited woman, with a clear memory, and told me many stories. She had never told me anything about her connection with powwowing, but then again, like many people of my generation, I had never directly asked. She did however, teach me an old remedy for hiccups – a condition to which I was prone as a child, because of a tendency to over-eat her delightful cooking. One was to take seven swallows of cold water in succession without breathing, and if it didn't work after trying it once, do it three times. I had understood that the numbers seven and three were significant, even holy according to some, but it was years before I had realized that this simple operation was a very basic, common form of powwowing. Although many powwow rituals involve elaborate prayers, the use of healing objects, or hand gestures, some rituals are as simple as my grandmother's cure for hiccups.

In 2006 I had the opportunity to learn to powwow from a traditional practitioner living just north of Kutztown. The woman who permitted me to learn from her (whose name I keep respectfully confidential) explained that although she could teach me words and procedures used in powwowing, everything had to be memorized. If I was unable to memorize the material or to recall it at will, then I was unfit to learn.

The majority of what I was to memorize were rounds of prayers in Pennsylvania Dutch along with a few in English, some for particular illnesses, and others as blessings for the body as a whole. Each set of prayers was accompanied by movements of the hands to physically inscribe the act of blessing, and remove an imbalance. I was taught prayers in three segments over three sessions. Each time I was seated on a chair facing east, and powwowed by my teacher, and I powwowed her in return to commit the lesson to memory.

Between each session with my teacher I was encouraged to practice the procedures in two ways. First I was to practice on an empty chair and simultaneously imagine myself seated upon it. Secondly, when I felt ready, I was to try sitting in the chair and learn to project my will outwards, and visualize practicing on myself. What I didn't know at the time is that I was being taught to conduct the rituals remotely, an essential component of the tradition, whereby a practitioner need not be in physical proximity to a person who is being powwowed.

Perhaps one of the most important things that I was taught is that although words and procedures can be learned, that there are some things that simply cannot be taught ('S gebt viel Dinge ass net gelannt warre kenne). On one hand this may on the surface appear to reinforce the old adage that there is no substitute for experience. At the same time, this also serves to remind anyone learning the tradition that every aspect is subject to some level of improvisation, and that there is a difference between actually powwowing, and simply going through the motions. Nevertheless, one must start somewhere.

Furthermore, I learned under the condition that if I were to transmit the information to others, I was bound to teach it the same way that I had learned, from a woman to a man, and vice versa, and purely as an oral tradition, not to be transmitted in any means by writing, or to be used for any objective outside of health and wholeness. This protocol was passed down to my teacher from her two male teachers, and to her teachers from their teachers, and so forth. This is the most common means that the tradition has been maintained over the centuries.

I was told that if I were to break such an agreement I would not only be unable to powwow effectively, but beyond this, I understood that to violate a teacher's trust would be to dishonor an elder as well as myself, and would be unbefitting of a healer. Such a compromise would also invariably set the tone for any subsequent use of the tradition, suggesting that what is obtained through dishonesty cannot be used for an honest purpose – essentially, the end does not justify the means.

Also requisite for learning to powwow is a willingness to use it for others. I began, somewhat self-consciously at first, to occasionally powwow for friends and family for a variety of ailments, as well as neighbors or anyone sent in my direction by word of mouth, and sometimes for complete strangers. Some found powwowing to be helpful and effective in addressing their concerns – in such cases, I can take absolutely no credit for any recovery or comfort, as I served merely as a conduit, and facilitator for a spiritual, and not purely physical, transformation.

Most of the people for whom I powwowed were dealing with conditions more complicated than purely physical afflictions, and these issues were frequently linked to spiritual and cultural concerns beyond the scope of conventional biomedical treatment. Everyone I've ever powwowed had either previously or concurrently received professional treatment from a doctor, and many had turned to powwow because of a distinct feeling that conventional medicine had not fully addressed their needs. It is true that like many other complementary or alternative medical systems, powwowing allows a person to participate in the act of becoming well in a way that may be deeply personal. Many of the people I have powwowed sought the experience for cultural reasons, and, because of the importance it held within their families, some found it deeply meaningful and healing. I have also powwowed for some concerns that were not specifically medical, such as one case for example, for a lost cat that returned home on the third day after the owner and I performed a ritual in the backyard based on directions in an eighteenth century manuscript from Lehigh County for recovering a lost horse. Like all traditions, powwow has continued to grow and change to meet the needs of people today.

Definitions of Powwowing and Elements of Its Practice

Pennsylvania's ritual healing traditions, known as powwowing or *Braucherei* in Pennsylvania Dutch, are recently experiencing a strong resurgence of interest as one of the oldest North American expressions of European folk belief that has survived to the present day. These distinctive ritual practices combine diverse applications of prayers, benedictions, gestures of blessing, and the use of everyday objects for the purpose of healing, protection from physical and spiritual harm, assistance in times of need, and assurance of positive outcomes in everyday affairs. These traditions have been passed by word of mouth and through written traditions from one generation to the next for over three centuries among the descendants of eighteenth-century German-speaking immigrants, known today as the Pennsylvania Dutch.

Although the word "powwow" is certainly Native American in origin, this term has also been used extensively since the eighteenth century to describe American healing practices of European origin. For better or for worse, powwowing is the most common designation today for the ritual traditions of the Pennsylvania Dutch. These practices are not to be confused with Native American traditions of the same name. Nonetheless, certain similarities with other traditional and indigenous healing systems may indeed be part of the reason that this term developed such a distinctive connotation in Pennsylvania.

Largely unknown outside of the communities in which these traditions are practiced, powwowing has remained in active use among the Pennsylvania Dutch to the present day and can be found in many places where the culture has spread across North America. Although its roots in the New World are the result of the massive transatlantic migration of German-speaking people from central Europe in the eighteenth century, powwowing is far from being a fossilized relic of a mythic, pre-industrial, agrarian past. Instead, as a vibrant expression of a dynamic folk culture, the survival of powwowing is evidence today of a legacy of adaptation and change. More subtly, its continued presence in modern society is an indication of a high-level of integration of ritual into the fabric of everyday life across many generations – an integration that ensured its survival and continued use in a rapidly changing society.

Although frequently construed as a purely esoteric, arcane, or covert practice, sequestered from the day-to-day lives of but only a select few individuals on the fringe of society, this perception is a fairly recent development in the history of powwowing, and the result of declining use in the home, in the garden, and on the farm. For many families no longer connected to the agricultural and domestic spheres that once united and shaped the culture, powwowing exists only in ancestral memory, as a precious heirloom that slipped away before anyone realized its importance. Some have forgotten that it was ever there at all.

In many communities, however, these traditions are still active, and participants in these practices are still living – both healers and those transformed by healing experiences. Stories continue to circulate and reinforce these experiences, as memories resurface of parents, grandparents, and great-grandparents, having been healed of childhood illnesses with simple ritual procedures, like passing an infant under the leg of a table for colic, or healing of a wart with a potato under the full moon. Some may recall specific rhymes or prayers, used to treat or prevent sickness, or of certain actions being performed three, seven, or nine times, and that ordinary objects, such as a dishcloth or a broom could have subtle uses beyond the mundane. Still others might remember that an everyday occurrence, such as the accidental dropping of a fork from the dinner table, could have special significance, or that the weather could be predicted using the breastbone of a goose.

Within communities where stories like these are still told (some far from Pennsylvania and scattered across the continent) knowledge and experience of powwowing is often still present, but very few know where to find it, or how to ask for it. Those who unwittingly stumble upon a powwow story within their family may struggle to fit such awareness into their lives. If narratives like these are kept secret, they can be a serious challenge to the next generation's sense of family identity, modernity, or faith, leaving important questions unanswered.

It is this very struggle for families to create meaningful narratives from stories of powwowing from previous generations that has provided the impetus for this exploration of Pennsylvania's healing traditions. This investigation is motivated by the lives and diverse accounts of everyday people, for these are the stories that are seldom told, and often ignored in favor of more salacious and scandalous tales. For this reason, this work will not focus exclusively on those aspects of the tradition that have been sensationalized in the media or the occasional tragic event that may still haunt our culture like the rural equivalents of urban legends. While there is much in the way of negative or misleading material about powwowing available to the average person in this age of information, there is also a tremendous amount of unexplored resources in stories that have never been committed to print, and in materials left behind by previous generations in the form of handwritten accounts in ledgers, papers tucked in family Bibles, and private manuscripts. Most important of all are the intangible aspects of the tradition, written in the hearts and minds of those who still maintain powwow practices as an active part of their lives – stories just waiting to be told.

Intentions and Purpose

This exploration aims to expand and enhance the dialogue of Pennsylvania's ritual traditions in four crucial directions, to better describe and interpret its relation to life, its range of accessibility, its diversity in form and practice, and its cultural origins.

First and foremost, this exploration will reach beyond the context of healing for a wider range of ritual expressions and applications woven throughout the domestic, agricultural, and religious spheres of life among the Pennsylvania Dutch. In order to establish a broader picture of powwowing, ritual procedures will be presented as a common theme in Pennsylvania Dutch experience and life – as opposed to a practice separate from the day-to-day. Powwowing is not separate from daily life. While powwowing is primarily a healing practice, ritual traditions also extend into farming, baking, hunting, fishing, gardening, and many other facets of life. It is also therefore necessary to demonstrate not only the way in which powwowing traditions have changed over time along with the structure of daily life, but also the way in these changes reflect the adaptation and development of the culture at large.

Second, I propose that the majority of ritual practices documented among the Pennsylvania Dutch over the last three centuries were not purely held under the purview of an elite class of practitioners, but rather in the hands of common everyday people. Rather than stress the secretive and esoteric aspects of powwowing to the exclusion of the domestic and agricultural applications, this work will aim to re-envision the relation of ritual in both the sacred and mundane spheres of life, and reframe it with a fundamentally more accessible narrative.

Third, this study will make every effort to present the character of powwowing as an inherently trans-cultural, polyethnic, and non-gender-specific ritual practice that embraces no one particular national, political, or religious agenda, but instead has consistently challenged contemporary notions of ethnic, geographic, and spiritual boundaries. This study will include practices and people who are of Irish, English, French, African American, Jewish, Native American, Latino, Roma, Greek, and Brazilian descent as essential fibers in Pennsylvania's colorful tapestry of ritual culture. On the other hand, this exploration will also provide evidence to suggest that Pennsylvania Dutch traditions, like those of many other cultures, have been occasionally both guilty of and subject to acts of cultural appropriation throughout the centuries, and these situations have contributed to some of the ambiguity and confusion concerning the early origins and the modern adaptations of powwowing.

Last, the European origins of powwowing will retrace the pilgrim's path from the rise of the veneration of saints in Roman Christendom to the Christianization of heathen Europe, which produced a winding labyrinth of liturgical and folk-cultural applications of benedictions in the Middle Ages. This study will explore the development of folk-cultural use of ritual, and follow these practices through times of crisis, witnessing its sanctioning and suppression during the Inquisition and Reformation. Ample European sources have laid dormant for far too long, obscured by the language barrier between American and German scholarship, with immense potential to provide a better understanding of how and under what circumstances European ritual traditions contributed to powwowing in Pennsylvania.

In addition, German sources reveal that many if not all of the crises concerning ritual traditions that arose in Pennsylvania and the United States, such as the effects of the rise of biomedicine on folk culture, and the sensationalism of ritual culture in mass media, are mirrored in their European counterparts on the other side of the Atlantic. Although this work will not aim to provide a comprehensive overview of present-day practices in Europe, my hope is that it will foster interest in further study abroad to discover the degree to which *Brauchen*, the predecessor to powwowing, may indeed be alive and well in Europe today.

Methodology

This exploration is the culmination of over ten years of active research in the field of Pennsylvania folklife, and most recently as part of my advocacy for the preservation of Pennsylvania Dutch folk culture and language at the Pennsylvania German Cultural Heritage Center at Kutztown University. My methodology combines a three-part approach to the gathering of information and sources:

I first began my work from an ethnographic model of participant observation in my own community and family, where I have collected first- and second-hand narratives in the form of oral histories and interviews, and studied with present-day, traditional powwow practitioners from Berks County. Oral histories referenced within this study will be identified by location and year, omitting all personal, identifying data out of respect for the privacy for my contacts, sources, and confidants. While powwowing is not a "secret" practice, it is one of many forms of social interaction that requires confidentiality and sensitivity.

Likewise, throughout this book, I will not include in my explorations any sensitive material that I specifically learned from living practitioners of the oral tradition, in keeping with the protocol communicated to me at the time that I learned to powwow. Likewise, a careful attempt has been made wherever possible to avoid the identification and direct citation of written materials which contain portions of the oral tradition that I learned, for two reasons:

First, the value of applying a methodological approach that is both culturally sensitive and consistent with the traditional framework of the teachings far outweighs any perceived benefits derived from the publication of sensitive materials, which are not essential to the description and study of the practice as a whole. Secondly, in every instance where I have come across published renditions of the prayers contained in the oral tradition, the presentation and application of this material has been inherently problematic, both linguistically and symbolically, to a degree that I do not recognize it as accurately representing a coherent and nuanced whole. In addition, a number of prayers and elements which have been essential to the ritual process among present-day, living practitioners, as well as my own experience, appear to have been entirely omitted or overlooked from all contemporary studies. I have no intention of publishing such "missing pieces," as it would constitute a form of cultural commodification.

For these reasons, the approach and interpretation of the tradition presented here will be informed by the oral tradition while making no direct or indirect quotations or references to sensitive materials as such. Furthermore, a reader who may have interest in learning more about the oral tradition is encouraged to forge a connection with a living practitioner, and in so doing, forge a valuable and transformative connection with the community and the culture at large.

This exploration, which features many original primary sources, will avoid the use of any personal information or images of present-day practitioners, for the privacy and consideration of my contacts and community. People who actively powwow tend to view certain kinds of documentation as intrusive, as rituals are performed for healing, not for educational demonstrations or for entertainment purposes. Therefore, images will appear of historical practitioners, rather than present-day people. I hope that readers will understand that this omission will ensure that research is conducted in a manner that is consistent with the community's values, as well as with current ethnographic ethics in mind.

Similarly, this work will avoid some of the more controversial elements of the discussion of present-day powwowing that is playing out in online forums and popular publications, which has recently found its way into academic discourse. While I am personally familiar with the individuals on both sides of a number of key issues, and have voiced some opinions in the past, I am, frankly, uninterested in taking sides in polarized debates and nebulous arguments over authenticity or legitimacy. I am much more interested in continuing to learn from my community about ritual healing experiences, than in taking sides in arguments that do not benefit the longevity of the culture and its traditions.

Parts of these arguments focus on notions of authenticity, and important questions about what is and what is not considered to be traditional. Other more personal divisions have formed over who should or should not be powwowing based upon their religious identities. These conversations include people of Christian, Jewish, and Islamic traditions, and a wide spectrum of neo-pagan, wiccan, and heathen orientations, as well as some that do not identify with any one particular religion. Across this diverse spectrum are individuals who have trained with older generations of powwow practitioners, and continue to teach others - albeit through new social and religious contexts. The internet, unavailable to previous generations, has also provided a digital platform for the dissemination of a wide variety of traditional, historical, adapted, and invented ritual practices, as well as some undercurrents of religious proselytizing, competitive self-promotion, and profiteering. For many contemporary people who self-identify as new generations of practitioners in the digital age, conflicting anxieties over the preservation of the tradition and the degree to which powwowing can be adapted to the needs and identities of contemporary society are at the forefront, but there is no one single, agreed-upon solution. Perhaps of greatest concern is the underlying question - who gets to determine the narrative of a folk tradition that simply cannot be owned, governed, or sanctioned?

At the heart of many of these debates are concerns over how a tradition can maintain a sense of cultural identity while persisting in an ever-changing and evolving world. My emphasis is not so much in putting forth arguments to support or place limits upon who is right and who is wrong, but instead exploring the ways in which the practice in its most essential forms is presently, and has been historically, inseparable from the language and culture of the Pennsylvania Dutch.

In addition to an ethnographic methodology, as a speaker of the Pennsylvania Dutch language, and an avid translator of rare, early German-language manuscripts, my work is conducted in part from an ethno-linguistic perspective, interpreting both literary and oral sources of current and historical perspectives on powwowing.

At the same time that I had begun to learn to powwow, I also had been immersing myself in the Pennsylvania Dutch language, through extensive community involvement with language preservation organizations to develop the ability not only to read, write, and translate, and but also to speak the language with anyone who would tolerate me. Although naturally in the beginning my abilities with the language were limited, the community responded positively to my persistence, and I came to understand that most of what I needed to learn was not to be found in books, but in day to day use of the language among native speakers. I also found that there were certain topics that were easier for people in Berks, Lehigh, Lebanon, and Schuylkill counties to discuss in the dialect, or at least in company with those who held the dialect in common.

Powwowing is one of those aspects of local experience that some will not speak of with outsiders, and knowing the language places a speaker of Pennsylvania Dutch on the inside of several layers of cultural boundaries. My experience is that powwowing, having been originally and firmly rooted in the ethno-linguistic context of Pennsylvania Dutch, is impossible to fully describe in English only. The language adds a different level of specificity in meaning and terminology to a conversation, with less ambiguity about the values placed on certain ideas.

For instance, in the most basic sense, the English term "powwow" generally holds a neutral connotation, as opposed to B*raucherei,* which is generally positive to speakers of Pennsylvania Dutch. On the other hand, to some monolingual English speakers, the controversial word *Hex* can also be neutral. In Pennsylvania Dutch, however, *Hex* (meaning either a witch or a curse) carries an extremely negative connotation, but *Braucher* (synonymous with a powwow practitioner) is positive rather than neutral, unless the context is one of humor or disbelief. Thus the same story told in Pennsylvania Dutch can have a drastically different feel and meaning when told in English to an English-only audience.

These meanings can also vary from community to community. For instance, a Pennsylvania Dutch speaker among the Old Order Mennonites will be likely to have a very different opinion of the word "powwowing" than a non-sectarian speaker of Pennsylvania Dutch belonging to a Lutheran or Reformed background in Berks, Lehigh or Lebanon County. The vast majority of my research has been conducted among the Pennsylvania Dutch descendants of the Church People, and this study is only peppered with experiences and anecdotes from the Plain People, without devoting significant space to the explorations of ritual traditions among the Old Order Amish or Mennonites. Although a family member is descended from a female healer among the Old Order Amish, who specialized in women's health (especially in treating postpartum hemorrhage), I will save this aspect of the cultural equation for a future study. This omission is not meant to diminish the importance of the Old Order communities, who are the primary bearers of the Pennsylvania Dutch language in North America. Although the population of sectarian speakers of Pennsylvania Dutch throughout the United States is over 300,000 and is growing at an exponential rate each year, there are currently no accurate numbers to indicate how many non-sectarian speakers of the language reside in Pennsylvania, Ohio, and other areas.

Although the language has been the subject of much research in recent years, there has been to date no recent study of powwowing by a speaker of Pennsylvania Dutch since Don Yoder in the 1970s. Prior to Yoder, the Rev. Thomas Brendle and Claude Unger produced their study in 1935, and over a century ago, and Edwin Miller Fogel collected over 2,000 dialect descriptions of rituals and beliefs in 1915. A contemporary study in context with Pennsylvania Dutch language is long overdue.

Third, my work continues in folklife and vernacular studies, with ten years of field work in documenting the ritual traditions, graffiti, folk art decorations, and the cultural significance of the Pennsylvania barn. I had received a research grant in 2008 from the Peter Wentz Farmstead Society in Montgomery County to systematically document all of Berks County's barns decorated with stars, popularly known as "hex signs" and create a photographic archive to preserve a contemporary view of today's cultural landscape for future generations – especially because, like powwowing, the tradition of painting barn stars was once perceived to be in a state of decline.

Part of my original motivation for conducting this research was to document, wherever possible, evidence of ritual traditions associated with the protection of the barn by means of powwowing, and to determine what relation, if any, these traditions had with the artistic traditions in the past and present. I had hoped that my first-hand experiences with powwowing would aid me in shedding some new light on the somewhat polarized debate concerning the symbolism of the barn stars - that is, whether they are "magical" or not. While I was able to document a wide variety of ritual practices associated with protecting barns, I found that in the core geographic region of the barn stars that there was no evidence to suggest that powwowers actively painted barns, and that to this day there are no barn painters actively powwowing. Occasionally, these traditions have cross-pollinated, and there are many examples of powwow blessings that incorporate images of stars – although usually these expressions are not so artistically developed as the barn murals produced in Berks and Lehigh counties. Instead, the traditions of powwowing and barn decorating are at best parallel expressions of the folk-culture, sharing in common a cosmological orientation and symbolism.

In all aspects of my work in local culture, whether in powwowing or folk art, my orientation has been one of community cooperation. When I began my barn survey in 2008, I asked permission to address an audience in Pennsylvania Dutch of over 500 speakers of the language at the Berks County *Versammling* (an annual language preservation celebration), in order to both announce the work that I was undertaking, but also to give the opportunity for the community to contribute and weigh-in on the process. As a result, I received a list of over 100 names of dialect-speaking barn owners, who were willing to support the project. Many of these same people have also shared with me their views and experiences with powwowing.

Just as I found that most of what I needed to know about speaking Pennsylvania Dutch was not to be found in books, so too was there some dissonance between working in the heartland of the Pennsylvania Dutch in *Alt Barricks* (Old Berks) and in surveying the literature surrounding powwowing traditions. So much of academic discourse has been focused on issues surrounding power, authority, and controversy, that subsequently the literature reflects these issues to the exclusion of a more compelling and complete view of the community's experiences with the tradition.

Ritual or Magical Studies?

Powwowing is frequently described as a folk-cultural practice of magic by academics, as well as in popular sources from outside of Pennsylvania Dutch culture. Although this word is often intended, in a neutral sense, to describe transactions with divine or spiritual forces for the purpose of creating tangible results by subtle means, this is not a word that is widely accepted in communities where powwowing is still practiced. Even in Pennsylvania Dutch, words such as *Zauberei* (magic or sorcery) are avoided, and carry strongly negative connotations, second only to *Hexerei* (witchcraft). Although popular culture has softened these words throughout recent history, associations of magic with powwowing can be highly offensive, and entirely counterproductive in discussions with those who see powwowing as an expression of religious piety.

Likewise, the word *charm* has its place within modern verbal ritual studies, but this word is largely unrecognized outside of academic circles or popular publications. While this word is in use in predominantly Anglo-American populations, it is absent in the oral traditions of Pennsylvania's communities.

Part of this has to do with the association of magic with deception, superstition, delusion, illegitimacy, or heresy. The use of the word *magic*, even in ancient times, has held a connotation of "otherness," and rather than being descriptive of a particular set of practices, tends to describe a broad range of generalized notions of what is not considered to be correct or real. In this usage, the term becomes exclusive, rather than particular. To the western mind, magic implies making use of spiritual forces in ways that are outside of the community's religious and ontological consensus, or as one nineteenth-century Pennsylvania law described it: "pretending to do the impossible" (see chapter II). In one sense, the category of magic implies a historical context of stigma, in a similar way that the term *superstition* expresses disapproval of someone else's beliefs, and is rarely used to describe one's own beliefs and cultural practices.

Furthermore, religion and magic are part of a spectrum of ritual expression that often defies simple categorization or distinction. What one culture may consider sacred, could appear magical or superstitious to another. For instance, to an outsider, the Roman Catholic Eucharist may appear to have all the features of a magical ritual performance - such as words of power (prayer, and the liturgical words of institution); the consecration of ritual elements (blessing of the wine & bread); use of ritual objects (the chalice, flagon and paten); the transformation of ordinary substances into potent spiritual materials (transubstantiation); practitioners (priests); and ritual timing (the liturgical calendar) - and yet, such a comparison with magic may be patently offensive to a Roman Catholic. Furthermore, magic is often relegated to practices which have little or no recognized hierarchy, institutional structure, or political power, or that which may stand contrary to such a hierarchy. Thus, institutionalized ritual is regarded as religion, and decentralized ritual is often subject to additional scrutiny. This does not mean however, that powwowing is a religion unto itself, but rather an expression of religious belief and cultural attitudes.

For the sake of this exploration, the word *magic* will be applied sparingly, and in context with its usage in historical sources. Rather than cloud the discussion with preconceived notions of what magic is or is not, this study will focus on the tradition of *Braucherei*, as an expression of ritual - a common feature to cultures across the globe.

Acknowledgements in the Field

Ritual studies continues to develop as an academic discipline, as scholars continue to redefine the parameters of ritual and its nuanced roles in human relationships and systems of belief. As an inherently interdisciplinary approach, the study of ritual brings together many sympathetic and disparate fields – archaeology and religion, theater and linguistics, history and anthropology, political science and folklife. This exploration is likewise necessarily diverse in its sources and scope, with an emphasis in folklife and religious studies. A number of significant scholars have proceeded me in blazing a network of trails surrounding the subject, and I am greatly indebted to these different perspectives.

Dr. David Hufford, in a wide range of highly significant essays and books, not only clarifies the need for more objective language in the research of healing belief systems, but provides an empirical model for interpreting belief-oriented health experiences. Dr. Barbara Reimensnyder interpreted powwowing in her native Union County as part of a network of community relationships, emphasizing that traditions are perpetuated by attitudes conveyed through relational narratives. Dr. David Kriebel built on field work with living practitioners, providing insight into the evolution of the tradition as a form of modern, faith-based alternative medicine, as well as a statistical analysis of the effectiveness of healing narratives and experiences.

I am most deeply indebted to my friend and mentor, Dr. Don Yoder (1921-2015) father of American Folklife Studies, and foremost advocate for Pennsylvania Dutch culture. Dr. Yoder's profound interest in powwowing was generously interwoven through his work in folk religion and folk medicine, and greatly enhanced by his study of the genealogy, foodways, material culture, oral traditions, and literature of the Pennsylvania Dutch. His earliest field work was conducted in the beloved valleys of his youth in Schuylkill County, but his passion took him abroad to Europe, and throughout the world, nurturing a global perspective on folklife and ritual.

My work with Don began in 2010, when I was sent on behalf of the Heritage Center at Kutztown University, to acquire an extensive collection of Pennsylvania Dutch language research materials for the university. My task was to sort the vast ocean of paperwork that Don had collected over the course of his lifetime – indeed the largest archive of Pennsylvania Dutch folklife research ever to have been compiled. As we sorted what seemed like endless waves of material over the course of many months, and then into the following year, we spent countless hours discussing his multi-faceted career and life-long research in religious and folk-cultural studies.

What I did not realize at the time, was that I was receiving one of the best quality educations that I ever could have hoped for, and within a few months Don Yoder began referring to me as his unofficial student. I had the benefit of spending more time with him one-on-one than any single professor with whom I've ever studied, and we built a profound and lasting friendship in the process.

Don mentored me through the research that eventually became my first book, *The Friend in Need: An Annotated Translation of A Pennsylvania Folk-Healing Manual*, published as the Heritage Center's first annual volume in 2012. Don also contributed a spirited foreword to my second work, *Hex Signs: Myth and Meaning in Pennsylvania Dutch Barn Stars* (2013), encouraging future exploration in the field.

After a long career, Don was actively engaged in selling books and manuscripts that he had acquired in over 75 years of collecting for a monumental work on powwowing. Although many of these works were offered for sale first to the Heritage Center at Kutztown University, they were respectfully declined under previous leadership as being beyond the means and scope of a small museum with limited resources. Rather than watch as these materials were scattered to the four winds through online auction services, I began to personally purchase any manuscript material that was put up for sale, and began building a research collection partially composed of materials from his jointly owned Roughwood Collection with Dr. William Woys Weaver. I named this research collection the Heilman Collection, in honor of my paternal grandfather, Robert Raymond Heilman of Lebanon (1931-2009). Although the collection began with materials from Roughwood, its contents have expanded at an exponential rate, with materials purchased from the Lester Breininger Collection, and other significant collectors and researchers.

Among the materials that Don sold were powwowing primary source materials that he had hoped to feature in his extensive work in process, advertised back in the fall of 1961 as Occult Pennsylvania, but later thoughtfully retitled as Powwow Healing. This work was originally billed as the upcoming annual volume of the Pennsylvania Folklife Society, a cutting-edge educational organization that revolutionized the study of folk culture and founded the oldest folklife festival in the United States at Kutztown.

Don Yoder's monumental work was anticipated for release in the spring of 1962, however, the Folklife Society's fall festival the previous year suffered a huge loss due to terrible weather, leaving the organization deep in debt on the brink of bankruptcy, and unable to found the folklife museum they had planned. Don was too preoccupied with negotiating the financial crisis and protecting the educational mandate of the society, that he never actually wrote his masterpiece, but continued to actively gather materials in the hope of one day completing the project.

As with many of the projects that are held closely to the heart, Don's powwowing notes and research grew ever wider in scope and content over the years as he accumulated more information – enough for several books. He re-envisioned his magnum opus several times as his awareness of the traditions grew, but he also became more distinctly aware of how much was yet to be discovered. As Don's research continued, and the project expanded, the finish line became farther from reach.

I asked Don once if he'd ever been powwowed, and he replied that he had not. It didn't exactly surprise me – Don was a Quaker, and, in another lifetime, early in his career he had been a Reformed minister. Although he was delighted by the liturgical elements of powwowing in an intellectual sense, it was not exactly his style of spiritual expression. I asked him if he'd ever want to be powwowed, and he politely replied, "Maybe." He'd had ample opportunities over the course of his career, and had personally known and interviewed many practitioners, including Sophia Bailer, "Saint of the Coal Regions," and William Beissel, who re-published an abridged translation of *The Secrets of Sympathy* (included unabridged at the end of this work). He had also interviewed practitioners in Brazil, such as Peter Schneider, a traditional *Braucher* who was bilingual in Portuguese and Hunsrücker German dialect. Nevertheless, as invested as Don was in his work, he preferred to keep an objective distance, and never participated in powwowing.

On his 91st birthday in 2012, Dr. Yoder asked me to continue his work, and told me that he intended to entrust the notes for his powwow book to my care, with the hope that it would result in the book that he had never written. With the prospect of continued collaboration, our hope was to regain some momentum for exploration of these traditions, and broaden the scope of ritual folk culture studies together.

Dr. Don Yoder passed away in the summer of 2015, while I was in the midst of preparing the first of a series of collaborative exhibitions in his honor through the Heritage Center at Kutztown, entitled *Powwowing in Pennsylvania,* at the Schwenkfelder Library and Heritage Center in Pennsburg. The exhibition, dedicated to his memory, featured many original manuscripts, books, and ritual objects that Dr. Yoder was originally instrumental in assembling, and had not been previously available to the public. Most recently, in 2017, the exhibition was greatly expanded to include a wide range of European objects illustrating the religious origins of powwowing, hosted by Glencairn Museum in Bryn Athyn, Pennsylvania. In keeping with Glencairn's mission, the exhibition invited a diverse audience to engage with religious beliefs and practices, past and present, with the goal of fostering empathy and building understanding among people of all beliefs.

This book will be one of many explorations of Pennsylvania's ritual traditions to culminate from the materials in the Heilman Collection, for, as Don Yoder would have agreed, there is more than enough for several lifetimes of research and investigation. My hope is that this material can be used for the benefit of the community, and to restore a sense of respect and wonder to the ritual traditions that were once commonly used to mediate life's challenges in Pennsylvania Dutch communities – framing life's ups and downs within a broader context of meaning, with the possibility of transforming ordinary experiences into expressions of cosmic and sacred proportions.

Conclusion

Although ritual traditions within the context of powwowing are used primarily for the purpose of healing, protection, and assistance in times of need, there are more subtle secondary functions of these traditions such as bringing people together, strengthening familial and community solidarity, and reinforcing a spiritual identity. Our modern, western world, often characterized by existential anxieties and concerns, is hungry for meaning and a sense of authenticity, yet at the same time opportunities to actively engage in communal and personal expressions of ritual have rapidly declined in American culture. Perhaps a deeper exploration of powwowing can provide the opportunity to more closely consider the value of ritual interactions as a means of creating meaningful dialogue within the social, spiritual, and domestic spheres of life.

There will be those who oppose the notion that anything of importance can be learned from examining the past and present traditions of powwowing - even some members of the Pennsylvania Dutch community - objecting on the grounds that such practices are better left behind as remnants of "superstition" or "unorthodox" belief. It is my hope that even those whose religious and cultural orientation may differ from the worldviews implicit in powwowing may graciously suspend judgement long enough appreciate the value of gaining a better understanding of the origins and development of Pennsylvania's distinctive folk culture.

For the past century or more, some have predicted the demise of these traditions as the inevitable result of the standardization of modern biomedicine, as well as the decline of the use of the Pennsylvania Dutch language in Southeastern Pennsylvania. However, no such extinction has actually taken place. Nevertheless, great care must be taken not only in ensuring the survival of the wisdom undergirding these traditions for future generations, but also in preserving the ethics, protocols, and structures of mutual respect that keep the tradition of powwowing culturally intact.

It is no longer acceptable to present this tradition as an accumulation of disparate cast-offs from previous stages of the culture's history and development, nor as an ethnically or religiously exclusive inheritance of only a select few – for the former is equally shallow as the latter is dangerous - but instead, as a living tradition with a vibrant past, and the potential for a dynamic and spirited future.

It is my hope that the process of remembering and reflecting on the significance of these ritual traditions, past and present, with a sense of openness and empathy will broaden the depth of our understanding of the culture's distinctive worldview, as an act both healing and fortifying to present and future generations.

+ + +
Patrick J. Donmoyer
April 25 2017
Am Markes sei Daag
The Feast of St. Mark

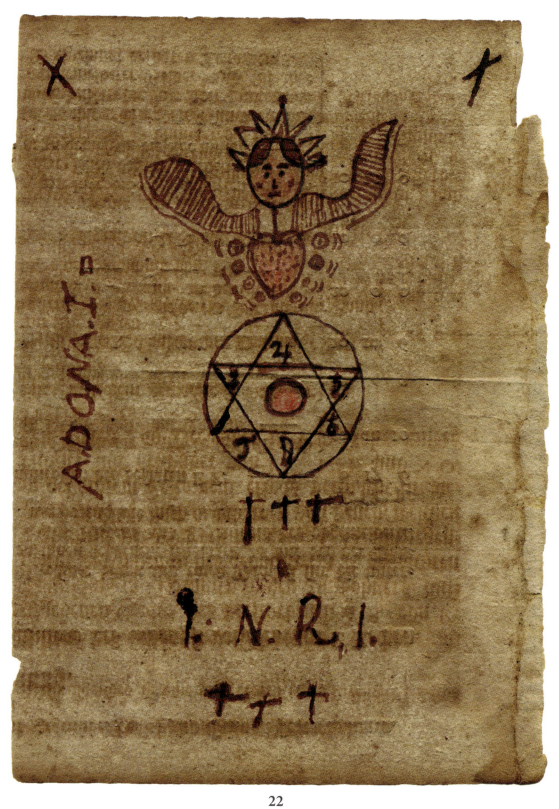

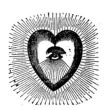  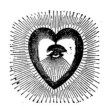

Chapter I
Ritual Traditions
of the Pennsylvania Dutch

Religious orders across the globe, transcending all lines of creed and ethnicity, engage in ritual as an active part of spirituality in practice, prayer, worship, and gathering. While the particular aesthetics and functions of ritual process are often unique to each faith experience, the use of ritual is also a unifying element in human experience, serving as an effective means to create and define meaningful interactions, spaces, and outcomes.

Ritual is by no means unique to the religious setting, as ritual practices interpenetrate all fields and levels of society, shaping and integrating the domestic, political, occupational, agricultural, and countless other social realms into a coherent whole. At the very same time that ritual is universal and ubiquitous, the performance of ritual within a specific context can serve to both delineate and reinforce a distinct sense of ethnic, cultural, national, or religious identity, revealing and emphasizing as many differences and divisions within humanity as there are similarities. Rituals can therefore serve to both divide and unify, to dissolve and to reconcile, to harm and to heal.

Pennsylvania's tradition of ritual healing known as powwowing, or *Braucherei* in the language of the Pennsylvania Dutch, is one of many vernacular healing systems in North America that combines elements of religion and belief with health and healing.[1] Informed primarily by oral tradition, powwowing encompasses a wide spectrum of healing rituals for restoring health and preventing illness among humans and livestock. Combining a diverse array of verbal benedictions, prayers, gestures, and the use of everyday objects, as well as celestial and calendar observances, these rituals are used not only for healing of the body, but also for protection from physical and spiritual harm, assistance in times of need, and ensuring good outcomes in everyday affairs. The majority of these rituals are overlain with Christian symbols in their pattern and content, comprising a veritable wellspring of folk-religious expression that is at once symbolic, poetic, and imbued with meaning worthy of serious attention and exploration.

In this traditional world view, warts can be cured with a potato and an invocation to the Holy Trinity by the light of the waxing moon. Verses of scripture are employed to stop bleeding from serious injuries. Burns are treated by blowing three times between cycles of religious invocations to dispel the heat from the body. A smooth stone from the barnyard can heal illnesses that prevent draft horses from working, and written inscriptions are fed to cattle to prevent parasites. The proper placement of a broom by the front door will protect from malicious people and spirits, and a pinch of dust from the four corners of the house when stirred into coffee will prevent homesickness. Farm and garden tools greased with the fat from frying *Fasnacht* cakes will ensure a prosperous growing season, and the ash from the woodstove sprinkled over the livestock on Ash Wednesday will prevent lice. Wild salad greens eaten on Maundy Thursday prevent illness and ensure vitality. Eggs laid on Good Friday are concealed in the attic for protection of the house and farm, and are especially good for removal of illness.[2]

All of these ritual procedures are classic expressions of the *Braucherei* tradition once widely practiced in Pennsylvania Dutch communities, and still continuing

---

Opposite page: An early personal protective powwow blessing produced in black and red ink on the verso of an unidentified, eighteenth-century Philadelphia printed estate document, featuring a winged angel with a burning heart and crown, associated with the mystical vision of the Sophia or feminine aspect of the Holy Spirit, popular among certain Pietist groups in early Pennsylvania. The angel oversees the six days of creation, depicted within the Star of David, with planetary symbols within each point and the sun in the center. However, Mars is missing, and replaced by a "J" - possibly an intentional inversion of martial influence as a protection from violence. The inscription I.N.R.I. (Iesus Nazarenus Rex Iudeorum - Jesus of Nazareth, King of the Jews) is a common protective inscription, flanked above and below with three crosses, symbolic of the Holy Trinity. *Adonai*, a Hebrew name for God meaning Lord, is inscribed on the left. Creases indicate it was folded and carried on the person. *Heilman Collection.*

today. These examples can either challenge or appeal to our notions of what is considered acceptable behavior for religious people, presenting a wide range of experiences that may overlap at times with formally-accepted, officially-sanctioned religious practice and those elements that may be relegated to a vernacular, or folk expression of religion.[3] Although these practices tend to be concentrated in the core region of southeastern Pennsylvania, they are not limited to the state, or even North America, and have been found in many places where the influence of the diaspora of German-speaking people has spread, including Southern Appalachia, the Ozarks, the Midwest, the Dakotas, Ontario, and even Brazil and Russia.[4]

As part of a spectrum of traditional health belief systems in the United States, powwowing within the Pennsylvania Dutch community is comparable to other folk-cultural and ethnic healing practices in North America, such as *Benedicaria* or "Passing" among Italian-Americans, Root-Work in the deep South, Santeria of the Caribbean and southern United States, *curanderismo* in the Southwest, "granny doctors" in southern Appalachia, and the healing traditions of the Cajun *traiteur*, all of which blend ritual, faith, and healing.[5] Despite obvious contrast with modern biomedical healthcare, these traditional healing systems are used in the present day as alternative and complementary medical practices that are blended with conventional care for the benefit of those who wish to engage a healing system that is sympathetic to religious and cultural values.[6] Powwow rituals provide the rare opportunity to examine the diversity of religious ritual in a healing context, and expand our awareness of the interrelation between official and folk-religious patterns.

OF WARTS AND WANING

Of all the powwow rituals that have been practiced in Pennsylvania up to the present day to restore health and healing, the most common of these are for the removal of warts. Ranging from trifling annoyance to painful excrescence, a wart is one of the most stubborn conditions encountered by the majority of people at least once over the course of a lifetime. Modern conventional medicine can also struggle to permanently prevent the return of warts, even after repeated treatments, some of which are painful or invasive to the patient. The non-invasive rituals used to treat warts among the Pennsylvania Dutch are some of the least complicated of all powwowing procedures in structure. These rituals combine poetic blessings, the use of a common everyday object such as a potato or a penny, and are scheduled according to the phase of the moon. Despite their simplicity, these rituals are perhaps some of the most integrated into aspects of everyday life, with far-reaching implications that overlap domestic, agricultural, and cosmic beliefs. This integration, coupled with a sense of universal accessibility – literally anyone can do it – has ensured the survival of these processes into the present day, despite substantial contrast with conventional biomedicine.

As a child, my first exposure to these beliefs was through my grandmother, who explained to me that her grandfather had powwowed away a tenacious wart on her hand when she was a young girl, using nothing more than a potato. His procedure was simple, and she recalled that under the full moon, he cut the potato in half, and rubbed each half on the wart. Then he put the potato back together and buried it beneath the downspout of the farmhouse. He quietly spoke words in Pennsylvania Dutch. Within a short while, the wart was completely gone.

It may come as a surprise to many that there is nothing particularly unusual about this experience among older Pennsylvanians. Although puzzling to an outsider, these types of common ritual involvements were neither scrutinized nor questioned to any great degree. It was not bothersome to my grandmother that she did not understand the words spoken by her grandfather, because the cure was understood to have been effective. Furthermore, she implicitly understood that as the potato rotted away, so did the wart.

Although the wart-cure is one of the simplest ritual applications of powwowing, the basis for how it is perceived to work is far more complex than appearances would suggest. In fact, this wart-cure provides a glimpse into a system of belief that expresses and embraces a whole worldview.

The phase and visibility of the moon are believed to be crucial for this process, as a beacon of cosmic order, and an agent of change, growth, and dispersal. Echoing principles delineated in the ever-present agricultural almanac, the moon, as it waxed to full, was believed to exert a particular force away from the earth, powerful enough to enhance the growth of ascending plants, such as corn or beans, as well as affect the rise of the tides, or the wetness and quality of wood when cutting timber, or even promote the growth of one's fingernails and hair. It is no wonder then that this lunar force was believed to assist in the transference of illness to the potato, which, when cut in half, has a cross-sectional profile that resembles the round, white, textured surface of the full moon.

However, close examination of the farmer's almanac would suggest that a proper potato crop was to be planted, not in the waxing moon, but when the moon is on the wane. This is when the moon's force was directed towards the earth, enhancing the downward growth of roots below the soil. By working against this commonly held principle and interring the potato in the waxing moon to cure a wart,

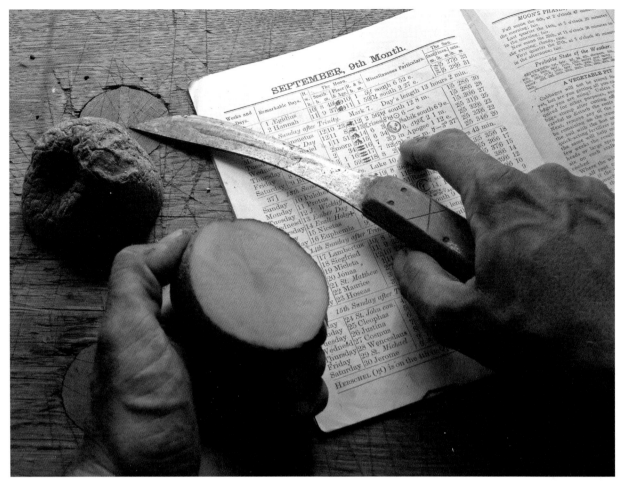

Removing warts by the light of the waxing moon with a potato is one of the most common powwow experiences in southeastern Pennsylvania.

it was believed that the potato would be more likely to rot away under the dampness of the downspout or below the drip-line of the eaves. This location represented the outermost boundary between the home and the outside world, separating that which is familiar from the unknown – a perfect, liminal place for the illness to be relegated until it is defused.

Although most recipients of ritual healing rarely hear the words that accompany these processes, because the blessings are often spoken *sotto voce*, or under the breath, these expressions are often descriptive of the ritual's mechanics and the desired outcome. The "moon prayer" that typically accompanies this wart remedy has been preserved in both oral tradition and written sources. One transcription, recorded in a doctor's ledger from 1830 in the Oley Valley, reads: *Alles was ich sehe das wachse, und was ich fühle das vergehe im Namen des Patri, Fillii et Spiritu Sancti* (All that I see may it increase, and what I touch, may it vanish, in the name of the Father, Son, and Holy Spirit). Other sources use the Pennsylvania Dutch words *zunemme* (to wax, increase) and *abnemme* (to wane, decrease), relating the withering of the wart with the waxing of the moon in an inverse relationship that reflects the direction of the moon's force of influence. The word *zunemme* also has a double-meaning: both "to wax" and "to take on" – as the moon itself is thought by some to actually take on the wart.[7]

These words could also be an echo of the words of John the Baptist: "He must increase, but I must decrease. He that cometh from above is above all: he that is of the earth is earthly, and speaketh of the earth: he that cometh from heaven is above all."[8] If this scriptural passage is indeed the origin of the words of the lunar wart cure, it would emphasize Christ's role as not only the redeemer of sins, but of the healer of physical ailments.

Verbal elements of powwow ritual, consisting of religious blessings and healing benedictions, are part of a memorized system of oral tradition, typically taught by a woman to a man, or vice versa. The rich imagery contained within these prayers, derived from scriptural and legendary narratives, is expressed in poetic rounds that are often metered and rhymed as part of their mnemonic function.

I learned a different variation of this moon-prayer from a traditional powwower in Berks County just over a decade ago, and since that time I have had many opportunities to use it for friends, relatives, and neighbors. It is one of many aspects of the tradition that was taught to me by word of mouth that I was instructed to never write down, and to only teach it to those who would wish to learn. I deeply respect these admonitions, and will not be committing any specific aspects of my experiences with the oral tradition to print. These words are in one sense like a precious heirloom – a sentiment that I've heard from many who learned these traditions from older family members. In a very real sense, at the same time, these prayers are part of a living tradition, and should not be regarded as a mere relic of the past.

Just like prayers belonging to officially sanctioned religious activities, powwow prayers and blessings incorporate invocations and supplications to divine forces and saints. However, the objectives in powwow rituals tend to be broader in scope, closely resembling prayers attributed to the comprehensive system of medieval prayers to the saints, used for concerns as varied as safe passage in a storm or finding an object that is lost. While all prayers are in a basic sense a form of communication and negotiation with divine forces, powwow blessings also serve as the script for a distinctive form of cultural and ceremonial performance, engaging both the patient and practitioner in a ritual context composed of elements that are at once mundane, cosmological, and sacred. Central to many of these ritual performances is the use of everyday objects. Such materials are incorporated into ritual in a manner that contrasts with ordinary use, but echoes the role that the object plays within a larger context – supporting the notion that an object imparts some measure of the sacredness of life.

Other forms of the lunar wart-cure involve the use of chicken feet,[9] an onion, a rind of bacon, a dishcloth, or a bone as the vector of illness removal.[10] In the last case, the bone is certainly not expected to rot away, like the potato, the feet, or the onion, but instead it is to be plucked from where it may lie in the barnyard, rubbed over the afflicted part, and then returned to the exact spot of ground from which it was taken. Similar acts of selecting, using, and replacing a stone are used for other disorders, such as sweeny (a form of muscular atrophy) or persistent nose-bleeds.[11]

Another type of wart-cure ritual involves the use of a penny to rub the wart, which when spent or abandoned at a crossroads, would transfer the wart to the next person who possessed it. With this ritual in mind, any objects left in the street were seen as suspect: "*Mer soll nix vun der Schtrooss uffhewe, es is verleicht gebraucht warre mit*" (One should pick up nothing from the street, as perhaps it was used to powwow).[12] In these cases, while the moon still plays a central role in the transference, the accompanying words are quite different. A man from the Kutztown area once told me that "the butcher bought my wart for a penny." This pronouncement echoes the Pennsylvania Dutch phrase used in such cases, *Ich kaaf dei Waartz fer ee Sent* – "I'm buying your wart for a penny."

Still other accounts suggest rituals involving the counting of the warts as a cure,[13] echoing the old belief that warts could be contracted by pointing at the stars and counting them.[14] This act, though seemingly harmless enough, and certainly not worthy of divine punishment by modern standards, can be contextualized in light of Biblical passages, such as Psalm 147, where counting the stars is a power ascribed to God alone.[15] Even in the passage in Genesis where Abraham's descendants are compared to the stars, the suggestion is that quantifying the infinite is beyond human abilities: "Look now toward heaven, and tell the stars, if thou be able to number them."[16]

Despite the fact that some folk-religious traditions, such as powwow, may resonate with patterns, sights, and sounds ascribed to earlier periods of a culture's or religion's development,[17] it is equally true that official expressions of faith are entitled to the very same privilege. But again, neither vernacular nor formal religion should be regarded as mere vestiges of the ancient, and instead, parts of a dynamic continuum of active relationships, informed by the past and working in the present.

Powwowing in Practice

The original word in Pennsylvania Dutch for these ritual practices is *Braucherei*, which literally from its German linguistic origin describes an accumulation of customs, ceremonies, traditions, and rites derived from *brauche* (to use, to need, to administer, practice, or employ), as well as *Breiche* (customs, ways, traditions) and *Gebrauch* (ceremony, custom, or ritual).[18] A female practitioner of *Braucherei* is called a *Braucherin* and a *Braucher* if male. In the present day, as the everyday use of Pennsylvania Dutch has declined in the core region of the Dutch Country, a practitioner is also called a "powwow doctor" or "powwower."

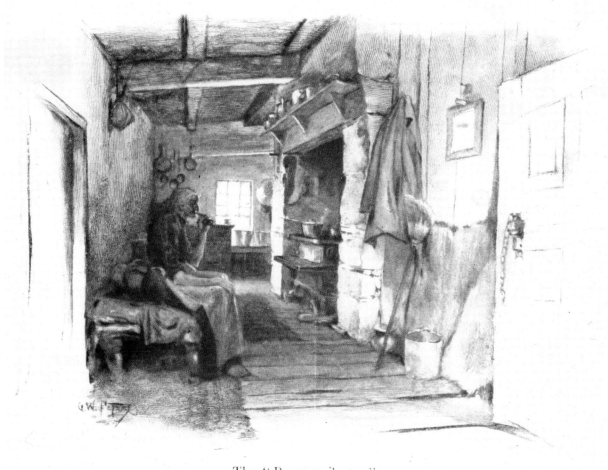

The "Powwow-doctor."

A classic lithograph of a Pennsylvania powwow practitioner by G. W. Peters, featured in Nelson Lloyd's "Among the Dunkers," in *Scribner's Magazine*, Vol XXX, No. 5, November 1901.

In some parts of the United States, a powwower is also called a "hex-doctor," which implies the healing of illnesses believed to be caused either unintentionally by a grudge, or deliberately by a curse, commonly known as a *Hex* in both English and Pennsylvania Dutch. Any maliciously-intended ritual activity that is used to harm an individual or livestock is called *Hexerei* (literally, malicious witchcraft).[19] Like the word hex-doctor, use of the term *Hexerei* can also be ambiguous, and in some areas of North America it is synonymous with the word powwowing; however, in Pennsylvania Dutch *Hexerei* always has a negative connotation. The powwower's role is not only to ritually cure unintentionally-occurring illness, but also to counteract the results of any malicious use of ritual that would produce a *Hex*.

Despite the variety of nuanced terminology for ritual practitioners, not everyone who powwows would identify him or herself as a practitioner, which inherently implies specialization or vocation on some level. Years ago, when powwowing was more common than it is today, a member of the family might powwow for anyone in the *Freindschaft* (an extended notion of the family, including friends and neighbors), and still not claim to be a practitioner. There are those who specialize in powwowing as an occupation, but such a thing tends to be controversial, as payment is usually neither specified nor required for assistance from a powwower. Reciprocity in ritual healing frequently takes the form of gifts of baked goods or free-will offerings left on the kitchen table. Although historically there have been powwow practitioners with highly lucrative practices, this is not common in the present day.[20]

Both of my paternal great-grandmothers could powwow, but neither would have considered herself to be a powwower in any formal sense of the word. Instead, both were familiar with common ritual cures that would have been known by many housewives of their generation. One of my great-grandmothers taught me a cure for hiccups when I was a child. The other lived on Hill Street in Lebanon, Pennsylvania, just a few houses down from a well-known powwower of the professional variety by the name of Reppert. In the 1930s and 40s, cars and horse-drawn buggies would line the street on a Sunday afternoon, when patients would come to see him. My great-grandmother would help out when the patients were too numerous, and she would powwow for those requesting assistance with childhood ailments, especially for "livergrown" children.

Livergrown is the English word for the Pennsylvania Dutch notion of being *aagewaxe*,[21] a condition once widely known across many early communities in America[22] and called by a variety of names, such as "hidebound" or "gripes." This disorder is one of many culturally-defined illnesses that do not readily fit the language of modern biomedicine. Equated with infant colic, this disorder is characterized by abdominal pains and cramps causing the infant or child to be fussy, downright inconsolable, or to have difficulty breathing. The belief was that these sensations were caused by the liver attaching itself to the inside of the body cavity, thus the word *aagewaxe* implies that which has "grown attached."

My great-grandmother powwowed for livergrown children with a common process involving the use of oil, which she used to anoint the child's sides with her thumbs. She would recite a prayer while employing a form of light massage.[24] Although no one in my family remembers the prayer, there are two commonly recorded prayers for this process. The first is spoken in Pennsylvania Dutch: "*Aagewaxe, geh weck vun meim Kind sei Ripp, yuscht wie der Grischdus aus sei Gripp gange iss*" (Livergown, depart from my child's rib, just as Christ got out of his crib).[25] Another blessing is derived from the standard German Luke 18:16: "*Und Jesus sprach, Lass die Kindlein zu mir kommen, und er segnete sie zu der selbigen Stunde…*" (And Jesus said, let the little children come unto me, and he blessed them at that very hour…).[26]

Like others who engage in powwowing, my great-grandmother was a devout Christian, whose remedies were sympathetic with her religious orientation. Her favorite hymn, *The Old Rugged Cross,* speaks volumes about her belief in the promise of a life beyond this world, provided by the transformative, healing power of Christ's suffering and death. The hymn expresses as sense of humility in following Christ's example, as a model for service to others. My great-grandmother was part of a community in which powwowing was a means to care for others in a culturally and religiously specific way, informed by many generations of healing experiences.

Customarily, powwowing is learned by word of mouth, as part of an oral tradition that is memorized, consisting of prayers, gestures, and ritual procedures. Some rituals are for specific illnesses, while others are part of a more comprehensive approach to bless and bring balance to the whole human body. The oral tradition comprises perhaps the single-most comprehensive cultural repository for ritual experience, and yet is guarded by protocol which determines the manner and frequency of how that information can be transmitted.

With very few exceptions, this protocol requires a male to learn from a female practitioner, or vice-versa (and usually the bulk of this oral material is in Pennsylvania Dutch). Although it is unknown how this alternating gender requirement developed, it certainly has contributed to a strong sense of gender equality in the tradition. Female practitioners are as common and known to be as effective as male practitioners, although occasionally there is some specialization among women for women's health issues. This gender requirement also excludes anyone from the practice with a tendency toward sexism – which would certainly be an obstacle to healing. When this tradition is passed down in families, it often skips a generation as it alternates. A grandmother might teach her grandson or a granddaughter may learn from her grandfather.

Rarely, when the tradition is held closely within a family, an exception to this gender-specific teaching can occur. Younger generations can sometimes gain firsthand experience by watching another family member powwow, without regard to gender. Sadly, it is much more common today to hear of such practices disappearing when a practitioner cannot find a willing pupil of the appropriate gender. As the language gap widens in southeastern Pennsylvania among the non-sectarian population, and older generations of native speakers of Pennsylvania Dutch are passing away, and few younger people are learning the language, the tradition has had to adapt in order to survive.

There tends to be a strong admonition against putting such memorized content into written form, except for personal reference. For many, learning to powwow implies a commitment to keeping the tradition in a fluid, intangible state that requires human interaction for continuation, and can be recalled only from memory. Dependence upon written materials is not looked upon favorably, and powwow practitioners do not read from manuals while working a cure. The only exception to this is the common use of a Bible, which is either held in the lap of a person receiving healing, placed under the chair where one is sitting, or held by the practitioner. The use of any book other than the Bible within the performance of a ritual procedure would be regarded as highly suspect, if not akin to idolatry.

While there are indeed many perceptions about why this aspect of the tradition may have developed, it reflects and reinforces the necessity of trust in communal bonds across many generations. It is also therefore difficult to commodify the tradition, and it cannot be bought, sold, or exchanged as a material good. This supports the notion that powwowing is not a service to be used for personal gain or remuneration, but rather as a gift from the divine, meant to be shared generously with others, and held in common by a community.

Nevertheless, a wide range of literary materials have developed both in Pennsylvania, and in Europe where the tradition originated, forming a parallel body of ritual practice that frequently cross-pollinates with its counterpart in oral tradition. Collections of prayers, recipes, and ritual procedures were recorded in private manuscripts from oral tradition, and some were passed down through family lines. Some printed healing manuals were largely derived from manuscript collections, and at the same time many personal collections of cures were derived from printed materials that had been in circulation for centuries. Likewise, some portions of the oral tradition have been included in both printed and hand-written materials, and some materials have also been memorized from books. It is therefore difficult to determine the exact provenance of many ritual procedures that turn up in sources on both sides of the Atlantic.

Powwowing is typically taught only under the condition that it be learned by a person who intends to earnestly use it to help other people, and not for the purpose of personal edification, curiosity, or intellectual and academic interest, especially if this were to lead to public scrutiny or publication of sensitive materials. Even such noble causes as historic or cultural preservation can be highly controversial if performed in a way that compromises a culture's values, and such efforts must be done with the utmost respect and ethical considerations.[27] As with any traditional practice, powwowing cannot be separated from the communities that it sustains, and therefore any efforts to engage or encounter this tradition as an outsider should begin by establishing meaningful connections with the community.

A Confluence of Cultures

While simultaneously affirming and challenging the values of present-day Americans, the religious origins of Pennsylvania's ritual tradition of powwowing are a direct result of the blossoming of the transatlantic religious exchange of eighteenth-century immigration prior to the American Revolution. German-speaking Protestants and Pietists, consisting of Lutheran and Reformed church members, Moravians, as well as the sects of Anabaptists, such as the Mennonites, Brethren, and Amish, and a very small minority of Roman Catholics crossed the Atlantic in a mass exodus, and escaped the turmoil and destruction following the Thirty Years War and Louis XIV's destruction of the Rhine. Pennsylvania's English Proprietor William Penn's open-door policies of religious tolerance provided an ideal destination not only for his own community of Quakers, but also for this religiously diverse group of German-speaking refugees from the regions of the Palatinate and Baden-Württemberg, as well as Alsace, Switzerland, and throughout the Rhine River Valley. Each of these religious communities migrated from central Europe and adapted to the cultural climate of North America to form New World identities.

As the most ethnically and religiously diverse of the original thirteen colonies, Pennsylvania provided the fertile soil for ritual traditions to flourish in the New World. Deeply rooted in the Roman Catholic consensus of the Middle Ages, revitalized by the post-Reformation mystical elements of Pietism among the Protestant population, the folk-religious climate of Pennsylvania was the new-world point of origin for a comprehensive system of beliefs that encompassed domestic, agricultural, and spiritual life. *Braucherei* in its original connotation implied customs, ceremonies, rites, and rituals that served to integrate these aspects of life into a coherent narrative.

Although the ritual practices of *Braucherei* are undoubtedly European in origin, the notion of powwowing – as the practice is known today - proceeds from a confluence of vastly different North American cultural forces. The term was originally appropriated from the Algonquian languages and incorporated into English by Puritan missionaries in 17th-century New England. In its original usage, the word *powwaw* among the Narragansett designated a medicine man, derived from a verb describing the actions of dreaming or divination for healing purposes.[28] Among the Puritans, this word took on a pejorative, and even sinister connotation, as the traditional medicine men and women were seen as obstacles to efforts to convert the native population in New England. Furthermore, because of this clash of cultures, the *powwaw* was associated with infernal practices of sorcery by the English, and such stories were

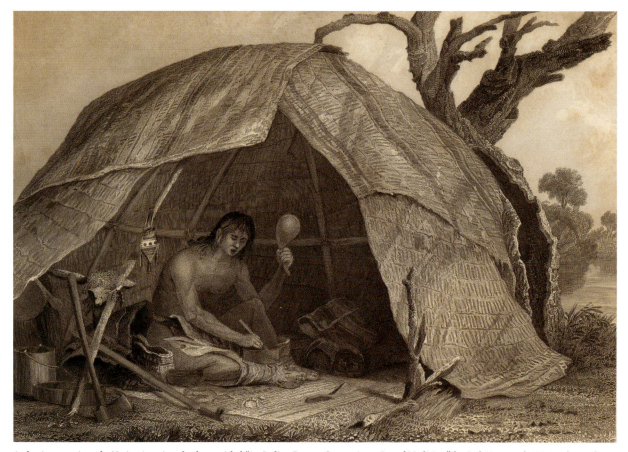

A classic engraving of a Native American healer, entitled "An Indian Doctor Concocting a Pot of Medicine," by Seth Eastman(1808-1875), a military mapmaker and illustrator of native American life while stationed at Fort Snelling Minesota. *Heilman Collection.* While powwowing in the Pennsylvania Dutch context is not Native American in origin, the word used to describe such practices was applied by speakers of English out of a sense of apparent similarity in the role of ritual in healing traditions from both cultures.

even included in mission correspondence by celebrated Puritan ministers Matthew Mayhew and John Elliot to Lord Protector of the Commonwealth, Oliver Cromwell.[29]

Based on this use of the word in early America, the term became synonymous with "magical rituals" in a derogatory sense, and the Native American word was applied by early English-speaking Pennsylvanians not only to describe the ritual practices of the Pennsylvania Dutch out of some apparent similarity in the process of ritual healing, but also to indicate a sense of judgment about the perceived "otherness" of these practices. Furthering this notion of scorn, the connotation of "noise" was associated with such ritual practices,[30] designating the non-English Native American and Pennsylvania Dutch languages as being unintelligible or meaningless.

One of the earliest recorded uses of powwowing in the Pennsylvania Dutch context appears in the memoirs of Pomeranian immigrant George Whitehead, who composed his transatlantic autobiography for posterity in the English language in Berks County, Pennsylvania in 1795. He recollects an experience from his early life as a servant in Pomerania, when a local hangman was asked to perform a ritual to cure him from the bite of a dog believed to have rabies. Whitehead describes his skeptical master's negative reaction to "powouring."[31] Despite its obvious anachronism on the lips of his European master, this citation indicates an already well-established Americanism just before the turn of the nineteenth century and confirms a sense of ambivalence in connotation – both as a widely accepted term for ritual healing, but also one that may come with a sense of judgment.

Powwow is the most common term for the tradition in the present day, and as the everyday use of Pennsylvania Dutch has declined in certain parts of Pennsylvania, awareness of the origin of the word powwow is also extremely limited. It is a common perception, despite copious evidence to the contrary, that the practice was derived from contact with Native Americans. Others, perhaps confused about the origins of the word powwow, have suggested that the tradition was based upon, or at least enhanced by, a desire to imitate or "play Indian," as a way for Americans of European descent to explore the exotic stereotypes of the indigenous experience.[32] Both of these perceptions of the practice are perhaps the result of a limited understanding, not only of the role and development of powwow as an English word in Pennsylvania, but also of the range of folk-religious experience in the United States - so much so that these types of non-sanctioned ritual practices are perceived to be out of place or exotic when practiced by Americans of European stock. These ritual practices are so frequently omitted and rarely discussed as part of the well-accepted narratives of early American and European history, that one can hardly begrudge bearers of the notion that powwow must have been borrowed from someone or somewhere else.

This idea of cultural borrowing, however, is wound in and through the *Braucherei* experience in both a syncretic and attributive sense, as even in Europe, rituals of Germanic cultural origin were once idealized as expressions popularly believed to have proceeded from Egyptian, "Gypsy" (Romani), Spanish, Roman, or Jewish sources.[33] While some of these influences are confirmed (such as occasional references to the Roman author Pliny the Elder), in general this form of cultural appropriation, especially that which concerned the Jewish or Romani element, says more about the idealized perceptions of the culture doing the borrowing, rather than any accurate representation of the culture from which certain ideas may or may not have actually been borrowed.

In most cases extra-cultural elements serve a particular function, while indulging a sense of exoticism. Some materials attributed to the Romani people (falsely believed to have come from Egypt, thus the name "gypsy" applied by non-Romani)[33] are thought to have great ceremonial and magical power, echoing the early twentieth century belief that "*Zigeiner kenne meh duh ass annere Leit*" (The gypsies can do things that other people can't).[34] Similarly, texts or sources derived from Jewish tradition and Hebrew language are believed to carry with them a sense of ancient biblical authority and power.[35] At the same time, objectification goes both ways, and can even become a means to condemn: some have blamed the diversity of early Pennsylvanian Christian ritual practices on the latent presence of a pagan or heathen frame of mind.[36] There are ancient precedents and origins of many religious practices, and certainly both official and folk forms of religion maintain some measure of this ancient influence.

This ambivalence about the religious origins of Pennsylvania's ritual traditions, and hesitancy to claim ownership in origin or practice, is not merely out of perceived exoticism, but especially the result of changes in doctrinal, theological, and institutional structures of religion, whereby change is part of an official and authoritative process, determining which aspects of religion will be endorsed, and what is to be discouraged. A general sense of "correctness" is associated with endorsement, while discouragement or prohibitive sanctioning determines what is considered "deviant," "unorthodox," or even "heresy."

On the other hand, folk religion, as a parallel trend of ever-changing, non-sanctioned religious experience, has a tendency to maintain some portion of that which has been discarded by orthodox religion, especially when those discarded elements are part of a cultural, regional, or ethnic expression linked to a community identity. For this very reason, Pennsylvania Dutch culture unconsciously maintained a certain level of historical Roman Catholic elements despite its predominantly Protestant culture. Invocations to the Virgin Mary and the whole hierarchy of specific saints for the healing of precise ailments, liturgical prayers such as the *Ave Maria* used within the context of penance, as well as the use of objects or places considered holy or sacred – these are just some of the ritual elements proceeding directly from a Roman Catholic past that were interwoven into Pennsylvania Dutch culture.[37] Although none of these elements are expressed within the corpus of officially sanctioned religious experience in the Protestant churches, and adherence to these practices may at times be invisible to the clergy, the membership of the churches may express these traditions in the home or other private venues where their role and ritual function within domestic, agricultural, and healing traditions is affirmed.

It is within the private sphere of life where these ritual practices gather momentum from generations of use, and are reinforced by family and personal narratives. Powwowing rituals are diverse in structure and performance, and are shaped by the people who use them and pass them on to future generations.

Although methods and procedures have varied considerably over three centuries of ritual practice within the Pennsylvania Dutch cultural region, the outcomes and experiences surrounding this tradition have woven a rich tapestry of cultural narratives that highlight the integration of ritual into all aspects of life, as well as provide insight into the challenges, conflicts, growth, and development of a distinct Pennsylvania Dutch folk culture.

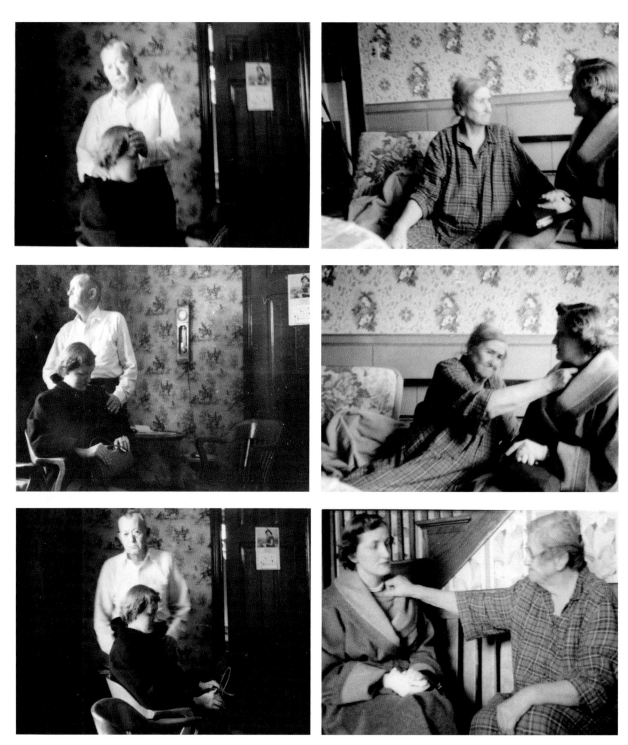

Snapshots from a series of undated, unidentified photographs from the papers of Dr. Don Yoder, featuring a series of early twentieth-century Pennsylvania healers in action. The same woman in each of the images, possibly a reporter or journalist, appears to have visited at least four powwow doctors, and some of the photographs emphasize the exchange of money in free will offerings. It is unclear whether the practitioners were aware that they were being photographed. *Pennsylvania German Cultural Heritage Center, Kutztown University of Pennsylvania.*

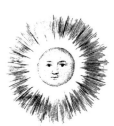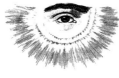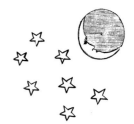

Chapter II
Faces of Powwowing
Healers, Practitioners, and Facilitators

Those who engage in the ritual expressions of powwowing are a diverse spread of people with a wide spectrum of roles. Ranging from those who employ only a few basic blessings or procedures to those who have mastered many, there are practitioners, facilitators, and tradition-bearers of various shades and degrees who powwow for friends and family, or serve their community by accepting clients from a wider geographic area. Although, as a folk tradition, there is no sense of clerical hierarchy governing the practice, with neither support nor sanctioning from medical or religious authorities, those who powwow in a more-than-occasional capacity often earn a reputation for inspiring confidence in those who seek them for healing.

A practitioner may actively create and facilitate a ritual experience for those in need – offering prayers, the laying on of hands, and elaborate ritual performances. These experiences may be outside of the realm of the ordinary for the patient, or they may resonate with sights and sounds that are at once familiar, and evocative of home. Alternately, a practitioner may merely suggest a course of action that is to be undertaken by another, allowing a patient to take matters into their own hands. Often these two modalities are blended to the effect that patients may seek assistance outside of their immediate situation, only to find that they must also play some role in the act of healing.

A classic example of both methodologies can be found in the standard wart cures, where a practitioner may be the one to apply the use of a potato, dish rag, rind of bacon, or other intermediary object to remove the illness. Such procedures are simple enough to be performed by anyone. Still, other practitioners may provide a detailed script that a patient must follow in order to enact a cure.

Following a series of detailed instructions, a gentleman from Lower Macungie effectively cured himself of a few irritating warts on his hands by employing the following procedure: He woke up before the sun, and while the dew was still on the grass, he made his way to the pig house on the family farm without speaking to anyone. He proceeded directly to the pig trough – an active trough, used daily by the animals – and he rubbed each wart three times on the rough surface of the trough. Then he walked out of the piggery and rubbed the warts three times on the dew covered grass. Then he hastened back to the house without speaking to anyone and without looking at his warts. He followed this procedure three times, on three consecutive days, and all the while ignored the warts. In his own words, he "forgot" about the warts, only to discover that when he remembered to examine his hands, the warts were gone.[1]

For those who are not up to the task of participating directly in their own ritual cure, two basic classes of practitioners have offered assistance to those in need. There are professionals, willing to accept a wide range of patients and clients from within their own community and from the outside. Still others powwow exclusively for friends and family, and only when asked to do so. Those who practice in a professional capacity are often willing to accept offerings at the patient's discretion, while anyone powwowing for a family member or friend is often unwilling to accept remuneration of any sort for the assistance.

Some people believe however, that one must seek assistance outside of their own direct family, in order for the cure to be effective. Although my great-grandmother Esther R. Heilman (1903-1999) could powwow, like many others who practiced for friends and family, she specialized in only a small number of cures, rather than a wide range. However, when her only son, my grandfather, was underweight as a young boy and did not seem to be thriving, my great-grandmother did not powwow him herself, but sent him to William H. Reppert (1881-1949), who lived down the street and powwowed for a wide range of disorders. My grandfather, Robert Raymond Heilman (1931-2009) was believed to have *Abnemme*, literally meaning in Pennsylvania Dutch "wasting" or "waning." Although some physicians have equated this illness with marasmus, caused by malnourishment, *Abnemme* was also believed to have a spiritual and emotional component which could also affect adults later in life and was akin to depression. My grandfather recalled being taken down the street to Reppert's home, in a room set aside for healing. An over-sized presentation Bible was handed to my grandfather, who was asked to take off his shirt and hold it against his chest, while Reppert softly recited prayers. The Good Book was so heavy that my grandfather recalled nearly buckling under the weight, as Reppert ran his cold hands down his back, gathering and removing the illness with sweeping gestures. My grandfather thereafter had a complete reversal of his symptoms and became a robust and healthy child.

William Reppert was widely known throughout the region for his work, which was regarded as a form of physical and spiritual care, and complementary to conventional medicine. His name was listed in the local Lebanon City directories, and the 1940 US Census as a "Faith Healer."[2] Even his World War II draft registration card described his healing activities. He charged no fees, administered no medicines, and according to one Lebanon contact, those who sought him out were not by any means opposed to conventional medicine.[3] In fact, Reppert was the second resort for stubborn complaints and disorders that had already been treated by conventional doctors. His work was not considered primary care.

One Lebanon contact, recalled visiting Reppert when her infant son had a severe case of open sores in the mouth from thrush, and although she took him to the doctor, the symptoms worsened. The infant was inconsolable, and was unable to be fed because of the ulcers. A neighbor gave her the contact information of William Reppert on Hill Street, and she took her son to him the very same day. Reppert was a mild-mannered man, with a soft voice. He brought her into a large room on the first floor of his home, where he kept his massive Bible on a table in the middle of the room. He asked her what was the matter with the child, and when she told him of the infant's trouble, without a moment's hesitation, he immediately opened his Bible and read a passage aloud in English about the healing of sores, possibly Job 5:18: "For he maketh sore, and bindeth up: he woundeth, and his hands make whole," or Matthew 10:7-8; "The kingdom of heaven is at hand. Heal the sick, cleanse the lepers, raise the dead, cast out devils: freely ye have received, freely give."[4] Reppert placed his hand upon the head of the child, and prayed quietly. When he was finished, he said, "Your son should be alright by tomorrow, but if not, visit the doctor again." As she left Reppert's home, the mother placed some money into a discrete basket positioned for such a purpose by the door. The following morning, anticipating another visit to the conventional doctor, she was delighted to find that the child's thrush was entirely gone.[5]

Reppert's repertoire of cures was not limited to childhood illnesses. When the Second World War broke out, and the draft was instated, many young men sought out Reppert when, for health reasons, they were barred from joining their peers in the armed forces. It was rumored that he had the ability to help one pass a physical examination, even with pre-existing conditions. One contact from Lebanon City recalled a young man in the neighborhood who had a heart condition and was devastated when he was not allowed into the army and could not serve his country. At a neighbor's suggestion, he visited Reppert, who powwowed him. According to my contact, the young man passed his physical examination, despite his previous rejection, and was allowed to serve in the military.[6]

Although Reppert had been a metal worker in his earlier years,[7] in his retirement, he supported himself with his healing practice. Despite his professional designation, he was by no means a profiteer, or unethical in his acceptance of cash. He set no fees, required no payment, and was generally regarded as generous with his time and energy. His patients believed fully in the efficacy of his cures and were more than willing to give offerings to him, in order support his practice and livelihood. Because

Above: The author's great-grandmother, Esther R. (Fox) Heilman (1903-1999) of Lebanon, Pennsylvania, who powwowed for livergrown children in the neighborhood and lived down the street from William Reppert.

powwowing is inherently a time-consuming and caring vocation, Reppert would never have been able to practice to the extent that he did, had he still been working a day job. In this sense, some powwowers became "professional" by popular demand.

Not all powwow doctors adhered to the same ethics regarding payment. Unlike Reppert, who operated out of his home, some practitioners traveled to meet their patients, which would be a costly and time-consuming venture. Dr. Joseph H. Hageman (1832-1905), who was known for a lucrative practice in the City of Reading, would also make house calls throughout Berks County.[8]

Isaac W. Zwally (1823-1899), a farmer and former teacher in Akron, Lancaster County, left behind a series of powwow ledgers,[9] outlining the geographic range of clients he served in Lancaster, Berks, and Lebanon Counties as a professional practitioner in the 1880s.[10]

Zwally's ledgers are extensive enough to suggest that when he was not farming, that he was actively powwowing large numbers of people, sometimes serving entire families all at once, and possibly traveling to his clients. While the majority his clients were from Akron, and neighboring Lancaster communities like Ephrata, Lititz, Millway, and Rothsville, there were also those from Lebanon, Annville, Schaefferstown, Prescott, and Jonestown, as well as Shillington, Sinking Spring, and other areas of Berks County.

Unlike some practitioners who specialize only in a few illnesses, Isaac Zwalley treated patients suffering from a wide range of illnesses and complaints, including dermatological concerns like tetter, eczema, corns, warts, and wildfire; psychological disorders such as hypochondria, nervousness, and fits; as well as a wide range of common ailments, from minor to severe: felons, sore eyes, tumors, rupture, catarrh, rheumatism, whooping cough, headache, asthma, dyspepsia, chills, epilepsy, palpitations of the heart, diarrhea, worms, cancer, and kidney disease.

What is unique about his registry of clients is that each entry consists of a date, the client's first and last name, their location, their illness or concern, and an x is placed next to each person that paid for their services.

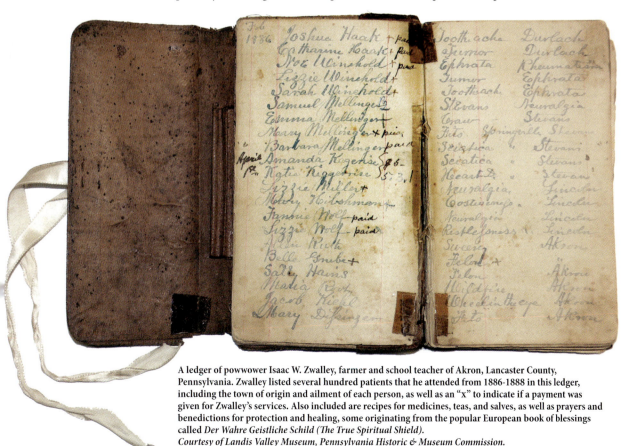

A ledger of powwower Isaac W. Zwalley, farmer and school teacher of Akron, Lancaster County, Pennsylvania. Zwalley listed several hundred patients that he attended from 1886-1888 in this ledger, including the town of origin and ailment of each person, as well as an "x" to indicate if a payment was given for Zwalley's services. Also included are recipes for medicines, teas, and salves, as well as prayers and benedictions for protection and healing, some originating from the popular European book of blessings called *Der Wahre Geistliche Schild (The True Spiritual Shield)*.
Courtesy of Landis Valley Museum, Pennsylvania Historic & Museum Commission.

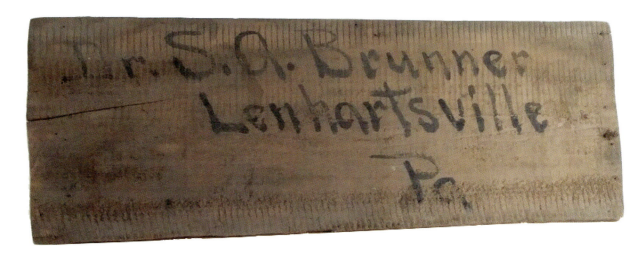

Original sign for the practice of Dr. Stanley A. Brunner (1884-1972) of Krumsville, near Lenhartsville, Berks County, Pennsylvania. "Doc" Brunner was a conventional family doctor, dentist, and powwow practitioner. *Private Collection.*

Powwow & Conventional Doctors

As one can imagine, those who powwowed in a professional capacity frequently found themselves on the wrong side of relations with certain conventional doctors who disagreed with powwow as a form of alternative medicine. These clashes with authority were common in the early twentieth century, when a period of cultural adjustment took place, with the rise of strict medical licensing laws, accreditation standards for medical schools, and in some cases, outright bans on certain genres of culturally specific folk medicine. As a result, some professional powwowers became entangled in legal disputes, especially if their client base was large, and monetary income was involved. Although the United States has become much more accepting of alternative and complementary practices in recent years, there was a time that medical societies and physicians actively worked to eradicate vernacular healing systems like powwow throughout the United States, and thus even on a local level, relations between official and folk practitioners of medicine were often tense.

A nonagenarian friend from Berks County whose father actively powwowed for friends and family recalled a confrontation that took place in the late 1930s during this period of conflict. It was Mother's Day, and both father and son were working at the local Shartlesville Hotel in northwest Berks on one of the busiest days of the year. A young woman bussing tables cut her hand on a broken glass, and the injury was severe enough that a doctor was called to attend her. The hotel staff feared for the woman's life, as she began to rapidly loose a significant amount of blood. As the doctor was some distance away, my friend's father offered to powwow her in the meantime. With her consent, he recited a biblical verse taken from the Book of Ezekiel chapter 16, verse 6, and passed his hand over the injury: "And when I passed by thee, and saw thee polluted in thine own blood, I said unto thee when thou wast in thy blood, Live; yea, I said unto thee when thou wast in thy blood, Live." The bleeding was said to have stopped immediately, and by the time the doctor had arrived some time later, the woman was already back to work, with an improvised bandage on her hand. The doctor, nevertheless, asked to examine the wound, which to his surprise was extremely deep, but was no longer bleeding or in need of stitches. Knowing full well the father's reputation with powwow, the doctor turned to him and said in the dialect: "*Ich wees was du geduh hoscht!*" – which means "I know what you did." and the implication was "…and I don't like it." Then the doctor left without speaking another word.[11]

Implicit in this interaction was the doctor's fear that if too much community credence was placed on such a practice, then powwowing could be mistaken for conventional primary care, or nurture anti-establishment sentiments about biomedical care. The perception among many physicians was that it could be to one's detriment to seek out a powwow doctor when critically ill or injured - not because powwow rituals were dangerous in any way, but that delaying necessary treatment could have dire consequences.

Not all doctors felt this way. In fact, some country doctors of Pennsylvania Dutch background were sympathetic to the cultural significance of the practice, and recognized that powwowing was used to treat a range of illnesses that were inherently difficult, even

An early nineteenth-century manuscript doctor's manual from the Oley Valley, Berks County, separated into chapters for *materia medica*, illnesses and symptoms, terminology in German and Latin, as well as several entries of *Sympathie* or sympathetic cures. The ledger includes incantations to remove warts and corns using the moon, stopping blood, soothing burns and other common cures. The writer made rare usage of Latin for the Trinitarian invocation, "*In Nomine Patris, et Fillii, et Spiritu Sancti*," – In the name of the Father, Son, and Holy Spirit – indicating a possible Roman Catholic influence in the creation of this work. *Heilman Collection.*

Also includes the SATOR square palindrome inscription, and instructions to write it on butter bread, and to eat it as a cure for rabies.

for conventional biomedical doctors. These were often chronic or ephemeral complaints that were interwoven with subjective cultural attitudes about illness. One country doctor who provided care on both ends of the spectrum, was the much-beloved Dr. Stanley A. "Doc" Brunner, whose medical practice stood at the crossroads of Old Route 22 in Krumsville, Berks County. Doc Brunner (1884-1972) was a trained conventional country doctor and dentist, who compounded and dispensed his own medicines, and was also known to powwow on the side.[12] I've spoken to at least half a dozen people presently living who were powwowed by Doc Brunner for warts. Although Doc Brunner was not by any means the norm, accounts of his prominent role in the community suggest that he was certainly not alone in his ability to care for his patients in both realms of the healing arts.

Another physician from western Berks, a Dr. James Livingood (1817-1891) of Womelsdorf, sent patients with chronic ailments to see his wife, who powwowed from their home in Womelsdorf.[13] According to one account, Dr. Livingood also powwowed for certain ailments himself, and was one of the teachers of Sophia Fessler Leininger, the mother of the celebrated Schuylkill County healer, Sophia Bailer.[14]

Evidence in early Pennsylvania doctor's ledgers suggests that Brunner and Livingood were not by any means anomalous, as historically many doctors appear to have had a foot in both worlds, bridging their academic training with their role among the people. This means that doctors had to have a firm grasp, not only of official notions of medicine, but of the way in which their patients perceived and described their concerns.

The prolific Johann Daniel Waldenberger of Manchester Township, York County, produced a highly organized and fully-indexed ledger in 1796. A conventional physician of his era, *ein "Doctor der Medicin und Vegetabeln"* (a doctor of medicine and botanicals), his ledger provides lengthy descriptions of illnesses and their symptoms, as well as detailed recipes and cures, separated into chapters for humans and animals. A number of his entries included powwow cures, including references to supernatural causation of illness in horses, such as *"wan's bezaubert iss"* (when a horse is hexed and unable to work).[15]

Wan Ros bezaubert ist:

Sind die Zeichen eines bezauberten Roses es henget den Kopff unter die Krippe und läßt die Haar im Mähn ausgehen und Schweifft es schwitzet und kan vor Mattigkeit fast keinen Schenkel heben zu diesem nimm Todtenbein vom Kirchhoff ein stuck Holz das daß Wasser ausworffen hat, dann nim ein neuen Irdenen Haffen thue drein ein Quart esig soffire drein, schabe ein wennig von dem Bein und holtz thue dieses auch drein rühre es wohl mit dem Holtz durch ein ander gieße es dem Roß ein du must ihm aber den Kopf wohl in die Höhe binden daß es alles verschluge schlag ihnm die Bug Adern und Schrankes in dem bein und holtz ihm etwas auf die rechte seite unter die Mahne daß übrige tragen wider an seinen ort wo du es genomen hast.

When a horse is hexed:

The signs of a hexed horse are such that it hangs its head below the manger and the hair comes loose from the mane. It sweats and drips, and from faintness can barely lift a leg. At this point, obtain the bone of a dead person from the church yard and a piece of wood from which the moisture has been removed, then obtain a new earthen pot, and pour into it a quart of vinegar, and scrape a little from the bone and wood and add this as well. Stir it thoroughly and blend it with the piece of wood. Administer it to the horse. You must tie the horse with its head upright, so that it swallows. Bleed the horse from the shoulder vein, staunch it with the bone and wood, at the right side under the mane. Then take what is left over and carry it back to the spot where you obtained it.

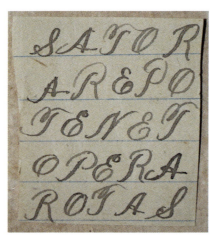

Schluckzettel (Edible blessing) ca. 1880, featuring the ancient Latin SATOR palindrome written on a 1" x 1" square of paper, intended to be fed to cattle to cure disease and protect from malicious spiritual forces. *Heilman Collection.*

Waldenberger also includes a ritual cure for rabies, suggesting that one write the exotic inscription "*x haga xx maga xx paga x*" on paper, and give it to the patient to eat – a type of cure called a *Schluck-Zettel* (edible blessing) when used for humans, and a *Fress-Zettel* for animals.[16]

Another sizeable conventional doctor's ledger from the 1830s in the Oley Valley of Berks County is organized in a similar manner, with whole chapters for symptoms, causation of illness, and lists in German and Latin for herbs and *materia medica*.[17] A chapter entitled "*Sympathie*," outlines seven powwowing rituals, including prayers for diarrhea, inflammation, warts, corns, bleeding, and wounds. Another powwowing entry cites the celebrated SATOR square palindrome from the Roman era and another cryptic inscription as cures for the bite of a rapid dog (see Chapter III). Each of these inscriptions was to be written on butter bread and fed to the patient in a similar manner to Dr. Waldenberger's *Schluck-Zettel*.

This unidentified ledger could be the work of Dr. Peter Y. Bertolett, Dr. Enoch Griesemer, or Dr. Francis Palm, all of whom are listed as physicians in the 1850 US Federal Census for Oley Township.[18] Perhaps a clue to the identity of the doctor is in the use of the Latin Trinitarian invocation concluding each powwow cure: *In nomine Patris, et Fillii, et Spiritu Sancti*. It is possible that the name Francis could indicate a possible connection to the small Roman Catholic contingency in Oley, a minority (roughly 1%) among the Pennsylvania Dutch, accounting for the writer's use of the invocation from the Latin Mass within the powwowing rituals.

Powwowing & the Clergy

Doctors are not the only class of citizens held in high esteem that have participated in ritual healing. In communities were such beliefs were common in rural parishes, Pennsylvania clergy occasionally participated directly in powwowing practices, as an extension of their pastoral care.

The Rev. Georg Mennig (1773-1851) was at one time the only ordained Lutheran minister residing in all of Schuylkill County, as well as a publisher of broadside instructions for powwowing, including a cure for erysipelas.[19] This celebrated and prolific pastor, whose tombstone boasts that "he preached 1633 sermons, confirmed 1733 and baptized 1631 people," administered communion to an astounding 19,680 people during his career. His influence in early Schuylkill County communities cannot be underestimated. Rev. Mennig's cures were used for generations after his passing, and his office lent credence to a practice that was openly condemned by some other clergy of his day.[20] Mennig's broadsides may have even influenced later published instructions on powwowing from the alleged hand of a Reverend Hill, who included a cure for epilepsy in both English and German, as well as German cures for the topical infections of ring-worm and tetter and a transcription of the biblical verse, Ezekiel 16:6 for stopping blood.[21]

Although Mennig's practices may at first glance appear to be contradictory to Lutheran doctrine, early Protestant sources suggest that there were strong precedents for such activities among the clergy in earlier phases of Lutheran faith expression.

Essentially, powwow doctors ministered to the sick using practices that were borrowed from earlier expressions of liturgical tradition. It should therefore be no surprise that some pastors participated in powwowing practices and that any form of sanctioning from the clergy would be valued by the laity. In fact, the names and reputations of ministers are generously interwoven through powwow narratives, with representatives in many denominations.

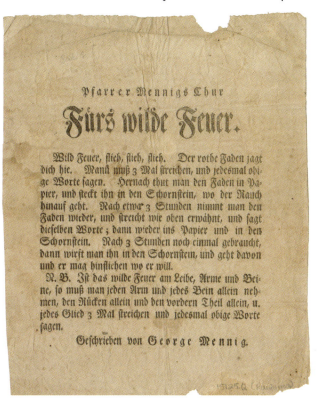

A mid-nineteenth-century broadside cure for erysipelas attributed to Rev. Georg Mennig. *Courtesy of the Library Company of Philadelphia.*

The Lutheran Rev. Mennig's powwow practice is mirrored by the Brethren minister Henry Schuler Long (1853-1918) of Franconia, Montgomery County, who was known to have carried written powwow prayers in the same notebook from which he preached his sermons.[22] The same is purported to have been true of the German Reformed minister Charles Gebler Herrmann of Maxatawny Township, Berks County, who compiled one of the most famous collections of German grave-side songs, *Sänger am Grabe* in 1842.[23]

On the other hand, his colleague William A. Helffrich (1827-1894), preaching in adjacent townships, was known to have openly discouraged his parishioners from visiting powwow doctors, and even postponed a home communion visitation on account of one parishioner's inclination to visit a powwower.[24] The Rev. Daniel Weiser indignantly criticized the activities of powwowing in his community, after repeated requests to have infants baptized – not as a sacrament to dedicate new life to the community of the church, but rather as a cure for infant colic – stating, "It is a marvel to us how any

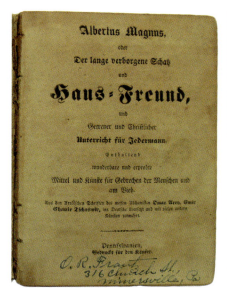
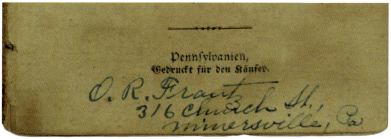

Powwowing manual printed ca. 1830, owned and inscribed by the well-respected Schuylkill County minister, Rev. Orville R. Frantz of Minersville (1868-1944). Serving the Reformed Church for 45 years at congregations in Summit Hill in Carbon County, Old Zionsville in Lehigh, and Minersville, Rev. Frantz was the clerk of the Schuylkill County Classis, and was secretary of the Reading Synod. It is unknown if Rev. Frantz actually powwowed, or merely kept the book for reference. It is notable, however, that Rev. Frantz indicated his ownership of the book with his name and home address, where he served the congregation at Emanuel Reformed Church. *Heilman Collection.*

Christian can ever walk in such direct opposition to the divine record."[25]

The Rev. J. Spangler Kieffer (1842-1919) contended with the same perceptions regarding baptism in his parish at Hagerstown, Maryland in 1886. A child suffering from *Abnemme* or marasmus was brought to Rev. Kieffer for christening, who was reluctant to argue with the parents about the purpose of the liturgical ritual. He baptized the child, but when he asked if he could borrow a pencil to record the birth and baptism in his church register, the parents refused on account of the fact that they were having the child powwowed too. They explained to him that they were unwilling to lend or borrow anything for nine days, or the powwowing would be ineffective.[26]

The expectation that the liturgy and the clergy inherently possessing healing qualities was the source of much annoyance for Dr. John George Schmucker (1771-1854), a founder of the General Synod of the Lutheran Church in America. Entirely by accident, after innocently examining a parishioner's wart, Schmucker was temporarily regarded as worker of miracles when the wart was spontaneously healed. One of Schmucker's contemporaries documented the incident: "The man declared that from that moment, it began to diminish until it disappeared altogether. His neighbors heard of it, and, for miles around, all who were affected with similar unnatural protuberances hastened to the "Pastor" to be healed…" Schmucker rebuked them all, and took great pains to convince the people that he was no healer at all.[27]

Such beliefs regarding the healing acts of clergy inspired one James Welsh of West Philadelphia, to impersonate a Roman Catholic priest in 1880, as a means to inspire confidence in his patients as a powwower.[28]

Apparently this tactic was used in many communities, as a Lebanon County doctor once decried: "When the charlatan appears in the character of a minister of the gospel, as is not unfrequently the case, in order to more successfully prey upon the weakness of human nature, what a degrading spectacle is presented to the eye of the Christian physician! He hardly knows whether to condemn or pity the unprincipled wretch".[29]

Of all historical ministers who opposed the practice of powwow, there was none so outspoken as the Rev. William B. Raber of the Pennsylvania Conference of the United Brethren in Christ. His 1855 treatise *The Devil and Some of His Doings* describes Raber's perception of the infernal illusions that deceived American society in his day, and includes a section on "Charms and Pawwowing." Raber condemns powwowing as being the work of the devil, even though he acknowledges that it is based on religious principles. Instead he says that it "belongs to paganism, from whence it came, and it is unworthy of an enlightened, leaving out of the question, a Christian community." Rev. Raber continues in a judicious tone:

> To cure by words and manipulations would be performing a miracle, and where would that supernatural power come from? The answer from every paw-wawer is, without conscience or comment – from the Lord. Well, let us see. The sixth verse of the sixteenth chapter of Ezekiel is used to stop bleeding, [When I passed by thee and saw thee polluted in thine own blood, I said unto thee, when thou wast in thy blood live, yea, when thou wast in thy blood live] by inserting the first name of the bleeding person before the word live. Now in that verse is a similitude of Jerusalem under a neglected, wretched infant. Apply that to an individual with a bleeding nose, or otherwise, and Holy Writ is violently wrestled out of its original meaning, by which a miracle is to be performed. Will God do such a thing? Is it in accordance

with his character as God, or commensurate with the truthful nature of his attributes? My dear reader! Such things are not from God. He cannot agreeably with his veracity as God, bless a wrong application of his Holy Word to perform a miracle.[30]

Rev. Raber's position is not so much a criticism of the use of scripture for healing, but the manner in which it is applied, and the aesthetics that create the ritual structure of powwow practice. This very criticism however, focuses on an excellent example of the adaptability of scriptural passages for the purpose of healing, despite the reverend's disagreement. The symbolic comparison of the city of Jerusalem to an abandoned, suffering infant "polluted" in its own blood that is described in the Book of Ezekiel, is used in powwowing to create yet another comparison, in this case of the bleeding person, who is often referred to as a "child of God" in powwowing prayers. This comparison is meant to apply scripture in a meaningful way to alleviate suffering and properly place the healing experience within a religious context.

Although Rev. Raber suspects that such an application of words is evidence of paganism and a corruption of biblical interpretation, on the contrary, this particular use of scripture is viewed as one of the simplest examples of biblically-based ritual healing among the Pennsylvania Dutch. This particular verse of scripture (shown below) was printed as a popular powwow broadside, and is sometimes found written out longhand among family papers, or marked in the margins of folio Bibles.[31]

Still other critics of powwow take a different perspective. Dr. J. H. Myers writes for the *American Lutheran* in 1870, and calls powwow "superstition" – except that he differentiates what he calls the "undeniable" healing resulting from the actual words that are used. Dr. Myers claims that the healing is actually achieved through the laying on of hands, and that the words were only a veneer that shrouded an otherwise sound, Christian healing practice.[32]

In each case, both Rev. Raber and Dr. Myers represent official denominational doctrines, and they judge

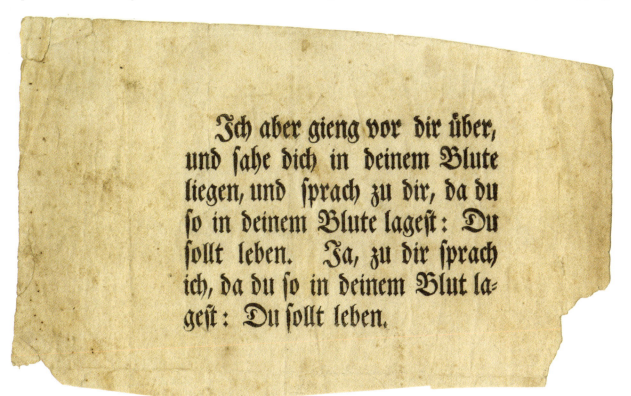

Ezekiel 16:6 Broadside remedy for stopping blood. ca. 1800. *Courtesy of the Library Company of Philadelphia*

The text is from Luther's translation: "When I passed by thee and saw thee polluted in thine own blood, I said unto thee, when thou wast in thy blood live, yea, when thou wast in thy blood live." This verse, which repeats the word "blood" three times, is used as a blessing to stop bleeding, wherein the sufferer's full baptismal name is inserted after each mention of the German pronoun "du" (you).

the practice of powwow based upon its divergence from their own religious expression, using similarity as their basis for determining its degree of correctness. Beyond this, both ministers redefine powwowing according to their own religious schematics and relegate the tradition to categories that fail to accurately describe it, portraying powwowing as either a devil-induced delusion or as an ignorant superstition. While the latter term is markedly less harsh, *superstition* is still a prejudiced term, implying beliefs worthy of denigration. Often the term is used to denote beliefs held by others, and is rarely self-reflective. While these forms of criticism are perhaps to be expected, such attitudes ignore the place of powwowing practice as part of a continuum of religious belief.

Powwowers in Public Office

Ministers are not the only community leaders to have engaged in powwow healing practices past and present. Even public officials have held such unofficial roles within the community, although accounts of their activities rarely appear in print.

John Henry Stump (1880-1949), three-time socialist mayor of Reading City, is fondly remembered not only for his political success, but also for powwowing away warts with a potato. A recent contact in Reading City recalled his brother's warts being taken off by Mayor Stump in the 1940s.

In 2012 I had the pleasure of meeting a Berks County man who powwows, and had formerly held the position of township supervisor (location withheld for privacy) for many years. As a well-respected person within his community, known for his honesty and pragmatism, his powwowing was discrete, but posed no threat to his reputation or public standing.[33] In fact, in 2017, he began to teach a local woman in order to pass his practice on to a new generation of healers.

As a young boy he lived with his family within the Greater Reading area sometime in the 1940s, and he had been taken to see a woman powwow doctor in West Reading for a case of childhood bedwetting that had persisted longer than the parents could endure. Conventional doctors were unable to offer any relief, so they visited a woman who was known for a high rate of success in treating such "nervous"

disorders. The woman powwowed him, but the main cure for his condition was to be fulfilled on his own, under her careful instructions. He was to go alone and unseen into a graveyard in the dark of night. Without talking to anyone about it beforehand, he was to find a freshly dug grave where a body had not yet been interred, and he was to urinate into the open grave.

Following what must have been a terrifying experience for the young boy, his bedwetting ceased immediately after his visit to the church yard. Some variations of this common ritual require that one do it at the time of the waning moon, without the aid of moonlight to illuminate the venture. The experience was so profoundly transformative to him, that when he grew older, he learned to powwow from the woman in West Reading, so that he could help others.

In his adulthood, he ran his own business had many opportunities to powwow for friends and neighbors. In all of his years of powwowing, one particular experience from decades ago resonates still strongly with him as an example of the power of powwow to alter the course of one's life.

HARRY I. GRUBER
SINKING SPRING, ROUTE 1, PA.

MONDAYS, 6 P. M. TO 9 P. M.
TUESDAYS, WEDNESDAYS, FRIDAYS, 9 A. M. TO 9 P. M.
SATURDAYS, 9 A. M. TO 3 P. M.
CLOSED THURSDAYS, SUNDAYS, HOLIDAYS

A business card, for the powwower Harry I. Gruber of Sinking Spring, near Reading, Pennsylvania, obtained by Don Yoder sometime in the 1960s. Gruber worked part time in the knitting mills by day, and powwowed in the hours remaining. *Heilman Collection.*

The son of a man who worked locally on the railroad was plagued with a terrible case of warts that covered his body from head to toe. These were no ordinary warts, but were drooping skin tags that consumed the surface of his skin. The boy was stigmatized by his appearance and had no hope for a normal life. The father of the boy was disheartened by the whole affair, as he had wasted time, energy, and money on a series of unsuccessful treatments from conventional doctors who were unable to permanently effect a cure. Surgical procedures used to treat the boy involved cauterizing, freezing, cutting, and the application of acids, all with minimal effect on his overall condition, and only serving to further torment the boy. The warts were so numerous that they could not possibly be removed in one treatment, and no sooner were they removed that they began to regrow.

My contact asked the father of the boy if he had ever had his son powwowed, and the father replied to the negative, stating that he did not believe that such treatments were effective. Eventually, after all else failed, he consented to having his son powwowed.

While my contact did not tell me exactly what version of the lunar wart cure he used for such an overwhelming number of warts, another not nearly as advanced case from Chester County recently required a sizeable quantity of potatoes, one for each wart.[34] After powwowing for the warts, he never saw the boy again – that is, until over a decade later when he had grown to a man.

My contact said he would never forget the day that he was sitting in a restaurant in West Reading, and a tall handsome young man, with a glowing complexion approached him and said, "You probably don't remember me, but I'll never forget what you did for me!"

Themes of community reciprocity run through many personal narratives of powwowing – stories of healing, teaching, learning, and transforming. For some, becoming a healer is the result of a recovery from illness,[35] for others it is a condition of birth, or in rare cases, a mixture of both.

Powwowing by Birthright

Although powwowing has been practiced over the centuries by people with a wide range of specializations and abilities, oral traditions describe particular circumstances under which one may be more inclined towards healing, or possess greater aptitude for the ritual arts. By virtue of birthright, a seventh son, whose father was a seventh son, was considered a rare and holy designation, portending supernatural abilities. Children born on Ember Days, reserved for fasting in the liturgical calendar, were allegedly able to see spirits. A "posthumous" child, who was born after the father's death, was believed to have healing powers superior to others, because of their connection with the world that lay beyond the grave.[36] And almost universally in European tradition, a child born with a caul, that is, with the amniotic membrane or veil covering the face, was believed to have uncanny abilities.[37] In some cases, the caul is saved, and later serves as an object of power for the individual. Called *der Wehl* in Pennsylvania Dutch,[38] this membrane can be likened to a funeral veil, and is symbolic of the passage between the worlds of the living and the dead.

Although the latter condition is extremely rare – about one in every 80,000 births – occasionally, stories surface of powwow doctors who were born with the caul. There is, however, none quite as compelling as the story of Harry Edward Swope (1882-1968), a well-known healer who worked in Hershey, Pennsylvania, who not only was born with the caul, but, later, was miraculously restored to life by a powwow doctor after being officially pronounced dead at the age of three.[39]

A great-granddaughter of Edward Swope recalled living with her family in the upstairs apartment on the second story of her great-grandfather's home, where, as a favored youngster, she was allowed to quietly witness Ed perform healing rituals for clients suffering from terminal illnesses. While she was young, her great-grandfather told her the story of how he learned to powwow from a woman who had raised him from the dead.

At the age of three, in 1885, Edward was seriously injured while playing with his older brother Clayton on a swing in the backyard, when he accidentally fell upon a rusted nail protruding from a board lying on the ground. Rapidly, the toddler began showing signs of a tetanus infection, and was diagnosed with lockjaw. Although Edward was pronounced dead just a few days later, he would never make it to the grave until 83 years later.

Above: early photograph of Ed Swope, around the time of his miraculous resurrection, ca. 1885. Right: A portrait of Ed Swope as a young man, possibly around the time that he learned to powwow. Courtesy of the family of Harry Edward Swope.

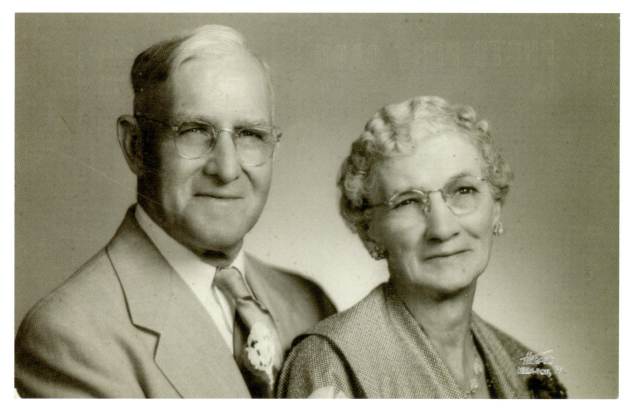

Family photograph of Ed and Bertha (Eckenroth) Swope, of Hershey, ca. 1950. *Courtesy of the family of Harry Edward Swope.*

On the day that his funeral preparations were to take place, as was the custom in those days, Edward's body had been laid out for a home viewing prior to embalming, and the family gathered to pay their respects. An old woman unfamiliar to the family came to the home, and asked, "Do you have a child that has recently died?" When the family replied to the affirmative, she asked if she would be allowed to pray over the deceased child. The family consented, and the woman went into the room alone where the body was laid. After some time, she emerged, and told Edward's mother, "your son needs you." His mother went into the room, and to her surprise, found him sitting up, and alive.

Although many scientific explanations could be conferred upon the incident, stories of Ed's miraculous resurrection received popular attention, and it was even covered in regional newspapers. Nearly a century later, when Ed's great-great-grandson was baptized in a nearby church in the fall of 1978, elderly members of the congregation still recalled Edward Swope, as the man who was raised from the dead.

The woman responsible for bringing Edward back to the land of the living was a local powwow doctor, whose name has been long forgotten, but the very same woman later became a mentor to Edward and taught him the healing arts. He grew to be a compassionate man, who never charged for his services to the sick, believing devoutly that whatever cures he could facilitate were a gift from God. His specialization was with the terminally ill, especially those who had reached the limits of conventional treatment, and were awaiting the inevitable. It is unknown whether or not Edward's experience with death and resurrection motivated him to care for people who were nearing the ends of their lives, but his reputation surely played a role in his expression of the tradition.

His wife, Bertha Eckenroth Swope, was also deeply religious, but she opposed his method of curing, and discouraged him from telling the tale of his extraordinary experiences. Edward's favorite great-granddaughter witnessed many of his powwowing sessions when she was only five or six years of age, but only when great-grandmother was away. If she was quiet and respectful she was allowed to sit in the very same room while he worked.

Edward powwowed in his study, where he kept his folio Bible open on his desk and he read from the scriptures as part of his ritual procedure. As a native speaker of the language, his healing words were always in Pennsylvania Dutch.

His great-granddaughter recalls a case where a woman with a massive inoperable growth of advanced cancer on her neck came to Edward for powwowing. He treated her many times, each time focusing his attention on the tumor, running his hands closely to her neck and jaw without touching her, and using a piece of string as if pulling and drawing out the illness from the woman's body. Edward's grand-daughter noticed a significant reduction in the size of the tumor, over the course of a number of treatments. Interestingly enough, a traditional way to remove a goiter or tumor was to pass the hand of a dead person over the growth.[40] Ed's reputation as a person who returned unscathed from death's clutches as a child may have earned him a stronger reputation as a healer.

When Edward passed away in 1968, he bequeathed a few of his personal powwowing items to his great-granddaughter. Among them was a German copy of Hohman's popular powwowing manual, *The Long Lost Friend*, as well as a cast concrete obelisk that once stood in the middle of Edward's backyard garden. The obelisk, measuring 20" high and 6" wide, has four sides featuring images of the sun, the full moon, the sun peeking out over rainclouds, and a bearded personification of the wind. The obelisk served an essential function in the latter years of Edward's powwowing. As part of his ritual practice, Edward would place written inscriptions under the obelisk, which rotted away in the damp earth, taking the illness with them.

ETHNIC DIVERSITY IN POWWOWING

Many practitioners, past and present, engage in practices, like Ed Swope, that are unique, and tailored to their individual preferences. Some may use specific locations, objects, or prayers that are idiosyncratic to their role or clientele. Other practices may reflect the identity of the practitioner, as certain individuals were believed to possess greater power to heal particular illnesses.

Such is the case for the black powwow practitioner Martin Springer (1862-1940) from Brecknock Township, Berks County, who was well-known in his community for visiting homes to treat mumps and whooping cough. Marty was a the son of the legendary Robert Springer, a man who escaped slavery and claimed to have been a wagon driver in the war of 1812, allegedly living to the age of 119.[41] Robert had established a homestead in the wooded border region where Brecknock meets Caernarvon Township, Lancaster County, and a number of formerly enslaved black families formed a hamlet there, known as Springerville or Brush Town.

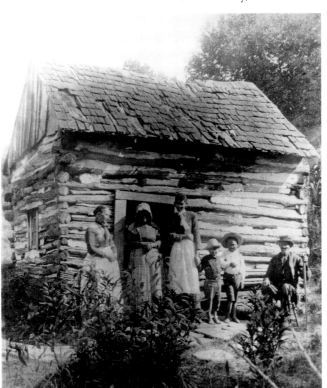

The Springer Family and their log home in Springerville, the earliest house in the wooded hamlet along the Berks-Lancaster Border. Robert Springer is seated, and Marty Springer is standing alongside his father. Courtesy of the Landis Valley Village & Farm Museum, Pennsylvania Historic and Museum Commission.

Marty Springer experienced severe discrimination in his younger years, and the local newspapers recorded a series of trumped-up accusations for of a number of crimes, everything from loitering, to horse thievery, and even marrying someone else's wife. Marty was also implicated in being part of a criminal cartel, which the local newspapers dubbed "the sassafras gang" (presumably on account of their dwelling in the forest). The supposed "gang" actually consisted of several witnesses and their families who testified against a white man, Joseph Spears who was the father of a child with Marty's sister Ellen Springer, both of whom Spears abandoned.[42] Spears was acquitted by a presumably white jury based on rumors about the mother's character, suggesting that she lived among thieves and criminals in the forest.

After testifying in the woman's defense, the "gang" consisting of Marty and his wife Margaret (who happened to be white), a black camp-meeting preacher, Rev. John Francis, and his wife, and two others identified as a white man and a woman of mixed racial background were all arrested for vagrancy while resting by the side of the road on their return trip home, and held in prison for weeks. Officers were sent to their homes, where they claimed to have found "no evidence of an honest means of support" – an attempt at circumstantial accusation of criminal activity. Without proof, everyone in the "gang" was finally released, except for Marty, who was held for further questioning about accusations of theft of some horses in Lancaster.[43] Despite Marty's experiences with discrimination and incarceration, he continued to live in the same community throughout his life.

Marty Springer was a master basket-maker, and the last resident of the settlement in the hills. His powwowing was unique to his role in the community as one of the few black residents, and according to local narratives, he employed a cure based in an old Pennsylvania Dutch belief that whooping cough and other childhood ailments could be cured by a kiss from a black man.[44] This belief was not unique to Berks County, and was documented in ten counties at the turn of the twentieth century.[45] Some claimed that the ritual was also a preventative measure, and was most effective if the child was under one year of age.[46] This ritual cure and vaccine certainly raises concerns about issues of racism and objectification of ethnic minorities. At the same time, it is difficult to interpret the procedure for people on both sides of the ritual experience based on today's values. Was such a ritual symbolically demeaning or empowering to Marty? Did Marty's healing role elevate his status within the community in times of otherwise tense national and local race relations?

Despite the complex context of racial tensions, it is important to also compare this ritual to other procedures, such as the notion that a posthumous child could cure whooping cough,[47] as well as a woman who has not changed her name by marriage (i.e. one who married a man with the same last name as her maiden name),[48] both of which were considered rare, exceptional circumstances. Was the ritual therefore suggestive of the idea that whooping cough was best cured by liminal figures outside of social norms, who walked the line between this world and the next?

Another common cure for whooping cough required drinking from a blue tumbler, and preferably one that did not belong to the family of the suffering child.[49] One could easily assume that the color blue is being used in a sympathetic manner for this cure, as the disease is called *Blohe Huschde* (the blue cough) in Pennsylvania Dutch, and another cure involves the use of a blue ribbon.[50] However, there is also another possibility relating to the use of blue glass bottles for exorcising or capturing spirits among black practitioners of Hoodoo in the south.[51] Hoodoo or root work, is a widely practiced system of healing, similar to powwowing, which developed in black communities in the south and blended West African and European traditions.

Hoodoo was certainly well established in Pennsylvania by the late nineteenth century, as evidenced by controversial personalities such as hoodoo doctor Joseph Littleton Teacle (d. 1891) of Philadelphia,[52] who later moved to West Chester, where his services were sought by urban and rural people of all ethnic backgrounds.

Doctor Joseph Littleton Teacle, a renowned hoodoo practitioner and healer of Chester County, Pennsylvania. From a fragment of the Philadelphia Newspaper, *The Evening Public Ledger*, Monday, November 23, 1914.

In Hoodoo traditions, "haint blue" is a color that is believed to be protective from malicious spiritual forces, and blue bottles can still be found hanging in trees in some communities in the south as a form of ritual protection of homes and yards.[53] Is it possible that drinking from a blue cup (perhaps the cup of a black practitioner) was related to the notion of the cure by a kiss?

According to oral history in Brecknock Township, Marty Springer was known to have embraced his role as a healer in the early twentieth century, and went around willingly visiting the families of children suffering from whooping cough. Some residents, even up until the present day, recall hearing positive stories about this particular way that Marty cared for the sick children in his neighborhood up until the year of his death in 1940. The perception among older white residents of Brecknock Township, many of whom still own exquisite examples of his craftsmanship in willow and oak baskets, remember that Marty was well liked in the community. Very little else is remembered about his powwowing activities, except for his healing kiss.[54]

Marty Springer's story is by no means unique, and powwowing was not unusual within black communities in Pennsylvania in the nineteenth and twentieth centuries. Although frequently characterized as an exclusive tradition, practiced only by the descendants of the first German-speaking immigrants, powwowing is not so much an indicator of ethnicity, but an expression of culture. Just as the Pennsylvania Dutch language was spoken by many Pennsylvanians, including African Americans,[55] so too is a broad spectrum of religious and cultural attitudes shared among many people and ethnicities within the Pennsylvania Dutch region.

At the same time that Marty Springer was powwowing in Brecknock as a secondary vocation, so too was Rufus Murray (1883-1940), a black powwower and gardener[56] in York, Pennsylvania. Rufus allegedly felt "a calling" to the tradition when he was a young man working in a shoeshine parlor in a hotel, and experienced some form of religious transformation.[57] His methods of treating the sick and afflicted were a syncretic blend of Pennsylvania Dutch, Hebrew, and hoodoo root-work traditions. Rufus' powwowing included the ritual use of the Psalms, and invocations of the Hebrew names of God, found in the *Sixth and Seventh Books of Moses*,[58] a work popular not only in Pennsylvania, but among hoodoo practitioners in the South (see Chapter V). Rufus also created ritual blessings which bear all the earmarks of root-work, with the use of specific herbs and roots, bound together with scriptural passages into bundles that were worn on the person for healing and protection.[59] Rufus received mild notoriety for his peripheral role in treating a mentally ill man, John Blymire of York in the late 1920s, who suffered from a perceived curse. Blymire and three accomplices later killed a colleague of Rufus named Nelson Rehmeyer in 1928, when they suspected that Rehmeyer was responsible for Blymire's misfortune.[60] Although the incident sparked international attention, and raised the ire of legal, medical, and religious institutions against powwowing, Rufus was never the target of any organized efforts, aside from some petty, critical journalism.

Around 1850 a black female practitioner, whose name has been lost to time, powwowed within about ten miles from Lancaster City, where she was known for having a vast clientele that traveled great distances to see her. She operated out her home, until the practice became too much for her private residence, whereby she commenced to practice out of a rented room in a hotel every Wednesday in Lancaster City. In addition to treating physical ailments, she was also known for being capable of compelling thieves to return stolen property, as well as counteract witchcraft. She was best known for a series of "miracles" which were performed remotely upon people whom she had never met. Although the details of these events were never documented, her critics suggest that her ritual procedures were all derived from German sources, and that she spoke them so softly that they could not be heard.[61]

People of many ethnic and racial backgrounds made use of German and Pennsylvania Dutch language in their powwowing practices. Third generation Irish-American Levi Laydom (1826-1902) living at Dicks Dam near Pinetown or New Chester, Adams County, kept an extensive manuscript of recipes, procedures and rituals of healing. As with most Americans, Laydom's background was mixed, and although his father was Irish and hailed from Maryland, his mother was a Chronister of Pennsylvania Dutch stock.[62] Laydom's manuscript reflected this blended background, and some of his cures were transcribed from phonetic pronunciations of German and Pennsylvania Dutch, and in other cases he provided literal translations of healing rituals in English. While it is not precisely clear if Laydom spoke Pennsylvania Dutch or not, the majority of his cures were in English, and many are dated:

> February 11 1859
> A cure for warts or other excrecents
> on the third day in the increace of the moon in the evening you see the new moon for the first time then take out your patent and putting your finger on the wart and looking up to the new moon say as follows: what I now look upon is increasing and what I now touch is decreasing after repeating this three times walk home again.

In this entry, Laydom provided the English version of the classic Pennsylvania Dutch lunar wart cure, and while no potato or other intermediary object plays a role, the words are the English counterpart to the German, "*Alles was ich sehe das wachse, und was ich fühle das vergehe.*" This cure expresses some ambiguity concerning the precise phase of the moon, as the words suggest that the moon is on "the increase"- meaning to wax, but reference to the "new moon" is used twice. This stems from the fact that the new moon is to be three days old at the time of the ritual, i.e. three days after new moon, when the moon begins to wax.

Laydom primarily cites herbal recipes, such as a salve made from soot and sweet cream applied with plantain

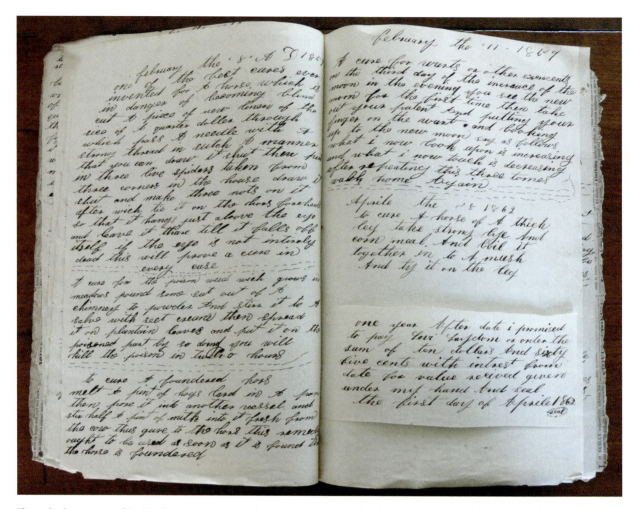

The medical manuscript of Levi Laydom, writen near New Chester, Adams County, in the 1850s and 60s. *Courtesy of Gregory Wonders and Family.*

leaves to poison ivy rash, or cornmeal mush applied to a swollen leg. On the other hand, his detailed powwowing remedies included both verbal and written blessings used for healing. His blessing for stopping blood is written in phonetic German, with pronounced Pennsylvania Dutch influence:

*Yasus Christus dires plude dos stilled de smartsen
und stilled dos plude
dos hildfed dear gut thare fother
gut thare sue gut thare hyeleghist omen.*

Jesus Christ's precious blood
that stops the pain
and stops the blood
this help thee, God the Father,
God the Son, God the Holy Spirit, Amen.

Another, for blowing burns appears in fragmented, phonetic German:

Host do de moundfyling othor brenen so blo ich der dri moal myen Autumn ins.

Hast thou the mouth-rot? So shall I blow my breath three times into thee.

Other blessings appear entirely in English:

A Cure for Burns:

When I am suffering with burning heart the Lord alone is my help he comes to me with kindness and takes away from [N.N.] hot and cold burnings the three highest names are then to be spoken and while doing so the injured part is to be blown upon three time the above to be repeated three times.

Both Levi Laydom and Marty Springer are certainly quintessential Pennsylvanians, from families of diverse backgrounds that acclimated over several generations to

Pennsylvania's unique cultural climate, and they are not alone in being remembered for generations as powwow healers. Another famous healer was Jacques Beauchamp (also spelled Grosjean, and other variations) or "French Jacob," eighteenth-century Alsatian immigrant[63] and owner of a pioneer trading post in Millersburg, Dauphin County[64] and eventually a series of grist mills, beginning in Buffalo Valley, present day Union County.

French Jacob was known not only to be a healer, but one to whom many miraculous acts, both benign and sinister, have been attached. He was known to perform all of the necessary functions of a powwow practitioner, including stopping blood, blowing burns, halting the spread of fire without water, and paralyzing snakes. But legendary narratives also gave to him the ability to transform people into animals, to become invisible to his enemies, and to conceal lodes of silver that no person could discover by ordinary means.[65]

Jacob eventually left Pennsylvania entirely, and moved to Kentucky, where he appears to have spent the rest of his days (others contend that he moved on to Missouri). Although much speculation concerning his milling enterprise, his descendants, and his final resting place has produced a multitude of conflicting genealogical narratives, it is generally agreed upon that French Jacob lived along the South Fork of the Licking River, where he continued his milling operations, and appeared on tax records in the late 1790s.[67] French Jacob's sojourn provides at least one documented example of the spreading influence of powwowing throughout the Pennsylvania Dutch diaspora in the eighteenth century.

Part-Time to Professional Powwow

Although it is evident that powwow practitioners have served in a variety of roles and occupations, everything from millers to basket-makers, from mayors to teachers, some practitioners blended their occupational and ritual activities in unique ways. Midwives, herbalists, pastors, farmers, barbers, blacksmiths, hoboes, and hangmen – people of all walks of life have specialized in ritual activities that serve an ancillary function for their primary occupation. For example, a midwife may specialize in ritually applied herbal compounds used to hasten or ease the pain of delivery, as well as blessings to ensure the safety and health of the mother and child.[68] A blacksmith or farrier may perform cures for horses and livestock, or fashion objects used in ritual applications (see Chapter VII). In some cases, however a person's occupation influenced the content or manner of their powwowing to such a degree that it contributed to a legendary persona.

One such man was Jake "*der Holzman*" (the woodsman), who was a logger, wood-worker, and *Braucher* in the hills surrounding Fredericksville, Rockland Township Berks County. Jake made use of wood in ritual applications, knowing the healing properties of bark, as well as the particulars of harvesting branches for dowsing, and in the creation of wound wood – sticks cut from a variety of trees and applied for the purpose of removing illness.[69]

In a similar manner to Jake's rural persona, an urban woman by the name of Catharina Margaret Hess (1799-1858) lived in the city of Reading and was sought far and wide for her healing reputation. She was known as "*Die Wascht Fraa*" (the Sausage Lady) in Pennsylvania Dutch, and as "*Die Wurst Frau*" among German-Americans.[70] because her husband, Johann Gottlieb Hess (1795-1850) was a butcher, and Catharina delivered his smoked bolognas to restaurants, hotels, and other customers. She also dispensed salves and herbal compounds from her single-story log home and sausage shop at 10th and Walnut Streets.[71]

Catharina emigrated from Germany in 1831 and had learned *Brauche* healing from her father, Johannes Kusterer, a *Bürgermeister* (chair of the city council) and master stone mason in Heimerdingen, Würtemburg.[72] She arrived and settled in Philadelphia with her first husband Johann Conrad Schmidt and seven children, but tragedy struck and Conrad was robbed and beaten to death in 1836. The family left the city and relocated to Reading.

Catherina's daughter, Catherine Margaretha Eberth (1826-1903) later received her mother's mantle as the second generation *Wascht Fraa,* but she did not learn directly from her mother. She learned from her husband, who served as an intermediary to transmit the oral tradition from the eldest *Wascht Fraa*, in keeping with the tradition of alternating gender.[73] The two *Wascht Fraa* collaborated until the mother's death in 1858. Catherina Hess was so beloved in Reading and the region, that her funeral was described as the most well-attended funeral that St. Luke's Lutheran Church had ever experienced, with standing-room only, and crowds waiting outside of the church.[74]

The younger *Wascht Fraa*, Catherine Eberth, then purchased a brick home on Walnut Street, from which she continued the family's herbal dispensary. A tin sign bearing the symbol of an apothecary, a mortar and pestle, advertised her practice.[75] Catherine was reported to be registered with the State of Pennsylvania as a physician,[76] and was listed as a "doctress" in the 1868 Reading City Directory.[77] It was rumored that the names of the *Wascht Fraa* were known by German-speaking people all across the Mid-Atlantic, and that they drew over 10,000 clients from the tri-state area with New York and New Jersey, serving people of distinction, such as lawyers, preachers, doctors, aldermen, merchants, judges, railroad men, and farmers throughout the region.[78] It was reported that she even supplied medicine and advice to people living in distant parts of the country, from Maine to California, and to the Gulf of Mexico, as well as for clients living in Africa.[79]

Despite her magnanimous reputation, she was arrested in April of 1890 on accusations from a local man, Charles Brown, who lost his thumb to gangrene.[80] He alleged that she charged him for powwowing, which resulted in the loss of his thumb, but Catherine refuted his claim, describing that he visited her four times to buy salve, but that she never treated him, nor would she ever charge for powwowing.[81] This incident neither shut down her business, nor sullied her status as one of two preeminent powwowers in Reading at the turn of the century, the other being Doctor Joseph H. Hageman (1832-1905), also a second-generation powwower in the Hageman family, who was known for a prolific practice located just a few blocks away on Elm Street (see Chapter IX).

Following her death, Catharine was memorialized as a beloved member of her community. Her minister, the Rev. F. K. Huntsinger, preached about her life of service and healing to a church full of people, comparing Catharine to the biblical Tabitha, an empowered disciple of Christ, who dedicated her life to helping others.[82] Eulogies and reflections appeared in local and regional papers, immortalizing the story of the *Wascht Fraa* in Greater Reading.

Catharine Eberth's adopted daughter, Katie Eberth (1861-1919), married a Reading pretzel baker, Andrew Denschellman (1858-1914), and carried the title of *Wascht Fraa* after Catharine Eberth passed away in 1903. Katie was the biological daughter of a young single mother named Sarah McDonough, who had given birth at the Eberth residence, presumably attended by Catharine as a midwife. Catharine and her husband Frederick had lost their only child as a baby, and they raised Katie as their own. Although a battle over inheritance ensued after Catherine's death concerning the unofficial status of Katie's adoption,[83] she eventually secured her inheritance by court order and continued the family practice until her death in 1919.[84]

Powwowing as Empowerment

Although it would appear that the *Wascht Fraa* dynasty may have originated as a non-professional practice, and only grew over time with many tales of success and increased exposure, the professional status of the family practice eventually placed Catharine Eberth in the unique position to serve as a spokesperson for the tradition at the turn of the century. At a time when the practice was increasingly under fire from medical and legal authorities, Catharine's reputation was like that of a local, living saint, and she provided some of the most succinct, yet detailed, public statements about the content and status of the tradition:

She says this is no more nor no less than a prayer to the Almighty, asking His aid, mercy and instruction. "Pow wowing" is based on certain texts found in Scripture, and also certain short addresses in the German language, which are known only to a few. These words are handed down from generation to generation, and are seldom if ever written. There are words especially arranged for burns, scalds, blood diseases, stopping the flow of blood and kindred ailments.[85]

Here we see that Catharine Eberth was not merely subject to the reporting of her region, but was able to speak for herself and define her work and role in her own words.

Catharina Eberth, second generation powwow practitioner in Reading, known by the title of *Die Wascht Fraa* (The Sausage Lady), after her mother, who was the wife of a butcher who delivered balognas throughout the city. Portrait from the *Reading Eagle*, July 26, 1903.

Through accounts like the *Wascht Fraa* and other trail-blazing female healers, the role of ritual healing is interwoven with stories of empowerment and perseverance through adversity in Pennsylvania communities. In the case of the immigrant Catharine Hess, *Brauche* was not only a means to acclimate to a new American society, in which certain traditional values were held in common with her point of origin. Powwowing was also one of the means by which she became a leading personality in the City of Reading, affording her a level of independence and respect that exceeded the societal expectations for women of her era. This sense of community distinction extended to her daughter Catharine Eberth, also a widow, a business proprietor and respected healer throughout the region.

This empowering trajectory from widow to healer, to community advocate occurs yet again half of a century later, through the work of Sophia E. Leininger Bailer (1870-1954), known affectionately in her day as the Saint of the Coal Regions. As a widow at the age of 35 living along the Swatara Creek in Tremont, Schuylkill County, Sophia Bailer (pronounced so-FY-uh)[86] was energetic to say the least, with a vibrant personality. She kept her own home, garden, and poultry well into her 80s, and was an avid singer, story-teller, performer in local theater, and a renowned healer.[87]

A native speaker of Pennsylvania Dutch, Sophia spoke English with a detectable Irish accent,[88] and her story was a culmination of the rich ethnic diversity of the coal region in the decades following the American Civil War. Sophia learned English among the children of mining families in the area, many of whom were Irish, or from a wide variety of other backgrounds.

A direct relation of Jacob Leininger, one of many people to discover coal in the region,[89] Sophia was born in Blackwood near the site of a massive coal breaker and railroad depot between the Sharp and Red Mountains.[90] Her father owned a profitable lumber business, but due to a rise in crime in the area, the family later moved from Blackwood to Tremont and purchased a farm.[91] With 14 brothers and two sisters, she grew to be a fierce and independent young woman. At the age of 19, she married a coal miner named James H. Gauntlett (1884-1905), and had a daughter by the name of Sophia P. Gauntlett.[92] Tragedy struck, and the marriage lasted less than a decade before James died in a mining accident.

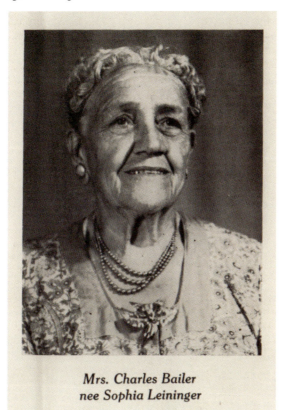

Mrs. Charles Bailer nee Sophia Leininger

Sophia (Leininger) Bailer, portrait ca. 1947, from her self-published history of *The Leininger Family: One of the Oldest in the State and Nation*, Tremont, Pennsylvania.

She was later remarried to Charles B. Bailer (1874-1945) of Tremont, a brick layer for a coal company.[93] They lived just down the street from her niece, Sophia E. (Leininger) Eberley, who later became her Aunt Sophia's apprentice in powwowing.

Sophia Bailer learned to powwow at the age of twelve[94] from her mother Sophia Fessler Leininger (1830-1904), originally from Womelsdorf, Berks County. Unlike many traditional healers, Sophia did not learn from a member of the opposite sex, as is typically a requisite for learning to powwow. Likewise, when Sophia passed her prayers on to her niece and name-sake, Sophia E. Eberley, she did so directly, without the use of a male intermediary, as was the case for the *Wascht Fraa*. She also wrote the prayers down, and even gave copies of them to her niece as a means of teaching the tradition.[95]

What made Sophia Bailer unique was not only her public presence as a storyteller, but that she was entirely open about her activities as a healer, with no qualms whatsoever about reciting the words, prayers, or procedures outside of a ritual context, even before a public audience. Contrary to the protocol employed by others in her field, Sophia Bailer held fast to no rules governing the transmission of the tradition. Aside from religious statements of piety, crediting only the divine for any success in her work, as well as a strictly free-will, gift-based exchange for her

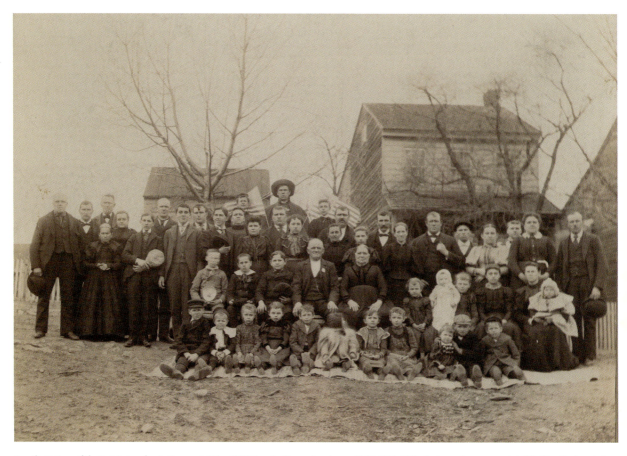

Family picture of the Leininger clan in Tremont, Schuylkill County, Pennsylvania, ca. 1870-1871. This photograph was annotated by Don Yoder, stating "Family of Sophia Bailer: She is the baby." *Pennsylvania German Cultural Heritage Center, Kutztown University.*

healing services, Sophia operated under a protocol as a healer that was minimal and straightforward.

Sophia Bailer used a number of words to describe her healing rituals, calling them alternately "blessings," "charms," and "powwow," although she preferred the self-styled term "calling a blessing," relating her work to the healing blessings of Christ.

> It's to Him I go, when I powwow for somebody. But today, I call it a blessing, the same as Christ did when He was on earth and went around and called the blessing with his disciples and called upon the sick. And that is what I call it. I don't give myself the honor. I'm only God's mouthpiece. [96]

Dr. Don Yoder produced a series of recordings for the Library of Congress of Sophia Bailer telling her story at the age of 83 in 1952, during which she expressed a wide range of beliefs, practices, and attitudes toward health and healing. Although he recorded many sessions with her, Dr. Yoder felt that he could have recorded Sophia Bailer for years without ever scratching the surface of how deeply she internalized her culture, taking her place among individuals who "encapsulate total traditional ethnic cultures, in their own minds and hearts."[98]

One of the many healing stories that earned Sophia her the title of "Saint" and a nearly-legendary status in her community was in response to an incident that occurred in a coal mine in Schuylkill Haven, when a man was injured so badly, that even doctors feared for his life. Don Yoder recorded Sophia's retelling of the story in her own words:

> There was a man hurt at the colliery and the doctor said he wouldn't live till he got home, that he'd bleed to death. And there was one miner there and he said, "I wish Mrs. Bailer was here." And they phoned in for me, and give me his name and I stopped it right away, with the help of God's words.

Opposite: Sophia Bailer's handwritten powwowing blessings, mailed to her niece and protégé Sophia Leininger (bottom right) in 1952. *Heilman Collection.*

Blude Stilla
deof ist dar und dalas
ist the Stant the vohase
vohase vohase gott ya gaben
hod Rodeslofa
Brode estas wosar drinka
feor estas Rodelofa
goullus goullus goullus goal
hund dona moul du mosa
hund hold dina mund
ous hod gott as shofen ond
dis hod gott os losen warden
fal tand blond blond ya
Bis uf dar Sund

Powvow for Rodelofa
unser haryases gate ever then lock
unser haryases kumt wetar und
shlost this rodelofa nedar
three high words
Pow vow for the Bota
Yosup gate ever ine acker are fonct
the dry harn warm, dar wicht is
wise thier onar is brow un dar drit
is rode du solst scharlagayen dode
three high words

Pow vow for such
bloder
Such bloder such dich
oder ich nam dar
doma un drickd dich
got father got son got
hilla giaht
Rode lofa
Brode hungerdt net
wasar durst net
fire list net
rode lofa und schwoth
wicha wick
Got

And when I passed by thee and saw tha
polluted in thine own blood I said unto
thee when thou waste in thy blood Live or
mam yea I said unto thee when thou wast
in thy blood Live

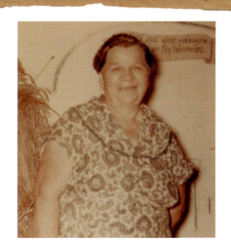

Mrs. Sophia Leininger
Tremont,
Penna.

This incident is an example of remote powwow healing by proxy – simply knowing the patient's name allows a healer to perform rituals from a distant location for healing and protection. Sophia also offered to record the words that she used not only for this particular instance, but to stop bleeding in general:

> I go down over the body, and I say:
> 'Jesus Christ's dearest blood
> That stoppeth the blood.
> In this help ------'
> Then I mention the person's name and I go down over.
> Then I say:
> 'God the Father
> The Son and the Holy Spirit
> Help to this. Amen. [99]

Sophia allowed these words to be recorded in English, but she used both English and Pennsylvania Dutch in her cures – sometimes interchangeably for the same cure. Sophia Bailer's words to stop bleeding are a well-known variation of a German language blessing, recorded by Johann Georg Hohman in his celebrated powwow manual:

> *Jesus Christus, theures Blut!*
> *Das stillet die Schmerzen, und stillet das Blut.*
> *Das helf dir (N.)*
> *Gott der Vater, Gott der Sohn,*
> *Gott der heilige Geist. Amen.*
>
> Jesus Christ, dearest blood!
> That stoppeth the pain, and stoppeth the blood.
> In this help you, (first name)
> God the Father, God the Son,
> God the Holy Spirit. Amen. [100]

Interestingly enough, Hohman's book foreshadows Sophia's remote use of the words with an introductory note, calling the words, "*Ein gewißes Mittel um das Blut zu stillen; es hilft, der Mensch mag so weit seyn, als er will, wenn man seinen Vornamen recht dabey spricht, wenn man für ihn braucht* (A certain remedy to stop bleeding—which cures, no matter how far a person be away, if only his first name is rightly pronounced when using it)."[101]

This particular method of stopping blood appears second only to the use of the biblical invocation taken from the sixth verse of the sixteenth chapter from the Book of Ezekiel, which Sophia Bailer also transcribed:

> And when I passed by thee, and saw thee polluted in thine own blood, I said unto thee when thou wast in thy blood, Live; yea, I said unto thee when thou wast in thy blood, Live.

Sophia Bailer's powwow writings contained two slips of paper with this verse written long-hand, and copied from the King James Bible. Another unique blessing for stopping blood is a rare variation of the blessing of the "Sacred Hour" of Christ's birth,[102] written in a phonetic hybrid of Pennsylvania Dutch, English, and old German:

> *Blutte Stille*
> *Deaf ist dar grund, selas*
> *is the stunt the whare*
> *whare whare gootd ya geben*
> *had.*
>
> To stop blood
> Deep is the ground, sacred
> is the hour the true
> true, true God did give.[103]

It is clear that although some of Sophia Bailer's powwowing prayers can be derived from published sources, the actual written materials that she owned were derived instead from oral sources and transcribed the way that they sounded to her, rather than copied verbatim from published books or written manuscripts. Sophia, known for her vivid memory, had taken these words to heart, and employed them effortlessly for the service of others.

The Healer as Local Saint

Although she may not have been aware of it, Aunt Sophia Bailer, "Saint of the Coal Regions", was following in the footsteps of one of Pennsylvania's most celebrated of all traditional healers, Anna Maria Jung (Young), known as Mountain Mary, or *Die Barriche Marriche*.[104] Mountain Mary's legendary persona is one of self-reliance, religious piety, and spiritual healing. Although it has been nearly 200 years since Mountain Mary's death, her grave is regarded as a shrine to the legacy of Pennsylvania's most celebrated powwow healer of the colonial era.

While there are some that doubt that Mountain Mary ever powwowed, it was widely accepted by the community in the years to follow that this was precisely the brand of healing she practiced.[105] Given the wide diversity of medicine deemed conventional in early Pennsylvania, a full range of possibilities existed for Mary to have blended elements of clinical, traditional, herbal, and religious medicine.

Anna Maria Jung died on Nov. 16, 1819, leaving behind virtually no documentation of her life and deeds, and yet the eulogies that sprung up within the decades to

Maria Jung (1749-1819), called Mountain Mary or *Barriche Mariche*, was a local Pennsylvania Dutch good neighbor and healer who was looked upon as a saint in the early nineteenth century. A multicolor woodcut print of Mountain Mary, possibly by Lehigh County folk artist Paul Wieand, showing scenes of her healing, farming, and her homestead located on the edge of the Oley Valley in Pike Township, Berks County, Pennsylvania. *Pennsylvania German Cultural Heritage Center, Kutztown University*

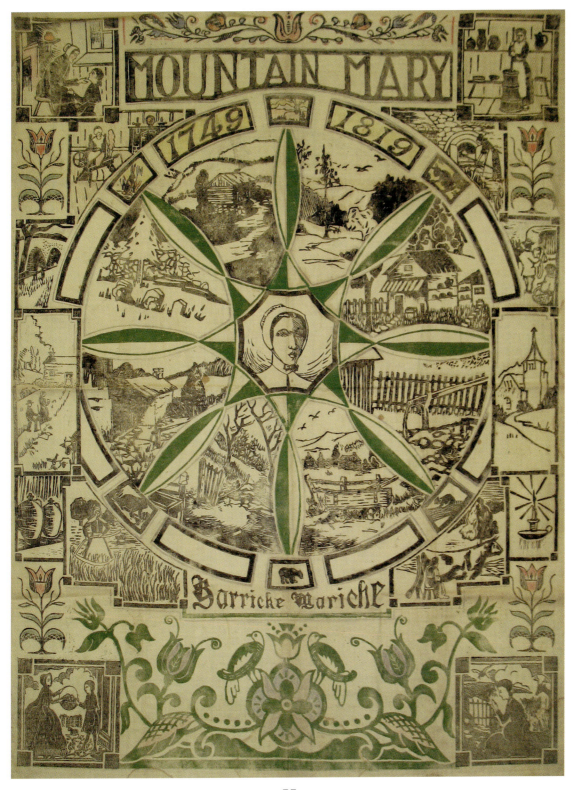

follow have characterized her as a hermit abbess of the valley, traveling far and wide to attend to the sick with her art of healing. These stories revealed a magnanimous spirit, and one that would capture the imagination of her community for generations to come.

Most telling are the writings of Philadelphia Quaker, Benjamin M. Hollinshead, who provided the sole surviving, narrative account of Mountain Mary while she was still living. He described her as a "hermitess" whose "remarks breathed a strain of devotional feeling which had a solemnizing effect upon the company, and the countenance of the speaker was one of the most benign I had ever beheld." He described her words as flowing with a spiritual fervor that she was unable to convey in the same tone in her secondary language of English, and so they relied upon a translator while she spoke her native German.[106]

Hollinshead recorded stories of Mary following her death, when neighbors said she was a "very intelligent and religious woman, and was visited by her neighbors to have her advice on their difficulties, which was often so judicious and far-seeing that she was thought by some to have a way of acquiring knowledge unknown to many."[107]

Although Hollinshead mentions nothing about her specific acts of healing, generations later many local people would regard her as a practitioner of traditional powwow folk healing, some even suggesting that entire lineages of powwow healers among the Pennsylvania Dutch claim Mountain Mary as their originator. Folklorist and storyteller Dennis Boyer's aunt, a powwower from Oley known as "*die Kefferli*" (The Lady Bug), claimed Mountain Mary as the originator of her lineage throughout the Oley *Freindschaft* (extended family) of practitioners.[108] Philadelphia journalist Arthur Lewis also alleged that John Blymire traced his York County lineage to Oley and Mountain Mary.[109]

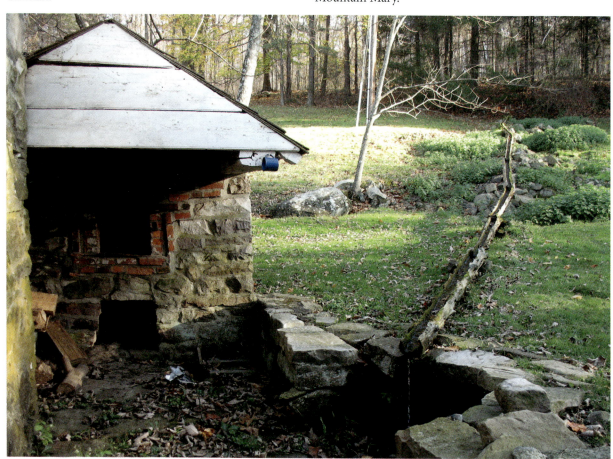

The original bakeoven and springhouse at the homestead of Mountain Mary, healer and hermitess of the Oley Valley, Pike Township, Berks County.

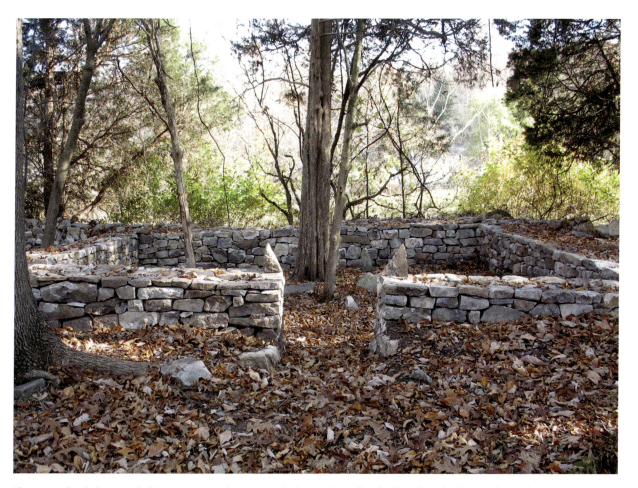

The graveyard at the homestead of Mountain Mary, where Mary and other members of her family are buried. Pike Township, Berks County.

In 1880, German American immigrant Ludwig August Wollenweber (1807-1888) would attempt to capture the narrative of Anna Maria Jung in a nationalistic melodrama entitled *Die Berg Maria*.[110] His image of her as a virgin Revolutionary War widow was purely fictional and written in the spirit of the American Centennial Exhibition held in Philadelphia held just five years prior to the publication. Moreover, Wollenweber's tale tells more about the brave deeds and revolutionary valor of Mary's fictional husband, Theodore Benz, than of Mary herself. Although the title of the work bears Mary's name, Wollenweber's character of Mary is demure and extremely passive - a woman defined by tragedy, exhibiting little to no agency of her own.

This appropriation of the local story into historical fiction of the Revolutionary Era held little sway over the hearts and minds of Pennsylvanians, who knew their local saint far better. Despite Wollenweber's depiction of Maria Jung as a widow, evidence suggests that she was never actually married.[111] However, her mother and widowed sisters lived in Oley nearby, and are buried in the family plot at Mountain Mary's homestead near Hill Church in Pikeville, where a springhouse and bakeoven are all that remain of her original home.

As a self-possessed woman in a period of history dominated by the voices and writings of men, the legends of Mountain Mary have coalesced into a persona revered much in the way of the regional and local saints of Europe. But how did this notion of sainthood develop among the Protestant Pennsylvania Dutch? And how are Pennsylvania's healing traditions an extension of veneration for the saints in Europe?

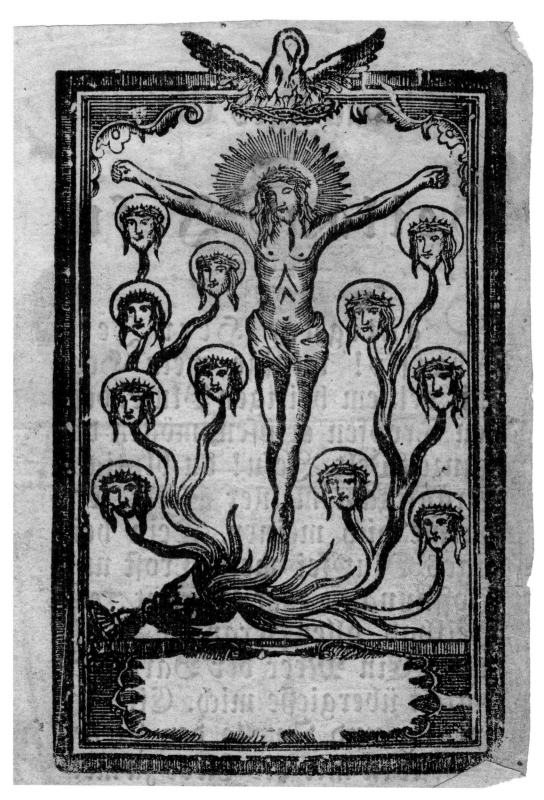

Chapter III
Euꝛopean Oꝛigins
Benediction, Blessing, Brauchen

Although the religious climate of Pennsylvania was decidedly Protestant from the onset, the early folk culture was still deeply rooted in centuries-old, pre-Reformation beliefs and observances, some of which are still maintained today as manifestations of ritual healing.[1] These attitudes and practices are often mistaken for theological or doctrinal castoffs from previous generations, rather than part of a distinctly European worldview, interwoven not only through the ages, but also throughout the total sphere of life.

During the Middle Ages, by the time that the culture of Christianity rose to ascendancy from the fall of the Roman world, Europe was already on a new religious trajectory that would serve to redefine the sacred and transform devotional practices. The development of the cult of the saints would be one of the defining factors in this transition, as the remains of the faithful departed and their devotional shrines replaced the civic centers of Roman life.[2] The remains and relics of the martyrs delineated a new spiritual topography that spread across Europe, plotting the routes of the pilgrimage, determining the sites of Gothic cathedrals, and consolidating religious authority.

These ancestors of a spiritual family, saints and martyrs, served not only as holy intercessors capable of touching the lives of mortals, but also as human faces that mediated contact with a heavenly, supernal reality.[3] Never before had Earth and the heavens seemed to so closely intersect. The saints were considered irrefutable evidence that the sacred could take physical form, and every physical manifestation of creation was the result of a spiritual counterpart. At the same time, the ever-growing hierarchy of the clergy merged with a heavenly order that encompassed the very choirs of heaven, the patriarchs and prophets, the Saints and Apostles, the Holy Family of Mary, Joseph and the Infant Christ, and above all, the ineffable mystery of the Holy Trinity.

However, the earth was also a realm of great peril, as the devil and the forces of darkness were given free rein to bring calamity and misfortune, illness and infirmity, pestilence and plague.[4] But the sufferings of humanity were not only to be relieved in the salvation of the afterlife, but in the restoration of the natural order and healing of the flesh through contact with the sacred.[5] Holy sites, objects, and people were the answer to this mortal conundrum, and served not as reminders of distant heavenly realities, but as proof of divine immanence.

Even when one's station in life did not permit direct contact with the sacrosanct, prayers and petitions to the saints could be offered to bless and assist in all earthly affairs and heal all infirmities. The Regensburg Cathedral was the earliest seat of widespread devotion to the much revered Fourteen Holy Helpers (*Vierzehn Nothhelfer*) which spread across Europe. These fourteen saints were helpers in times of need or distress (*Noth*), and were called upon by common people to intercede in times of sickness, death, plague, famine, and danger from fire. Blessed inscriptions on paper and fabric as well as medals stamped with the images of the saints could be worn on one's body to guide and protect in daily life, on journeys, and in times of war.[6] A sacred calendar, reflecting the movements of the heavens as beacons of cosmic order, synchronized the days, months, and seasons with a cyclical pattern of veneration and devotion. Each saint received their own feast day and every transition in life was given a special liturgical rite and benediction – from birth to death.[7] The health of a person extended beyond his or her physical body, to include family and neighbors, home and farmyard, barns and livestock, fields and crops, and seamlessly joined a universal order that stretched

Opposite Page: *Andächtiges Gebet zu unserm Heiland Jesu* (Devotional Prayer to our Savior Jesus), 1864, Ofen, Budapest. A classic German emblematic tract, containing a devotional prayer for spiritual and physical healing, making use of the imagery of the blood and wounds of Christ. The emblem on the cover depicts the mystery of the Eucharist, with Christ's presence in the wine of the chalice. At the top is the symbol of the Pelican feeding her young from a wound in her breast - an allegory for the sacrifice of Christ, common also in Pennsylvania folk art. *Pennsylvania German Cultural Heritage Center, Kutztown University of Pennsylvania.*

to the four corners of the earth, and was reflected in all creation.

This concept of the sacred was so integrated into all aspects of life and proved to be so incredibly stable that even when the rise of the Reformation and Renaissance would shake Europe to its very core, this cosmic arrangement persisted and colored later expressions of religious piety and everyday life by shades and degrees. Even centuries later, after changes in theology, science, fashion, and economy, prayers that appeal to the saints would continue to describe these heavenly hierarchies:

> Today I rise and tend to the day which I have received, in thy name: The first is God the Father †, the other is God the Son †, the third is God the Holy Spirit † – Protect my body and soul, my flesh and my life, which Jesus, the Son of God himself, has given to me; whereupon shall I be blessed, as the Holy Bread of Heaven that our loving Lord Jesus, the Son of God, had given to his disciples. When I go out from the house over the threshold and into the streets, Jesus † Mary † Joseph †, the Holy Three Kings, Caspar †, Melchior † and Balthasar † are my travel companions – the Heavens are my hat and the Earth is my shoes. These six holy persons accompany me and all that are in my house, and when I am on the streets, so shall they protect my journey, from thieves, murderers, and malicious people. All those who meet me must have love and value for me. Therefore help me God the Father †, God the Son †, God the Holy Spirit †, Jesus, † Mary, † Joseph, † Caspar, Melchior, Balthasar, and the Four Evangelists be with me in all my doings, trade and commerce, going and coming, be it on water or land, before fire and inferno, they will protect me with their strong hand. To God the Father †, I reveal myself – to God the Son †, I commend myself – in God the Holy Spirit †, I immerse myself. The glorious Holy Trinity be above me, Jesus, Mary and Joseph before me, Caspar, Melchior and Balthasar be behind and beside me through all time, before I come into eternal joy and bliss, help me Jesus, Mary and Joseph. Caspar † Melchior † and Balthasar †, pray for us now, and in the hour of our death. Amen.[8]

This Powerful Prayer (*Ein sehr kräftiges heiliges Gebet*) originates in the city of Cologne, at the Cathedral dedicated to the Three Kings, but was used and published just before the turn of the twentieth century in Kutztown, the heart of the Pennsylvania Dutch Country.[9] This prayer may seem about as far removed from the rational theology and humble piety to be expected of the Lutheran and Reformed congregations as could be imagined, that is, until one compares it with other prayers associated with powwowing, where rituals may conclude with making the sign of the cross three times, followed by the Ave Maria in series with penitential recitations of the Apostles' Creed and the Lord's Prayer.[10] While the latter two expressions were certainly at the core of Protestant expressions of faith, nevertheless this ritual context was wholly foreign to the offices of the Protestant churches.

Despite the implications of such Roman Catholic elements in Protestant communities, the Pennsylvania Dutch had certainly not forgotten that the celebrated image of Dr. Martin Luther graced the inside covers of not only their German Bibles, but also early Pennsylvania prayer books, hymnals, catechisms, and even their children's spelling-books and grammars.[11] The spirit of the Reformation that inspired the transatlantic migration was hardly forgotten in the New World, and Pennsylvania, founded as a colony with no state-mandated religious requirements, was a perfect place for religious expression to flourish.

It would appear that these vestigial elements of Roman Catholicism within folk culture did not merely survive in spite of Protestantism, but were fundamentally transformed and possibly invigorated by it. As the prayers to the saints and a reverence to their shrines and relics were removed from the official realm of Protestant expression, it was within the home that these traditions continued to grow and change into a fundamentally new creature, no longer informed by the doctrines and reinforced by the sanctioning of the official Protestant churches – but thriving nonetheless as a familial form of devotion. For Protestants that embraced Luther's notion of the "priesthood of all believers," the Reformation placed a new sense of empowerment into the hands of the people and perhaps inadvertently revitalized a sense of folk religious expression.

The early Christian martyrs, largely forsaken by Protestant authorities, make their appearances throughout the oral and literary ritual healing traditions in Pennsylvania. Prayers for burns were used in Pennsylvania invoking St. Lawrence, martyred on an iron griddle, and prayers to St. Blaise were used for menstrual complications. St. George and St. Martin were invoked to thwart highway robbers, and St. Cyprian against curses and malicious people.[12] The "Three Holy Women," Saints Elizabeth, Brigid, and Matilda, were invoked to cure swelling.[13] The Biblical saints, patriarchs, and protagonists receive equal treatment, each with their specialized invocations: the Virgin Mary for extinguishing fire and healing burns; and St. Peter for binding and releasing thieves. The names of the four Evangelists were used to bless the body against illness and danger. The "Three Holy Men," Shadrach, Meshach and Abednego, were invoked to cure inflammation, and their "song" in the fiery furnace was good to protect from destruction by fire, storms, infant convulsions, and the bite of a mad dog.[14]

These unofficial traditions served to nurture parts of the human experience that no longer had a place within public, post-enlightenment Protestant expression, especially under the careful watch of Lutheran and Reformed clergy, many of whom were educated at

Drei-Königzettel (Three Kings Broadside), late eighteenth century. *Heilman Collection.*

A European broadside of the Three Kings Prayer, which was later republished in Pennsylvania, most notably, in Kutztown by Urich & Gehring ca. 1880. This prayer developed in the wake of veneration of the Three Kings following the moving of their legendary remains to the cathedral in Cologne. The prayer appeals to the Three Kings, symbolized by the initials C†M†B† for protection against natural disaster and the predations of the wicked.

Below right: An eighteenth-century, European copper engraving of The Fourteen Helpers in Need (*Die Vierzehn Nothhelfer*), embellished with foil and paper, depicting a circle of the fourteen saintly helpers, surrounding the infant Christ. *Heilman Collection.*

Below: Ein Sehr Kräftiges Gebet (A Very Powerful Prayer) ca. 1880, Urich & Gehring, Kutztown
Don Yoder Collection, Pennsylvania German Cultural Heritage Center, Kutztown University.

A rare Kutztown broadside blessing, attributed to the Three Kings and the cathedral dedicated to them in Cologne, Germany. The concluding words in the central column ask for assurance both now and in eternity, echoing the last lines of the Roman Catholic Hail Mary, "…nunc, et in hora mortis nostrae" - "Now and in the hour of our death."

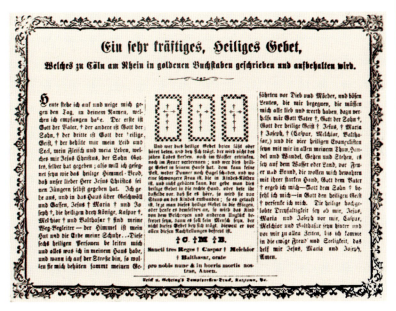

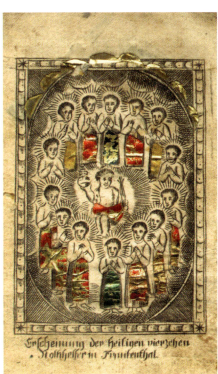

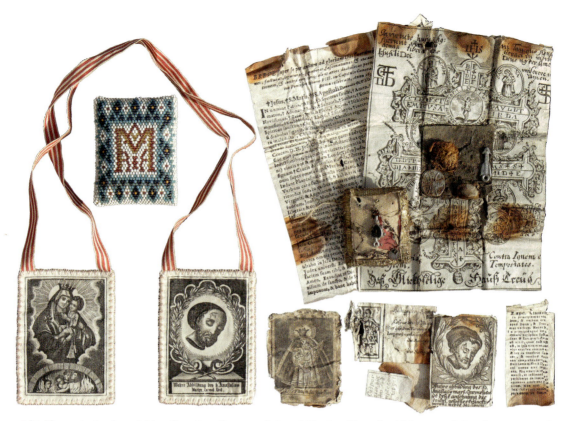

Above right: The contents of an eighteenth-century European letter of blessing (*Breverl*) which was sealed and worn on one's person. *Above left:* A scapular worn around the shoulders with images of the saints, as well as an unopened *Breverl*, highly embellished with the beaded monogram of the Virgin Mary. *Heilman Collection.*

European universities, further dividing them from their North American parishioners. Non-ordinary experiences with spirits and the supernatural, illnesses believed to be caused by grudges or sin, even the possibility that calamity could be caused intentionally by the envy of malicious people – all of these experiences and perceptions no longer fit the Protestant climate, yet were never successfully expunged from the worldview of the people. Rituals and prayers for healing, protection, and assistance served to mitigate these concerns and integrate such narratives into a coherent and meaningful undercurrent that has served the needs of Pennsylvanians for centuries.

Although the original aim of the Reformation was to fundamentally challenge the authoritative structures of Rome that mediated humanity's connection to the divine, the resulting Protestant discourse, as both a spiritual and an intellectual movement, became increasingly centered on the use of reason and rationalism to debate rival factions, revise the tenets of faith, and expunge those elements of Roman Catholicism that had accumulated in the medieval era and were based in tradition, rather than biblical literature.[15] Aside from the primary doctrinal debates concerning the nature of salvation and concerns about abuses of power, to the Protestant movement all aspects of religious experience were suddenly under scrutiny for evidence of perceived contamination from papal authority, even symbolism, iconography, and especially the role of the saints.

Luther's Large Catechism, a central document for Lutherans, equates the veneration of saints with sorcery:

> Consider what in our blindness, we have hitherto been practicing and doing under the Papacy. If anyone had toothache, he fasted and honored St. Apollonia [lacerated his flesh by voluntary fasting to the honor of St. Apollonia]; if he was afraid of fire, he chose St. Lawrence as his helper in need; if he dreaded pestilence, he made a vow to St. Sebastian or Rochio, and a countless number of such abominations, where everyone selected his own saint, worshiped him, and called for help to him in distress. Here belong those also, as, e.g., sorcerers and magicians, whose idolatry is most gross, and who make a covenant with the devil, in order that he may give them plenty of money or help them in love-affairs, preserve their cattle, restore to them lost possessions, etc. For all these place their heart and trust elsewhere than in the true God, look for nothing good to Him nor seek it from Him.[16]

While the traditional Roman Catholic veneration of the saints was attacked for its extra-biblical and legendary facets, Dr. Martin Luther warned against wholesale iconoclasm in regard to the saints, advocating that those saints who were biblical in nature should be maintained for their inspirational and didactic role as models of a Christian life.[17] Despite this concession, there were serious consequences of this new theology. To undermine the traditional reverence for the saints was to potentially initiate the unraveling of an entire worldview in which the supernal hierarchy of heavenly beings had the power to touch and change the lives of humans. This is not to say that Protestants in any way dismissed a relationship with the divine, or even the angels, but holy agents with human faces were replaced with a much more remote, abstract, and cerebral conception of the divine. This transition was only partially successful.

In addition to the scriptural arguments against non-biblical saints,[18] Protestant leaders were also distinctly aware that the destruction of the cult of the saints would dismantle the power structures that had evolved around the tombs, shrines, and relics of the martyrs and disrupt this expression of popular piety throughout Europe, as well as redefine the very nature of the sacred that originated in Roman Christianity. It was not only the folk culture that struggled with these changes; it was the very leadership of the Holy Roman Empire.

Even the Elector of Saxony, Frederick III, The Wise, who protected Martin Luther while he penned his revolutionary vernacular translation of the Bible, was intimately connected to the cult of the saints and the power that it represented. It was well known that by the time that Luther released his German New Testament in 1522, Frederick owned over 19,000 holy relics of Christ and the saints, including one thumb of St. Anne, straw from Christ's holy manger, a twig from the burning bush of Moses, and even a vial of milk from the Virgin Mary![19]

Frederick's relics were housed in the All Saints Cathedral in Wittenberg, where they were displayed each year on the second Sunday after Easter between 1503 and 1523, and vast sums of money were culled from pilgrims and nobles alike, who were granted indulgences for public veneration of the relics. These indulgences were part of an elaborate system designed to provide exemption in the afterlife from time spent in Purgatory prior to entry into Heaven. Ironically Frederick III put an end to his collecting following the 1517 controversy of Luther's *Ninety-Five Theses on the Power and Efficacy of Indulgences*, and following Frederick's death less than a decade later, the relics were dispersed and destroyed in the wake of the iconoclastic fervor that swept across the German territories.[20]

But while overt display of images of the saints were discouraged in Protestant lands, poetic, prayerful invocations of the saints remained written in the hearts and minds of Protestant people, who eventually made their way to the New World.

Martin Luther & Ritual of the Reformation Era

As the central figure in the Reformation, Luther is often assumed to have been the living embodiment of Protestant doctrine and therefore to have been the primary proponent of the rational theology that so characterized the shift from the Roman Catholic consensus of his era. While the theology of Lutheranism certainly bears the mark of its originator, Luther himself held a much more complex view of the relation of humanity to the divine than is often reflected in the Augsburg Confession. As a mystic, Luther's worldview shaped some of the very attitudes that would later come under criticism in Protestant theology.[21] Discussions of spirits and the supernatural causes of natural phenomena were some of the highlights of Luther's *Table Talks*

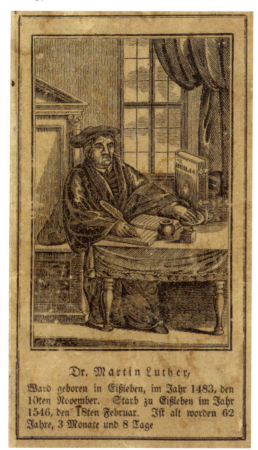

Martin Luther translating the Bible into German. A classic engraving of on the cover of an ABC-Book by Philadelphia printers Schäfer and Koradi, ca. 1830. *Pennsylvania German Cultural Heritage Center, Kutztown University.*

(Tisch Reden), a publication of informal discussions held between Luther and his closest friends and colleagues.[2] While these documents were never intended as the basis for church doctrine, they are revealing of the attitudes and beliefs commonly held in Luther's time.

Luther was unshakably certain, for instance, that the devil and his demonic servants were active agents of destruction in the world, causing calamity, storms, and illnesses - and he considered himself to be a primary target. Not only did he believe that his physical illnesses were the result of continual spiritual struggles with the forces of darkness, he also asserted that doctors were of no avail in such circumstances. Luther also reinforced the old Roman Catholic notion that illness could be the direct result of sin or possession by evil spirits. Although Luther admitted that scientific medicine and the aid of devout physicians were indeed gifts from God, he maintained that clergy were more effective as healers of spiritual illness.

In a broader sense, Luther was warning that spiritual disorders could not be healed by purely physical means, but more specifically, he was referring to specialized rites that were used by clergy for the purpose of driving away the influence of evil. Such formalized rites in Luther's day were part of the Roman Catholic liturgy, where exorcism was a crucial part of the ritual of baptism, consecration of holy water and salt, and the blessing of the sick.

I cast you out, unclean spirit, in the name of the Father, + and of the Son, + and of the Holy + Spirit. Depart and stay far away from this servant of God, N. For it is the Lord Himself who commands you, accursed and doomed spirit, He who walked on the sea and reached out His hand to Peter as he was sinking. So then, foul fiend, recall the curse that decided your fate once and for all. Indeed, pay homage to the living and true God, pay homage to Jesus Christ, His Son, and to the Holy Spirit. Keep far from this servant of God, N., for Jesus Christ, our Lord and God, has freely called them to His holy grace and blessed way and to the waters of baptism...[24]

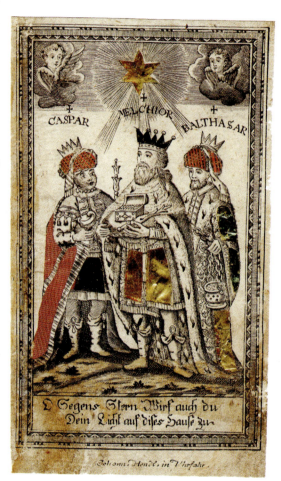

The Three Kings Blessing (Drei-Könige-Segen), a copper engraving embellished with fabric and paper, depicting the Three Kings Caspar, Melchior, and Balthasar standing under the star of Bethlehem. The inscription reads "O Blessed Star, cast thy light upon this house." The Three Kings appear extensively in both officially sanctioned and folk-religious blessings throughout Europe and Pennsylvania. Johann Hendl, Urfahr, Linz, Austria. *Heilman Collection.*

These highly elaborate exorcism rituals are not limited to Roman Catholicism and were also once part of Protestant expressions of faith. Dr. Martin Luther's first vernacular translation of the Baptismal Rite of 1523 incorporates such elements as exorcizing evil spirits from an infant by blowing under the eyes three times, anointing the ears and nose with the minister's spittle, and the use of salt (which was actually put into the child's mouth), along with more formally accepted elements such anointing with oil, and making the sign of the cross. During the period of adjustment in the development of early Protestantism, these elements were eventually removed from the liturgy.[25] Each of these procedures appears centuries later, preserved within Pennsylvania Dutch folk practices: blowing is used to exorcize fire from a burn, and salt is a substance commonly believed to neutralize misfortune and repel evil. Both saliva and oil were historically part of powwow practice and were applied in the healing of certain childhood ailments such as colic. Ubiquitously, the sign of the cross is used as a central feature in most powwow healing rituals to bless parts of the body that are afflicted.

These beliefs and practices were already firmly established among the laity in Luther's day and in the centuries to follow among Protestants, as evidenced by reports from clergy of wandering *Teufelsbanner* - folk practitioners who ritually exorcized *Krankheitsdämonen*[26] - spiritual forces responsible for illness.[27]

Luther was also distinctly aware of a broad spectrum of folk ritual cures, and again in his *Table Talks* described the common belief that three toads when skewered and left to dry in the sun can draw the "poison" out of tumors. Luther even described certain remedies that are effective only when applied by nobles, such as holy water applied by the Elector of Saxony, Frederick III. Luther also believed strongly that religiously-rebellious humans could harm their neighbors through malicious ritual means. He describes certain people (usually women) who could by infernal powers cause milk, butter, and eggs to spoil so that the food would drop to the floor when one tried to eat it, and that anyone who chastised such people for their deeds would fall victim to the plagues of the devil. Luther described that even his own mother struggled with a neighbor who was known to curse infants so that they would cry themselves to death and cursed a clergyman with a deadly illness that no remedy could cure using the dust from his footprints. When asked about the proper recourse for such behavior, Luther cited scripture, and reminded his colleagues that in the Old Law, the priests cast the first stone at such malefactors.[28]

In his famous Epiphany sermon of 1522, Luther spoke out against the use of religious ritual for the purpose of magic, sorcery, and divination. The feast of Epiphany (*Dreikönigstag*) celebrates the veneration of the Christ child by the Three Kings, described in the second chapter of the Gospel of Mathew as wisemen (*Weiser*), and called "Magi" in the Latin Vulgate Bible - literally meaning magicians or diviners of astrology. In order to clarify what this title implies for the Gospel reading, Luther carefully described eight forms of magic condemned in the book of Deuteronomy:[29]

1. Those who use divination (*Weissager*) to see the future, whom Luther compares to false prophets in league with the devil.
2. Those that practice augury (*Tagewähler*) and read omens in order to determine the best days and times for certain human activities.
3. Diviners (*Geistgenossen*), who seek treasure by means of consulting the devil through mirrors, crystals, rods, etc.
4. Witches (*Hexen*) in service with the devil, who steal milk, create storms, ride goats and brooms, fly with their cloaks, strike down people with curses, as well as cripple and wither their bodies, kill infants in the cradle, curse members of the body, etc.
5. Enchanters (*Beschwörer*) who bless animals and people, charm snakes, enchant steel and iron, see much, levitate, and work wonders.
6. Fortune-tellers, (*Wahrsager*) to whom the devil speaks, to reveal to what is lost or predict the future.
7. Sorcery (*Zauberei*), to deceive people with illusions and other things of the devil.
8. Necromancers, who consult wandering spirits (*wandelnden Geister*) and the dead.[30]

Most striking about Luther's classification however, are the descriptions of the witches and enchanters.[31] The malicious activities of the former are itemized at great length, with no uncertainty about his disdain. Surprisingly, the latter are presented in language bordering on the laudatory, and perhaps, at worst, merely ambivalent. In fact, aside from augury, the enchanters are the only category whose power Luther did not ascribe to the devil.

Luther's original word *Beschwörer* (also spelled *Beschweerer*) does not fit nicely into an English definition. Translated alternately as "charmer" or "conjurer," the verb *beschweeren* can mean to "adjure," "exorcize," "swear an oath," or "enchant."[32] Centuries later, these German terms would be used interchangeably within the language and terminology of powwowing in North America.

In Luther's treatment of *Beschwörer*, there is no doubt that he was referring to a class of healing practitioners. This omission of direct condemnation may have been intentional, so as not to condemn folk-cultural practices that may have been considered traditional within Luther's own community and congregation.

It is difficult to ascertain Luther's precise perspective on the nature of enchanting based solely upon his text. Sermons are inherently performative, and the very act of preaching is part of public discourse. There is no indication in the homily of how Luther delivered this description to his congregation, and his tone would have supplied additional meaning. Nevertheless, without any further clarification, this sermon was later circulated in the form of a religious tract against Roman Catholic use of ritual.[33] Was his lack of condemnation of enchantment a form of tolerance? What effect did Luther's view have upon the Lutheran clergy and laity?

Although a lack of condemnation certainly does not prove to be the same as an outright endorsement, centuries later in Pennsylvania, the Lutheran population would play a strong role in the integration of rituals formerly belonging to the Catholic liturgy into the everyday lives of the Pennsylvania Dutch. While some influential Reformed ministers spoke out against such practices, a number of Lutheran ministers were actually known to powwow and remained in good standing with their congregations and synods. A classic example is the Rev. Georg Mennig who is known to have published broadsides with instructions for powwowing, which unabashedly bore his name (see Chapter II).

Regardless of the nuances of Luther's perspective on enchanting, the adaptation of liturgical ritual into the realm of non-sanctioned expression has always been subject to criticism and debate. Notions of legitimacy tend to focus on the difference between the sanctioned use of liturgical ritual and its appropriation for other purposes - especially personal gain, or undermining the authority of ecclesiastical leadership. This appropriation of religious ritual took place on many fronts, which produced a broad spectrum of devotional and healing practices in both folk and popular culture, as well as in the upper echelon of academic and clerical circles where elements of the liturgy informed practices associated with ceremonial magic. This latter category was specifically forbidden and condemned as sorcery, while ritual practices among the folk tended to occupy a less publically visible role in society. Nevertheless, non-sanctioned forms of ritual would later come under fire in the era of witchcraft persecution, when a broad spectrum of folk cultural expressions - everything from curing with prayer to the administering of healing salves - fell under suspicion for heresy and the influence of the devil.

Inquisition, Witchcraft & Exorcism

Although the era leading up to the Reformation is often celebrated for cultural, scientific, and social advances, Europe was deeply embroiled in a series of dark inner conflicts. Not only would Europe experience centuries of bloodshed over religious ideals, but on a domestic level, both ecclesiastic and secular authorities turned their attention to rooting out and prosecuting witchcraft and heresy.

While there is insufficient space in this brief summary to discuss the complex cultural forces and social conflicts that produced these proceedings throughout Europe, it is important to note that the historical record from this period provides extensive documentation of folk-religious and ritual practices - some of which were sanctioned, others merely tolerated, and many the subject of cruel interrogations. While the accounts are often problematic in that testimonies are flimsy and confessions were produced under the pain of excruciating torture, nevertheless this period of cultural crisis can provide tremendous insight into the folk-religious ritual practices and cultural climate in the centuries preceding the mass exodus of German-speaking people from the Rhineland to Pennsylvania.

It would be imprudent and inappropriate to directly equate Pennsylvania's ritual culture to the epidemic of mass hysteria that characterized this period - with accounts of witches' flights, profaning of the Mass in the witches' Sabbath, worship of the devil, and the wildest of confessions extracted by means of torture. What is most relevant from this era of crisis to the development of the Pennsylvania folk culture is the application of a wide variety of anti-witchcraft practices that were employed by Catholics and Protestants alike, among both clergy and the laity, during this period. In well-described manuals of exorcism written by prestigious clergy, the structure and rules governing these practices are outlined, and in these works are not only the forerunners to powwowing in Pennsylvania, but also direct citations of identical practices, attitudes, and ethics later appearing in ritual practices in North America.

According to inquisition records, an estimated 40-60,000 people during the early modern period were accused of witchcraft, interrogated, tortured, and executed.[34] These numbers include people of all ages, social statuses and religious affiliations including children of only a few years of age.[35] The demographics were disproportionately representative of women, who were the primary target of such allegations. The courts that orchestrated these atrocities were Catholic, Protestant, and secular, although the social and religious tensions between these institutions frequently exacerbated an already tumultuous political climate. Just as the Reformation's roots can be traced to the religious unrest in Germany at the turn of the sixteenth century, so too is Germany, and, more particularly, the Alpine region, the epicenter for the rise of witchcraft executions in the period of counter-reformation that followed.

Although laws in the early modern era often forbade the use of blessings for treating humans and animals among the laity, the practice was widespread and difficult to sanction.[36] Although a number of healers and healing practices are highlighted in the records of witchcraft trials, it is unclear to what degree such practices roused the attention of authorities in secular and ecclesiastical courts. Nevertheless, such proceedings record blessings used in Tyrol in 1645 for gout (*Vergichtsegen*), the three-fold blessing for stopping thieves (*Diebsegen*), as well as blessings also attributed to the Saints including the Crown Blessing to St. Magdelena (*Krongebeth*) and the Blessing of Saint Jacob (*Poppensegen*), and even the creation of blessed bundles anointed with Baptismal water for protection (*Chrismbündlein*). One woman of Remlingen in Lower Franconia was arrested in 1621 after healing a boy of worms with the *Dreyerlei Würm-Segen* (Threefold Worm Blessing), and was forced to recite all of the healing blessings she used, as well as the names of all of the individuals in her community from whom she learned her blessings.[37] While this case is unusual, it shows that healers were by no means immune to witchcraft accusations even though their methods were traditional.

Centuries prior, early medieval Christianity had put an end to witch hunts as being contrary to Christian doctrine,[38] and punishment for witchcraft was minimal. This was in part an effort at stabilization of medieval

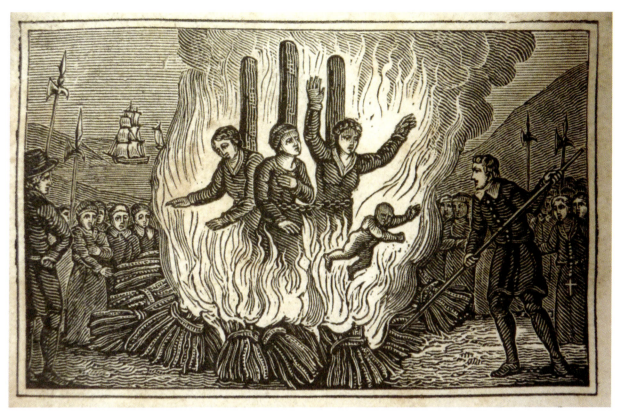

Punishments for those accused of heresy and witchcraft were particularly horrific in Early Modern Europe, a time when many religious sectarians, socially marginalized people, and their family members of all ages were tortured and executed by fire. Engraving of the Guernsey Martyrs, burned as heretics in 1556, from *Fox's Book of Martyrs*, 1830, Philadelphia. *Heilman Collection.*

society, which had retained many aspects of its pagan roots and customs. Ironically, witch-hunts were by no means the invention of Christianity, but were common and particularly brutal across ancient pagan Europe prior to the spread of Christianity.[39] However, the Christian era is responsible for establishing witchcraft as a form of heresy, as opposed to the pagans, who held no such legalistic notions, and only punished witches when they were perceived to have caused harm to another person.

The establishment of witchcraft as a form of heresy punishable by death was a new development for Roman Catholicism in the fifteenth century, authorizing the Inquisition to combat not only the rise of sectarianism, but also any ritual behavior not sanctioned by the Church. This policy was expounded in *Summis desiderantes affectibus*, Papal Bull of Innocent VIII in 1484, which mobilized two Dominican friars Heinrich Kramer (1430-1505) and Jacob Sprenger (d. 1495) to initiate a new phase of the Inquisition specifically targeting the alleged epidemic of witchcraft in southwestern Germany and Austria:

In some parts of upper Germany, as well as in the provinces, cities, territories, regions, and dioceses of Mainz, Koln, Trier, Salzburg, and Bremen, many persons of both sexes, heedless of their own salvation and forsaking the catholic faith, give themselves over to devils male and female, and by their incantations, charms, and conjurings, and by other abominable superstitions and sortileges, offences, crimes, and misdeeds, ruin and cause to perish the offspring of women, the foal of animals, the products of the earth, the grapes of vines, and the fruits of trees, as well as men and women, cattle and flocks and herds and animals of every kind, vineyards also and orchards, meadows, pastures, harvests, grains and other fruits of the earth; that they afflict and torture with dire pains and anguish, both internal and external, these men, women, cattle, flocks, herds, and animals, and hinder men from begetting and women from conceiving, and prevent all consummation of marriage; that, moreover, they deny with sacrilegious lips the faith they received in holy baptism; and that, at the instigation of the enemy of mankind, they do not fear to commit and perpetrate many other abominable offences and crimes, at the risk of their own souls, to the insult of the divine majesty and to the pernicious example and scandal of multitudes...[40]

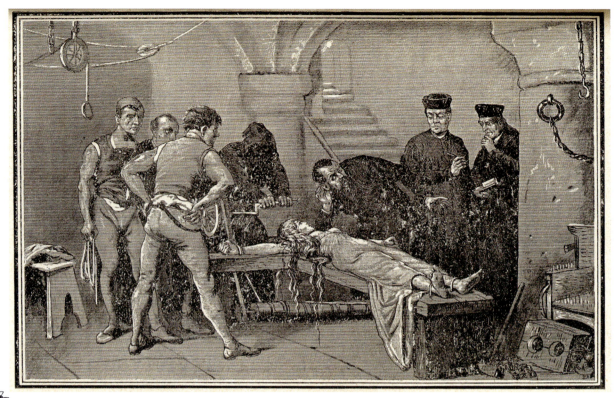

Confessions extracted by means of horrific torture in witchcraft prosecutions. Lithograph from Carl Lempen's *Geschichte der Hexen und Hexenprozesse*. 1880, St. Gallen. *Heilman Collection.*

This document authorized Kramer to commence on his campaign of witchcraft prosecution, and set the precedent that belief in the irrefutable reality of witchcraft became part of officially sanctioned church doctrine. Furthermore, disbelief in witchcraft or any resistance to the efforts of the inquisition was, by default, a form of heresy punishable by death. Although Kramer's brutish methods were rejected by local authorities,[41] he went on to publish the most infamous manual of exorcism and anti-witchcraft, entitled *Malleus Maleficarum* (*Hexenhammer* or *Hammer of Witches*). Building on the torments described in Pope Innocent VIII's decree, Kramer expounded his theories that women were in fact responsible for communities suffering at the hands of witchcraft:

> [All witchcraft] is governed by carnal lusting, which is insatiable to them, and for this reason they even cavort with demons to satisfy their lust... For intelligent men it appears to be reasonably unsurprising that more women than men are found to be tainted with the heresy of sorceresses... Blessed be the Highest One, Who has down to the present day, preserved the male kind from such disgraceful behavior, and clearly made man privileged since He wished to be born and suffer on our behalf in the guise of a man.[42]

Kramer's work was not well received by his learned contemporaries, who described him as obsessed and deranged.[43] Nevertheless his work was extremely popular and highly influential in secular courts throughout the centuries to follow, and inspired the adoption of execution by fire as punishment for witchcraft in the *Halsgerichtsordnung* (code of law for capital crimes) of Charles V in 1532.[44] The *Malleus* contained instructions for identifying *maleficia* or harm caused by witches, standards for interrogation and prosecution, as well as how to lawfully heal through exorcism those who are afflicted.

According to Kramer and his contemporaries, witches were able, through discourse with demons, to cause sickness, calamities, storms, crop failure, and infertility. Because of the notion that demons were at the command of witches and present in the workings of misfortune, all illnesses were regarded as possible manifestations of demonic possession.[45] The remedies prescribed for such maladies in the later portions of Kramer's text provide insight into the well-established culture of exorcism officially sanctioned by the church. Naturally, as an inquisitor, Kramer advocated that exorcisms should be under the purview of the clergy. However, he was also well aware that, like many religious practices, use of these methods among the laity was inevitable, and likely to be employed in nonsanctioned circumstances.

The *Malleus* outlines Kramer's criteria for the lawful use of exorcism among the laity:

> When some work takes place by the virtue of the Christian religion, for instance when someone wishes to help a sick person through some prayer or blessing involving Holy Words… this person has to consider seven conditions, and if they are fulfilled, it is considered a lawful blessing. If it takes place in the manner of an adjuration by the virtue of the Divine Name and by the virtue of the famous works of Christ relating to His Nativity, Passion, precious Death and so on, through which even the Devil is defeated and cast out, these blessings, chants and exorcisms are called lawful and those who put them into practice can be called exorcists, or lawful enchanters."[46]

This description affords some measure of sanctioning for activities among the folk, providing that the following are satisfied: (1) Neither overt nor indirect invocation of demonic forces are permitted; (2) Benedictions shall contain no names of unknown entities, so as not to conceal the nature of an invocation; (3) There must be no use of incantations or prayers that include fictitious elements; (4) There must be no seals or characters other than the sign of the cross; (5) No faith is to be placed on the particular manner of the creation or enactment of a blessing that has nothing to do with reverence for God; (6) That the use of divine words and scripture should be used in reverence for God, and that the desired effect is sought from God or from the Saints, who derive their power from God; (7) The effect of such practices must be placed in the hands of God, who determines the correct outcome. Such incantations are determined to be lawful, "provided that the attention is fixed only on the sacred words and the Divine virtue."[47]

As to the efficacy of using such words, Kramer cites St. Thomas Aquinas: "The words of God are not less holy than the Relics of the Saints." He continues and suggests some of the religious content that can be used in such lawful exorcisms and incantations:

> … according to everyone it is permissible for people to carry the Relics of Saints with them reverently. Therefore, in whatever way the name of God is ritually invoked, whether through the Lord's Prayer, the Hail Mary, His Nativity and Passion, the Five Wounds, the Seven Words that He uttered on the Cross, the Triumphal Placard [I.N.R.I.], the Three Nails, or the other weapons of the Church militant of Christ against the Devil and his works, these will be altogether lawful and hope can be placed in them when the effect is entrusted to the will of God, provided that it is only the Holy Words and the virtue of God that are being respected…[48]

This listing of approved religious content for use in incantations and prayers for the purpose of healing by exorcism perfectly describes a wide range of prayers used in powwowing in Pennsylvania. These very inscriptions turn up in the written blessings produced en masse by Dr. Joseph H. Hageman of Reading, Pennsylvania until just after 1900, over 400 years after Kramer's publication.[49]

The Malleus goes on to describe:

> These Holy Words serve not only to rescue but also to heal those who have been affected by sorcery. Words with a particular ability to rescue the places of humans and domestic animals are the Triumphal Title of Our Savior, "Iesus + Nazarenus + Rex + Iudeorum" so long as they are inscribed in the manner of a cross on four sides of the place, or if the name of the Virgin Mary or of the Evangelists or the words of John, "The Word was made flesh" are added. [50]

Although Kramer set the tone for both witchcraft prosecution and legitimate use of ritual for exorcism, he was by no means the only author to do so. What is significant

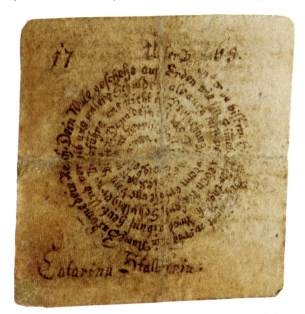

A miniature inscription of the Lord's prayer, spiraling inward clockwise, and bearing the name of Lancaster County resident Catharina Stauffer and the date 1769. Measuring no more than 1" square, the inscription shows evidence of having been folded into an even smaller ¼ size, whereby it was likely concealed within her personal effects as an amulet. While Catharina Stauffer's precise intentions are unrecorded, this practice is identical to traditions documented in the Middle Ages when such inscriptions were considered lawful means to secure protection from spiritual and physical harm. The inscription is evidence of the continuation of these practices in Pennsylvania, even among the plain communities. The inscription was likely produced by a skilled calligrapher with the use of a magnifying glass, and was found by Dr. Don Yoder among the family papers of the Konigmachers of Ephrata. *Courtesy of the Landis Valley Museum, Pennsylvania Historic and Museum Commission."*

about Kramer is the support he received directly from the Pope to incite the widespread use of violence to suppress witchcraft as a form of heresy.

These practices were not without criticism. The Protestant jurist Johann Georg Gödelmann considered such Roman Catholic exorcisms to be akin to enchanters (*incantores* or *magi*) who use ceremonies, the names of God, the Virgin Mary and the saints to drive out evil spirits from people, livestock, and houses.[51]

Although both Protestants and Catholics employed the use of exorcism, Protestants were critical of papal authority to sanction such activity. Martin Luther, for instance, purportedly cured a woman possessed by demons by kicking her to show disdain for the devil.[52] Tensions between Protestants and Catholics played out in witch trials as well, and the Counter-Reformation benefitted from such prosecutions as an opportunity to reclaim lands lost to Lutherans. Infamous Catholic inquisitor Balthasar Ross of Fulda in Hesse, calling himself *Malefizmeister*, executed 250 people. This was done, under the auspices of Catholic Prince-Abbot Balthasar von Dernbach, who returned from exile and sought to reinstate his rule by prosecuting his Protestant opposition. Ross was personally compensated for each execution, and he was later thrown in jail himself for corrupt extortion, and beheaded.[53] Interestingly enough, the inquisitor's title *Malefizmeister,* as a combination of Latin and German roots, was synonymous with *Hexenmeister* – one who exercises power over witchcraft. Among speakers of English today, this term is often misused and conflated with a practitioner of *Hexerei*, when in fact, the term *Hexenmeister* was used by exorcists on a folk-cultural level to designate the counter-witchcraft activities of an exorcist or healer.[54]

Malefizmeister Ross may have been corrupt, but his compensation for prosecution was commonplace for the time. Judges, executioners, guards, and torturers were paid handsomely for their services, and prominent families paid tributes to powerful judges to assure that they would be immune to accusations. When the accused parties were rich, confiscations of property and wealth were added to the coffers of princes and the ecclesiastical estates. Exorcists were equally susceptible to the lure of profits, and many Catholic and Protestant practitioners were suspected of preying upon the families of the sick.[55]

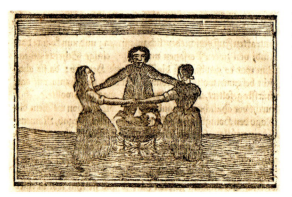

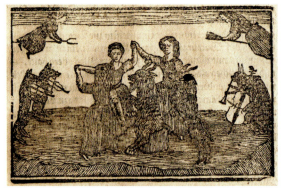

Popularly imagined scenes of witches gathering to eat a child (above), and the Witches' Sabath on Walpurgisnacht (below). Woodcuts from Heinrich Ludwig Fisher's *Buch vom Aberglaubens (Book of Superstitions)* 1791, Leipzig. Heilman Collection.

Over a century after Kramer, Girolamo Menghi, exorcist and demonologist, wrote two of the most authoritative works on the subject of exorcism,[56] entitled *Flagellum Daemonum (Scourge of Demons)* in 1576, which was expanded and released as *Fustis Daemonum (Bludgeon of Demons)* in 1584.[57] This work appeared when witchcraft prosecutions were at their height, and provided a manual on how to correctly identify the signs of witchcraft, and how to apply the necessary ritual cures through the advice of an experienced exorcist.

Menghi presided over exorcisms himself, including a case in 1582 in Bologna, where a local parish priest was confined to his bed for months with an unidentifiable sickness. After searching his bedding, they found numerous diabolical items of unspecified varieties concealed, which were burned. A month later, after the priest had not recovered, a similar search was conducted, and again similar concealed items were found. Menghi advised that demons were responsible for placing these items unbeknownst to the sufferer, and repeated searches were necessary.

Menghi advised the creation of *Brevia* or written blessings to cure cases like the parish priest. One was to take a small amount of gold, frankincense, myrrh, exorcised salt, olives, blessed wax, and rue, and put the ingredients into folded papers marked with three crosses, and to place one at each bedpost. He includes numerous inscriptions based on the names of God or scriptural verses to be written and hung on the neck of the afflicted person.

At great length, Menghi writes of the ethics of the exorcist, who should not use sorcery to defeat sorcery, nor transfer the curse to another, or invoke the demon by name to remove the illness. Furthermore, as it was not lawful for an exorcist or priest to practice medicine, one must consult a doctor about medical remedies. This sharp division between the disciplines of exorcism and medicine, recognized that the two practices were treating the same person, but in different ways, suggesting that exorcism functioned in a manner consistent with complementary medicine.[58]

This emphasis on ethics was to avoid the abuse of power among exorcists, who occupied a position of public trust within the framework of late medieval and early modern society. Franciscan doctor of theology, Valerio Polidori further expounds these ethics, stating that one should not specify a particular payment for services, but that alms that are freely given may be accepted. The exorcist is to be firm in faith, and whatever success he receives is attributable only to God, not to his own credit.[59] Such ethical codes outlined for exorcists in the works of Menghi and Polidori are identical to expectations still applied to the role of the powwow practitioner in Pennsylvania, demonstrating a common current in these manifestations of folk-religious healing.

Despite a number of the commonalities in practice, function, and ethics between the lawful application of exorcism and folk ritual expression, the quintessential conflicts between such practices were not so much based in the particulars of content, but in sanctioning, authority and power.

Blessing in the Early Modern Era

In the centuries that followed the Reformation and Inquisition, practices such as spiritual healing, exorcism, and anti-witchcraft measures continued to grow and evolve among Protestants and Catholics alike. Although attitudes towards healing and exorcism would undergo a great deal of change within the structure of church authorities, among the folk, such practices continued unfettered by larger conflicts centering on confessional differences. Although two parallel branches of ritual practices also developed at this point in time along the lines of creed reflecting changes in the upper strata, cross-pollination on a folk-cultural level between members of different religious groups played an important role in the dissemination of ritual practices throughout Europe that were a hybrid of Roman Catholic and Protestant traditions. Practices of both denominations would later influence the tradition of powwowing in Pennsylvania.

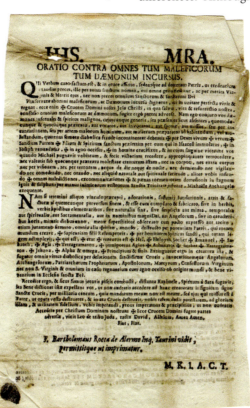

Latin *Prayer against Witches and Demonic Attacks*, a rare, late 17th-century Roman Catholic protective document attributed to Fr. Bartholomaeus Rocca Palermo Inq[uisitor] of Turin. The broadsheet is printed on both sides with blessings attributed to St. Vincent, invocations of the Latin, Greek, and Hebrew highest names of God, and passages from the Gospel of John on the verso. The document was folded, sealed with wax, kept in a square metal cover and carried for protection. *Heilman Collection.*

Among Catholics, veneration of the saints and their healing relics flourished with a renewed vigor in the wake of the Counter-Reformation. Where actual relics were inaccessible to the common person, a wide range of commercially produced devotional and protective items fed the need of the masses to engage with the sacred. Although printmaking enabled the dissemination of the literature of the Reformation through publications and tracts, printers also fueled the veneration of the saints through their increasingly sophisticated prints and engravings.[60] Elaborately printed images and documents, often alleging sacred origin, were associated with the shrines of particular saints and sold to pilgrims and devotees as empowered objects to be carried on one's person or kept in the home. These objects played an important role in the development of religious

71

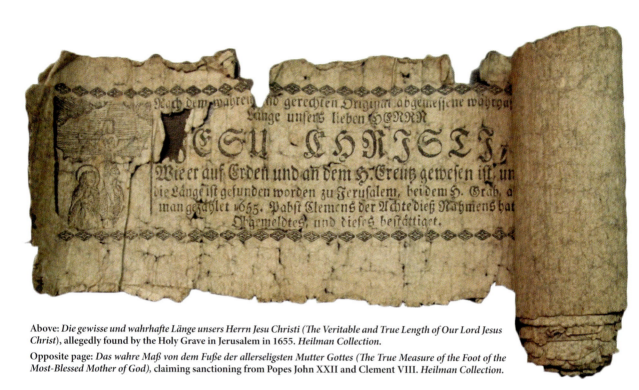

Above: *Die gewisse und wahrhafte Länge unsers Herrn Jesu Christi (The Veritable and True Length of Our Lord Jesus Christ)*, allegedly found by the Holy Grave in Jerusalem in 1655. Heilman Collection.

Opposite page: *Das wahre Maß von dem Fuße der allerseligsten Mutter Gottes (The True Measure of the Foot of the Most-Blessed Mother of God)*, claiming sanctioning from Popes John XXII and Clement VIII. Heilman Collection.

healing traditions in a variety of ways, both in terms of the specific contents of curative prayers and inscriptions, as well as the use of objects in ritual healing.

One class of widely accessible objects of religious devotion were those promising a "true measurement" of the bodily dimensions of Christ and the Virgin Mary, known as *Die gewisse und wahrhafte Länge unsers Herrn Jesu Christi* (*The Veritable and True Length of Our Lord Jesus Christ*), and *Die gewisse wahrhafte rechte Läng und Dicke unser lieben Frauen Maria* (*The veritable and True Length and width of Our Dear Lady Mary*). The *True Length of Christ* claimed to have been discovered at the Holy Grave in Jerusalem in 1655, and sanctioned by Pope Clement VIII.[61] These took the form of ribbons or rolled bands of paper believed to accurately portray Christ's height or Mary's girdle, and were printed with protective and inspirational prayers that were carried on the person. The earliest of these date to the 14th Century,[62] but were most widely circulated in the eighteenth and nineteenth centuries. Other variations claimed the true measurement of Mary's footprint, the side-wound of Christ, or the length of the nails used in the crucifixion. These images were also created for other saints such as saints Sixtus, Leopold, Franz, John, and Barbara.

Christianity cannot lay complete claim to this tradition of quantifying the legendary body of a divine agent in order to consecrate the object of measurement. Ancient Egyptians used the Holy Cubit of the god Thot as a sacred standard for measurement,[63] and later among the ancient Hebrews, Joseph's Cubit became the standard.[64] Just as Christian women used *The True Length of Mary* as a protective amulet in childbirth, so too in the Holy Land, expectant Palestinian Jewish women measured the temple wall with a piece of silk string, and then wound the string around their hips to ensure a safe delivery.[65]

For those who could not afford to purchase such printed copies of the *True Length*, ribbons, string or strips of cloth were used to measure the width of doorways of shrines, so that such strings could be carried home and used for healing.[66] It is small wonder then that the use of lengths of string can be found in healing traditions across Europe, among German, Spanish, Italian, and French populations, as well as in North America, among the Pennsylvania Dutch and the French Creole of Louisiana, and similar practices are found among American Jews.[67]

The *True Length* is one of many Roman Catholic traditions that emphasizes the sanctity of objects that have been ritually blessed, either by proximity or ceremony, and applied to prints which were mass produced. In the spirit of the hotly disputed sale of indulgences, a wide range of printed broadsides from the turn of the sixteenth century onward offered prayers for healing, exorcism, forgiveness, deliverance from disaster, and for the release of souls in purgatory. Such commodities often bore the spurious marks of sanctioning by popes, cardinals, bishops, and inquisitors, yet were condemned by authorities in Rome.

Letters of heavenly origin, known as *Himmelsbriefe*, allegedly written by the hand of God and delivered by means of angels to the sites of cathedrals across Europe, were printed as broadsides for the buyer and attributed to miracles at Magdeburg, Cologne, and St. Germain. These letters provided concise admonitions for righteous living, and offered blessings to those who observed their tenets, and additional blessings to those who copied the letter or allowed it to be copied by others.[68]

As early as the 4th century, bishops outlawed the use of hand-written Letters of Heaven, and Charlemagne issued a decree against them in 789,[69] yet Gutenberg's invention of the printing press enabled widespread distribution in many languages. The earliest printed Himmelsbrief is the St. Michaelsberg text published by Johan Schobser of Munich in 1500,[70] a document which Martin Luther condemned as fraudulent.[71] The circulation of Letters of Heaven would later come to a peak in the eighteenth and nineteenth centuries during the time of mass European emigration to North America, where they would become widely popular in German and English.

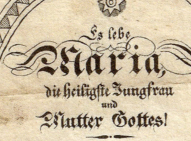

A Letter, that was written by God Himself and was let down at Magdeburg. It was written with golden letters and was sent from God by an angel... it shall be given to whoever will copy; whoever condemns it shall be forsaken of God.

He who labors upon Sunday is damned; therefore, I command you not to labor upon the Sunday, but go regularly to church, but do not ornament yourselves; you shall not wear false hair and not follow pride; of your riches you shall give unto the poor; share abundantly with them and believe that this letter was written by my own hand, and was published by Christ himself; and that you do not like unto unreasoning beasts; you have six days wherein to do all your work, but the seventh (namely that is the Sunday) you shall keep holy; if you do not then I will send war, famine, pestilence and sorrow among you and shall punish you with many plagues. Also, I command you every one, whether he be young or old, small or great, that you never work late on Saturday; rather that you repent of your sins that they may be forgiven; lay up neither silver or gold; follow not after the lusts of the flesh and of matter; remember that I have made you and can destroy you, rejoice not that your neighbor is poor, have the more patience - or charity - with him that it may be well with you; you children honor father and mother, so that it may be well with you on earth; he who does not believe this and keep it, is damned and lost; I, Jesus, have written this with my own hand; he who denies it and ridicules it, that same person shall have no help to expect from me; whoever has this letter and does not publish it, he is accursed from the Christian church; and if your sins were as large again, if you repent and are sorry, they shall be forgiven you; whoever does not believe it shall die

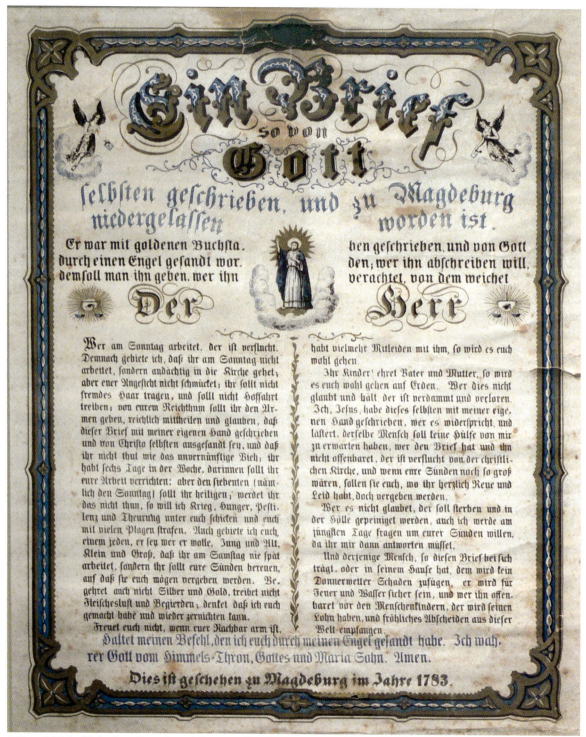

A *Himmelsbrief* or "Letter from Heaven" containing a text allegedly written by the hand of God and dropped down from the clouds by an angel in the German city of Magdeburg in the year 1783, promising blessings and protection from storms, fire, floods, and illness. Printed by Augustus Kohler, Philadelphia, ca. 1860. *Heilman Collection.*

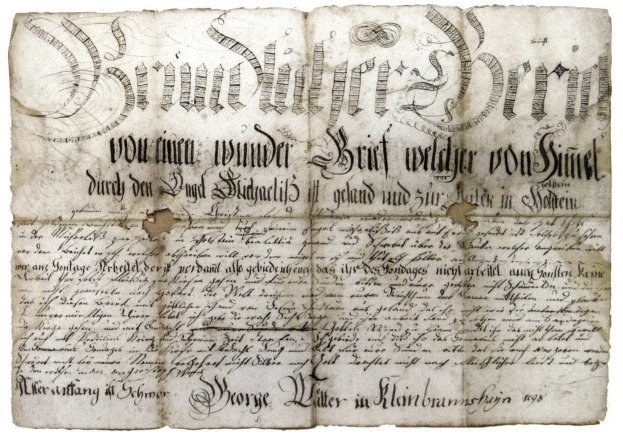

A hand-written *Himmeslbrief*, entitled *Grundlicher Bericht* (*A Detailed Report*), transcribed by George Wälter of Klein Braunshain, in Thuringia, Germany, dated 1798. *Heilman Collection*.

and be punished in hell; also I shall ask about your sins at the judgment day, where you then must answer; and that same person who carries this letter with him, or has it in his house, he shall not be harmed by thunder storms, he shall be safe from fire and water; and whoever publishes it to the children of mankind, he shall have his reward and shall have a happy departure from out of this world; keep my command that I have sent you by my angel. I, truly God, of Heaven's Throne, God's and Mary's son. Amen. This transpired, at Magdeburg, in the year 1783.[72]

The *Himmelsbrief* is part of a diverse genre of documents catering to popular interest in extra-biblical revelations,[73] which contain narratives and details not found in the Biblical canon. The *Himmelsbrief* in particular suggested that not only was God continuing to speak in present times outside of context of the church, but that messages from the divine were directly accessible for inspiration and protection without being mediated by the clergy. This notion of accessibility made the *Himmelsbrief* widely popular among German Catholics and Protestants alike. Despite the fact that clergy spoke out against them on both sides of the confessional divide, the long period of domestic and political instability brought on by generations of religious wars caused letters of protection to increase in popularity.[74]

Another eighteenth century protective letter of Roman Catholic origin was the *Seven Holy Bolts of Heaven* (*Sieben Heiligen Himmelsriegel*) allegedly delivered to a pious hermit by his guardian angel, and sanctioned by the high clergy (*hohe Geistlichkeit*) in Cologne in 1750. This series of exhortations outlines the crucifixion narrative of Christ and concludes with the "Seven Words" or last statements made by Christ on the cross. These seven statements unlock the symbolic "bolts" which open the gates of heaven:

> O Jesus! Thou hast unbolted the heavenly gates for us with thy holy bitter suffering and death…. Thou remained alive for three hours on the cross, and spoke seven powerful words, afterword thou, O my dearest Jesus, didst depart on the holy Cross. O my Jesus, with all thy holiest bitter passion and death and with thy seven holy sayings on the cross will I, N. N., in God's name, fasten my body and soul forever.[75]

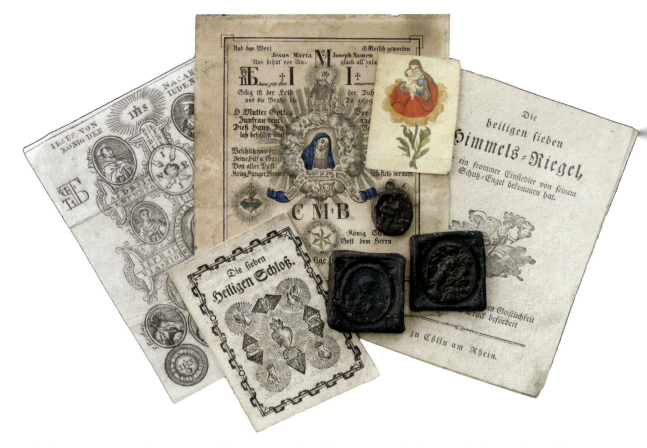

Clockwise from the right: European *Breverl* (Austrian dialect for a little protective letter) featuring the Caravaca Cross, eighteenth century; colored etching *Glückselige Haussegen* (Sacred House Blessing) with the Virigin Mary and the initials of the Three Kings, CMB, and the *Segen-Stern*, a six-pointed star with the letters IEHOVA spread across the points, nineteenth Century, Munich; small *Gnadenbild* (Holy Image) of the Virgin Mary, which was physically touched to the Holy Image of the Virgin Mary in Passau, Lower Bavaria, eighteenth century; *Die heiligen sieben Himmels-Riegel (The Seven Holy Bolts of Heaven)*, a protective prayer allegedly given to a hermit by his guardian angel, Cologne, Germany; three Fraisen-Steine (Epilepsy Stones) cast from zinc with images of the saints, carried by epileptics for deliverance from seizures; *Die sieben Heiligen Schloß (The Seven Holy Seals)*, a seven-fold prayer for protection, claiming to have been printed "on the German press in Jerusalem," nineteenth century. *Heilman Collection.*

The bolts of heaven therefore represent a liminal threshold not only between the earth and heaven, but a safeguard between the bearer of the letter and all imminent danger.

> Whoever carries with them *The Seven Holy Bolts of Heaven*, from this person all evil spirits and demonic apparitions must depart by day and night. And in whichever house *The Seven Holy Bolts of Heaven* lie imprinted, no thunderstorm will strike down in this house and it will be spared from all fiery inferno. And when a woman is in the pain of childbirth, so then take *The Seven Holy Bolts of Heaven* and lay them upon her breast or back so she will give birth without pain and she will be pleased with a healthy infant… And whichever person carries with them *The Seven Holy Bolts of Heaven*, to this person will Christ reveal the certain time before the end, the very hour when he must die. However, when one prays *The Seven Holy Bolts of Heaven* on seven Fridays in succession, no terrible sickness will come into a house in which the Seven Holy Heavenly-Bolts are kept.[76]

The Seven Holy Bolts of Heaven were often printed in as chapbooks along with other popular prayers and narratives, such as *Our Dear Lady's Dream* (*Unserer lieben Frauen Traum*), an apocryphal account of the Virgin Mary's premonition of the crucifixion of Christ.[77]

> As the Holy Virgin was asleep on the hill at Bethlehem, the Son of God, her dear Angel came to her and spoke to her:
> 'My dearest mother, are you asleep or awake?' She said, 'I was sleeping and you have awoken me and I have dreamed terribly. I have seen that you were captured in a garden, bound with cords and lead from Caiaphas to Pilate and from Pilate to Herod, that they struck your holy head and crowned you with thorns and led to you to the courthouse. A timber was laid upon your shoulder, and you were led out

of the city up a high hill, and hung upon a cross, so high, that I could not reach you. Your holy side was pierced through, and out flowed blood and water and it dripped from you. Afterword You were taken from the cross, and laid in the earth and buried as a dead man, and my heart could have burst from such great pain.'

Jesus spoke thusly to her, 'My dearest Mother, it is a true dream that has come to you. Whosoever contemplates on this dream or carries it with them, they will remain free from all evil things, and will not die suddenly, also will not pass from this world without receiving of the holy sacraments. I and Thou, dear Mother, will be at his final end and we will lead his soul into the heavenly kingdom.'

The Roman Catholic church outlawed this apocryphal narrative, as well as *The Seven Holy Bolts of Heaven*,[78] adding them to an ever growing list of banned prayers and texts based on the notion that such documents promoted unfulfillable promises of protection and salvation. Despite this condemnation, *Our Dear Lady's Dream* and other popular blessings and prayers were commonly included in personalized, handwritten prayer books and missals, alongside transcriptions of the liturgy of the Holy Mass. *The prayer of the Seven Holy Seals* (*Sieben Heiligen Schluss-Gebet*) in addition to being a popular broadside depicting seven symbolic locks, was often transcribed as a closing prayer for such personalized texts.[79] This prayer, like *Our Dear Lady's Dream,* made some heavy promises of protection, excepting that this prayer of *The Seven Holy Seals* was alleged to keep a person from passing into eternal damnation if prayed on their deathbed.[80] These views were theologically problematic, as they objectified words and prayers as inherently sacred and powerful in and of themselves, as opposed to regarding prayers as supplications and petitions directed to the power of the divine for assistance and salvation. Instead, such books and the prayers they contained played a dual role as amulets in addition to texts used in daily devotions.

Although prized by Catholic parishioners, such hand-copied prayer books containing forbidden texts, were regarded by the church as works of sorcery.[81] This notion was further advanced by the fact that some prayer books were filled with exotic characters and seals accompanying prayers to the saints and the archangels.[82] Although such symbols were influenced by Christian interpretations of the mystical Jewish devotional practices associated with the Hebrew Kabbalah, the use of such practices among Christians was equated with *Zauberei* (sorcery) and looked upon with suspicion by authorities.

Handwritten prayer books containing forbidden texts were not the only works under scrutiny by the church. *Der Wahre Geistliche Schild (The True Spiritual Shield)* was a widely circulated prayer book in Catholic and Protestant lands, comprising a litany of banned prayers allegedly sanctioned by popes, cardinals, and bishops, such as *Our Dear Lady's Dream*. The work was produced throughout the eighteenth and nineteenth centuries in Germany and Austria, usually bearing the spurious imprint of 1647 with a variety of locations, such as Prague, Vienna, Mainz, and even Reading, Pennsylvania. Some editions claim sanctioning by Pope Urban VIII while others attribute the work to Pope Leo X,

The seven seals of the archangels of the days of the week, from *Andachtiges Seelen Regal, Bestehend ein Morgens-, Abends-, Mess-, Beicht-, und Communion-, dann Divers anmüthige-Gebether! 1797.* Austrian manuscript prayer book belonging to Sexaphin Antoni Oberdorfer. *Heilman Collection.*

77

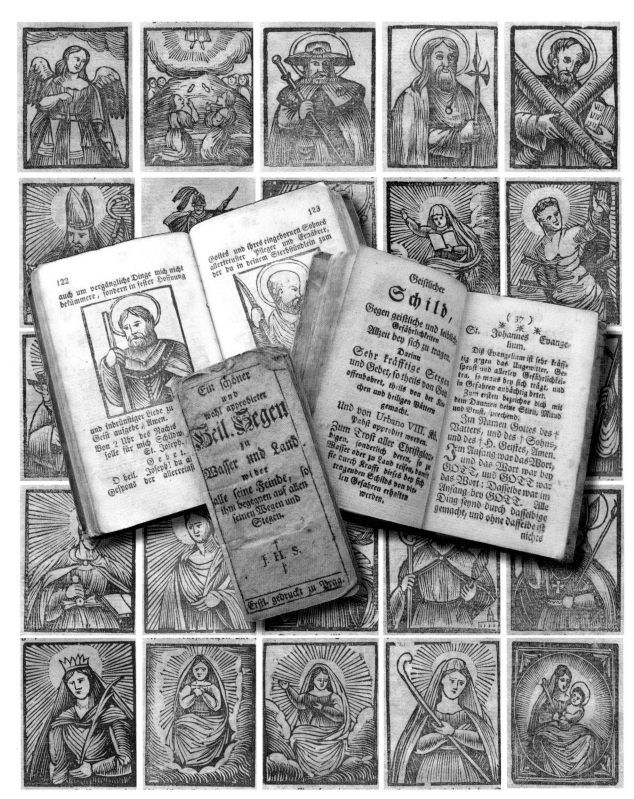

but all editions promise the owner and bearer of the work protection from "spiritual and bodily danger."[83]

The work begins with the first fourteen verses of the Gospel of John, instructing one to make the sign of the cross with the thumb over the forehead, mouth and breast before commencing the recitation of the Gospel, as a protective measure "against storms, spirits, and all danger."[84]

> In the beginning was the Word, and the Word was with God, and the Word was God. The same was in the beginning with God. All things were made by him; and without him was not anything made that was made. In him was life; and the life was the light of men. And the light shineth in darkness; and the darkness comprehended it not. There was a man sent from God, whose name was John. The same came for a witness, to bear witness of the Light, that all men through him might believe. He was not that Light, but was sent to bear witness of that Light. That was the true Light, which lighteth every man that cometh into the world. He was in the world, and the world was made by him, and the world knew him not. He came unto his own, and his own received him not. But as many as received him, to them gave he power to become the sons of God, even to them that believe on his name: Which were born, not of blood, nor of the will of the flesh, nor of the will of man, but of God. And the Word was made flesh, and dwelt among us, (and we beheld his glory, the glory as of the only begotten of the Father,) full of grace and truth.[85]

The gospel recitation concludes with "*God sei Dank*" (Thanks be to God), and the making of the letters I.N.R.I. with the thumb on the forehead once again, while speaking:

> Jesus of Nazareth, King of the Jews: This triumphant title of Jesus Christ the Crucified be between me and all my enemies, visible or invisible, that they cannot approach nor harm me, neither in body nor in spirit. Amen.[86]

The litany continues with a long invocation of the names of God in Latinized Hebrew and Greek, and it was used for protection from sorcery and physical harm, claiming sanctioning by Pope Urban VIII in 1633 or 1635 during the time that the Thirty Years War ravaged Central Europe.[87]

> *Jesu † Maria*
>
> *Im Namen Gottes des † Vaters, und des † Sohnes und des † heil. Geistes. Amen.*
> *Gott Heloem, Gott Tetragramation, Gott Antoni, Gott Sabaoth, Gott Emalluel, Got hagios, Gott Othios, Gott Ischroos, Gott Jehova, GOTT Mesiia, Gott Alpha und Omega....*[88]

European broadside of *Our Dear Lady's Dream*, alledging protection and salvation to the bearer of the inscription. Folds indicate it was concealed and carried in the owner's personal belongings. Heilman Collection.

Although Pope Urban VIII could not have possibly written the contents of *The True Spiritual Shield* and his successors condemned the book, the false appearance of licensing through the holy offices of the church lent a sense of credibility to the prayers to a wide readership. Some of the prayers are attributed to Pope Leo X, Pope Marcello II, Pope Alexander I, as well as Bishops in Jerusalem, Salamanca, and Antioch; even the Council of Trent in 1545 is invoked to sanction the *Blessing of Zachariah* (*Zacharias-Segen*), an abbreviated inscription derived from the Psalms carried for protection against the plague.[89]

As an addendum to *The True Spiritual Shield*, a section entitled *The Spiritual Shield-Vigil* provides a round of prayers attributed to the 24 patron saints of each hour of the day, along with woodcuts of each saint, and the admonition to heed the words from the Gospel of Matthew 24:42: "Watch therefore: for ye know not what hour your Lord doth come," and Mark 13:33: "Take ye heed, watch and pray: for ye know not when the time is."[90]

Der Wahre Geistliche Schild, Heiliger Segen, und Geistliche Schild-Wacht (*The True Spiritual Shield, The Holy Blessing, and Spiritual Shield Vigil*), three editions of the classic compilation of European seventeenth-century benedictions, prayers, and blessings for protection from danger, evil spirits and plague. These works, while largely unknown today, were once frequently recorded in manuscript form throughout Pennsylvania and used for powwowing, as well as printed in Reading and Erie, Pennsylvania, as well as Cincinnati, Ohio. The two open, hard-backed editions were owned by Pennsylvanians, and the one on the right was likely to have been printed in Reading, Pennsylvania. Heilman Collection.

The Spiritual Shield compilation also served as a vehicle to cloak the sale of a far more controversial book within its contents. Printed between the main text of *The True Spiritual Shield* and *The Spiritual Shield-Vigil* was the most popular of all European works of ritual healing and protection, *das Romanus-Büchlein* (*The Little Book of Romanus*). When printed with the *True Spiritual Shield*, the text of *Romanus* appeared instead under the title *Heiliger Segen* or *Holy Blessing, For the Use of Pious Christians to be Safe from All Danger, By Which Both Man and Beast are Often Delivered*.[91]

The earliest known imprint of *Romanus* from 1788 bears the image of a tonsured saint in robes, carrying a cross in one hand, and a miniature cathedral in the other. The saint, although not identified in print, is accompanied by the inscription, "This book protects man and beast from misfortune and sickness, danger from fire and water, theft, injury from weapons of all sorts, as well as sorcery, both in the home and abroad."[92] The work was printed in Glatz, a city in Lower Silesia, now part of present-day Poland. Although the book is attributed in title only to "Romanus," literally meaning "Roman," there is no consensus as to whom this name precisely refers. Some have suggested St. Romanus Caesarea who was martyred at the turn of the 4th century. One problem with this notion is that there are eight such saints named Romanus from the period of early Christianity,[93] and the book gives no indication of which, if any, of these saints are the inspiration for the title. St. Romanus Ostiarius, a companion of St. Lawrence, is a possible candidate, whose feast day is maintained in the Roman Catholic liturgical calendar on August 9th.

The most convincing evidence for the namesake of the *Romanus* text, however, is for Saint Romanus of Condat, a fifth century hermit, responsible for founding monasteries with his brother Lupicinus in the Jura Mountains along the border of France and Switzerland. He is buried at Romanum Monasterium (*Romainmôtier*) in Canton Vaud, Switzerland. Saint Romanus continues to be venerated in the Catholic and Protestant liturgical calendars on February 28th well up until the present day.[94] Most telling however, is that he is often depicted holding a church building in his hand, as a founder of monasteries. The earliest known printing of *Romanus* from Glatz features the saint with his characteristic identifier of the church in hand, although this images is also identical to the image of Saint Dominick, founder of the Dominican order, included in some editions of the *Spiritual Shield*.

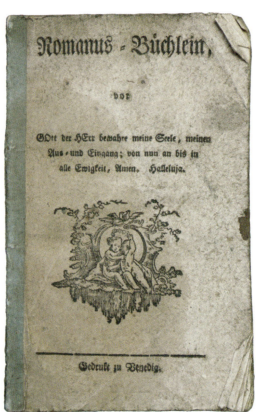

Late eighteenth-century collection of blessings, *The Little Book of Romanus* (*Romanus-Büchlein*), bearing the false imprint of Venice, Italy. Heilman Collection.

St. Romanus of Condat was also venerated as a healer and worker of miracles. According to legend, in the year 460 on a pilgrimage to the tomb of Saint Maurice, St. Romanus was shown hospitality by two lepers living near Geneva, who allowed him to stay overnight. When the lepers were miraculously cured the following morning, word spread throughout Switzerland and the region. Upon Romanus' return trip through Geneva, he was greeted by a massive procession of magistrates, clergy, and throngs of people honoring the healing miracle that had taken place.[95]

This narrative alone, coupled with the Saint's identifying symbol of the church, has not satisfied some European critics, who have suggested further possibilities for the origin of the title of *Romanus* such as famous German lawyers and statesmen,[96] but these associations are an unlikely fit for such a book of ritual healing. Later editions confuse the issue further, depicting Saint John the Baptist on the cover, without any specific mention of Saint Romanus.[97] Another nineteenth-century edition titles the work "*Aprobirtes Romann-Büchlein*," claiming to have been "published by a famous Jesuit in 1796 in Prague."[98] This latter title may also have been derived from a compounding in the imaginations of the folk with the title of *Romanus* and the *Rituale Romanum*, the standard ritual liturgical order of the Roman Catholic Church.

Even more perplexing is the fact that the contents of *Romanus* were republished in an American powwow manual, entitled *Der lange Verborgene Freund* (*The Long Lost Friend*) first compiled in 1819 by Johann Georg Hohman, who claims that his work was derived from a "*Zigeuner-Buch*" (Gypsy/Romani Book).[99] The term Romani is an adjective describing the language and ethnicity of the Roma or Romani people, and was not likely to be in common usage in Germany during the time that the *Romanus* collection was first published. It is equally unlikely that Hohman was aware of such a term in 1820, despite the word's usage in the early nineteenth century among speakers of English.[100]

The *Romanus* collection opens with two classic prayers that outline two distinct forms of healing and protective blessings.[101] The first, in the spirit of the heavenly letters, promises protection by means of invoking sacred protectors. The latter form is based in non-literary, oral recitations of poetic, apocryphal narratives used as a ritual blessing.

> A Morning Prayer, which one must pray before going on a journey, so that it shall protect the person from all misfortune:
>
> I, N. (here speak your full name), will go on a journey today; I will walk upon God's path, and walk where God himself did walk, and our dear Lord Jesus Christ, and our dearest Virgin with her dear little babe, with her seven rings, and her true things. O thou my dear Lord Jesus Christ! I am thine own, that no dog may bite me, no wolf bite me, and no murderer secretly approach me. Save me, O my God, from sudden death. I am in God's hands, and there I will bind myself. In God's hands I am bound by our Lord Jesus' five wounds, that each and every gun or weapon may do me no more harm than our Holy Virgin Mary's virginity was harmed by the favor of her spouse Joseph. After this say the Lord's Prayer three times, the Ave Maria three times, and the Creed.[102]

Although this traveler's blessing is comparable to other prayers in *The Spiritual Shield*, the majority of healing prayers in *Romanus* are apocryphal in nature, with poetic expressions of hypothetical biblical events. The second prayer in *Romanus* is a classic ritual for healing a child suffering from thrush (*Mundfäule*), involving the prayerful recitation of an apocryphal discussion between God and Job, and the action of blowing three times into the mouth of the child while invoking the Holy Trinity. The details of the prayer are only loosely suggestive of the biblical accounts of Job's affliction with sores in the Book of Job,[103] but the legendary conversation is scripted in such a way as to allow the suffering child and the healer to enter into the narrative and participate in the cure of the illness. The pious Job's suffering and subsequent healing are to serve as a symbolic corollary to the illness and recovery of the child:

> Job went out upon the land, he held his staff in his hand, then the Lord God appeared to him, and said unto him: Job, Why grievest thou so? Job said: O God! Why shall I not grieve? My throat and my mouth are rotting away. Then spoke the Lord to Job: In yonder valley there flows a spring, which shall heal thee N. N., thy throat and thy mouth, in the name of God the Father, and of the Son, and of the Holy Spirit, Amen.[104]

This particular prayer dates back at least to the 12th century and was produced in many variations, including similar narratives featuring Peter, Mary and other saints instead of Job.[105] Although its content is essentially Christian, the apocryphal format of this legendary prayer is ancient in origin. The prayer is not based in a literal rendering of the Book of Job, as its style and performance as a ritual is ultimately derived from early European ritual traditions that made no use of sacred writings of Christian scripture. This latter form of blessing is intended to be memorized and recited orally, as opposed to the opening traveler's prayer, which was frequently hand-written and carried as a blessing.[106]

These two basic types of blessings, both recited and written, oral and literary, form the basis for European ritual healing and protective traditions. However, it was the spoken word which inspired a highly developed system of performative healing traditions in Europe, known as *brauchen* (to heal with blessings). As this tradition was in its earliest form a primarily oral tradition with little dependence upon literature, the practice employed distinctive methods of transmission whereby a man must learn from a woman, and a woman must learn from a man[107] claimed by some to date to ancient Teutonic traditions.[108] This traditional means of learning the contents of verbal blessings continues even today in Pennsylvania.

BRAUCHEN, BESPRECHEN, BEPISPELN

In the original German, *das Brauchen* refers to both the practice and the action of healing, and implies a traditional means of employing a ritual cure. The verb *brauchen* has a wide variety of implications, everything from "to need," "to make use of," or "to employ," as well as the particular connotation with healing, "to practice healing; to treat."[109]

The etymology of *Brauchen* in Europe and *Braucherei* in Pennsylvania is somewhat shrouded in mystery. *Brauchen* has been linked to a much older, albeit unknown, word that is preserved in the related Latin words, *frui* (to enjoy) and *fructis* (enjoyment, product, fruit, profit),[110] but there are also a number of other similar words from Celtic roots that suggest a connection with ritual. In Spanish, the suspiciously similar words, *bruja* and *brujeria* imply, respectively, "a user of magic" and "a spell or sorcery," and in Portuguese, the same definitions apply to *bruxa* and *bruxaria*, as well as Catalan *bruixa* and *bruixeria*,[111] as well as *bruèissa* in Occitan, and *bruisha* or *brouche* in the dialect of Gascony.[112] Although many sources suggest the origin of these words is unknown in Romance languages, such words are all likely to be derived from Celtic roots, and related to *breou* (sorcery, charms) and *bre* (witch) in Breton, Middle-Welsh *brith-ron* (magic wand), and Old Irish *brichtu* (charms), *brigim* (to light up), and the name Brigid (shining one).[113]

Given the complex and often pejorative associations with defining terms like magic, sorcery, and even charms throughout the ages, it is likely that all of these terms originally referred to ritual traditions specific to earlier cultural modalities that have been lost to time. The related German word, *Brauch*, implies a custom, a practice, a ritual, or a ceremony,[114] but within a folk-cultural context, it is synonymous with healing by means of employing a ritual blessing.[115] Just like in Pennsylvania, a European female practitioner is a *Braucherin*, and a male is a *Braucher*.

As blessings within this context are specifically verbal, this notion of *brauchen* – to heal with a spoken blessing (*Segenspruch*) – is found in regional dialects across Germany, but each locality developed very specific, nuanced ways of describing this verbal process. In addition to *brauche* (to administer healing or to treat) in the Pfalz, one also finds *pischbere* (to whisper) and *murmele* (to murmur),[116] suggesting a soft ritualized tone, *sotto voce*. In Wittgenstein, in the south one finds *bepispele* (to whisper), and *beschwatze* (to invoke), *bespreche* (to invoke/bespeak) and *bekrispele* (to rustle) in the North, as well as *sann* (to bless).[117] In other cases, one's healing abilities were expressed in idioms, such as "*Hä kann wos*," or "*Dea wees wos*" (one who knows something),[118] or one who "*mehr können als Brot essen*" (knows more than how to eat bread, i.e. more than the common person).[119] This is comparable to idioms in Pennsylvania where it is said of one who powwows: "*sie kann meh wie Brot esse*" (she can do more than eat bread).[120]

Despite all of these epithets for the act of healing and blessing, more specific terms were actually used in ritual applications. In the Pfalz, certain ailments were "blown away" (*wegblasen*) as in the case of burns, throat ailments, and eye troubles; worms were "destroyed" (*töten*), and colic was ritually "dismissed" (*abthun*).[121] Although whispering, murmuring, and treating were used in a general sense, each ailment was engaged in a manner that produced a robust system of describing illnesses, their causes, symptoms, and cures.

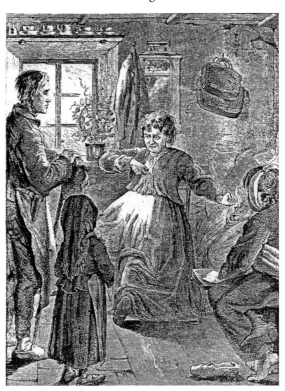

Nineteenth-century German engraving of a rural Palatine healer or *Braucherin* performing a ritual cure. Don Yoder Collection, original source unknown. Pennsylvania German Cultural Heritage Center, Kutztown University of Pennsylvania.

It has been suggested, that all of these words were used as a means of ritual discretion, that is, alternately fearing that naming the practice would have negative consequences,[122] or that such words were used in place of more unsavory words like "magic" (*Zauberei*),[123] which would have been punishable by state and religious authorities. While there is some merit to both of these explanations, even the word "to bless" was suspect to authorities if used outside of sanctioned circumstances.

For instance, the *Polizeiordnung* (Police Order) of Saxony in 1556[124] criminalized the use of blessings containing exotic words, and laws in Wittgenstein in 1573 set the early precedent for illegalizing the "blessing of man and beast" (*Segen an Menschen und Vieh*), on the grounds of likening it to "superstition" (*Aberglauben*) and "sorcery" (*Zauberei*). Such laws also benefited and protected the conventional doctors and apothecaries of the times.[125] Local and regional laws such as these remained in place for centuries, and prosecutions of healers accused of witchcraft continued well into the eighteenth century.

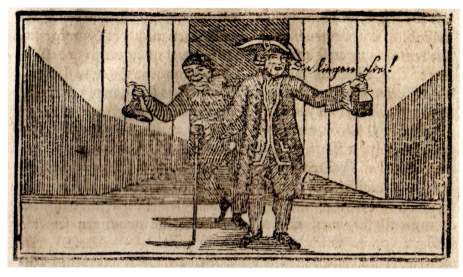

An eighteenth-century European *Wunderdoctor*, accompanied by a clown, performing a medicine show for the public sale of patent medicine, stating "Da liegen sie" (There they are). Fischer's *Buch vom Aberglauben,* 1791. Heilman Collection.

Despite such persecutions, the practice of *Brauchen* was widespread, and by the time that mass emigration to the North American continent among German-speaking Protestants and Anabaptists commenced in the eighteenth century, a significant body of oral tradition would begin to be imparted to the New World. As evidenced in works such as *The Spiritual Shield* and *Romanus*, the literature of ritual healing and blessing was already well-established and robust. Although such works were essentially illegal in Europe, they were nonetheless brought to Pennsylvania where they were not only tolerated, but also became highly influential in Pennsylvania folk culture. As German-speaking people continued to emigrate to North America well into the nineteenth century, ritual traditions were by no means isolated between the continents, but part of a continual process of cross-pollination.

Criticism of Brauchen

Throughout the time of emigration and thereafter, an equally robust genre of criticism appeared in the popular press, in the form of tracts, broadsides, almanacs, and chapbooks. Many of these works provide detailed accounts of European practices that mirror the development of powwowing in North America, and highlight similar conflicts with legal, academic, and religious authorities.

With the development of academic medicine, *Brauchen* was subject to new forms of legal disputes, as many doctors opposed such practices and offered public criticism of any medicine outside of the realm of the learned elite. While old laws such as the 1573 *Polizeiordnung* condemned *Brauchen* on the grounds of comparison to witchcraft, other terms came to dominate the denigration of the practice of *Brauchen* on an intellectual level, such as *Quacksalber* (Quack), *Wunderdocktor,* (Miracle Healer), *Gsundbeter* (Prayer-Healer), and so forth. Although these words were used in the upper strata of society, they were not used by the people who employed blessings for healing,[126] but instead appeared largely in the language of those who opposed the practices.

Much criticism centered on the development of a new class of imposters of folk healers at the end of the seventeenth century, who aimed to capitalize on the public sale of remedies and salves in the theatrical manner of the medicine show. Such traveling charlatans known as *Marktschreiern* (market-criers) and *Wunderdoctoren* (miracle-doctors) were accompanied by a clown (*Hans Wurst*), a whole troupe of clowns for comic relief, or a "wild man" in furs to lend credence to a peddler of miracle herbal cures from the wilderness.[127] These so-called miracle-doctors relied on the spectacle they produced to sell their medicines to eager buyers. Such performances relied upon providing the appearance of knowledge of traditional healing methods akin to *Brauchen* or even techniques employed by adherents to mesmerism to impress their audiences and create the illusion of credibility. Even the phrase *Gott allein die Ehre* (Glory to God alone) was appropriated by such miracle-doctors, who attributed their cures to the power of the divine.[128] Although such spectacles were in no way related to the practice of *Brauchen*, the performances and the resulting sales of dubious medicines provided fodder for public ridicule of folk healing.

Ironically, one of the most impressive chapbooks decrying the deceptions of the *Wunderdocktor* capitalized upon public interest in the supposedly clandestine techniques employed in *Brauchen* by publishing detailed descriptions of traditional ritual procedures and supplying

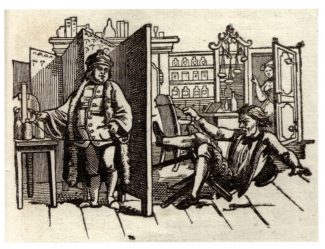 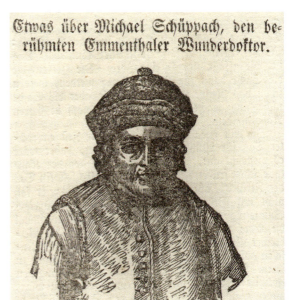

The humorous satire of Swiss "*Wunderdoktor*" Michael Schüppach, the famous practitioner from Emmenthal, featuring a comical view of his consultation room, where, by means of a screen, he decieves his patients. A portrait of the *Wunderdoktor* (right) accompanied the *Bauern-Kalender auf das Jahr 1853, Langnau, bei Friedrich Wyß*. Heilman Collection.

critical commentary. An alleged medical doctor, aggravated by his competition from traditional healers and known only by the *nom de plume* "Doctor Medicus," compiled what would appear at first glance to be a work of healing blessings, but was actually an educational work against such practices.

On the outer cover, the work was entitled *Der Hausarzt und die Hausapotheke, welche in allen Fällen Hulfe schaffen, oder die Kunst in 24 Stunden sein eigener Arzt zu werden* (*The Domestic Doctor and House Apothecary, Providing Assistance in All Circumstances, or the Method to Become Your Own Doctor in 24 Hours*), but the inner cover sported a scandalous title, catering to occult interests: *Der kluge und geschickte Wunderdoctor, oder die großen Geheimnisse der Sympathie, nebst der Zauberkunst des Docter Faust. Neu herausgegeben von Docter Medicus.* (*The Clever and Skillfull Wonder-Doctor, or the Great Secrets of Sympathy, Together with the Magic Art of Doctor Faust. Newly Compiled by Doctor Medicus.*)

Despite Dr. Medicus' deception, the buyer was able to purchase a work that would enable dabbling with traditional healing blessings, and depending upon their level of literacy, the buyer still may have been convinced that they had purchased a work of ritual healing, or even sorcery. The work was printed in 1830 in Reutlingen by J. N. Enßlin, a publisher that was responsible for printing copies of *The Spiritual Shield* and other classic works, but also distributed his works through Blummer & Gräter's Bookstore in Allentown, Pennsylvania.[129]

Dr. Medicus' descriptions of *Brauchen* in eighteenth and nineteenth century Germany are exceptionally detailed, albeit, on occasion, distastefully biased:

> The genuine and proper miracle-doctor is ordinarily a depraved person, who is too stupid or too rotten to support himself by any other honorable means, and because of this he is impudent enough to extoll his skillfulness in the healing arts to the common folk and deceive misfortunate sick people out of their money and lives with his corrupt cures. Of his profession, he ordinarily tends to be a knacker, a herdsman, a peddler, a shepherd, a tinker, and so forth; although no less often counted among the barbers, the surgeons, traveling doctors, harness-makers, Tyroleans, veterinarians, apothecaries, executioners, and old women; - to all of these people it comes easily to cure an illness in 24 hours or at most until the 9th day with the help of God, claiming to be a panacea for the incurable. Why wonder then, that they are held in high esteem by the honest and credulous rural folk? The common man believes their pomposities, and holds their promises and pretenses of impossible things as truth, and despises a skilled doctor, because he is no worker of miracles.

While this scathing account portrays the common person of his era as gullible and susceptible to the wiles of charlatans, Dr. Medicus also confirms many facts known about the nature of rural and urban practitioners, and their position in society. Although Medicus demeans the occupations he lists, the fact is, that many who received the title of *Braucher* for their healing practices were practicing not as a primary occupation, but as a function of certain perceptions about their trade. Herdsmen and shepherds were believed to possess greater knowledge about the workings of nature and the body,[131] while blacksmiths, tinkers, and other tradesmen were valued because of their knowledge of metallurgy and its relation to the creation of metal religious votives used in healing practices.[132] Barbers, veterinarians, and harness makers, along with farriers, were valued for their skill in treating animals and humans, as well as in *Aderlassen* or the letting of blood.

At the extreme, executioners and their equipment, the gallows and the sword, were believed to hold special healing powers due to their relation to sanctioned execution – an echo of ancient human sacrifice. Executioners' swords, having taken many a criminal from this world, were believed to heal by means of removing (i.e. executing) illness in a similar manner.[133] The noose was likewise valued, and cut into pieces to be sold at high prices to cure everything from toothache, epilepsy, and childhood illnesses.[134]

On the other end of the spectrum of healing practitioners were the farmers, midwives, and even some Capuchin friars, who by virtue of their close connection, respectively, with the earth and plants, fertility and birth, the holy and sacred, were valued for their knowledge of healing, blessing, and protection.[135] In all of these cases, the traditional understanding is that no monetary fee could be charged for a blessing, and, in some cases, no verbal statement of thanks was allowed, otherwise the blessing would not be effective.[136]

Dr. Medicus continues with condemnations of individuals who use such knowledge for profit and deception:

> The genuine and proper miracle-doctor is regarded as better than the scientific doctor. Utilizing credulity, ignorance, and superstition, these possessions of the simpleminded that hardly ever will be eradicated, he deceives and cheats the people, pulls the wool over their eyes, and tells of outrageous miracle-cures. He declares how each and every illness proceeds from a supernatural cause, being the result of bewitching, the wiles of the Devil, and the movements of the heavenly bodies, as well as how one must drive away the following illnesses solely through sympathy: Epilepsy (*fallende Krankheit*), sweeny (*Schwindsucht*), catalepsy (*Staffsucht*), erysipelas (*das heilige Ding*), palpatations of the heart (*Herzgespann*), St. Vitus' Dance (*Veitstanz*), marasmus (*Dürrsucht*), styes (*Schussblatter*), mouth-rot (*Mundfäule*), frostbite (*kalte Frieren*) and cancer (*Krebs*). His repertoire of splendid virtues are ranked as follows: 1.) Benedictions (*das Segensprechen*); 2.) Fumigation (*das Räuchern*); 3.) Exorcisms (*das Bannen*); 4.) Preparation of various amulets (*das Fertigen verschiedener Amulette*); 5.) Deception and unabashed lying; and 6.) Diagnosis by urine (*Urinbeschauen*). The first five characteristics are commonly learned, impudence and secretive practices being the primary objective, while urine diagnosis in contrast requires yet a certain gadgetry and cleverness, as the following narratives will obviously demonstrate…"[137]

Dr. Medicus claims to have obtained a long series of healing blessings from a *Wunder-Docktor*, also a knacker (*Schinder*) by trade in Odenwald. Many of these blessings were derived from *Romanus*. The miracle-doctor's procedure for treating Erysipelas is compared to Dr. Medicus' conventional methods:

> To the miracle-doctors are known the best remedies for Erysipelas (*die Rose, den Rotlauf, das heilige Ding*).
>
> He recognizes erysipelas by the inflammation that in each case spreads across the surface of the skin, and when the patient experiences burning pain on the spot. The miracle-doctor is highly effective in curing erysipelas. He is fetched to the patients, who have such advanced cases, where the face, or a hand, or any other limb, where the "Holy Thing" (*das heilige Ding*) has taken hold, is completely fire-red, and covered over and over with blisters, as though they were burned. They experience shivering, heat, restlessness, headache, and even a fever. Many times the face is so thickly swollen on one side that one cannot see the eyes. To him this is a trifle, and he speakes thusly:
>
> *Es gieng eine weiße Frau über das Land,*
> *Die hatte einen Brand an der Hand*
> *Brand Du sollst stille stehn*
> *Du sollst nicht weiter gehn*
> *Du sollst heilen wie ein frisches Ey*
> *Das zähl ich N. N. Dir zur Buß*
> *Das dein Rothlauf weichen muß.*
>
> There goes a white woman over the land,
> she holds a fiery brand in hand,
> Brand, still shalt thou stand,
> Thou shalt go no further,
> Thou shalt heal like a fresh egg,
> This I reckon to thee N. N. as penance,
> So that thy Erysipelas must vanish.[138]
>
> He repeats this for 3 days, one after the other, and orders that the sick person be kept in a state of mild perspiration, though without overheating or strong enough to make them sweat. Also the sick person must avoid meat and wine. Instead he should diligently drink elder tea. If one has the erysipelas on the head, a warm foot-soak has often done a good service.
>
> The Wonder-Doctor even further often rendered much harm, because one should use no fatty or oily substance, or spread anything wet upon it, whereby the Erysipelas will strike again, and spread into the lungs, or become gangrenous, or create fetid sores, and so forth. He would have often done better, if he had ordered nothing at all, except to lay a soft wool or a little sack of elder upon it, whereupon by the seventh day, the skin will become yellow, and the surface will peel off by the glassful.[139]

Medicus includes another blessing to heal erysipelas:

> *Die heilige Mutter Gottes*
> *Ging über den Nora*
> *Dort wollte Sie*
> *Rothlaufenkraut brechen.*
> *Das Kraut ist gebrochen*
> *Die Worte sind gesprochen*
> *Das zähl ich N. N. Dir zur Buß*
> *Daß Dein Rothlauf weichen muß.*
> *Im Namen + + +*

The Holy Mother of God
Went over the Nora
She wanted there to
Pluck Herb-Robert
The herb is broken
The words are spoken
This I reckon to thee N. N. as penance
That your Erysipelas must vanish
In the name of [God the Father, Son,
and Holy Spirit] + + + [140]

Dr. Medicus explains that the miracle-doctor employs this latter remedy also for animals, but that he professionally recommends the use of *Fieberrinde* – Jesuit's bark, or *cinchona*, china bark - both given to the animals internally, or applied with a compress, by boiling it and the bark in water. For each cure involving the use of a blessing, Dr. Medicus counters with a botanical remedy.[142]

Unlike the meticulous criticisms of Dr. Medicus, other critics took a stab at discrediting these traditions in a more scathing and satirical light. For example, *der Freimüthige Volkskalender* (*The Straightforward People's Calendar*) by Austrian almanac maker Eduard Breier offered a three-page parody of a new edition of *Romanus*, featuring satirical narratives of attempts to use rituals described in the book. One such account, the author claims, was shared regarding a seamstress from the Riegengebirge, in Silesia:

> A woman named Schneider owned a male and female goat. One day, when the female goat's milk had dried up, Mrs. Schneider assumed the goat was hexed. She wrote out a blessing from *Romanus* in order to feed it to the goat, but while she was preparing her midday meal, she forgot about the blessing. It accidentally fell into her husband's sauerkraut, whereby he ate it. From the moment forth, Mr. Schneider took on the behavior and qualities of the goat, and bleated – and who knows, whether or not Mr. Schneider would have given milk, had he been milked.[143]

Editor Breier continues with an analysis of a blessing used to create a hazelwood rod that can be used to ritually punish a witch or malefactor remotely from a great distance. This involved dedicating a hazel rod (see Chapter VII), calling the name of the malefactor, and flogging a coat or hat, so that the person receives the blows vicariously. The editor voices frustration that the publisher of *Romanus* did not include his name on the title page, whereby the editor would have tested the ritual by invoking the name of the publisher in order to give "the rascal what he rightly deserves."[144]

Breier's accounts concluded his satire with a remedy for stupidity:

> To become sensible: take the *Romanusbüchel*, burn it, and scatter the ashes to the four winds, and say the following words three times "get thee behind me Satan, so that I may become smart and sensible!" and thus shall the first rational action have been committed.[145]

Interjecting humor into such critical texts formed a sub-genre of eighteenth and nineteenth century literature dealing with all manner of traditions that came under scrutiny with the rise of the Age of Enlightenment, and deemed "superstition."[146] On the other hand, the work of some critics mounted not so much an assault on folk-cultural beliefs, but instead provided thorough literary documentation of the traditions.

The Poetry of the Blessing

As a counterpoise to Breier's scathing editorials, the beauty of Dr. Medicus' chapbook against ritual healing is that although he objects strongly (and occasionally in a vitriolic manner) to *Brauchen*, he preserves the prayers and blessings intact, and with better renderings than some published versions in actual healing manuals. For instance, he cites a lyrical variation of the *Merseberg Incantation* for healing a sprain:

> Als unser Herr Christus ritt zu Jerusalem ein,
> Stieß sich sein Eselein an einen Stein
> Und verrenkte sich den Fuß und das Bein;
> Nun gehe Ader zu Ader und Bein zu Bein
> An die rechte Statt,
> Wo sie vorhin gelegen hatt'.
> Im Namen Gottes des Vaters + + + Amen.
>
> As Our Lord Christ rode into Jerusalem
> His donkey stumbled on a stone,
> And sprained the foot and the bone.
> Now go vein to vein and bone to bone,
> In the right place,
> Where they previously laid.
> In the Name of God the Father... + + + Amen.[147]

This variant of the celebrated blessing from Merseberg appears to be uniquely corrected in rhyme and meter, unlike other versions, which are less inclined towards poetic expression. The earliest version of this blessing is one of the oldest surviving written samples in the German language, from the 10th century. It has since been translated in standard German, English, Dutch, Norwegian, Finnish, Swedish, Estonian, Polish, Czech, Slovenian, Serbian, Russian, Belorussian, Ukrainian, and other languages.[148] The original tenth-century text features a pantheon of pagan gods, as opposed to Christ, the Virgin Mary, or other saints and biblical figures. In translation from the original Old High German, it reads:

> Phol and Wodan rode into the woods,
> There Balder's foal sprained its foot.
> It was blessed by Sinthgunt, her sister Sunna;
> It was blessed by Frija, her sister Volla;
> It was blessed by Wodan, as he well knew how:
> Bone-sprain, like blood-sprain,
> Like limb-sprain:
> Bone to bone; blood to blood;
> Limb to limb as they were glued.

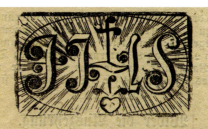

A European tract of prayers for fever, worms, sties on the eye, consumption, and stopping blood, attributed to a healer, named Dr. Riegel of Bürgenland, Austria. His remedy for consumption involves drinking red wine poured over a consecrated cross three Fridays in succession. The collection proudly displays the Roman Catholic symbolism of the monogram of Christ (IHS) and the sacred heart. *Heilman Collection.*

While the characters vary considerably from the biblical reference to Christ's arrival in Jerusalem, the format of the healing description "bone to bone" is essentially the same, encouraging some to question whether the origin of such lyrical blessings as a genre proceed from a pagan rather than Christian source. Like many aspects of religious concepts and rites, the borrowing and appropriating of content is not unique to Christianity, but ubiquitous to religious experiences throughout the world. However, the Merseberg blessing is unique among texts from the Middle Ages for the breadth of pagan personae included in the text at such a date.

A 9th-century healing blessing used to rid the body of worms, likewise appears in later variations used in *Brauchen*. Translated from Early Low German, the text describes a progression of removing the illness from the body of a horse:

Depart, worm, with your nine young,
Depart out of the marrow into the vein,
Out of the vein and into the flesh,
Out of the flesh and into the skin,
Out of the skin and into the hoof.
Then say the Lord's Prayer three times.[149]

There is little or no religious content in this blessing aside from the closing line, suggesting that, again, the blessing predates the Christian element. The Christian invocation appears to be supplied as an addendum to the blessing, rather than central to its content. This does not, however, mean that the blessing was simply a cloaked pagan practice, but rather, that the blessing found a continuity of use among both Christian and pagan traditions during early periods of transition in Europe.

Perhaps surprisingly, this notion of mutual use among Christians and pagans is further corroborated by the motif of the worm, representing a personification of an unknown cause of the illness. The notion of *Krankheitsdämonen* (illness-causing spirits),[150] although ancient in origin, was later applied with equal fervor by Christians who identified the "worm" with the "serpent," or "dragon," as a personification of the devil.

A simple formula, citing the dragon as the cause of erysipelas, demonstrates the belief that when the cause of the illness is destroyed, the symptoms immediately vanish.

Die Rose und der Drach
Die gingen miteinander zu Bach,
Der Drach ertrank,
Und die Rose verschwand.
Im Namen Gottes des Vaters, des Sohns,
un des heiligen Geistes. + + +

Erysipelas and the dragon
Went together over the stream,
The dragon drowned,
And Erysipelas vanished.
In the name of the Father, Son,
and Holy Spirit. + + +[151]

Such spirits of illness were once believed to travel solo and in cohorts, seeking humans to devour. A manuscript from rural Saxony, maintained in the private papers of a minister, Ernst August Gröbel (1783-1854), Rector of the Kreuzschule Dresden, features an elaborate blessing for exorcizing inflammation, gangrene, and erysipelas. The blessing is scripted like a conversation between Christ and an infectious cohort:

Unser Herr Jesus ging über Land
Da begegnete ihm Rotlauf, Kaltbrand, un wilde Feuer.
Jesus fragte es, wo willst du?
In einen Menschen.
Was willst du da thun?
Dem Menschen sein Fleisch un Blut zu verderben.
Unser Herr Jesus sprach:
Des sollst du nicht thun.
Alle Glocken haben geklungen und
Alle Evangelium sind gesungen
Alle Messen sind gelesen,
Die soll der Mensch genesen. + + +

Our Lord Jesus went out upon the land
There he met inflammation, gangrene, and erysipelas.
Jesus asked: Wither goest thou?
Into a mortal, they replied.
What wilt thou do there?
Spoil the mortal's flesh and blood.
Our Lord Jesus said:
This you shall not do.
All bells have been rung,
All Gospels have been sung,
All masses have been read,
And these shall revive the mortal. + + +[152]

Christ's rebuke of the cohort of illnesses is a common motif in European healing blessings, referencing the healing miracles of the Gospels, and in particular the healing of the demoniac in the fifth chapter of Mark. In this classic narrative, Christ addresses the spirits, asks their name, and commands them to depart.[153] In the Dresden manuscript, however, Christ authorizes the ringing of the church bells, singing (reading) of the gospels,[154] and the reading of the mass to intercede, banish the illness, and bring the mortal back from the brink of death.

In other cases, Christ's healing takes a more literal form, and a blessing for healing a sprain from the Oberpfalz depicts Christ plying common remedies:

Es ging ein Hirsch über eine Heide,
Er ging nach seiner grünen Weide,
Stößt seinen Fuß an einen Stein,
Verstauchte ihm ein Bein;
Da kam der Herr Jesus Christ
Und schmierte es mit Schmalz und mit Schmer,
Daß es ging hin und her.
Im Namen + + +

There went a deer over the heath,
It went towards its green meadow,
and turned its foot upon a stone,
and broke a bone.
Then came our Lord Jesus Christ
And anointed it with lard and salve,
So it went here and there.
In the name of the Father, Son, and Holy Spirit. + + +[155]

This blessing however, was accompanied with a series of important instructions that the healer must pass the index finger of the right hand over the sprain and each time blow over the sprain. Then without speaking, make a compress in the form of a band from a sack filled with rye flour, and bind it onto the sprain, above and below. The one who receives the sprain must be treated in this manner by a woman who bore two sons.[156]

Although the significance of the two sons is uncertain, it can be likened to a statement that appears repeatedly in the oral traditions of Europe, concerning the impossibility (according to Roman Catholic tradition) of Virgin Mary bearing a second son. Blessings used to stop blood (*Blut-Stillung*), stop bullets (*Kugel-Abweissung*), quench fire (*Feuer-Segen*), and stop enemy forces (*Stellung für die feindliche Gewalt*) often aim to halt immanent danger in the name of the Virgin Mary by presenting an apparent impossibility: "…*so seyd ihr an der Erden gebannt bis die Mutter Christi gebieret einen andern Sohn*" (…so shalt thou be fixed upon the earth, until the Mother of Christ bears another son).[157]

This notion of overcoming adversity by presenting an impossibility is one of many motifs in ritual blessings that operates under the notion of analogy, beginning with statements such as "like unto…" (*als wie*), and "so truly as…" (*so wahr als…*), and this occurs in both positive and negative (impossible) forms.

An old and well-used manuscript from Nürnberg, Germany, with entries written by practitioners spanning three centuries, cites numerous nineteenth-century blessings with simple analogies:

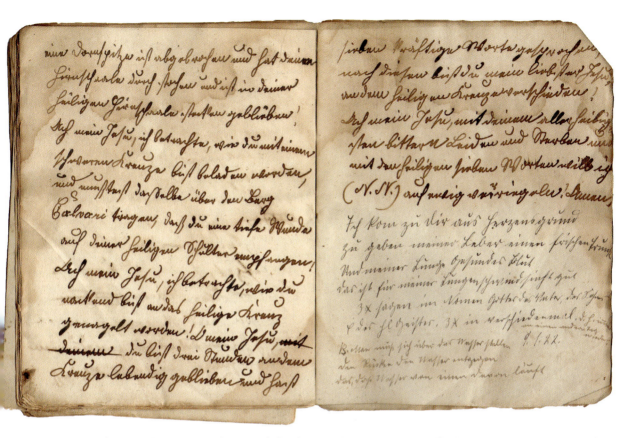

European manuscript from Nürnberg, Germany, featuring the handwriting of several generations of healers spanning three centuries. The earliest entries are from the late eighteenth century, and the most recent is dated 1922. *Heilman Collection.*

Weich Rippen-Gerip,
Wie das Pferd aus Krippen frißt! + + +

Vanish colic
Just as the horse eats from the manger! + + + [158]

This can be compared to a blessing to remove a stye from Zwenkau, Saxony:

Blatter fall aus dem Aug
Wie der Regen aus der Trauf!
Im Namen Gottes des Vaters, des Sohns, und des heiligen Geistes. + + +

Stye fall out of the eye,
Just as the rain falls from the eaves!
In the name of the Father, Son, and Holy Spirit. + + + [159]

While some analogies invoke simple certainties of commonplace evidence of cause and effect, such as the appetite of a horse being fed or the dripping of the rain from the roof, other analogies reach to religious and heavenly certainties. Another from the Nürnberg manuscript cites the surety of a minister or priest in performing their spiritual role:

Blatter vergehe, und nicht zerbrich,
Wie der Pfarrer das Evangelium spricht! + + +

Stye depart, and do not rupture,
Just as the minister preaches the gospel! + + + [160]

This blessing can be compared to another from Altenburg, which takes the analogy a step closer to divinity:

Blatter fall vom Aug gschwind,
Wie unser Herr Christus am Kreuz verschied.
Das sage ich dir N. N. zu gut
Im Namen Gottes des Vaters, des Sohns,
und des heiligen Geistes. + + +

Stye, fall from the eye quickly,
So [surely] as Our Lord Christ died on the cross.
This I say for the good of N.N.
In the Name of the Father, Son,
and Holy Spirit. + + + [161]

Other analogies reach to celestial forces, as indicated in a blessing to banish epilepsy, which compares the peace of heaven to the body free from the illness:

Fahr aus Gicht, alle böse Gesicht,
Fahr naus in wilden Wald, fahr nein in wilde Bäume.
Drinnen sollst du reißen und zehren,
Sollst mir N. N. mein Fleisch und Blut nicht verzehren.
Friede im Himmel, Freude auf Erden
Friede in meinen Fleisch und Blut
Gleichwie das heilige Firmament am Himmel thut.
Das helf mir N. N. Gottes des Vaters, des Sohns,
und des heiligen Geistes. + + +

Depart Epilepsy, and all evil visages,
Depart into the wild wood, depart into the wild trees,
Therein you shall tear and consume,
So that you shall not consume N. N. my flesh and blood.
Peace in Heaven, Joy on Earth,
Peace be in my flesh and blood,
Just as the Holy Firmament in the Heavens.
This help me N. N. in the name of the Father, Son,
and Holy Spirit. + + +

As with many blessings which compel illness to depart through sacred analogy, the illness is directed where to go, such as into the wild wood, the deeps of the sea, or into a deep well:

Jesus und die Atter ging über Land,
Und unser lieber Herr Jesus Christus
hatte die Blatter in der Hand,
Da kamen sie zu einem Brunn:
Die Atter ertrank,
Die Blatter verschwand,
Das zähle ich dir zur Buße
Im Namen Gottes des Vaters, des Sohns, un des heiligen Geistes. + + +

Jesus and the serpent went over the land,
And our dear lord Jesus Christ held the stye in hand,
They came to a well:
The serpent drowned
The stye vanished.
This I reckon unto thee as penance,
In the name of the Father, Son,
and Holy Spirit. + + + [163]

In this blessing, the world "*Buß*" (penance) does not merely apply to the Roman Catholic sacrament in which sins are forgiven through absolution by a priest following confession. Within the context of healing, it relates the forgiveness of sin to the healing of the illness. Thus the absolution of sin is the healing of the soul and echoed in the physical body.[164] In some regions, the word *Büßer* is synonymous with a healing practitioner or *Braucher*,[165] implying the interplay of spiritual forces, capable of restoring balance in the physical body, as well as in situations of illness and adversity. The practitioner in the folk context acts as the restorer of balance, both specifically for the supplicant, and universally, as the particular needs of the individual are considered part of a greater universal order.

This notion of penance is repeated in a popular broadside entitled *Eine wahre und approbirte Kunst in Feuers-Brünsten und Pestilenz-Zeiten nützlich zu gebrauchen* (*A Veritable and Approved Method Useful To Employ In Times of Pestilence and Conflagration*), widely circulated in Europe and Pennsylvania in both printed and manuscript forms.[166] The document begins with a narrative account in the year 1714 in Prussia of six Romani men condemned to death, the eldest of whom, a man of eighty years, performs a miracle, and saves the city from a devastating fire. The provenance of his *Feuer-Segen* (Fire Blessing) was attributed to an enigmatic persona – "the Christian Gypsy King of Egypt" – a figure whose legend is rooted in the mistaken association of the Romani people with Egypt.[167] This notion is further compounded by the belief that the Three Kings from the East, Caspar, Melchior, and Balthasar, were the ancestors of the Romani.[168]

> One must walk around the fire three times, so that the sun riseth behind him, and speak the following:
>
> Thus art thou welcome, thou fiery guest, seize no further than what thou hast; this I reckon to thee as penance, in the name of God the Father, the Son and the Holy Spirit. I command thee Fire, by the power of God, that doth all and createth all, thou wouldst stand still and go no further, so truly as Christ hath stood in the Jordan, where the Holy Man John baptized him. This I reckon to thee Fire as a penance in the name of the Holy Trinity. I command thee by the power of God, thou wouldst lay down thy flames, so true as Mary maintained her maidenhead before all women, this she hath maintained so chaste and pure, stop here thy flames, Fire. This I reckon to thee as a penance, in the name of the Holy Trinity. I command thee, Fire, thou wouldst lay down thy heat, by the precious blood of Jesus Christ, that he hath shed for us, for our sin and misdoing. This I reckon to thee, Fire, as penance in the name of God the Father, the Son and the Holy Spirit. Jesus of Nazareth, a King of the Jews, help us out of this fiery-strife and guard this land and border, from all plague and pestilence.
>
> Whoever hath in his house this saying as previously recorded, by him no conflagration will break out nor arise. Also in the same way, if a pregnant woman carrieth this letter with her, neither sorcery or evil spirits can harm her or her baby. Also the house will be safe against the infestation of plague.[169]

The *Feuersegen* of the Gypsy King is one of many protective letters addressing issues of unjust sentencing, with the promise of ritual deliverance. Just at the elderly Romani man is the hero of the story, so too is the servant of Count Phillip of Flanders, who is sentenced to death in another ritual narrative blessing where no weapon can harm him because of an inscription he carried.[170] These stories highlight the continuing tension between the bearers of ritual traditions and secular and ecclesiastical authorities.

The aforementioned Nürnberg manuscript features an elaborate protective blessing against unjust sentencing in Europe, describing the role of the healer within a larger sacred framework that is distinct from secular authority:

Vor Gericht
Der Herr ist mein Hirte,
Der Himmel ist mein Hut,
Die Welt ist mein Gewandt,
Die Erde ist mein Schuh.
Komm ich vor das Amtshaus,
Sahen es drei Tode:
Sie hatten Köpfe wie Töpfe,
Der erste ist dumm,
D. 2. ist Stumm,
D. 3. hat keine Zunge.
Im Namen
Gottes Vaters Sohnes
und des Heiligen Geistes, Amen. X X X

Before the Court:
The Lord is my shepherd,
Heaven is my hat,
The world is my imagination,
The earth is my shoes.
I come before the courthouse,
I see three dead men:
They have heads like pots,
The first is a fool,
The second is dumb,
The third has no tongue.
In the name of God the Father, Son,
and Holy Spirit. X X X [171]

This blessing consists of two parts, the first of which eloquently articulates the medieval worldview: Christ as shepherd, with the protective heavens above, the solid earth below, and all of creation as a cloak. But the second paints a dark image of the secular courts envisioned as harboring "dead men," witnesses with heads like pots. This description of the witnesses is not merely random. It is derived from an old ritual means of uncloaking clandestine malefactors in the community by carrying a bundle of ground-ivy to church on the 1st of May, whereby the malefactors in the community will appear in church with pots on their heads that are invisible to everyone, save the bearer of the ground-ivy.[172]

Such accounts, just like the *Gericht-Segen*, appear to indicate the perspective that the forces of good and evil are at work in all aspects of society, but that appearances are deceiving. While all human institutions, religious or secular, were believed to be subject to such infernal infiltration, the *Braucher* appealed to the divine for incorruptible forms of justice. Such divine justice would overcome all human evil, illness, or infirmity. Such notions of divine justice and virtue play a role in the language of the blessing, allying the will to be healed with Christian virtues:

Auf Christi Grab, da stehn drei Lilien,
die erste heisst die Gottheit,
die zweite ist Gerechtigkeit,
die dritte ist dein eigener Wille,
dass dein Schmerz, dein Blut steht stille. + + +

On Christ's grave stand three lilies.
The first is called divinity,
The second is justice,
The third is thy own will,
that thy pain, thy blood shall stand still + + +[173]

While the poetry of these blessings draws upon Roman Catholic and ancient symbols of healing, these blessings were used widely by Protestants, who liberally borrowed elements from across a wide spectrum of religious attitudes. In a sense, the decentralization of ritual practices, influenced by the Reformation's empowerment of the laity, produced a wide and diverse literary content in the verbal expressions of blessing. But while the symbols and content of liturgical tradition were free for the taking, and while the blessings were freely performed with no schedule of fees, the words themselves were often carefully guarded. Prayers were treated with a level of discretion proportional to their degree of sacredness. Families passed down prayers like precious heirlooms, maintaining them as oral tradition for centuries.[174] Printed or handwritten compilations were brought to the New World, second only to the family Bible. More important than any physical object, book, or evidence of *Brauchen* brought to the New World, were the stories, attitudes, and oral traditions that allowed the practice to continue and thrive on a new continent.

BRAUCHEN & TRANSATLANTIC EMIGRATION

The oldest surviving handwritten collection of blessings and remedies known to have made the transatlantic voyage to Pennsylvania from the Rhine River Valley is attributed to Christophell Thommaß (Christoph Thomas), a corporal in an undocumented military force defending the Rhine from Louis XIV's campaign in 1713.[175] According to his diary, wherein he kept roll calls from 1713-1714, Thomas was stationed at Schwetzingen on the west side of the Rhine near Mannheim. Evidence in the diary suggests that he was in the cavalry, listing among the contents of an inventory of his gear two pistols, a mantle and a rapier, as well as a horse.[176] There are no military records after July of 1714, just a few months following the Treaty of Rastatt on March 6th. Either during or after his time in the military, the journal was used to keep an extensive collection of over 304 cures, ranging from herbal compounds, poultices, decoctions, salves, teas, and tinctures. At the very end of the book, only just over half a dozen of these constitute rituals employing verbal blessings and invocations, while the remainder are only ritual in the sense of prescribed procedures that suggest more than mere *material medica* from their content and scope.

The first of these the blessings, listed at the back of the journal, is intended to protect from the bite of a rabid dog: *"Ierum Korum Kaffra Koddafra."* This phrase is doubtlessly at least in part derived from the phrase *abracadabra*, rendered here *"Kaffra Koddafra."* This ancient healing blessing was used to cure fevers among the Romans and was written in both Latin and Hebrew letters. The descending triangular shape that is formed in the letters was believed to mirror the dissipation of the illness:

```
A B R A C A D A B R A
 A B R A C A D A B R
  A B R A C A D A B
   A B R A C A D A
    A B R A C A D
     A B R A C A
      A B R A C
       A B R A
        A B R
         A B
          A
```

The earliest recorded reference to the use of *abracadabra* is from the Roman poet and statesman Serenus Sammonicus (d. 211) from the turn of the 3rd century, who included it in a work entitled *Liber medicinalis* as a cure for fever. However, its origins have been contested as having been from Greek, Latin, Aramaic, Arabic, Chaldean, or Hebrew. A widely debated theory suggests that the word is Latinized from the ancient Hebrew *abar ka dabar* meaning "it shrinks like the word." In this manner, whether written or recited, with each drop of a letter, the fever is believed to gradually subside. [177]

Another version of Thomas's phrase is rendered in Latin characters directly below the previous inscription in German script: "IRUMX RRIUM X OFFRU MX RUSSO FF RUMX.[178] Although only identifiable with the previous passage by proximity, this garbled passage is characteristic of blessings that have been transmitted repeatedly in oral and written forms, and recorded by writers with varying degrees of literacy.

Thomas's second entry of this variety is also aimed at achieving protection from wild animals:

Undiehr ich duh dich winnen
Ich will dihr dein Maull zu binen.
In Nahm des X X X

Beast, I shall overcome thee.
I will pin thy mouth closed.
In the name of the [Father, Son, and Holy Spirit] XXX[179]

Thomas's writing is highly idiosyncratic and likely related to his use of regional dialect. Another blessing is for ridding cattle of worms:

Vor die Wurm an den rind Fih:
Brauge hast du die
wurmlein klein du
stickts gleich zwische
fleish oder beÿ du sey
gleich schwatz brou weis
bloh kroh grun gehl
oder rot du sollst gleich
sein in der Erste stund
Doth + + +

For worms in cattle:
Say (*Brauche*): hast thou the
Little worms? Thou
Art now embedded between
Flesh and bone. Be thou
Now black, brown, white,
Blue, gray, green, yellow,
Or red, thou shall now
Be in the first hour
Dead. + + +[180]

This unusually colorful variation of the *Würm-Segen* invokes all worms of all varieties – each color representing symbolic correspondences to symptoms of illness: red suggests inflammation; white, yellow, and green are the colors of purulence; and black, blue, brown, and gray, represent mortification and gangrene.[181] In many classic blessings, the illness is called "worm," when in fact, this harkens back to the old notion of demonic personification of illness. Such blessings may have been used to treat any number of illnesses, especially infections which were correctly perceived to be the result of invasive pathogens. While bacteria and viruses were yet unknown, their symptoms were attributed to the "worm." This gives rise to the culturally defined illnesses of the period, known as *Zahnwurm* (toothache and gingivitis), *Fingerwurm* (whitlow), and the dreaded *Herzwurm* (heartworm, consumption).

Another illness addressed in Christoph Thomas's manuscript that was equally mysterious at the time is called *Feibel* among horses, characterized by the swelling of the glands by the ears[182] and, eventually, fever from infection within the body cavity.[183] This disease, most closely resembling advanced cases of equine "strangles,"[184] is a highly contagious bacterial infection of the lymph glands. Thomas's cure, like the previous for worms, is in the form of a verbal blessing:

Vor die Feilbel der Pfehrt
Mehr Pfehrt hast du
die feilbel im Leib
fahr aus dem Lein in
daß fleisch, auß dem fleisch
in die Haut, auß der Haut
in die Harr, auß der Haar
in der wind. Halt dich dei
gotteß Mutt ihr lieb Kind. + + +

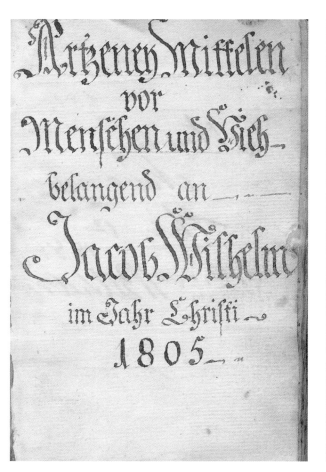 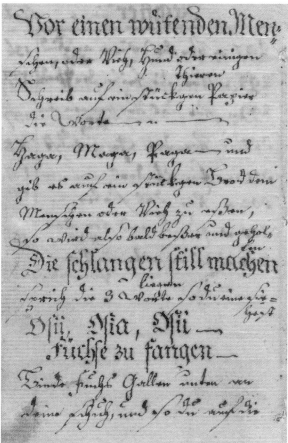

Above: The powwow book of Jacob Wilhelm formerly owned by Corporal Christophell Thommaß, and inscribed by Johannes Ernst Spangenberg. Courtesy of the Northampton County Historical and Genealogical Society Archives.

For the strangles in horses
Mare, horse, thou hast
the strangles in thy body.
Depart from the body into
Flesh, out of the flesh
into the skin, out of the skin
and into the hair, out of the hair
and into the wind. Keep thine own,
[as] the Mother of God [kept] her dear child. + + +[185]

    Little is known about the author outside of the text of his journal. Church records within the region indicate that a "Christoph David Thomas," son of Balthasar and Ursula Maria Thomas, was baptized on July 18th, 1677, at the Lutheran Church of St. Katharina in Schwäbisch Hall, Baden-Württemberg.[186] The same Christoph David Thomas was married to Anna Dorothea Metwen on January 3rd, 1689, at the Lutheran church in Eckartsweiler, in Ohringen. If the same Christoph David Thomas is the author of the manuscript, it would have made him thirty-seven at the close of the war. Although nothing is known about his or his family's whereabouts after 1714, an inscription on the front flyleaf indicates that the book was purchased from Thomas by Johan Michael Koch of Weinheim, just sixteen miles north of Schwetzingen, where his journal indicates that Thomas was stationed in 1714 as part of a personal guard (*Leib Compagni*). Koch immigrated to Pennsylvania aboard the Ship *Robert & Alice* in 1742, and settled in Durham Township, Northampton County. There he attended the same church with the family of the powwow healer Jacob Wilhelm (1744-1821), who eventually came into possession of the journal of Christoph Thomas in 1805, and had it elaborately inscribed with his name, with the addition of a few additional cures.[187]

    This inscription was written by none other than Johannes Ernst Spangenberg (1748-1814), celebrated scrivener, teacher, and artist of elaborately illuminated Bibles and certificates of Northampton County. Spangenberg was the schoolmaster for the Lutheran

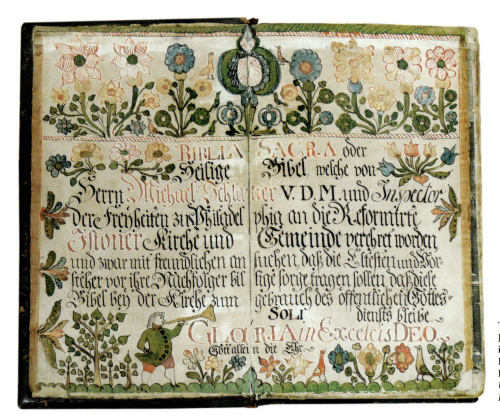

The fraktur unscription by Johannes Ernst Spangenberg in the pulpit Bible of the First Reformed Church of Easton. *Courtesy of the First United Church of Christ, Easton, Pennsylvania.*

and Reformed Union congregation at Easton, and was the illustrator of the pulpit Bible given to the First Reformed Church by the Reverend Michael Schlatter, organizer of the first Reformed Synod in Pennsylvania.[188] Spangenberg's work as a scrivener ranged from legal documents to decorative certificates, and at least three known works relating to powwowing.

The inscription on the flyleaf of the Christoph Thomas journal indicating ownership by Jacob Wilhelm in 1805 was but a small portion of Spangenberg's contribution to the work. His meticulous script also fully indexed 304 of Thomas's entries. Spangenberg added four additional entries, including a blessing to paralyze a snake utilizing the words "*Osii, Osia, Osii*"; a recipe to catch foxes with fox-gall rubbed on one's shoe soles; how to bait a trap with chicken fat or fox-gall; as well as a classic blessing to be eaten to cure rabies in humans, livestock, and dogs by means of the phrase "Haga, Maga, Paga" written on a piece of paper and consumed with bread.[189]

Another slightly more extensive work from the hand of Spangenberg is a manuscript entitled *Merkwürdige Dinger zugehörig an Johannes Stecher* (*Extraordinary Things Belonging to Johannes Stecher*). This manuscript contains a total of seven entries, including three identical to those written for Jacob Wilhelm in 1805. Four additional entries include one for casting bullets that contain equal parts lead and "falling stars" or asafetida to increase accuracy; two for stopping thieves; and another for catching deer. The latter is a lengthy invocation:

*Es stehen 3 Lilien auf unsers Herrn Gottes Grab,
die 1ste ist Gottes Muth,
der andere ist Gottes Blut,
die 3te ist Gottes Will,
Hirsch steh still
so wenig als Jesus Christus ist
von dem Kreutz weggelauffen,
so wenig solt du mir von der stätt laufen,
das gebieth ich dir bey den 4 Evangelisten
und Elementen des Himmels,
du seyest ein Fluß oder Schuß
in Gericht oder Gesicht,
so beschwörr ich dich
bey dem jüngsten Gerichts,
daß du still stehest und nicht weiter gehest,
bis ich alle der Sternen ansehen
und die Sonne giebt ihren Schein,
also stelle ich dir dem lauffen und springen ein,
das gebiethe dir Gott der Vatter, Gott der Sohn
und Gott der heilige Geist und
dieses 3 mal gesprochen.*

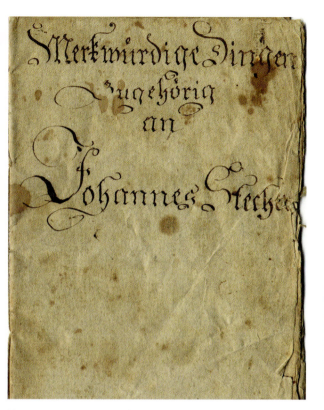 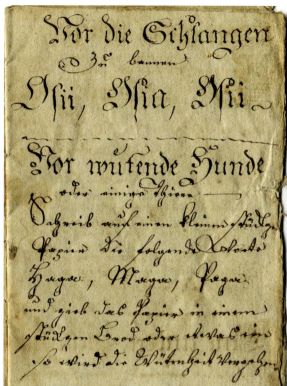

The powwow manuscript of Johannes Stecher of Forks Township, Northampton County, written by Johannes Spangenberg, bearing nearly identical contents to an addendum in Jacob Wilhem's powwow book. *Pennsylvania German Cultural Heritage Center, Kutztown University.*

There stand three lilies on our
Lord God's grave, the first
is God's valor, the second
is God's blood, the third
is God's will.
 Deer, stand still,
Just as little as Jesus Christ
Walked from the Cross,
So little shalt thou
walk from this spot. This
I command thee by the Four
Evangelists and elements of
Heaven, whether there be force
Or shot, in court or
Countenance, I bind thee
Until the crack of doomsday,
That you stand still and go
Not further, until I look
Upon all the stars, and the son
Gives up its shine, therefore
I halt thee from running or jumping,
This I command thee, in the name of
God the Father, God the Son, and
God the Holy Spirit,
And say this three times.[190]

Stecher's manuscript is undated, but it appears contemporary to Wilhelm's, with a similar layout for the inscription. Johannes Stecher (1765-1823) and his wife Catharina (1778-1854) (nee Schweitzer) lived in Forks Township, Northampton County, where they had two daughters and one son. Both Johannes and Catharina are buried in the Forks Cemetery in Stockerton.[191]

Although the provenance of the blessings in Stecher's manuscript is unknown, all evidence points to Johannes Ernst Spangenberg as scrivener of both the Wilhelm and Stecher manuscripts. This begs the questions: was Spangenberg the compiler of these ritual instructions, and did he produce these works upon demand for customers?

One additional piece remains of Spangenberg's ritual writings – an undated, decorated sheet inscribed with the celebrated SATOR square palindrome, framed with an elaborate border of flowers.[192] This square of 25 letters reads the same forwards and backwards, up and down, and has been documented in ritual use since at least 79 AD, when it was preserved at Pompeii.[193] Although Spangenberg's rendering is atypical, it is not entirely uncommon to find many variations.[194] The traditional arrangement is:

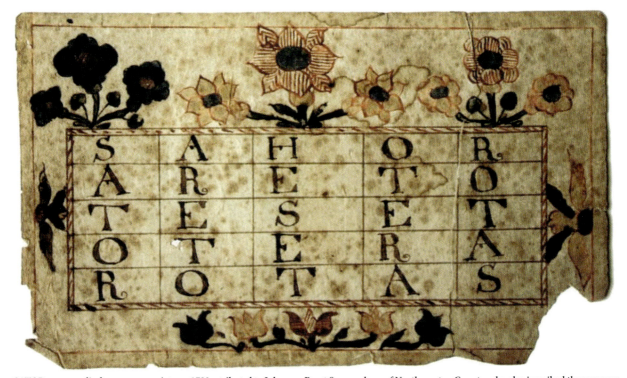

SATOR square palindrome manuscript, ca. 1790, atributed to Johannes Ernst Spangenberg of Northampton County, who also inscribed the powwow manuscripts of Jacob Wilhelm and Johannes Stecher of Northampton County. *Courtesy of The Earnest Archives and Library.*

```
S A T O R
A R E P O
T E N E T
O P E R A
R O T A S
```

This enigmatic square has baffled scholars for centuries, and there is still no single agreed-upon translation of the simple Latin arrangement. Some point to the fact that the letters can be rearranged to form a cross, reading *Pater Noster* (Our Father) in two lines, vertical and horizontal, intersecting in the middle at the letter N:

```
            P
            A
      A T   O
            E
            R
P A T E R N O S T E R
            O
            S
      A T   O
            E
            R
```

The two pairs of A and O represent the Alpha and Omega, the beginning and the end of the Greek alphabet, signifying the infinite nature of the divine in the Book of Revelation: "I am Alpha and Omega, the beginning and the ending, saith the Lord, which is, and which was, and which is to come, the Almighty."[195]

This Christian rendering has led to the belief that this square was used as an encrypted message by the early church,[196] while others point to a cosmological rendering of its literal meaning.[197] Lines 1, 3-5 form the Latin sentence *sator tenet opera rotas* (the sower holds the wheels with effort), a poetic statement evoking the sower as a ritual practitioner or farmer, who by means of effort, is able to render the cyclical "wheels" of the cosmos useful for productive purposes.[198]

This meaning, however, has been complicated by the word *arepo*, which has been the source of much disagreement. Some claim that it is a proper name, while still others argue that it is an entirely made-up word used merely to complete an otherwise flawless palindrome.[199]

In keeping with the poetic nature of the square, another interpretation is that *arepo* is a contraction of two words used in a prepositional phrase, one of which is adapted: *a repo*, or "from the bank." While normally the word would read *repa* being a feminine noun, the conventions of Latin poetry often allow for the adaptations of words to fit meter, rhymes, and syllabic structure.[200] In this case, a feminine word is inflected with a masculine ending to complete the palindrome: "The sower holds the wheels from the bank with effort." Thus, *arepo* provides a setting for the cosmic sower, a liminal space between earth and water, to harness cosmological forces for the benefit of humanity.

Although it is unlikely that Spangenberg was aware of the subtleties of the SATOR square when he penned his illustration, he was mostly likely acquainted with the fact that the palindrome was used in both Europe and Pennsylvania for ritual healing and protection. For instance, *Romanus* suggests that the words can be written on paper and administered to cattle to eat as a protective ritual against malicious spiritual forces, and that the inscription can be written on both sides of a plate which can be used to extinguish fire without water. Such plates have turned up in early Pennsylvania Dutch communities on English pewter.[201]

In all of the early Pennsylvania evidence, whether in the transatlantic journey of the healing journal of Christoph Thomas or the appearance of the SATOR square in ritual objects and art, the forms and functions of Pennsylvania's ritual traditions are by no means unique to the North America, but part of a broad European diaspora. At the same time that cultures, traditions and identities have continued to diverge between the two continents, ritual traditions on both sides of the Atlantic continue to reflect their shared origins. While these North American ritual traditions trace their lineage to Europe, so too does Europe find examples of rare and exceptional glimpses of the Old World in Pennsylvania that have all but vanished in Europe.

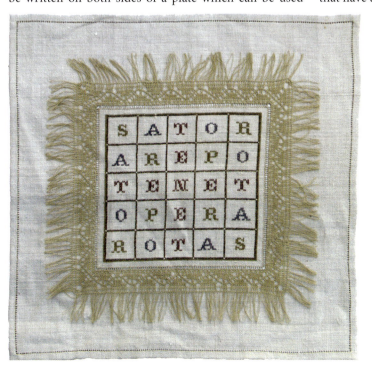

Plate with SATOR Square Inscription.
Pewter Plate made ca. 1800 by Thomas Compton, London, inscription date unknown.
Nancy and Abe Roan Collection, Courtesy of the Schwenkfelder Library and Heritage Center.
John George Hohman provides instructions in his popular powwowing manual The Long Lost Friend (1820) for extinguishing fire without water by using a plate inscribed with the SATOR square palindrome on both sides. The plate was to be thrown into fire in order to ritually extinguish the blaze in times of emergency. This early pewter plate was purchased at a yard sale by Abe Roan, and after cleaning it, revealed the SATOR inscription on both sides.

Right: A twentieth-century SATOR needle-point handkerchief made by a woman in Soyen, Bavaria, who produced a wide range of traditional embroidered *Spruchtücher* (inscribed cloths) as house blessings and for personal protection. The lace border was added later by an artist in Mühldorf, Bavaria at the request of the former owner, Dr. William Woys Weaver. This piece demonstrates that such traditions did not merely come to Pennsylvania, but continued to be maintained in Europe centuries later. *Heilman Collection.*

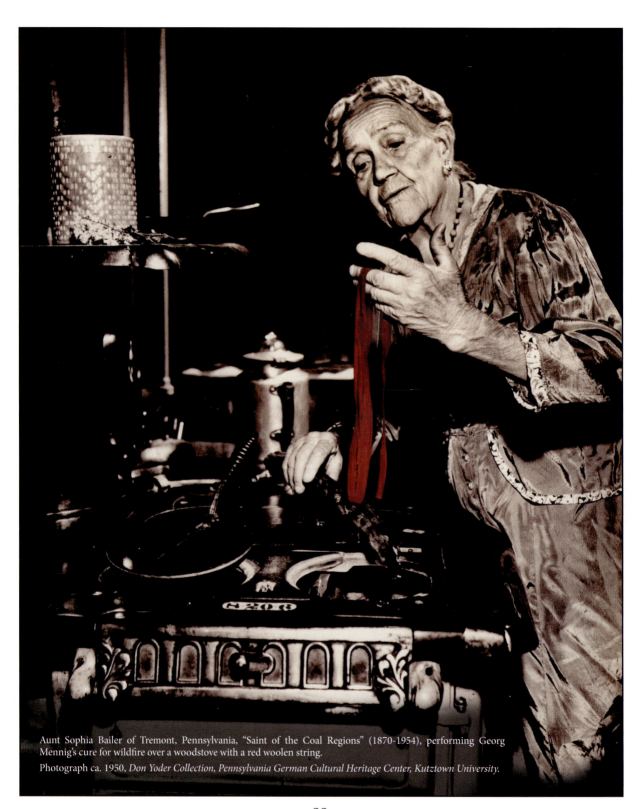

Aunt Sophia Bailer of Tremont, Pennsylvania, "Saint of the Coal Regions" (1870-1954), performing Georg Mennig's cure for wildfire over a woodstove with a red woolen string.

Photograph ca. 1950, *Don Yoder Collection, Pennsylvania German Cultural Heritage Center, Kutztown University.*

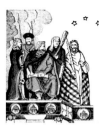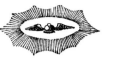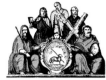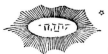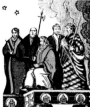

Chapter IV
Healing, Cosmology & Faith
Ritual Space & Performance

Rituals are actions, not merely mundane, but symbolic, expressing a broader system of relationships that interpenetrate all fields of life. While inherently performative and participatory, ritual practices also define and reinforce social relations and articulate attitudes towards humanity's relationship to cosmic and religious forces. This is especially true within the realm of ritual healing, where health and well-being are not only described in physical terms, but also within a broader social and spiritual context.

Ritual healing traditions provide a script for engaging in performative dialogue with life's challenges in a way that not only reflects such attitudes, but creatively establishes a space and state of being conducive to producing profound change. While such transformations are at least partially a function of a participant's beliefs, these changes are nevertheless considered to be real changes taking place on physical, emotional, and spiritual levels. Therefore, the ritual performance of powwowing is both instructive of a way to operate within a set of religious and social modalities, and an effective means of describing and communicating those values through experiences that are highly meaningful to those who participate. Thus healing ritual plays a dual role of both expressing religious or social identity, as well as sustaining and defining a broader set of relationships.[1]

For the Pennsylvania Dutch, powwowing rituals appeal to forces beyond the normal scope of human control with the hope and expectation of influencing outcomes. This is not unlike the essential functions of prayer within some official religious settings, but the nuances of such interactions are markedly different. While powwowing is based in the notion that healing is the result of divine will, precisely how such transformations are initiated is a matter of human intention. Such an interplay ascribes vastly different degrees of power and significance to the actions of the individual and the divine, proportionate to their roles on both a micro and macrocosmic scale.

Many practitioners firmly believe that the source of all healing power is divine, and all of aspects of existence share a divine source of origin, with some measure of relation to one another. Within a ritual setting these relationships are explored through the use of spoken words and objects, gestures and actions, conducted by particular people, according to certain timing and repetition, within specific settings and venues.

Although the relationships that undergird this ritual process can be understood as symbolic, these beliefs reflect a specific form of relationship, known as sympathy, an ontology that interrelates all manifestations of existence by subtle, cosmic relationships. As an ancient philosophical and pre-scientific doctrine, this concept was widely accepted throughout the Middle Ages into the Early Modern Era until the time of the Enlightenment, when it was discarded by the scientific community, but persisted on the esoteric, and folk-cultural level in ritual practice.[2] Based ultimately upon the notion of the divinely created universe, this doctrine contends that all manifestations of the material and invisible worlds are connected by subtle relationships. Attributes and sensory qualities assist in the delineation of these affinities for both physical and immaterial entities, and reveal patterns that can be put to use for the benefit of humanity.

Within the sympathetic and folk-cultural worldview, these material aspects range from the stars to the soil, and everything in between – a potato, a broom, a lock of hair, a pitchfork, an egg, a coal shovel, a pig trough, the house, the wagon, and the barn.

The more subtle immaterial aspects include human emotions, thoughts, alliances, kinship – but the correspondences are rarely linear. Colors, materials, shapes, fragrances, temperatures – each property and descriptor expresses a greater significance beyond its literal meaning.

While the implications of the sympathetic worldview are vast, the practical applications are quite specific and traditionally defined. This means that although ritual reveals broader notions of cosmic and religious systems, it is problematic to presume the existence of one unifying and overarching system, rather than many smaller, overlapping systems interrelating, challenging and reinforcing patterns of belief. The specifics of interacting with these systems are not necessarily harmonious, but also contrasting in tense interrelation. It is important however, to avoid systematizing ritual elements beyond the degree to which participants would conceive of them.[3]

This study will not seek to forcibly unify these rituals with a pre-existing framework, whether esoteric, religious, ancient or otherwise. Instead, a number of ritual features and specific elements will be examined in terms of function, by identifying key components that illustrate not only the ways in which a given ritual was expected to work, but also how the ritual affirms beliefs concerning how the cosmos is perceived to operate.

Forms of Ritual Performance

While not all powwow rituals are scripted in a literary sense, instructions for ritual performance are part of learned patterns passed from generation to generation, and intended for continued use. As a primarily oral tradition, ritual instructions in powwowing emphasize the role of spoken words as well as ritual performances that include actions, gestures, objects, timing, repetition, and specific settings, as well as human and animal participants. The majority of these features are commonplace, but their placement within a ritual context links their mundane roles to a greater awareness of belief in a sacred and cosmic reality.

Not all powwowing rituals employ words, or uniformly emphasize all aspects of ritual expression for each procedure. Some rituals include words but no objects, while others may include gestures and objects with no use of words. Thus powwowing is expressed in varying degrees of complexity, and some have suggested that a general sense of specialization increases among practitioners with the number of ritual elements employed in performance.[4] While this observation is certainly true in an analytical sense, it is not a view that is generally expressed by practitioners or patients of powwowing, who tend to view ritual as a whole, with the complexity of a ritual having no bearing on its efficacy.

Powwowing can be as simple as passing an infant three times around a table leg to cure colic,[5] or stopping a nose-bleed by lifting a stone from the ground, allowing three drops of blood to fall into the spot, and immediately replacing the stone.[6] While these ritual procedures have no accompanying prayers, there are varying degrees of participation: the colic cure requires at least two people to safely pass the infant around the table leg, but the nose-bleed cure can be performed solo. Both involve the use of objects that are commonly available, but the table is likely to be found indoors in a kitchen or dining-room, as opposed to the cure for a nose-bleed, which can be utilized anywhere that a stone can be found embedded in the ground. Both of these rituals utilize repetitions of three, a number that prominently features in ritual performance. Even when no words are spoken, the number three serves as a form of silent short-hand for invoking the Holy Trinity or the Three Highest Names; The Father, Son, and Holy Spirit.

On the other end of the spectrum, there are very few complex rituals that do not involve the use of at least some words. These take the form of prayers, exorcisms, and invocations addressing spiritual forces. The spoken word is perhaps one of the most important components of many rituals, and it often serves to connect the beliefs of the practitioner and patient with the ritual performance. This is especially true for blessings, benedictions, or prayers which invoke sacred concepts or holy entities, such as the Trinity, the saints, or archangels. These statements serve to focus the mind of the practitioner on divine operations, and, if spoken aloud, engender a state of being in the patient conducive to healing transformation. However, such prayers are not meant only for the humans involved in the ritual, but appeal directly to spiritual forces that are believed to be actively working in the ritual space along with the people.

Some rituals make use of blessings or benedictions which consist of invocations of positive spiritual forces that are asked for assistance, healing, and protection. A statement of intention is made with a wish for a positive outcome, and although a blessing is established, there is no promise that such desired outcomes will be assured or granted.[7]

A common written powwow blessing, used for protection, and for the blessing of a home, states: *Daß alles bewahret sey, hier zeitlich und dort ewiglich* (All this be protected, here in time, and there in eternity), and concludes with the sign of the cross three times. Several versions include variations of the inscription I. N. R. I. Blessings such as these conform closely to standards in churches for liturgical blessings used in a variety of circumstances such as asking for protection in times of danger or calamity. Other basic powwow blessings simply call or invoke the names the Four Archangels, the Four Evangelists, the three holy men, Shadrach Meshach and Abednego (or Hananiah, Mishael, and Azariah), or other saints as a request for assistance in earthly affairs

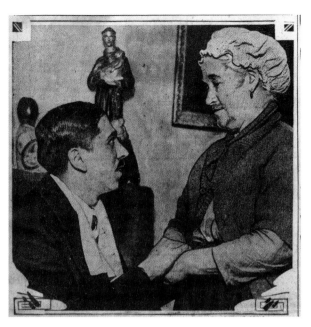

Newspaper clipping of powwow healer, Mrs. Anna Maria (Schmidt) Furst (1858-1938) laying hands upon a male patient in York Pennsylvania. Anna Maria and her husband J. Frederick Furst were Roman Catholics and first-generation German-Americans, born in Prussian and Bavaria. Her activities were highlighted in the city edition of the *New York Evening Journal* on December 8, 1928, amidst the media attention on powwowing during the York "Hex Trials" (see Chapter IX).

The commonality here is that blessings bestow a sense of connection with divine forces and aim to influence earthly affairs, while at the same time the recipient of a blessing yields to divine will, without assurance of a positive outcome.

An early nineteenth century ritual cure employed for an unknown, unidentified ailment blends the language of the blessing with a prayerful request for divine intervention:

> *Bist du gesund worden und Gott so führe ich wieder zu Gott dem Vater, Sohn und heiligen Geist, ich weiß nicht wiedir geschehen oder was dir gebricht, darum so helf dir Vater, Sohn und heiliger Geist, unser Herr Jesus Christus gern, und sollst du sowohl gesegnet sein, als der Kelch und der Wein, und daß heilige Brod, daß unser Herr Jesus Christ am hohen Donnerstag zu Nacht, seinen Lieben Jüngern anbat, dazu helfe dir der Name, der dir den Tod am Stamme des Kreuzes gelitten hat.*
>
> Hast thou recovered health and God? So I lead thee back to God the Father, Son and Holy Spirit. I know not what has befallen thee, or what ails thee, therefore so help thee Father, Son and Holy Spirit. Our Lord Jesus gladly blessed, and shalt thou blessed be, as the chalice and the wine, and the holy bread, that our Lord Jesus Christ offered to his beloved disciples at night on Maundy Thursday. Therefore, help thee in the name of him who suffered for thee death upon the cross.[10]

Although similar to blessings, prayers used in Christian churches, such as those included in the *Book of Common Prayer*, typically follow a petitionary style, whereby a series of specific requests are made for divine assistance. Such petitions aim to balance hope for good outcomes while resigning one's self to the notion that divine forces work independently of human agency and are not bound to deliver requests by prayers. At the same time, prayer offers the opportunity for individuals and communities to engage in dialogue with the divine in order to not only make requests, but to identify personal and communal objectives for the good of the community. While this form of petitionary prayer is the norm in sanctioned Christian settings, it is rare within the context of healing rituals. This lack of petitionary prayers in powwowing sets the practice apart from other forms of faith healing used by Pentecostal and Evangelical denominations in the United States.

More commonly, a blending of blessings, requests, exorcisms, and scriptural passages produce poetic invocations to divine forces. These forms of prayer are typically recited softly in a voice that is barely audible. If spoken aloud by the healer and heard by the patient, these inspirational words could produce a profound effect upon the hearer. The following blessing, used for a sore throat makes use of quotations from the New Testament Letter of Paul to the Romans:[11]

> *Vor Halsweh, nehme ein wollen Band, winde es fünfmahl um den Hals, und sage jedesmal folgende Worte:*
>
> *Den mich verlanget dich zu sehen auf daß ich dir mittheile etwas Geistliche gabe, dich zu stärken, im Namen Jesus des gekreuzigten, sollen diese Schmerzen von dir weichen, Gurgel und Hals sind Gott geweiht, von nun an bis in Ewigkeit.*
>
> For a sore throat, take a woolen band, wind it around the neck five times, and each time say the following words:
>
> For I long to see thee, that I may impart unto thee some spiritual gift, that thou may be strengthened. In the name of Jesus the Crucified, shall these pains depart from thee. Throat and neck, ye are consecrated unto God, from now on until eternity.[12]

Other powwowing rituals involve the language of the exorcism, addressing the illness directly as a willful entity, and commanding it to depart:

> *Ihr Schmerzen ich banne euch, verweise euch, treibe euch zurück, laß diese Glieder Ruh und Frieden, sei auf den höchsten Berg verweisen und in das tiefe Meer versenkt. Maria hat Jesus in Schmerzen geboren, hierdurch gehn alle Schmerzen verloren, im Namen der Schutz Engeln.*
>
> Ye pains, I banish you, I rebuke you, I expel you. Let these limbs have rest and peace. Be ye expelled to the highest mountain and sunk into the deepest sea. Through Mary's pains was Jesus born, therefore all pains will be forlorn, In the names of the Guardian Angels.[13]

The invocation is to be made each time after calling the baptismal name of the afflicted person five times, perhaps corresponding to the five wounds inflicted upon Christ on the cross. In each of the last two examples above, the poetic blessings are accompanied by instructions beyond the use of words only.

The simplest of verbal forms, such as the ritual to stop bleeding with the recitation of the verse of scripture from Ezekiel 16:6 employs words but no objects, and can be performed without accompanying actions or gestures. The ritual can take place anywhere, and can even be performed upon one's self. Another basic verbal formula invokes the Three Kings, Caspar, Melchior, and Balthasar, to calm young or unruly livestock, by saying: "Caspar take thee, Melchior bind thee, and Balthasar lead thee, in the name of the Father, Son, and Holy Spirit."[14] Overall, there are relatively few examples of powwowing that involve words only, without the use of accompanying gestures such as making the sign of the cross, or passing a hand over the ailment. Although numerous powwowing books and private manuscripts may document ritual words with no accompanying instructions, it is crucial to remember that such documents were created with varying degrees of implicit or unspoken assumptions regarding the use of words within a traditional format. For instance, the use of gestures or motions with the hands may be taken for granted as commonly understood ritual functions, without explicit inclusion in written documents.

Such gestures may be rarely recorded, but are frequently applied at the discretion of the practitioner according to their individual methods. Ritual actions consist of gestures and motions of the hands, postures and positions of the body, the use of breath, or gestures with an object. Body postures may involve facing certain directions such as towards or away from the rising sun or the home, as well as standing, kneeling, or sitting in certain locations or liminal spaces, such as standing in the doorway, or hanging a finger out the window to cure whitlow, or kneeling in front of the bakeoven to remove inflammation.[15]

Powwower and farrier of the Tulpehocken, Conrad Raber describes the use of the bakeoven for curing inflammation from the rash erysipelas:

> **Bake as much as you want, and then do the following carefully: Place the person before the opening of the bakeoven, hold fast to the base of the head and shovel the coals out over [and away from] them. So do this 3 times, so shall the inflammation soon subside.**[16]

While the act of throwing hot coals over and away from the person's body is certainly the most expressive part of the performance, equally important is the fact that the practitioner holds the base of the head of the patient while doing so. Although the location of the illness on the body of the patient is not specified in Raber's text, it is clear that the illness must be drawn out of the head, by means of the non-dominant hand of the practitioner, who carefully uses the shovel in the other. The procedure suggests that the illness passes through the practitioner's body and exits by means of the dominant hand, drawn by the heat of the coals. Not only are the coals operating in sympathy with the inflammation, but the head too is aligned with the element of fire and the sign of Aries according to the common farmer's almanac, ubiquitous among the Pennsylvania Dutch.

This particular alignment of ritual actions with the zodiac is consistent with the image of the cosmic man of signs, typically illustrated on the inside of the back cover of the farmer's almanac, depicting the progression of the zodiac upon the human body beginning with Aries at the head, and Pisces at the feet.[38] Although to a casual observer this common diagram would seem to imply that the appropriate time for treating illnesses would be when the afflicted part corresponds to the position of the moon within the sign, however, this is not the case. In fact, the opposite is true: the almanac advised not to treat the part of the body that is afflicted with disease when the moon is in the corresponding sign - otherwise it was considered dangerous![17]

A fragment from an eighteenth century edition of Albertus Magnus' *Book of Aggregations,* containing chapters on midwifery, as well as the virtues and properties of stones, animals, birds, and herbs. *Pennsylvania German Cultural Heritage Center, Kutztown University of Pennsylvania.*

These words are echoed in a cautionary poem attributed to St. Albert the Great, widely distributed in North America and Europe:

Wer Arzney sich gebrauchet dar,
Und nicht der Zeichen wohl nimmt wahr,
Auch seine Sach nicht richt darnach,
der Leib gern, was kommt, Ungemach,
hüt dich, nicht laß das Glied an dir,
so das Zeichen die Adern rühr,
wie die Figur ausweiset gut,
so bleibt schon in gutter Hut.

He who would require medicine here,
and doth not choose the true sign well,
also his part not right therefore,
the body receives what misfortune befalls.
Hear, bleed thou not the part of thee,
as the vein the sign doth affect,
as the figure revealeth well,
thus remaineth one well in good keeping.[18]

The use of the image of the cosmic man compares the patient's body to an ideal, celestial body, suggesting that actions performed by and upon the body echo the movements of the heavens – for good or for ill.

Unlike Raber's description of holding the base of the head, ritual operations with the hands can involve little or no contact with the patient such as passing the hands over the body without touching, making the sign of the cross, as well as manipulations of the illness with physical actions resembling pulling, cupping, or capturing. Physical contact with the patient is not universally applied in powwowing, but such instances may include rubbing, stroking, the direct laying on of hands, or even light massage.[19]

Blowing or inhaling features strongly in rituals for burns or infections such as thrush. For burns, breath is directed over, across, and away from the burn in order to soothe the pain and ritually dispel the heat. While these procedures are usually accompanied with words, the action of blowing is so dramatic and performative, that such ritual cures are commonly referred to as "blowing for burns."[20] Treatments of the oral bacterial infection of infant thrush may utilize breath in either of two forms – either the practitioner inhales through their hand cupped around the infant's mouth to ritually suck out the illness, which is then exhaled away from the body, or the breath is directed into the mouth of the child three times,[21] suggesting an enacted form of invocation of the Holy Spirit.[22]

A friend from Shartlesville, Berks County, recalls his grandmother powwowing the children in the family preventatively with another form of exhalation – that of blowing smoke. She would gather the leaves of jimsonweed, and lay them out in the sun to dry on brown paper bags. The leaves were then packed into her tobacco pipe, and she would blow the smoke over each of the children to prevent illness.[23] In the Kutztown area, another contact recalls an aunt blowing the smoke from a smoldering corn cob over a patient for the removal of illness.[24] This can also be compared to the ubiquitous use of smoke as a home remedy, which was once commonly used to irrigate the ear canal of one suffering from a painful infection or sinus congestion.

The smoke derived from culturally specific plants is also administered over hot coals, by means of blowing across the person or animal being treated, in a form of ritual fumigation:

Wann ein Haupt Vieh, in einen Bösen Wind kommen oder Von bösen Leuthen Verunreind Worden, so nimm 3 Wacholder schoos, 3 Häslein schoos, und 3 stäudlein rauten, das thu alles auf ein Pfann Voll feuriger Kohlen, dass es ein rauch gibt, beräuche das Vieh 3 mahl damit alle mahl in 3 höchsten Namen das übrige gibt man dem Vieh im gesegneten Saltz und gundelreben, zu essen, so kommt es wieder zu recht.

When a head of cattle comes in contact with an evil wind (spirit) or contaminated by an evil person, then take 3 shoots of juniper, 3 shoots of hazel, and 3 sprigs of rue, then place them all on a pan full of hot coals, so that it creates a smoke. Fumigate the animal 3 times, and each time in the 3 Highest Names. Whatever is left over of the shoots, feed it to the cow with blessed salt and ground ivy, so that all will be right again.[25]

As with the use of exhalation or blowing of smoke by means of a pipe or pan, actions and gestures often involve the use of ritual objects such as a string, a stone, roots, an egg, an onion, a broom, or any number of domestic, agricultural, botanical, industrial, or sacred objects.

Everyday objects symbolically link domestic and agricultural narratives with healing transformations, either through transference of qualities from the object to the patient, or by serving as a receptive object to remove illness or infirmity from the patient. An object can serve both functions, and in some cases simultaneously. A stone is used in remedies for equine atrophy (sweeny) where it is rubbed over the horse's shoulder and then either tossed over the barn, or placed back where it was found. In one variation of the ritual, the stone is to be taken from the cellar, where no sun shines, and it must be used in combination with blowing three times over the affected limb, on three Fridays mornings in succession before, during, and just after the full moon, without speaking to anyone. The stone must be returned to its place in the cellar after use.[26] While this ritual appears to demonstrate an act of transference of illness to the stone, the accompanying words in some cases indicate that the stone is simultaneously transferring healing properties to the horse.

A blessing to treat equine sweeny (atrophy), using a stone that is rubbed over the afflicted muscle, and later thrown over the barn or into a body of water. From the papers of Nathaniel Fernsler Krall, Rexmont, Lebanon County. Courtesy of Anna Mae Grubb. *Heilman Collection.*

A cure from the papers of Nathan Fernsler Krall (1867-1944), a farmer from Rexmont, Lebanon County, describes the ritual:

> *Fleish und Blut und Mark und Bein und Swein sind harter als ein Stein.*
> Flesh and blood, marrow and bone, and sweeny are harder than a stone.[27]

It is the stone's quality of hardness that restores tone to the horse's muscle, and the same basic function is true for many remedies believed to result from the lack of certain sufficient qualities or weakness. In rituals used for illnesses of excess such as growths, tumors, fevers, or inflammation, the illness is typically transferred to an object such as a potato, a rind of bacon, roots, a string, or a dishcloth.

At the same time, an object's role in mundane activities often indicates some measure of the object's symbolic potential for ritual significance. For example, a dishcloth plays a role in remedies for homesickness, especially among resident hired farm or house workers, when a drink is poured discretely through the rag and is served to the worker. Because the rag comes into direct contact with the family's dishes, some essential quality of the new home enters into the worker, who then will not pine for their place of origin.[28] The same idea holds true for feeding scrapings of the wooden surface of the dinner table to a dog so that it will not stray.[29]

The dishcloth is also a perfect illustration of how an object's properties are multidimensional and rarely linear. Although the dishcloth plays a role in remedies for homesickness, the rag is also used in a similar manner to a potato in some wart cures,[30] or for other discrete purposes. In Centre County, a dishcloth slipped secretly into a hunter's clothes without their knowledge, is believed to bring luck to the hunter.[31] This may stem once again from the notion of the rag carrying some beneficial essence of the house and home.

On the other end of the spectrum, this idea of the dishcloth as a carrier of the home and family's essence could be applied in a manner contrary to the well-being of the home from which it proceeds. An anecdote from Lebanon County describes a woman whose bread always seemed to burn, even under her careful watch and much to her chagrin. The woman believed this was due to a grudge she held with her neighbor. So a dishcloth was stolen from the neighbor's wash-line, and cut into three pieces. Three holes were bored in the lintel of the bake-oven. A piece of the rag was put into each hole, and plugged up. The woman's baking was never again subject to disturbance.[32]

The dishcloth ritual begs the question of how such an outcome is perceived to be achieved. Did the action of stealing the neighbor's dishcloth and concealing it suggest or symbolize a tipping of the balance of power between the neighbors and their grudge? Did the cutting and sequestering of the rag suggest ritual mutilation or sacrifice as a means to harm or disempower the neighbor? Or, from another perspective, is it possible that the woman's bread was always burning because she was forgetful or preoccupied by the conflict with the neighbor? Was the ritual performance merely a process of instilling intention and mindfulness in order to transform the woman's state of being while baking? While it may be tempting (and possibly useful) to analyze healing narratives from a reductionist perspective, such ritual experiences must also be considered at face value in order to better understand the woman's frame of reference and the story's cultural implications. Only when the reality of the experience for the bearer of the narrative is taken into account, can the story continue to function within its ritual and cultural context. Stories of ritual healing are not merely retold for enjoyment or analysis, but as a means to reinforce and perpetuate the role of ritual in the community as powerful means of transformation.

Unlike everyday domestic objects like the dishcloth, ritual objects may also be considered part of a sacred context, as holy or distinct from the mundane because of their consecration on holy days, or by proximity to the church and its liturgical functions. Eggs laid on Good Friday are eaten for health, or hidden within the home for protection from fire and lightning (see Chapter X). Herbs gathered on Green Thursday or Ascension Day are valued for their enhanced medicinal qualities. Items set out on the windowsill overnight on Christmas Eve, such as water, salt, or bread, are believed to cure fevers, while three types of food (typically salt, flour, and butter) are put out on the windowsill overnight on New Year's Eve and consumed on New Year's day in order to ensure that you will never run out of these foods over the course of the year.[33] Straw was placed out in the barnyard overnight on Christmas Eve and fed to the cattle on Christmas to prevent illness, as such straw would collect the sacred Christmas dew.[34] The dew could also be collected on the same night with a bowl or loaf of bread on the windowsill, and consumed as a preventative against illness throughout the year.[35]

Holy objects and substances may also be related to liturgical consecration or holy spaces, such as the grease from church bells to cure deafness,[36] or baptismal water to ease the pain of infant teething.[37] In some cases, what remains of the sacred host after communion is placed in the home for blessing and protection,[38] but above all the Bible itself plays a role as a sacred object used for healing and protection.

Ritual objects of power are those personal objects created or adapted exclusively for their role in ritual applications such as stones used to cure insomnia, canes used for dowsing or healing, mirrors for divination, or ritual knives used for protection (see Chapter VIII). Other significant ritual objects are those that must be found, begged, borrowed, or even stolen, in order to be effective such as a found horseshoe, begged nails used to ritually compel thieves to return stolen property, or begged pieces of wood used to punish a witch responsible for a cow going dry.[39] Other objects are empowered with written verbal blessings or inscriptions, and may contain Biblical verses, sacred names, or ancient inscriptions.

Just as sacred ritual objects may be empowered for use by their dedication at certain holy days or times, so too are many rituals enhanced by timing and frequency. A number of powwowers preferred to heal on Fridays, echoing the religious significance of Good Friday, especially the first Friday after the new moon. Two highly prolific healers, who treated scores of people each Friday, were Dennis Rex of Slatedale, and Dr. John H. Wilhelm of Raubsville.[40] John Wilhelm's practice was inherited by his son Eugene, who regularly treated over 100 people on a single Friday. An estimated 400 people would line up outside of his home when the new moon fell on a Friday.[41] Other rituals were timed by certain times of day or hours such as before dawn to remove warts or freckles with dew, or after dark in a graveyard to cure bedwetting,[42] or

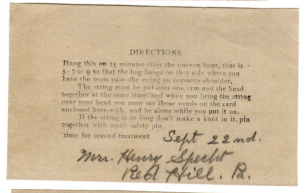

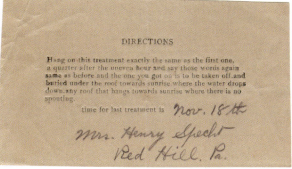

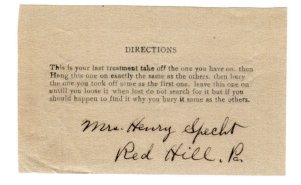

Healing procedures outlined by an unknown practitioner in Montgomery County for a patient suffering from pain: Mrs. Mary Malinda (Karver) Specht (1850-1929), buried at Red Hill Lutheran Cemetery. The three dated sets of directions were to be used in succession, according to an unknown powwow doctor. In each case, the patient is to take a bundle containing previously agreed-upon contents, and hang it on the body closest to the location of the pain 15 minutes after the striking of an uneven hour, and recite the invocation of the Holy Trinity indicated on the little card (top). The bundles are to be buried under the eaves of the roof towards the rise of the sun, indicating that the bundles were believed to absorb the patient's pain. Courtesy of Joyce Clemmer Munro, *Heilman Collection*.

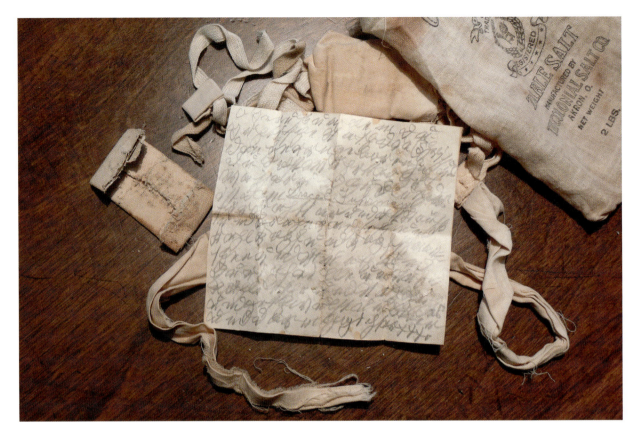

A bag of prepared written blessings prepared by one of the famous powwow doctors of Raubsville, not far from the legendary healing site of *Hexenkopf* in Williams Township, Northampton County. *Courtesy of Ned and Linda Heindel.*

in an uneven hour for curing fevers.[43] Other rituals are performed on saint's days such as feeding three cloves of garlic to humans or animals on St. Martin's day to prevent the power of a *Hex*,[42] or cutting of brush or unwanted facial hair on St. Abdon's day to prevent it from growing back.[44]

Other powwowing rituals make use of certain repetitions and timing such as healing processes scheduled on "three successive Fridays in the witness of the moon, as it waxes to full and wanes,"[45] or repetitions of three, four, five, seven, or nine times – sacred numbers with diverse symbolic implications: such as three for the Trinity, the Three Kings, or the Three Holy Men (Shadrach, Meshach and Abednego); the Four Evangelists (Matthew, Mark, Luke and John), and the Four Archangels (Raphael, Gabriel, Uriel, and Michael); five for the Five Holy Wounds of Christ (his hands, feet, and side), and the five-fold division of human kind in the five senses, and the number of digits on each hand and foot.

Such ritual scheduling and repetition is further enhanced by placement and space, including areas specially designated as familiar (the home, the barn, the property), or public (a roadside, a churchyard), or liminal (a property line, a threshold, a crossroads). Such designations often overlap such as in the case of a churchyard or cemetery, which can be considered both public and liminal, as a nexus of the worlds of the living and the dead, the sacred and the mundane.

While certain familiar spaces represent the home and family such as the hearth, the garden, or the bakeoven, other familiar spaces represent the transition from public to private such as the front door, or the eaves of the house. For wart cures involving the use of a buried potato under the eaves, it is notable that this space is as close as one can be to the outer spheres of life, while still being under the roof of the home. According to some, this location was once considered to be where protective spirits of the home dwelled and the closest that evil spirits could come to the house, and no further.[46] This notion may undergird the use of the attic or garrison space under the roof of the house as a location for protective blessings or objects such as Good Friday eggs.

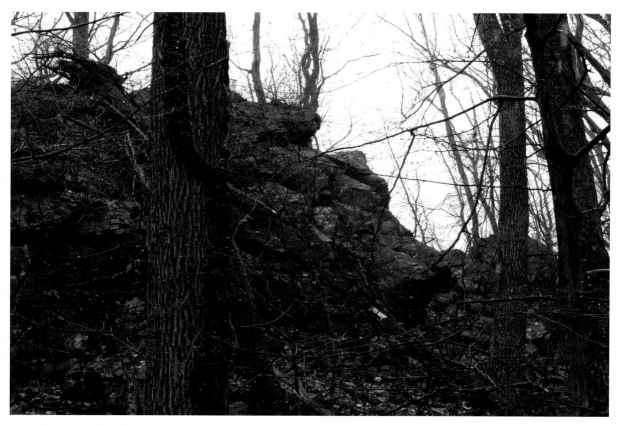

A view of one of many "profiles" seen in the legendary *Hexenhopf* (Witches' Head) of Williams Township, Northampton County. The rocky outcropping was used as a ritual site for transference of illness by generations of powwowers in the region.

Aside from the eaves, other liminal spaces are also favorable for depositing objects or substances used in powwowing such as the outhouse or the manure pile. Such spaces may be simply regarded as dirty, but they are also understood to be the site of decay or composting - a space for essentially neutralizing an illness. "*Alles Uebel soll vergehen wie Staub und Mischt, wo das Uebel herkommt, soll es wieder hinziehen*" (All evil shall pass away, as dust and dung. From whence the evil cometh, so shall it return).[47] In many a European *Bauernhof* (farm complex), the manure pile was bordered by a square enclosure that shared one corner or an edge with the home, and it was the location for depositing any household or agricultural waste that would eventually become useful compost. Even the runoff from the box was saved and used as fertilizer.[48]

In some cases, the soil itself is used as a site for ritual disposal. A friend once lived on a farm near Lenhartsville, Berks County, and had experienced some marital problems. His wife went to see powwower Charlie Thomas, who lived in the nearby town of Hamburg. Thomas suggested that a curse was responsible for the couple's woes. He recommended that the husband have three acres of their land plowed and to take their wedding bed, a valuable antique constructed of walnut, out into the middle of the three acres and burn it. The ashes were then to be scattered and plowed into the soil to destroy the curse, which the wife believed was plaguing their marriage. My friend did as his wife was directed and had three acres plowed. They never did have their bed burned, however, for the marriage did not last long enough to complete the ritual.[49]

Other specific locations and geological features were used in a similar manner as site of ritual deposit, and there is no site more renowned for the purpose than the legendary Hexenkopf Hill of Williams Township, Northampton County.[50] This rocky outcropping and associations with ritual activities – both healing and witchcraft – have been the subject of controversy and speculation for generations. It is known, however that a significant lineage of *Braucher* including Johann Peter Saylor (1721-1803), Jacob Wilhelm (1744-1821), and their descendants lived within the vicinity of the base of the mountain for generations, and used the site as a place to transfer illnesses into the rocky crags of the *Hexenkopf* (Witches' Head). The name of the hill is derived from the appearance of the rock formations, parts of which are likened to the jagged profile of a withered face. This name and reputation inspired stories of witches dancing on the summit and numerous urban legends far removed from healing narratives.

Unlike the healing sites of old Europe defined by the legends of saints and their miracles, Hexenkopf hill is reminiscent of the peak of the Blocksberg in the Harz mountain range in Northern Germany, where, according to local mythology, witches gathered throughout the centuries to conduct annual ceremonies.[51] Similar stories are told about a number of locations throughout the Dutch Country, including Hexenkopf in Northampton and *Hexebarrich* in Windsor Township, Berks County. Although the latter site has no known stories of ritual healing attached to it, the possibility does exist that the hill may have held similar significance as a ritual dump for illnesses or curses, hence the name, which has a dual meaning – Witches' Hill or Curse Hill. The latter is quite likely, as the township only named the road which runs along the ridge in English in the 1970s, and decided upon the translation "Witchcraft Road."[52]

Not all sites of ritual deposits take on such a sinister connotation. In fact, most sites used for disposing of illness or curses are by nature intended to dilute, dissipate, or immolate the negative effects of illness. Flowing water is featured in rituals involving cleansing or reducing of inflammation, and in some cases, the water must flow in a particular direction such as towards the rising sun.

An early nineteenth century remedy for complications with eyesight suggests a complex interplay of repetition, locations, and orientation, so much so that the function of the water could easily be overlooked, not only as a means for cleansing, but as a means for dilution of the salt and the disease:

> For weak and blurry eyes, go to flowing water before sunrise, and wash the eyes five times with the left hand, and each time say the following words, and then throw a handful of salt into the water. Then take seven steps backwards and then go home forwards. Do this three days in succession:
>
> *Wie dieses Salz wird vergehen,*
> *Sollen meine Augen heller sehn,*
> *Christus ist der helfen kan,*
> *Hiermit fangt der Seegen an.*
>
> As this salt shall disappear,
> So shall my eyes be clear.
> Christ is he who can help me,
> Herewith begins the blessing.[53]

The action of the flowing of the water is not unlike other rituals that suggest the use of the chimney, stove, or bakeoven as a location for the disease to be either burned by the fire, or dissipated by the smoke. The action of the smoke, which has the ability to "cure" meat, is also seen as a stabilizing and curative measure for human illness.

In some cases, illness is not merely deposited at a place but fed or given to an animal or human. Just as warts can be sold for a penny and cast by the side of the road to be contracted by the next person to pick up the penny,[54] so too can illnesses be given to animals such as pigs, dogs, or fish. When warts are rubbed on a pig trough, the illness is ingested by the pigs, who digest the illness, much like the vegetable and agricultural scraps that are mainstays in their diet. The pigs also correspond to the biblical healing of the demoniac, when Christ commands a multitude of demons into a herd of swine.[55] Pigs are not the only farm animal used in this manner, as one remedy for jaundice used in Brazilian *Brauche* involves urinating on nine kernels of corn and throwing them to the chickens.[56]

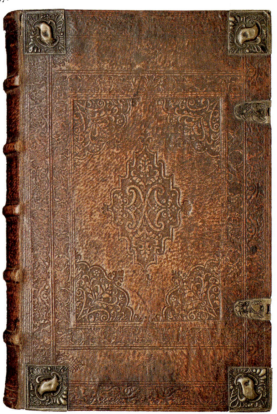

Historically and in the present day, some powwow practitioners have required or suggested that the patient to hold a Bible during ritual treatment as a symbolic acknowledgement of belief. Occasionally, these were pocket New Testaments, while others used large folio bibles like this 1778 Basel Bible. *Pennsylvania German Cultural Heritage Center, Kutztown University of Pennsylvania.*

The retired Lutheran minister and *Braucher* Frederick A. Weicksel (1867-1948)[57] powwowed for warts by rubbing them with spit, saying "Let's give those to the fish."[58]

But just as swine, chickens, or fish are seen as bottom-feeding animals that consume waste, other animals are valued in ritual traditions for their discernment such as dogs. An old form of divination used to determine whether or not an illness is terminal involves the use of a rind of bacon rubbed on the feet of a critically ill person, or a crust of bread rubbed over the gums. If the dog refuses to eat the bacon or the bread, then it portends certain death for the sick person.[59]

Animals play a variety of roles in ritual process, whether wild or domesticated. They can serve ancillary functions, like the divinatory role of the dog above, or, just like people, they can provide *materia medica* for a ritual cure or procedure. When living, animals can provide substances for ritual purposes in the form of hair, saliva, and excrement, or if an animal is deceased or butchered (especially for farm animals), a ritual may require a bone, hide, or fat. Animals are also frequently the recipients of healing, and there is little distinction between the treatments provided to humans and animals.[60]

While humans and animals may be treated for illness in a similar manner, their active roles facilitating ritual performance are understandably of an entirely different nature. It is generally agreed, that both the practitioner and patient must share some degree of commonality in religious, cultural, or cosmic belief – although the finer points of this notion of shared belief are subject to very different perspectives.

Belief: Prerequisite or Preference?

Some practitioners require their patients to share their particular religious orientation, while for others it is merely the belief in a higher power, without adherence to one particular faith.[61] Among older residents of Berks County, I have encountered the perception that anyone can be powwowed, but only if they believe in the efficacy of the practice. These prerequisites, either specific belief in God or the belief in the value of the tradition, have both theological and practical implications, and raise a number of significant questions: Does an obligatory belief in God suggest that a member of another faith or a non-believer is unable or unfit to receive blessings from the divine in a ritual encounter? What happens if a person is willing to participate in a powwowing ritual, but has no prior experience with the tradition? If a believing person does not benefit from a ritual encounter does this imply a crisis of faith? Do these rules suggest that God's blessing is an exclusive experience?

These problematic notions of necessary beliefs are further compounded by the incorporation of the idea of the placebo effect into common parlance in the present day, suggesting that results obtained from ritual healing are exclusively the self-fulfillment of expectations held by the patient. Such ideas are a common feature of discussions about powwowing in the present day, even among older generations of Pennsylvania Dutch people who firmly believe that powwowing works. Such blending of traditional and scientific concepts is an indication of changing dynamics within the culture's attitudes towards the nature of health and healing, and an example of how traditional systems adapt to modern thinking.

This exploration will neither defend nor espouse the notion of a single "correct" position on the interrelation of belief to the benefits of ritual process, and will make no claims concerning the efficacy of powwowing. There are, however, significant factors that suggest that powwowing and other vernacular health belief systems are part of a far more complex equation than what is solely expressed in such belief-oriented requirements or in relation to the placebo effect.

For instance, if powwowing is entirely dependent upon doctrinal beliefs, why are such a disproportionately large number of powwowing narratives concerned with infant and childhood ailments? Infants and toddlers are not able to engage in doctrinal discourse, much less provide detailed statements of belief. The same would invariably hold true for animals.

Furthermore, why are so many documented rituals focused on veterinary medicine, if positive results from powwowing are merely the results of self-fulfilling expectations of cause and effect? While the effects of conditioning are certainly applicable to domesticated animals that are raised and trained within contexts created by humans, anecdotes of animal treatment with traditional, ritual medicine often reveal complex and even contradictory attitudes held by the owners of the animals and the practitioners that treat them.

In 2014, a Lebanon County cattle owner shared an anecdote of veterinary powwowing from the 1970's when her whole family was assisting with dehorning a number of cows in their herd. This process can cause mild to severe bleeding from the horn, which can be controlled under normal circumstances, but can also be life threatening if complications arise. As in previous years, the family called a powwower to come to the farm when they struggled to control the bleeding of three cows. The powwowwer agreed to stop the blood, but asked that anyone who did not believe in powwowing to leave, because it would make the process more difficult. The powwower treated the cows by means of a blessing, and two of the three immediately stopped bleeding. The third continued to bleed despite the practitioner's repeated attempts, at which time she turned to the family and said: "There is someone here who does not believe. I need you to please leave." The father sheepishly walked away from the spectacle, and the powwower tried one last time. To the family's surprise, the bleeding stopped instantly.

For the owner of the cattle, this story indicated that it was the belief of the owners that was relevant to the healing of the cows. This attitude is confirmed by the nineteenth century horse doctor Isaac Leib of Manheim, Lancaster County, who recommended that one must use the owner's name when stopping blood for an animal, with the following blessing:

> Three holy virgins went walking. The one is bleeding, the second is dropping, and the third is stopping. In the beginning was the Word, and the Word was with God, and the Word was God; the same was in the beginning with God, and by the same Word we command that all veins must stop which are now bleeding, with the three holy names.[62]

Similar stories have been told of infants being healed on account of the faith of their parents. This perception that belief may be required of a responsible party or of witnesses of a ritual, rather than from the recipient of healing, suggests that the collective faith of a group affects the outcome. The fact that the practitioner treating the bleeding cows was perceived to be only partially effective due to a group of witnesses that were incompletely harmonious with powwowing indicates that witnesses may have a higher level of agency than mere passive reinforcement of the powwower's work, and are at least partially responsible for empowering a ritual experience. This idea may find its origins within biblical statements of Christ, concerning the nature of collective prayer, from the Gospel of Matthew:

> Verily I say unto you, Whatsoever ye shall bind on earth shall be bound in heaven: and whatsoever ye shall loose on earth shall be loosed in heaven. Again I say unto you, That if two of you shall agree on earth as touching any thing that they shall ask, it shall be done for them of my Father which is in heaven. For where two or three are gathered together in my name, there am I in the midst of them.[63]

In this sense, the powwower may be perceived to not only serve as a channel for divine healing directly from God, but also a means to gather or even amplify healing power through a collective ritual experience. Variable perceptions of the role and function of belief may, therefore, be directly related to the desire to enforce a sense of mutually-shared religious conviction in a ritual setting.

Prerequisites for belief appear for all practical purposes to be the preferences of certain practitioners and are by no means uniformly enforced. As an additional consequence, these rules also set into place certain protections for the practice against potential acts of appropriation by those who would seek to employ powwowing outside of the bounds of the cultural and religious context of the tradition. At the same time, such rules invariably set the tone for healing experiences and provide insight into perceptions of how the powwowing rituals were expected to function within the context of belief.

Cosmology of the Ritual Blessing

Although terms like worldview, structures of belief, and cosmology are not by any means a normal part of the vocabulary of powwowing, it is not uncommon to find ritual instructions, prayers, or benedictions that refer directly to the cosmos and the belief in a divine presence in the forces of creation. An elaborate manuscript inscribed for Regina Selzser of Jackson Township, Lebanon County, in 1837 describes a benediction for treating snakebite and begins with such a statement:

> Und, Gott, had, alles, erschaffen, was, im, Himmel, und, auf, erden, ist, und, alles, war, gud, nicht, als, allein, die, schlange, had, Gott, verflucht, verflucht, solst, du, bleiben, schlangen, geschwülst, ich, stelle, dich, gift, und, schmertz, ich, döde, dich, zian, dein, gift, zian, dein, gift, zian, dein, gift, amen, X X X. Regina Selzser 1837

> And God created all things in heaven and on earth, and everything was good, except for thee, Snake, which God cursed, and cursed shalt thou remain. Swelling I halt thee, poison and pain, I destroy thee. Withdraw thy poison, withdraw thy poison, withdraw thy poison, Amen, [in the name of God the Father, and of the Son, and of the Holy Spirit X X X. Regina Selzser 1837

Above all other aspects of the ritual process described above, the opening declaration, derived from the first chapter of the Book of Genesis, immediately places the afflicted person within an ordered, sacred universe. Conversely in the statement which follows, the incident of the snakebite and the resulting physical affliction are identified with an aberration of creation.[64] This cosmic dissonance resonates not merely for the afflicted person present at the time of the ritual's performance. Framed through the expression of religious truth, the experience takes on a larger dimension of the universal pain of a fallen humanity. It would be reasonable to posit that these statements, which identify the source of the natural world as the work of a supernatural creator, are intended to overcome the cause and effect of the natural world with the truth of a higher supernal reality (i.e. the Trinity, represented by "XXX," which abbreviates the three highest names and the liturgical gesture of the sign of the cross three times).

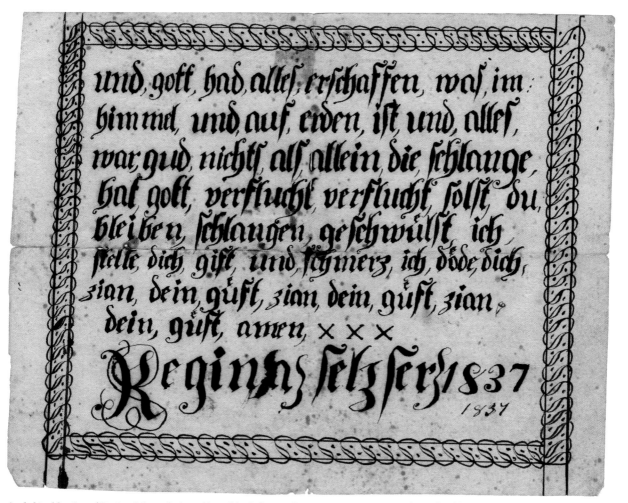

Snakebite blessing of Regina Selzser, Jackson Township, Lebanon County, 1837. Former Roughwood Collection. *Heilman Collection.*

It is equally relevant to consider the popularity of macrocosmic theology among the Pennsylvania Dutch at the time of the recording of this ritual, when common household prayer books in the nineteenth century included the works of mystics such as Johann Arndt, whose works were printed locally in Allentown [65] and Philadelphia, the latter of which was published by none other than Benjamin Franklin. The application of macrocosmic interpretation would offer that suffering is alleviated through the experience of the creator being present in both the cause and the effect, an awareness which is transformative, mitigating what theologian Paul Tillich would later call "the consequences of existential estrangement," that is, ultimately in this case, the estrangement of man from the divine.[66]

While this particular snakebite ritual is based in biblical literature, it does not directly make use of any particular method of ritual curing which is described in biblical passages such as the curing of the snakebites of the people of Israel by Moses, who received specific instructions concerning how to do so directly from God in the wilderness.[67] However, numerous rituals that make use of direct scriptural quotations and processes reflecting the miracles of Christ are a central theme and source of inspiration for *Braucherei*. Sophia Bailer described this form of healing as "calling a blessing," likening it to the acts of Jesus and the apostles.[68] In a sense, Christ was seen as the model for the spiritual healer, using words, exhalations, spitting, touch, written symbols, and applications of healing agents.

Although Christ used no elaborate scripted prayers comparable to powwowing, his use of Aramaic language in certain healing acts evokes a sense of ceremoniality. Christ raises the daughter of Jarius from the dead, and utters

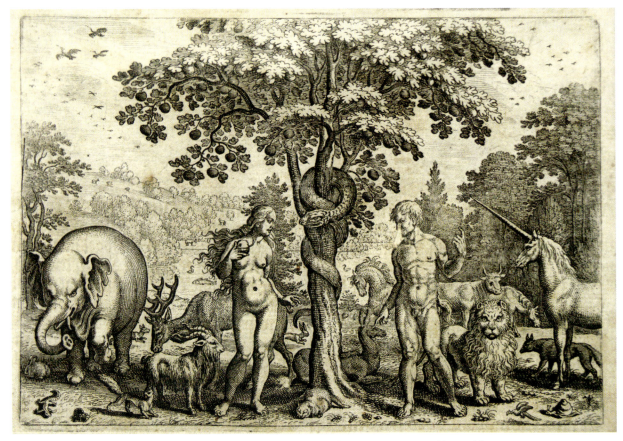

Temptation of Adam and Eve in the Garden of Eden by the serpent, engraving from the 1704 Merian Bible, Frankfurt am Mayn.
Courtesy of the Evangelical and Reformed Historical Society, Lancaster, Pennsylvania.

the words "Talitha Koum," meaning "little girl arise."[69] He heals the deaf-mute by uttering a deep sigh, and exclaims "*Ephphatha*" – "be opened."[70] Especially in the latter case, Christ's exclamation can be understood as a statement of power, as opposed to a command to the deaf man, who is unable to hear Christ's words until his ear is opened.[71] It is unknown why the author of the Gospel of Mark preserved these healing words in the original language, while the rest of the Gospel is in Greek, but their presence in the healing narratives is distinct and powerful. Johannes Deigendesch, an executioner who published works on veterinary medicine in Lancaster, suggested the ritual use of the word "*Ephatha*" combined with other treatments in order to relieve constipation in a horse, thus reflecting his knowledge of both the meaning of the biblical phrase, and its use in "opening."[72]

References to Christ healing with words appears extensively in powwow manuals,[73] as well as in accounts of Sophia Bailer, who emphasized the power of words by referring to herself as "The Lord's mouthpiece."[74] In other healing acts of Christ, he uses the imperative, commanding demons to depart,[75] and calling to Lazarus to come out of the tomb.[76] Christ also commands the leper to "be clean!" and his words are combined with a gesture of healing, as Christ reaches out and touches the leper.[77]

Elsewhere, Christ heals simply by laying his hands on sick people.[78] The healing power not only in Christ's physical body, but in his clothing, is described in the story of the woman suffering from hemorrhage who touches his garment and is instantly healed.[79] This happens again in Gennesaret, when the ill "besought him that they might only touch the hem of his garment: and as many as touched were made perfectly whole."[80] The apostles are later regarded similarly, as handkerchiefs that were touched by St. Paul were used to heal the sick and cast out demons.[81]

It is clear however, that Christ was by no means the author of this form of healing with hands, as the story of the prophet Elisha curing the Syrian captain Naaman of leprosy suggests. Elisha commands Naaman to wash in the

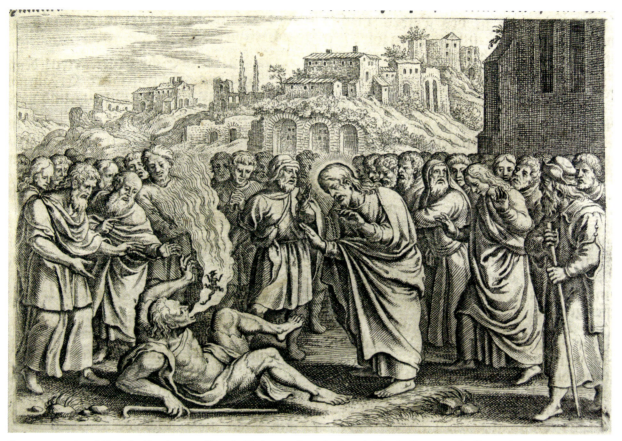

German engraving of Christ healing the man afflicted with demons, from the Gospel of Mark, Chapter 5. The illness is leaving the man in the form of a visible entity, exiting by means of a wind from the mouth. From the 1704 Merian Bible, printed at Frankfurt am Mayn by Johann Phillip Andreas, from the Kurtz family in Pennsylvania. *Courtesy of the Evangelical and Reformed Historical Society, Lancaster, Pennsylvania.*

River Jordan, but Naaman is surprised, saying, "I thought, He will surely come out to me, and stand, and call on the name of the LORD his God, and strike his hand over the place, and recover the leper."[82] Naaman's words reveal that this form of healing was widespread across many ancient cultures, and not unique to the Hebrews.

The ritual actions of Christ and his use of healing agents is controversial, because just like his words of power, it is generally assumed that his divine nature would allow for healing to take place without any need for ritual procedures. Why then, does Christ spit and touch the deaf-mute's tongue, or place his finger in his ear?[83] Or why does he bother to make mud with his spit to anoint the blind man before requiring him to wash in the pool of Siloam?[84] Regardless of the authors' original intentions for these seemingly ritual procedures, such actions not only resonate with healers on a folk-cultural level, but also within the context of the liturgy, where spittle is still used by some Catholics in the sacrament of baptism.[85]

Perhaps most controversial is Christ's often overlooked inscription of unknown characters upon the ground to dismiss an angry crowd bent on stoning an adulteress.[86] While the typical interpretation is that the message of his words tugged at the conscience of the crowd - "He that is without sin among you, let him first cast a stone at her" – it is also evident from German Bible illustrations from the eighteenth and nineteenth centuries that the popular interpretation held that Christ's inscription was equally responsible for the diffusing of the situation.[87]

Although the theological implications of Christ's miracles are open to debate, these healing narratives directly inspire healing procedures combining words, exhalations, and other actions such as this procedure, inspired by direct quotations from the Gospel of Mark:[88]

> **For a wen in the eye, blow nine times into the eye, and say the following words each time, and place the person for whom thou tryest on the threshold of the home:**

113

Above: Rhyming cure for burns and inflamation, invoking the elements of fire, water, and wind, ca. 1880. *Heilman Collection.*

Right: A copy of an original broadside compiled ca. 1880 and published by William A. Woomer. The broadside includes two cures in both English and German variations, including an alternate version of the rhyming cure for burns appearing above in manuscript form. William A Woomer served as a private in the Civil War in the 17th cavalry of PA, Co. E. A William Woomer is listed in the US Federal Census in 1870 and 1880 (b.1819) living in the vicinity of Jackson Township, Lebanon County. *Heilman Collection.*

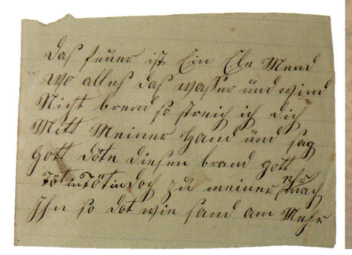

Jesus said, What wilt thou that I should do unto thee? Lord, that I might receive my sight. It be so, see! In Jesus' name thine eyes shall become bright, pure, clean, clear, as the moon and stars in the firmament of heaven.[89]

This familiar story is combined with a progression of ritual procedures, including blowing nine times into the eye, each time repeating the biblical blessing, and placing the person on the threshold of the house to perform the cure.

Less specific healing narratives of Christ's cures are echoed in verbal blessings used for powwowing everything from bleeding to burns and from hernias to sprains, as described in detail in cures such as this one for a sprain:

Für Verrenkung streiche mit der Hand dreymal über den wehen Theil des Körpers und sage jedesmal folgendes Worte:

Christus machte Lahme gehen, Todte machte er auferstehn, So heile denn dein Verrenken, In die Tiefe soll es versenken, Jesus allein heilet Kranken, Ihn allein soll man danken - im Namen des Vaters, des Sohnes und des Heiligen Geistes.

For a sprain, pass thine hand three times over the affected part of the body, and each time say the following words:

Christ hath made the lame to walk, the dead to rise: thus may thy sprain heal. It shall descend into the depths. Jesus alone healeth the sick, and to him alone shall one give praise, in the name of the Father and of the Son, and of the Holy Spirit.[90]

In these latter forms, the healing acts of Christ are asserted as statements of divine truth, against which no disease can prevail. This notion of positioning a religious statement against physical affliction, or likening a particular doctrinal statement to the removal of illness, is consistent with healing applications of sympathy.

Sympathy

In *Braucherei* prayers and benedictions, verbal statements serve to invoke sympathetic relationships, with religious language or celestial imagery:

Christ upon the cross was hanged, and thy bone is sprained. It harmed him not, thus shall thy sprain harm thee not, in the name of God the Father, Son, and Holy Spirit.[91]

May [the bullet] turn away from me, powder and lead, as the sun turneth away from the moon.[92]

Whether the intention was to subordinate earthly experience to religious doctrine or to contextualize it within a macrocosmic view, it is true that many of these statements containing religious symbolism point to a sense of mutability in the physical world. It is equally common to find statements such as the previous sympathetic injunction of a bullet, which point to the certainty of the celestial sphere and earthly elements of divine creation. The same applies to the following cure for burns:

Das Feuer ist ein Ele Mend,
Wo alles das Wasser und Wind nicht brend,
So streich ich dich mit meiner Hand,
Und Sag Gott döte diesen Brand.
Gott töt in, töt in, doch zu meiner Ehr,
Mach ihn so dot wie Sand am Mehr.

The fire is an element
Which burneth not water and wind,
Thus I pass over thee with my hand,
And ask God to destroy this burn,
Destroy it, destroy it, though to my honor,
Make it as dead as the sand by the sea.[93]

Burn cures often make use of blowing over the afflicted part of the body three times,[94] physically invoking the element of air to remove the heat of the burn. The use of the four elements is not to be thought of as functioning independently of the divine, but rather through divine direction such as this remedy for menstrual cramps recorded by Peter Schlessman (1769-1828) from Bethel Township, Berks County in 1816:

Vor den Kramb, Ein plauen wollen fatam den soll man 3 m[a]hl drum pinden: Das feier und das waser ging durch der Engel Gasse da kam unsere liebe Jungfrau und dät das feier beschlisen und lass das wasser flisen.

For Cramps, [take] a blue wollen string, then one shall wrap the string around [the afflicted person]:

Fire and water flow through the angel-path, then came our dear Virgin, and she would extinguish the fire, and let the water flow.[95]

In each of the previous two instances, the properties of the elements are believed to regulate and establish balance within the body of the person, as is intended here for painful menstruation, where the fire is likened to the pain of cramps; the water, the establishment a regular flow. Although there exist rituals for regulation of both the congestion of menstrual flow and the overabundance of flow in other collections of benedictions,[96] this particular ritual is less specialized in its written composition.

One of the classic everyday objects that finds its way into myriad healing rituals is common string, ribbon, or cord. Used for a broad spectrum of ailments ranging from inflammation to menstrual cramps, the string varies in color based on how it is used, and what illness is to be removed. For instance, a red string is used to remove the inflammation from the dangerous skin infection erysipelas, known among the folk as "wildfire." The red of the string relates the color of the fire of the inflammation in a like-attracts-like scenario.

Notably, the use of color in Peter Schlessman's cure for cramps, likewise expresses a sympathetic alignment between the blue woolen string and the elemental quality of water in order to re-establish a healthy flow from the body. In each of these cases, the linear, directional, connective quality of the fiber suggests a movement through or away from the body, or a passage from one point to another.

This action can pertain to the withdrawing of an illness, as well as the regulation of normal bodily functions. In an overarching sense, the string is a visualization of the subtle connections between all things.

The string's composition is usually silk or wool, and most rituals specify that it has to either have been previously unused for any other purpose, or that it has to have been begged or borrowed rather than purchased. In most rituals, the string is either used to measure the afflicted person's body or wrapped around the person. By measuring the person, essentially the image or qualities of the person have been transferred to the string, serving as a proxy for removal of the illness. Depending on the nature and elemental correspondence of the illness, the string could be disposed of in a chimney, or tossed down a well. In other cases the string might be wrapped around a fence post until it rots away.

A classic example of the use of red string is in ritual descriptions of drawing out the inflammation of erysipelas or wildfire (*Wildfeier*). Erysipelas is an acute bacterial infection of the skin characterized by extreme inflammation and swelling that would rapidly spread, earning it the dialect names *Rotlaaf* – literally "the running redness," or *Wildfeier*. Prior to the use of antibiotics, erysipelas is estimated to have claimed over one-third of those who contracted it,[97] and conventional physicians often struggled to provide relief. The esteemed Lutheran circuit-rider Rev. Georg P. Mennig (1773-1851), who also ministered to his community as a powwow practitioner,[98] commissioned the printing of a broadside featuring a ritual cure for "wildfire" or erysipelas.

Mennig's procedure made use of a red string to remove the illness and was widely practiced throughout the Dutch Country. His cure called out to the illness animistically and asked it to depart:

Wild Feuer, flieh, flieh, flieh. Der rothe Faden jagt dich hie!
Wildfire, flee, flee, flee. The red string chases you away![99]

Mennig's instructions continue that one must pass the string three times over the afflicted person, and each time say the indicated words. Thereafter, one must tuck the string into a piece of paper and hide it in the chimney, where the string would be smoked by a fire. After three hours, one should take the string again and perform the procedure a second time, then place the string back into the chimney. After another three hours, the process is to be repeated once more, and then the string is cast up into the chimney. The illness will depart when the string falls where it will. The instructions conclude with a *nota bene*, that if the wildfire has afflicted the body, the arms, and the legs, one must pass the string three times over each limb, the legs, the back and the front of the person, and say the words each time.[100]

Some variations of Rev. Mennig's cure include the notion of drawing the heat from the inflammation with a rhyming couplet of commands for both the string and the illness. A ritual procedure recorded by Conrad Reber (1778-1817), a *Braucher*, horse doctor, and farrier from Tulpehocken, Berks County, suggests the following words to accompany the same actions as Mennig:

Rother seiten fatem zick, zick, zick.
Wilth Feuer flick, flick, flick."
Red silk string, draw, draw, draw,
Wild fire fly away, fly away, fly away.

Interestingly enough, Reber's use of "Zick, Zick, Zick" is a contracted echo of earlier forms of the command *"zieh an dein Gift"* (withdraw thy poison) included in the aforementioned ritual for snakebite, and also included in later renderings as "Zing, Zing, Zing!"[101] These three variations demonstrate the difficulties of preserving oral tradition in writing, because truncated, abbreviated, or corrupted forms are inevitably preserved in mistranscription for posterity. Likewise Reber's "Flick, Flick, Flick" is a contraction of the dialect phrase "*Flieg weck*" (Fly away). In these examples, it is apparent that some instances of what may be perceived as magic words are ultimately derived from grammatically correct phrases lost in transcription.

Another variation from Kuztown Pennsylvania suggests the phrase:

Rodar Fadem zieg, zieg, zieg,
Wildes Fier fleag, fleag, fleag.

While these words are spoken, the red string is to be tied into a loop and passed over the body of the patient.[102]

These remedies proceed from an ancient idea that like attracts like: that a red string, representing fire, could be used to attract and remove the fiery skin infection. Likewise the smoke from the chimney would carry away the illness as it is extinguished. Furthermore, the ritual is framed as an animistic dialogue between the practitioner and the disease, indicating that the infection was ultimately believed to be caused by an invasive spirit, a folk belief that foreshadows the later discovery of biological pathogens.

Although Mennig's ritual is scripted as a basic form of exorcism, typically powwowing prayers command the illnesses to depart by the authority of a higher source of power. Yet the procedure endorsed by Rev. Mennig is decidedly devoid of specific Christian references. One explanation for the absence of explicit Christian imagery in certain examples of powwow praxis is that an invocation of the Holy Trinity customarily concludes each ritual. Beyond this, the expectation is that such rituals function as part of a broader network of sacred relationships, and that the practitioner who performs the ritual serves only as a facilitator or intermediary. This notion is echoed in one of the most widely circulated powwow manuals, attributing the following words to St. Albert the Great: "...*aber nicht durch mich, sondern durch Gott Vater, Gott Sohn und Gott heiligen Geist...*" – "but not through me, rather through God the Father, God the Son, and God the Holy Spirit."[103]

Although explicit verbalization of Christian themes is absent in Mennig's cure, elements such as the red string have the potential to implicitly undergird the ritual with meaning within a Judeo-Christian framework, as red string appears in Biblical descriptions of healing rituals throughout the Old Testament. For instance, a ritual for cleansing the house of a person healed of leprosy, another dangerous infection of the skin, is described at the opening of the fourteenth chapter of the Book of Leviticus:

> The Lord said to Moses, 'These are the regulations for any diseased person at the time of their ceremonial cleansing, when they are brought to the priest: The priest is to go outside the camp and examine them. If they have been healed of their defiling skin disease, the priest shall order that two live clean birds and some cedar wood, scarlet yarn and hyssop be brought for the person to be cleansed. Then the priest shall order that one of the birds be killed over fresh water in a clay pot. He is then to take the live bird and dip it, together with the cedar wood, the scarlet yarn and the hyssop, into the blood of the bird that was killed over the fresh water. Seven times he shall sprinkle the one to be cleansed of the defiling disease, and then pronounce them clean. After that, he is to release the live bird in the open fields.[104]

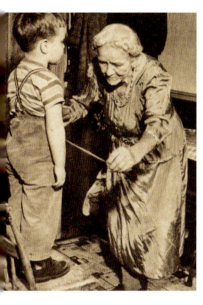 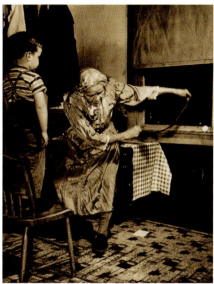 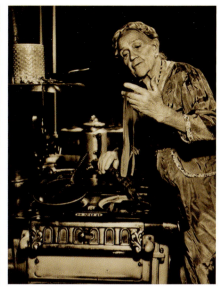

Aunt Sophia Bailer, Saint of the Coal Regions (1870-1954) ca. 1950, photographs by Don Yoder. *Pennsylvania German Cultural Heritage Center.*

"Aunt" Sophia (Leininger) Bailer, *Braucherin* from Tremont, Schuylkill County, participated annually in the Kutztown Folk Festival, discussing her powwowing techniques, or as she called it, "Calling a blessing." Sophia Bailer was an energetic and amicable person who helped in many ways to transform the public perception of powwow practitioners in the twentieth century. Sophia represented her culture well, and reminded the public that many grandmothers in the Dutch country powwowed for common ailments and were well received in a positive light. This series of photographs depicts Sophia demonstrating the common powwow ritual for curing *Wildfeier* or erysipelas, an inflammatory infection of the skin. The process requires the use of a red woolen string.

(Clockwise From Top Left:) First, she transfers the illness to the string, by drawing it along the body; After accumulating the illness in the woolen string, Aunt Sophia sweeps the string away from the body three times, while addressing the illness and commanding it to depart from the child: "*Wildfeier, Wildfeier, Flieh, Flieh, Flieh! Der rote Fadem jagt dich hie, hie hie!*" (Erysipelas, Erysipelas, Fly, fly, fly! The red string chases you away, away, away!); After the removal of the illness from the body, Aunt Sophia "smokes the string" by holding it over an open burner on her wood-fired kitchen stove. This action serves to neutralize the illness; Aunt Sophia hangs the sting on a line above the stove, but she does not fasten it. The wool must fall before the boy can be rid of his ailment; When the wool has fallen to the floor, indicating that the child has begun to recover, Aunt Sopia carefully sweeps the string into a dustpan; The woolen string is burned in the kitchen stove, as a final measure.

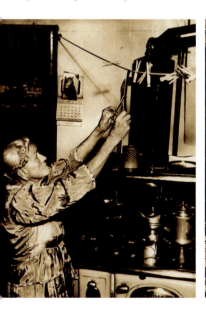 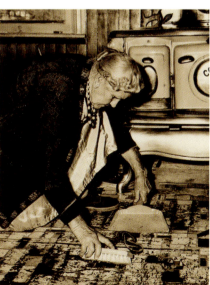 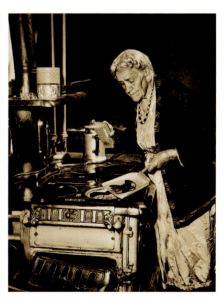

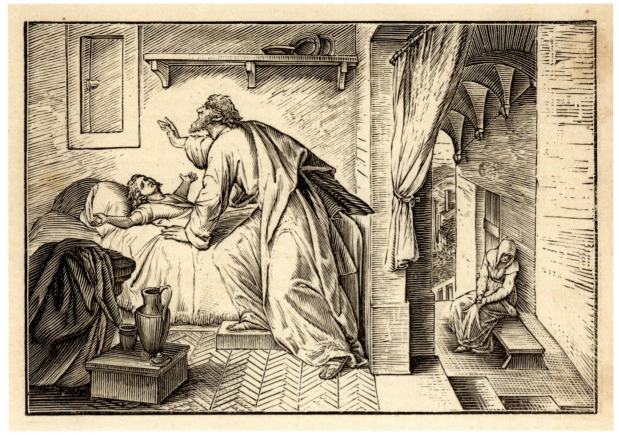

Elijah resurrecting the son of the widow of Zarephath by measuring or stretching himself over the child. Engraving by Julius Schnorr von Carolsfeld, in the bilingual *Bibel in Bilder or the Bible in Pictures*, printed in Philadelphia by Ignatius Kohler. *Pennsylvania German Cultural Heritage Center, Kutztown University.*

Red string appears again in the Book of Genesis, at the birth of Zerah and his twin brother Phares; when Zarah's hand emerges first from the womb, the midwife ties a red string around his wrist.[105] In the Book of Joshua, a red cord is hung in the window of Rahab's home in Jericho as a signal to the Israelite forces to spare her life.[106]

"The Scarlet Thread" is also a popular metaphor used in sermons to relate the gospel narratives of Christ to themes of sacrifice and redemption throughout the Old Testament. This Christian sense of continuity builds upon the notion that Christ was present at the time of creation as suggested in the Gospel of John and foreshadowed by the Prophets.[107]

This meaning is consistent with the symbolism of the Middle Ages, when a baptismal cloth called a *birrus* was placed upon the head of the child to retain the chrism (baptismal water), which had a red thread woven into the white fabric to symbolize Christ's Passion.[108]

Thus the red string of Mennig's cure could be synonymous with the Biblical "Scarlet Thread," as a symbol of Christ and his sacrifice. If the red string were to symbolize Christ in powwowing, the string is imbued with a form of agency, as a means to drive out illness, and is an echo of Christ's healing miracles in the gospel narratives when his garments serve as an intermediary for healing.[109]

It is entirely possible that Mennig's cure was inspired by the use of ribbons or bands of fabric blessed at holy shrines in Europe and provided to the sick for healing or the legendary *True Length of Christ* allegedly discovered in the Holy Tomb.[110] Although Mennig's ritual does not specifically state that one is to be measured with the string or ribbon, this is precisely how Sophia Bailer employed the same ritual in 1950, when she allowed Dr. Don Yoder to photograph the process. Thus the measurement of the patient, as a means of transference of the illness, is not unlike the transference of divine blessings to the band of cloth that measured the *True Length of Christ*. In both cases, some portion of the body's essence is present in the measurement.

This notion of transference of qualities through measurement is present in a wide variety of powwow cures. Pennsylvania German folklorist and Reformed Minister Thomas Brendle likens this idea of transference to the Pennsylvania Dutch word *abnemme*, meaning "to take off."[111] In some cases, the ritual removal of an illness is actually referred to as "a take off," even in areas outside of Pennsylvania.[112] The word also has a secondary meaning, "to wane," which also describes a wasting disease known as *Abnemme,* and equated with marasmus in children or muscular atrophy in adults. The cure again involves the use of a string, which is used to measure the body and its proportions. Sometimes the sufferer's height is compared to the width of their outstretched arms, or the height versus the measurement of the foot multiplied by seven. In each case, these are classic human proportions, and if the measurements do not add up, the string is disposed of outside so that when it rots away the illness also departs.

A similar idea is present in the miraculous healing of the son of the widow of Zarephath when Elijah stretches himself out upon the dead child:

> And he said unto her, Give me thy son. And he took him out of her bosom, and carried him up into a loft, where he abode, and laid him upon his own bed. And he cried unto the LORD, and said, O LORD my God, hast thou also brought evil upon the widow with whom I sojourn, by slaying her son? And he stretched himself upon the child three times, and cried unto the LORD, and said, O LORD my God, I pray thee, let this child's soul come into him again. And the LORD heard the voice of Elijah; and the soul of the child came into him again, and he revived.[113]

COMPREHENSIVE RITUALS OF THE BODY

While much emphasis is placed on the use of words and their meanings, activating an emotional, cerebral, or spiritual engagement with the ritual process, it is equally necessary that the ritual and its transformations reside within the body, as the primary site of ritual transformation. Powwowing rituals are not merely believed, they are felt and internalized. As a mutually inhabited space, ritual healing is not merely something that happens to a person seeking a restoration of health, but a dynamic encounter whereby both healer and patient are challenged and depart from the experience changed.

For the patient this means that the body must be receptive to the intentions of the practitioner, and the practitioner is sensitive to the body of the patient. Both the patient and the practitioner, however, are subject to forces greater than themselves, and it is in this shared, ritually defined space where both experience the workings of the divine.

Like Sophia Bailer's description of being the "mouthpiece" of God, practitioners throughout the generations have described their role in facilitating a healing experience as being that of an "instrument," a "channel," or "conduit" for the Holy Spirit. Therefore, because the healer is not acting alone, but as an agent of the divine, no credit is due for effectively facilitating a change in the patient's state of being. Instead many practitioners see the ritual process as a means to glorify God.

For the patient the experience may be transformative, but for the practitioner, it is visceral. Some practitioners I have personally known report the ability to feel the patient's imbalance or sickness echoed within their own bodies, while others have described the experience of briefly taking the illness upon themselves, or of feeling sick after working on patients with advanced or terminal illnesses. Following completion of the ritual, some feel exhausted or emotionally affected, according to the severity of the patient's illness or state of being.

While many rituals focus on specific parts of the body such as the location of the inflammation in Mennig's cure or the ribs of a livergrown child, there are also comprehensive rituals that address the body as a whole. Although each part of the body is blessed, the procedure is not merely a blessing for each part, but an elaborate ritual performance that places the body within a sacred space as a means to address the whole person – body, mind and spirit. Such procedures are comprehensive, with rounds of specialized prayers for each region of the body, as well as accompanying physical actions employed by the practitioner for the removal of imbalance and the invoking of divine presence.

Although there are many ritual forms used in this manner, I was taught a particular, comprehensive sequence that invariably begins with a patient requesting assistance. I was given the advice that a practitioner can offer, but the patient must always ask. This indicates that it is truly the wish of the patient to be powwowed, as opposed to merely going along with someone else's suggestion. From the very beginning, the patient is expected to take an active part of the process, rather than merely passive.

When an agreeable time and place is determined, the space is prepared and established for the ritual. For some, the best location is a kitchen, a parlor, a back porch, or the barn, either at the property of the patient, the practitioner, or a friend. In some cases, practitioners have special spaces set aside such as an outbuilding or study, but this varies considerably.

This process can also take place outside in open air, day or night. Working outside can be particularly helpful for addressing certain illnesses, which may need to be traditionally timed according to the phase and visibility of the moon. If, for instance, the practitioner has been asked to address a wart, a tumor, goiter or other growth, it may be important for the ritual to take place outside in a place where the moon is visible. Thus the ritual sequence is flexible enough to incorporate other specific ritual elements as needed.

If the patient is able to sit, a sturdy chair is positioned facing east, often in the middle of a room or outdoor space so that the practitioner can move freely around the chair. The patient must be seated without crossing their arms or legs in a relaxed and open posture. Otherwise the patient may stand, but the directional orientation is still the same.

This easterly significance is reflected in a number of religious practices throughout the ages and is reflected in the notion that Christ's second coming will be from the east, as suggested in the Gospel of Matthew: "For as the lightning cometh out of the east, and shineth even unto the west; so shall also the coming of the Son of man be."[114] This passage echoes the vision of Ezekiel, "And, behold, the glory of the God of Israel came from the way of the east: and his voice was like a noise of many waters: and the earth shined with his glory."[115] This east orientation has been reflected in the direction of prayer for Christians, as well as some Jews, who pray facing east towards Jerusalem in most of the west, as well as Muslims who face Mecca. Likewise, in Ezekiel's descriptions of the temple, the steps to the altar face east,[116] and many altars in European and American cathedrals are approached from the east. Only some of the early Pennsylvania Dutch churches face an east, such as the 1806 Bindnagel Lutheran Church along the Swatara Creek in Lebanon County, in which the pulpit and communion table face east. Others such as Belleman's 1815 Union Church in Mohrsville, Berks County, face south, but the gravestones outside face east, as is customary, thus linking the easterly orientation to the notion of resurrection. The symbolism of the resurrection and the rising sun is significant in many healing rituals.

The practitioner provides a Bible to the patient, or the patient may have one of their own, to either hold in their lap or to carefully place under the chair. The practitioner must ask the patient "Do you believe?" – a straight-forward, but multidimensional question that, if answered in the affirmative, gives the practitioner permission to proceed. The same phrase will be asked in Pennsylvania Dutch by some, like one Schuylkill County contact: "*Duhscht du glaawe?*" This is not so much a test to determine any one particular religious orientation, but an affirmation of the sincerity of the patient. A simple yes, allows for the ritual to move beyond the initial stages of preparation and commence with performance.

The practitioner begins with the soft recitation of an opening blessing and the full baptismal name of the patient while facing east in front of the patient. Although I have both witnessed and participated in this process hundreds of times, I have only heard the words spoken aloud on occasions when the process is being taught. In all other cases, the words are spoken like a whisper.

Following the invocation, the practitioner turns clockwise to face the patient, and passes their hands from the crown of the head to the soles of the feet three times, hovering just inches from the patient's body. The practitioner may kneel for this portion of the ritual, as I have always done, as it allows for ease of motion, and minimizes the need to sustain uncomfortable, bent postures. These first three passes are not only part of a blessing, accompanied by spoken prayers, it also the time when the practitioner essentially scans the body for imbalances.

This diagnostic technique is based in a keen sensitivity that the practitioner develops through experience. The practitioner's hands do not actually touch the body, but feel for disturbances in both the body and the spirit. Some practitioners describe sensations of heat or coolness concentrated at certain locations along the body, while others have experienced vibrations or tingling at the site of imbalance.

Ironically, although this practice closely resembles other complementary and alternative therapies with robust vocabularies to describe healing exchanges such as Reiki, powwowing is somewhat tacit, and rarely explicitly described in terms of manipulation of "energy," "light," or "polarity." Instead imbalance in the body is described in somewhat dualistic terms as either heat or cold; excess or lack, and these qualities are manipulated by practitioners' hands and the invocation of the Trinity: "*Im Nahme Gott der Vadder, der Suh, un der Heilich Geischt.*" Nevertheless, a healer from Schuylkill County frequently remarks that her use of "active prayer" (her alternative to the word powwowing) is "just like Reiki."[117]

Following the initial three passes over the body, the practitioner walks around the chair to a position behind the patient, where a series of prayers commence,

Opposite page: Snapshots from a series of undated, unidentified photographs from the papers of Dr. Don Yoder, featuring an early twentieth-century Pennsylvania healer "trying" for a female patient. The sequence shows a progression from top to bottom, with broad sweeping motions to remove imbalance from the body. *Pennsylvania German Cultural Heritage Center, Kutztown University of Pennsylvania.*

blessing each part of the body from top to bottom, front to back, all the while moving only in a clockwise direction. The practitioner's hands hover over the parts of the body in succession, and each part of the body is sealed with the sign of the cross with either the thumb or the fore and middle fingers. This portion of the process is fluid, and characterized by gentle sweeping, stroking, and passing motions that are highly variable and tailored to the style of the practitioner.

With each pass of the hand, a recitation of the appropriate blessing follows. Such motions with the hands are meant to simultaneously perform several types of specific functions including additional scanning, blessing, and removal of imbalance. This latter function appears in the form of intermittent use of gestures like pulling, cupping, and sweeping away from the body at the site of imbalance. Such removals are used for everything from removal of the heat of inflammation to reducing muscular tension. Movements are also specifically tailored to certain parts of the body, as well as the particular function of certain organs. Some practitioners use large upward sweeping movements across the body with both hands for the lungs, following the direction of an exhalation, while movements along the abdomen and digestive tract follow the direction of evacuation. Several general rules appear widespread: For the limbs, all removal is towards the extremities of the fingers and toes. All imbalance is removed and directed away from the core of the body, as the perception

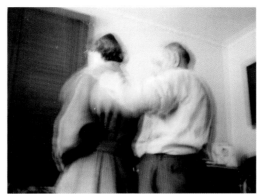
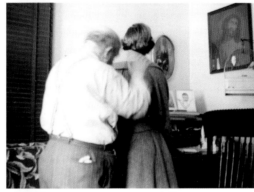
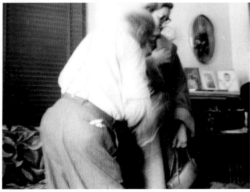
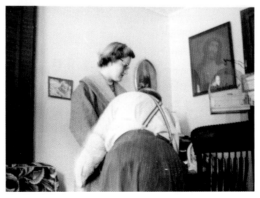

is that illnesses can be "driven deeper" into the body.[118]

While some practitioners mirror their motions between right and left hands, others use their hands independently of one another, or with different functions. I have known several practitioners who insisted that the right hand was for blessing, and the left hand was for removal – even though the motions of each hand were performed in mirror image. In this case the right hand sweeps clockwise, and the left counterclockwise, with differing roles for the right and left hand, respectively, as active or receptive. The active hand blesses, while the receptive hand removes. However, the sealing of each part of the body with the sign of the cross is invariably performed with the right hand, and usually with the thumb or index and middle fingers.

Because the practitioner's hands play such an important role in attending the body and facilitating the removal of illness, numerous forms of ritually cleansing gestures are used to rid the hands of any residual imbalance as an after-effect of the ritual. Frequently, the practitioner will shake off or wring their hands, or flick their fingers periodically throughout this portion of the ritual, as well as during the initial scan. Some practitioners frequently touch the floor to "ground" any unwanted residual illness, or will wash their hands in running water between sessions.

This act of ritual cleansing is particularly important following the identification of key areas of imbalance where specialized prayers and rituals are performed, tailored to the type and severity of the illness. At the site of such disturbances, in addition to gestures of stroking, pulling, stretching, gathering, or even winding up the illness, inhalation or blowing may be used, especially in cases of inflammatory illnesses. In some cases, illnesses that have been gathered by the hands of the practitioner are not merely shaken off, but thrown or dismissed to the west – the direction of the setting sun, symbolic of disappearance of the illness. Such removals are followed by sealing of the afflicted part of the body with the sign of the cross.

This whole comprehensive process is completed in three rounds, with removals limited to three per round, and a short break in between each round. Each session of three rounds is usually scheduled on the same day of the week for three weeks, or a day or so early if the exact day is impossible.

Like many of powwowing rituals, this elaborate process does not require the practitioner to be physically near to the patient, and can be performed remotely. For the patient, this means scheduling an appointment over the telephone[119] or some other means of communication, and following the practitioner's instructions to sit facing east just as they would if the ritual were taking place in person. The practitioner has two general means of performing the ritual remotely – either by physically enacting the whole process over an empty chair that is facing east as if the patient were present, or alternately sitting in the chair facing east, and enacting the ritual in spirit by projecting their will to the patient. This latter method is a form of trance, whereby some practitioners experience leaving their bodies for periods of time to attend to the patient.[220]

Such non-ordinary experiences among practitioners are equal and opposite to the healing experiences of those who are treated by powwowing remotely. A woman from Lebanon County who suffered from chronic swelling in her legs explained to me that during a series of remote powwow sessions, she could feel the presence of the practitioner there with her, even though he was in Berks County. She not only felt relief from the pain of the swelling, but she also distinctly felt sensations as if the practitioner's hands were actually hovering just inches from her body.

Remote work in powwowing is by no means common among all practitioners, and many prefer face-to-face direct interaction. Interestingly enough, some methods of learning to powwow are inextricably related to remote work, as one has the ability to use remote techniques in the learning process as a means to practice memorized ritual procedures.

Learning and Teaching is Ritual

Just as the prayers, actions, and timing of powwowing are elements of a ritual performance, so too is the act of learning to powwow part of a ritual experience. Learning the prayers and procedures employed for healing and protection is carefully orchestrated under specific circumstances, defined by timing, repetition, oral recitation, discretion, and gender specificity.

In addition to the usual custom that a man must learn from a woman, and vice versa, the learning process is structured over a series of sessions dedicated to gradual memorization. This memorization is crucial for a future practitioner who must be able to recall the verbal components of the ritual at will, and be able to apply them appropriately in times of need.

Learning sessions are typically scheduled much in the same way as a series of healing sessions on consecutive weeks, with the exception that the number of sessions appears to vary depending upon the teacher. Some have suggested that the prayers are learned over as many as ten installments,[222] while others have learned in as few as three. At each learning session, the teacher recites the prayers and blessings for the apprentice,[223] who must be able to memorize them in manageable installments. Some teachers are only willing to say each part of the ritual once, while there are others that repeat them multiple times, but only in one session. It is possible that the latter makes for less variation in the oral tradition over time, as a repetition of three may provide additional assurance that the student has heard the prayers correctly. If a student hears the prayers only once, the likelihood of mishearing is far greater. Some present-day powwowers with whom I am familiar recalled being expected to repeat the prayers back to the teacher, allowing the teacher to correct their pronunciation or content. Despite the carefully orchestrated nature of the ritual of teaching and learning, of the nearly dozen powwowers that I've personally known, no two people describe this process exactly the same. In fact, some appear to have learned with virtually no structure at all.

In my own experience with a traditional healer near Kutztown, I learned over the course of three sessions, and memorized a long series of prayers that varied in length and were distributed unevenly throughout the sessions. In each session, I learned both verbal blessings, their use, and the accompanying actions. In some cases, the blessings were short enough to learn more than one per session. I memorized the prayers line by line as a form of call and response, and they were each repeated three times. The bulk of the prayers were in Pennsylvania Dutch, but some were in English.

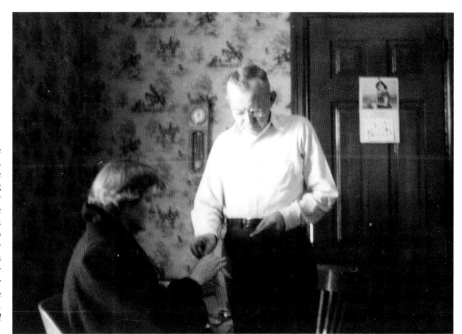

A powwow doctor making change for a client, from a series of undated, unidentified photographs from the papers of Dr. Don Yoder, featuring a series of early twentieth-century Pennsylvania healers in action. The woman in the images, possibly a reporter or journalist, appears to have visited at least four powwow doctors, and some of the photographs emphasize the exchange of money in free will offerings. It is unclear whether the practitioners were aware that they were being photographed. *Pennsylvania German Cultural Heritage Center, Kutztown University.*

During each session, my teacher powwowed me, and taught me new portions of the rituals. Beginning on my second session, I was also expected to demonstrate what I had learned in the previous session in order to confirm that I was taking the process seriously, and so I would powwow my teacher.

Between sessions, I was encouraged to practice what I was learning in a few ways. For the blessings, prayers, and oral portions of the tradition, I could practice through rounds of silent repetition in order to commit the words to memory. In order to review the full orchestration of the ritual process, I was encouraged to practice in two ways. First, I could place a chair in a discrete location facing east, and by imagining myself passively sitting in the chair, I would physically enact the whole procedure as though I were in two places at once. When I felt more confident with the specifics, I could try the exercise in reverse, by actually sitting in the chair, and imagining myself outside of my body, actively performing the rituals. This latter form of practice is not unlike certain forms of visualization meditation, aiming to project one's will outside of the body. The goal of these types of exercises are to leave lasting impressions in one's physical, mental, and spiritual make-up, so that one is no longer merely following prescribed actions, but internalizing them.

At any time during these sessions, at my teacher's discretion, the process of learning could have been ended had I not fulfilled my obligations. I had only a few rules by which I was asked to abide: No discussion of the tradition was to take place for whimsical purposes. One should not powwow after drinking any amount of alcohol, and under no circumstances should one powwow a person who is intoxicated. I was only to powwow when I was feeling physically well, and not when sick or otherwise compromised. One additional rule did not apply to me, but was a warning for women to avoid powwowing during the time of menstruation.[224] I was only to powwow when necessary for the benefit of others and not for monetary remuneration. I was not to teach anyone else except through the same protocol that I had learned. I was to commit the rituals to memory and not to write them down.

Although many accounts describe the learning and healing process as being a deliberate act of secrecy,[225] this tends to be overstated. Any healing practitioner, whether in conventional biomedicine or culturally-specific, vernacular forms, exercises discretion as an essential part of the healing experience, whether this is in protecting the privacy of a patient or in particular aspects of therapeutic process and proprietary information. While all modern biomedicine operates under strict adherence to laws protecting a patient's right to privacy and informed consent, medical professionals are also discrete about their practice and are not likely to teach an aspiring healer, unless certain criteria are met such as medical school and licensing. Although, most vernacular healing systems are not standardized in this manner, powwowing presents criteria for learning that is culturally-defined and, at the same time, subject to variation.

The fact that many practitioners recite prayers under their breath, *sotto voce*, may at first appear to substantiate this notion of secrecy, but this assumes that the goal is concealment – rather than any number of possible reasons for speaking softly, such as discretion or humility. The use of silence, or soft speaking, is by no means foreign to prayer or other meditative, contemplative spaces. In fact, Christians could easily justify the act of speaking softly in prayer through the example of Christ:

> And when thou prayest, thou shalt not be as the hypocrites are: for they love to pray standing in the synagogues and in the corners of the streets, that they may be seen of men. Verily I say unto you, they have their reward. But thou, when thou prayest, enter into thy closet, and when thou hast shut thy door, pray to thy Father which is in secret; and thy Father which seeth in secret shall reward thee openly.[226]

While the English translation of this passage uses the word "secret," the intention here is not secrecy for the purpose of concealment, privilege, or power, but humility and integrity. For powwow practitioners who take this to heart, it may also suggest that the content of the words is between the practitioner and God, rather than between the patient and the practitioner. The content, through years of use and repetition, certainly serves to focus the mind of the practitioner on the work being performed. This does not necessarily imply that the patient is not affected by the experience of the sound of the prayer being whispered, or that intentionally silent portions of the experience do not in some way contribute to the aesthetics of the ritual space. On the contrary, such features of the ritual may contribute positively to a patient's state of being and encourage contemplation or restfulness, as an ancillary aspect to a healing transformation.

In the same manner, solo rituals also make use of silence and consist of acts performed privately before sunrise, and without speaking to anyone such as cures involving collection of the morning dew for the removal of freckles, warts, or growths.[227] Such silence can be compared to fasting for religious purposes, which requires abstaining from a set of normal activities in order to facilitate a different state of being, and to set a ritual activity apart from a mundane experience.

Payment as Ritual

In the same way that silence or whispering can be viewed as having broader implications in powwowing beyond notions of mere secrecy, so too do rules concerning reciprocity play an important role in ritual negotiations. A strong taboo exists concerning payment of a practitioner for services rendered, or according to a set fee schedule. Such prohibitions are no small part of powwowing's formerly widespread reputation of accessibility and affordability among the frugal Pennsylvania Dutch. However, in practice these limitations on reciprocity do not necessarily mean that no money or goods are exchanged, and there is no one uniformly accepted way of interpreting this rule.

Many powwowers will gladly accept some form of payment in the form of material favors, and such things are especially appreciated if they consist of baked goods, produce from the garden, or delicacies from the farm such as smoked meat or raw honey. Farm work or favors in kind were also accepted in some communities.[228] Others will indeed accept cash, especially if the practitioner travels, or expends their own resources in efforts to assist a patient, but the exchange should in no way be made much of – no price is to be placed upon the encounter, no change is to be made, and no promises or obligations are to result from the giving of money. A typical procedure in previous generations was to leave money on the table or place it in a discrete place. William Reppert (1881-1949) of Lebanon kept a basket by the door for freewill offerings,[229] and the retired Lutheran minister Frederick A. Weicksel (1867-1948) would hand his patients a bible following treatment, into which they could slip a dollar bill if they would so choose.[230] In the cases of both Reppert and Weicksel, they were hardly entrepreneurs, but, instead, were seniors living on fixed incomes.

Some have rationalized this cultural attitude as purely a by-product of concerns over medical licensing,[231] and fears of prosecution for fraud.[232] While, this part of the equation was certainly a reality for practitioners in the twentieth century, especially for those who may have derived a significant amount of money from powwowing, there are other factors that long predate concerns over medical licensing that continue to play a strong role in the negotiation of reciprocity, not only in powwowing, but in everyday life.

For instance, there are those who strongly believe that powwowing does not work if it is treated like a business and a price is set for treatment.[233] This is not merely an ethical concern, but one based on related ideas that suggest paying for something may nullify its effect. This belief plays out in both positive and negative forms in social interactions and powwowing. Objects used for powwowing are usually, begged, borrowed, or taken without paying – suggesting that an object's ritual function is compromised by paying for it.[234] This type of thinking is parallel to other social interactions, such as in the giving of gifts. For instance, it was once customary that if a friend or acquaintance gave you a plant as a gift, you were not to say "thank you" or pay for it, for it was believed that the plant would not grow.[235] The belief may stem from the notion that gifts are often connected with notions of obligation or guilt, and warning that friendships which are overextended by excessive giving may become unhealthy or competitive.

Others, suspecting that gifts may be given as a pretense for a curse, will exchange a penny or some nominal coin in order to nullify any negative influence or sinister ritual effect from the gift. This was once especially true of pins, which like gifts of knives or other sharp objects, were believed to ritually sever a relationship unless something was given in return.[235] Thus, for some, providing payment was a sure way to cancel the effects of ritual behavior, regardless of whether positive or negative outcomes were expected be derived from powwowing.

On the other hand, there are also powwowing narratives that highlight the belief that some form of compensation is necessary for an effective cure.[236] Such payments or gifts are not specified by price, but nonetheless reflect a sense of respect and awareness of the healer's time and efforts. In some cases, the outcome of a ritual healing is perceived to be directly related to the generosity of the patient, and stinginess can be cause for failure or delay.

In an early twentieth-century story from the Fredericksville Hotel in Berks County, a powwower was slighted when, after assisting the proprietor with an illness, was treated to a glass of beer in consideration for his services. The proprietor was stingy, however, as the glass was significantly smaller than a normal portion. Thus when the ailment was better, but not entirely gone after three sessions, the proprietor publically shamed the *Braucher* one day in the barroom for his slow-working cure. The powwower responded by saying that he could have easily cured the illness the first time around had the owner shown the courtesy of a standard glass of beer, remarking "a little cure, for a little beer."[237]

In communities of North Dakota Russian-Germans (*Volga-Deitsch*), payment for *Brauche* is expected, however, such payments are typically placed in church offering plates, paying tribute, in a sense, to the role of the divine in healing outcomes.[238] Part of the hesitance among the Pennsylvania Dutch to place monetary value upon a healing ritual stems from the belief that any outcomes of powwowing are the result of encounters with the sacred. The *Braucher* serves as an intermediary, but the transformations are attributed to God. Just as it is discouraged for a powwow practitioner to set a price for services to the community, so too is it problematic to assume that a practitioner's acceptance of a donation or free-will offering suggests that cures can be purchased or commodified.

As with numerous ethical stances in powwowing, biblical narratives provide some level of precedent for rejecting the equivalence of monetary value with spiritual healing: After Elisha cures Naaman's leprosy, he refuses payment. "As the LORD liveth, before whom I stand, I will receive none. And [Naaman] urged him to take it; but he refused."[239] By this, Elisha asserts that the gifts of God are not to be sold or assigned a value. Instead Elisha's servant Gehazi secretly accepts the goods from Naaman, whereby Elisha rebukes him, and Gehazi receives Naaman's leprosy:

> Is it a time to receive money, and to receive garments, and oliveyards, and vineyards, and sheep, and oxen, and menservants, and maidservants? The leprosy therefore of Naaman shall cleave unto thee, and unto thy seed for ever. And he went out from his presence a leper as white as snow.[240]

Accounts in the Gospel of Matthew likewise admonish healers from acceping money. Christ sends his disciples out to do good works in the community, with strict instructions:

> And when he had called unto him his twelve disciples, he gave them power against unclean spirits, to cast them out, and to heal all manner of sickness and all manner of disease… And as ye go, preach, saying, the kingdom of heaven is at hand. Heal the sick, cleanse the lepers, raise the dead, cast out devils: freely ye have received, freely give. Provide neither gold, nor silver, nor brass in your purses…[241]

After Christ's death and resurrection, the apostles continued his work, providing numerous precedents for healing, including the rejection of monetary remuneration for receiving spiritual gifts of the Holy Spirit. Among many descriptions of healing miracles through the laying on of hands, the Book of Acts describes an encounter with a newly converted Christian, and former sorcerer named Simon of Samaria, who attempts to purchase spiritual gifts of the Holy Spirit from Peter and John:

> …when Simon saw that through laying on of the apostles' hands the Holy Spirit was given, he offered them money, Saying, Give me also this power, that on whomsoever I lay hands, he may receive the Holy Spirit. But Peter said unto him, Thy money perish with thee, because thou hast thought that the gift of God may be purchased with money…[242]

This injunction also resonates with perspectives concerning the process of learning to powwow, suggesting that monetary compensation for learning to facilitate acts of healing is forbidden. In one sense, this correlates to the ethic of oral transmission for the tradition, which stresses face to face interactions and discourages not only the commodification of healing prayers and processes in the form of publications, but also the reliance on such publications rather than committing ritual practices to memory. Nevertheless, a wide range of instructive powwowing literature for sale has served to promote the tradition, as well as simultaneously challenge and reinforce some of its core values.

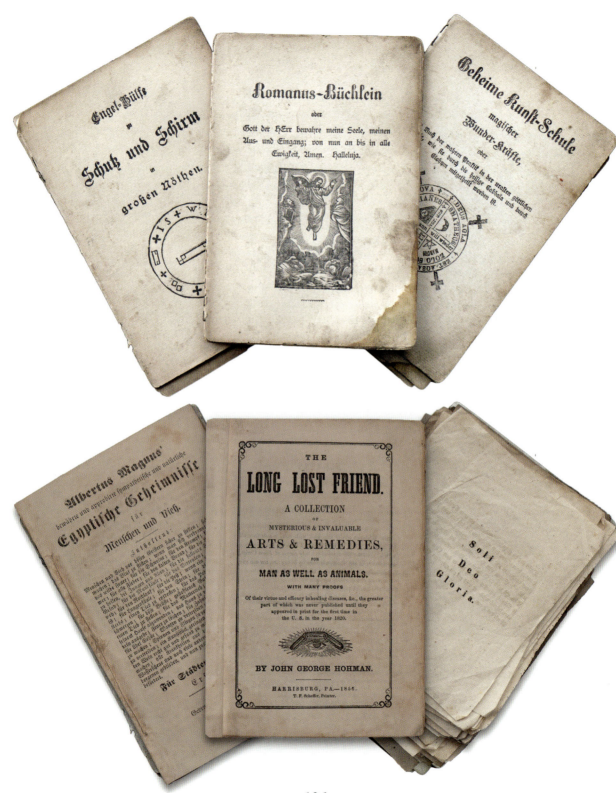

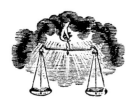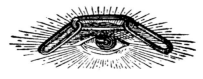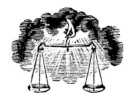

Chapter V
Ritual Literature
Manuscripts, Books, Broadsides

The rituals and techniques employed by powwow healers are informed by generations of oral tradition; however a wide range of literature has accumulated on the subject in Pennsylvania, and most of this material is derived directly from European sources. Personal manuscripts, broadsides, almanacs, chapbooks of household and veterinary remedies, and voluminous collections of benedictions and blessings all play a role in the literary record of ritual practices in Pennsylvania and wherever powwowing spread with the migration of the culture throughout North America.

These works contain instructions for ritual procedures in varying levels of detail, ranging from simple healing and protective benedictions to elaborate descriptions of complex processes scripted for performance with words, symbolic actions, objects, *materia medica*, and directions for timing and setting. Many of the simplest instructions lack any sense of context and are recorded in a manner that leaves much of the ritual performance to rely upon implicitly assumed prior knowledge from the reader, or open to the possibility of individual interpretation. Although many works spuriously claim to be from authoritative literary voices such as St. Albert the Great, Aristotle, Pope Leo X, or Moses,[1] others are simply anonymous, deriving their allure from the suggestion of mysterious origins. For a handful of successful, published powwow manuals, local Pennsylvania authors and compilers made no attempts to conceal their identities and developed their books and pamphlets for a general audience.

No matter how seemingly authoritative or widely accessible such works have been, a strong taboo discourages the use of literary sources for powwowing beyond personal reference, and reading from books other than the Bible in ritual performance is viewed negatively. This attitude regarding what is allowed or preferable within the bounds of ritual space, is not condemning of written or printed sources. Instead, tradition suggests literary works contain words and instructions that should be internalized by the practitioner through memorization and employed fluidly for the benefit of another, rather than being read directly from a scripted source. Otherwise, one runs the risk of inadvertently creating the appearance that such books - rather than divine forces – empower the ritual process. Incorporating a book in such a manner would seem to suggest that the book is a powerful component of the ritual as opposed to an instructive text. The idea of ritually powerful books is commonly associated with *Hexerei*, rather than with powwowing. The only book which does not provoke such concerns in ritual space is the Bible and, in some rare cases, a prayer book or hymnal.

In addition, although the taboo associated with recording the oral tradition in writing has created a sense of ambivalence towards ritual literature, it is important to recognize the undeniable interrelation between written, printed, and oral material. These three parallel traditions are mutually interrelated, with variations of oral traditions appearing in print, manuscripts copied from printed works, and oral traditions both memorized from and preserved in private manuscripts. It is generally agreed that written and printed sources were derived at some point in history from oral traditions that had not been previously part of a literary corpus. However, printed works have been in circulation for centuries, and written sources have recorded similar practices as early as the 10th century.[2] Thus, the oral tradition of today can claim hybrid origins, rather than a purely linear, oral provenance.

The earliest known work of powwow ritual procedures written in Pennsylvania is the 1775 manuscript

Top: Three of the most popularly distributed German-language ritual manuals in Europe and parts of South America, *Engel-Hülf zu Schutz und Schirm in großen Nöthen* (Angelic Assistance as Shield and Guard in Times of Great Emergency), *Das Romanus-Büchlein* (The Little Book of Romanus), *Geheime Kunst-Schule magische Wunder-Kräfte* (Secret School of Ritual Arts and Magical Miraculous Powers).
Bottom: Thee most significant Pennsylvania powwowing manuals, Albertus Magnus' *Egyptische Geheimnisse* (Egyptian Secrets of St. Albert the Great), *The Long Lost Friend*, and Dr. G. F. Helfenstein's *Secrets of Sympathy, or Soli Deo Gloria* (Glory to God Alone).

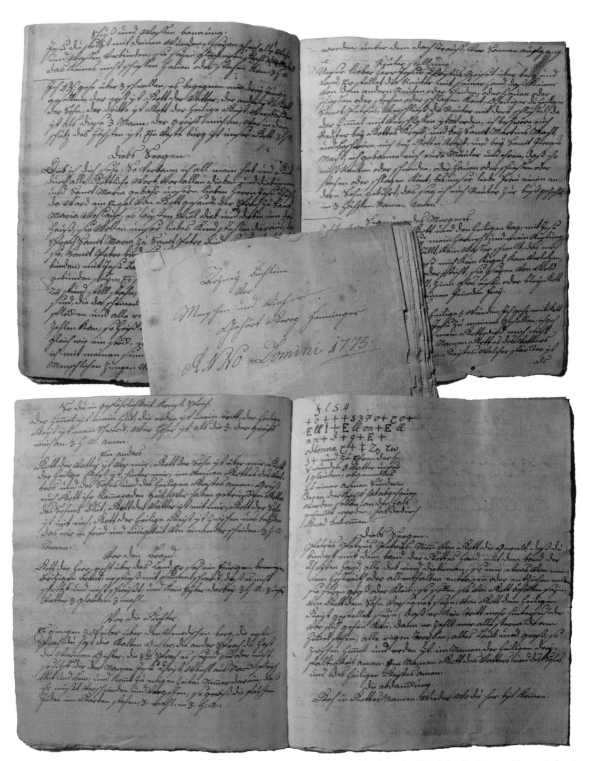

Arzneÿ Büchlein für Menschen und Vieh, Gehört Georg Henninger, ANNO Domini 1775 (Little Book of Medicine for Man and Beast, Belonging to George Henninger, in the Year of Our Lord 1775). Albany Township, Berks County. *Heilman Collection.*

of Johann Georg Henninger (1737-1815). Henninger was an Alsatian emigrant and the son of a weaver Johan Martin and his wife Anna Catharina (Fuchs) Henninger, born on April 13th, 1737, in the small town of Hatten, just a mere ten miles west of the Rhine River. In 1763 he crossed the Atlantic aboard the ship *Chance*, and made his way to Albany Township, Berks County, where it is likely that he penned his manuscript.[3]

Henninger's work consists of two parts: The first is a series of lengthy transcriptions from a European medical booklet, *Kurzgefasstes Arzney Büchlein für Menschen und Vieh* (*Little Book of Medicine for Man and Beast*), allegedly first printed in Vienna[4] and later reprinted at the Ephrata Cloister in 1791. Henninger's manuscript was produced prior to this American publication and contains 51 entries for horses, 22 for cows, and 79 for humans, with copious additions not found in the Ephrata imprint.[5] Henninger's second half is the most significant, consisting of twenty-seven rare, previously unpublished blessings used for stopping blood and convulsions, healing burns, calming fevers, protection from calamity and criminal violence, and compelling thieves to return stolen property. He also includes inscriptions to be carried on one's person to avoid false accusations, prayers for invisibility in times of danger, and instructions for creating a ceremonial knife marked with nine crosses used in rituals for protection.[6]

One of the simplest entries in Henninger's manuscript consists of a classic three-fold poetic blessing to stop bleeding:

Blut-Stellung: Es stehen 3 rothe Rosen am Himmel
Die eine ist gut, die ander stellt's Blut, die dritte heilt's gut.
3. H. N.

A cure for bleeding: In heaven stand three roses red, The first is good, the second stops the blood, the third heals it good. In the Three Highest Names.

Henninger's Trinitarian blessing employs a poetic, non-scriptural, religious statement, whereby earthly troubles are overcome by heavenly, celestial forces, and it concludes with an invocation of the Father, Son, and Holy Spirit. A unique blessing "for invisibility" is also included in Henninger's text. This religious blessing was not intended for mischief, as one could easily assume, but instead it was a protective measure, so that anyone wishing harm upon the user would be unable to see:

Heut tritt ich über diese Schwell,
Christus Jesus mein Gesell,
Die Erd mein Schu,
Die Himmel mein Huth,
Die heilige Engel mein Schwerd,
Der mich heut siehst, ist mir Lieb und Werth,
Sondern meine Feind müssen Verblenden,
Daß sie mich an keinen Orten noch finden,
Daß gebe mir Gott und liebe Frau

Woran daß ich greifen, dem muss ich gleichen.
15 Vater Unser, 5 Glauben, 3 Mahl.

Today I step over the threshold, Christ is my comrade, The earth is my shoes, and the heavens are my hat, The holy angel is my sword. Only those who love and value me will see me today, Otherwise my enemies must be blind, that in no place shall they see or find me, this be granted to me by God and Our Dear Lady, that whosoever I engage, I shall match them. 15 Our Fathers, 5 Creeds, 3 times.

A careful reading of the original German renders a poetic series of metered, rhyming couplets, and the blessing concludes with four lines of cross-rhyme. The rhyming serves both poetic and utilitarian functions because it allowed for ease of memorization. This mnemonic function is found in a wide range of religious prayers intended for recitation from memory in both official and folk-religious settings. It is notable that Henninger's blessing concludes with instructions that are also part of the rhyming scheme, including fifteen recitations of the Lord's Prayer and five of the Apostles' Creed, repeated in three rounds. While Henninger himself was a Lutheran and attended church in Grimsville, Berks County, his material is clearly derived from a well-established oral tradition that predates the Reformation and retains the marks of its Roman Catholic origins.

In contrast, Henninger also included a blessing against criminal violence that includes the opening line from Luther's classic Protestant hymn, "*Ein' Feste Berg ist Unser Gott*" (*A Mighty Fortress is Our God*). In this application, the "mighty fortress" is invoked as a protective shield to counteract physical and spiritual harm. This echoes other uses of Protestant hymnody for ritual purposes such as the classic song "*Herr Jesu dir leb ich, Herr Jesu dir sterb ich, Herr Jesu dein bin ich todt un lebendig...*" (Lord Jesus, I live to thee, Lord Jesus I die to thee, Lord Jesus, I am thine, in death and in life...), which was incorporated into blessings to safeguard one against danger.[7]

In addition to verbal blessings, Henninger also incorporates sympathetic procedures with decidedly religious overtones:

Vor alle Fieber, Dreÿ Freÿtag vor der Sonnen aufgang, in ein fliessend Wasser baarfuss, gegen Sonnen aufgang gestanden, den rechten voran gestellt, und gesprochen, Wasser ich tritte, Herr Jesu Christ ich bitte, gib mir von deinem Fleisch und Blut, das ist vor alles sicher und gut. + + + 3 Glauben, 3 Vatter Unser.

For all fevers, three Fridays before the rising of the sun, stand barefoot in flowing water [facing west] away from the rising of the sun, with the right foot extended forward, and say: Water, I kick thee. Lord Jesus Christ, I bid thee: give to me of thy flesh and blood, which for everything is sure and good. + + + 3 Creeds, 3 Lord's Prayers.

Henninger's blessings to be used against criminal violence are benedictions to ensure protection from guns, highwaymen, and bullets. These invocations brought from the Rhineland highlight concerns for personal safety in times of political and domestic turmoil and were equally applicable to the anxieties of settlers in the early American scene. One of these blessings includes an entourage of saints, including saints George and Martin, who are not frequently included in other powwowing materials, suggesting an early European provenance:

> Unser Herr Jesus Christus reiset über Berg und Land, Er stellet die Reuter mit seiner Hand, dass keiner von dem andern Reuten oder scheiden, oder hauen oder schiesse oder stechen oder schlagen kont, O heiliger du heiliger Sanct Petrus, verschliess die Reuter mit dem Schlüssel da der Himmel mit verschlissen ist werden, ich beschwöre euch Reuter beÿ Gottes Kraft und beÿ Sanct Martins Macht, und beschwöre euch beÿ Gottes Krafft und beÿ Sanct Georgis Macht, ich gebanne euch eure Mäuler und Ohren, dass ihr nicht Reuten oder schneiden, oder hauen oder schiessen oder stechen oder schlagen könt, bis unser liebe Frau einen andern Sohn geburt, das sag ich euch Reuter zur Buss gezehlt, in 3 Höchsten Namen Amen.

> Our Lord Jesus journeys over the mountains and lands, and he stoppeth the riders with his hand, so that none of the others can ride or depart, cut or shoot, stab or strike. O saints! Thou saint Peter, lock the riders with the keys with which the heavens are locked. I adjure you riders by the power of God and by the might of Saint Martin, and I adjure you riders by the power of God and the might of Saint George. I bind thee thy mouths and ears, that ye cannot ride or depart, cut or shoot, stab or strike, until our dear Lady beareth another Son. This I reckon unto you riders as penance, in the Three Highest Names, Amen.

Other blessings in Henninger's collection are clearly meant for use in times of war. One particular procedure invokes the story of Christ's release of the captives in the land of the dead,[8] which is described in the Apostles' Creed and dramatized in the Roman Catholic legend of the "Harrowing of Hell" as Christ's triumphant storming of the infernal gates:

> N: N: Zeuch hin in den Streit, Wie Gott der Herr, der die Thür der Höllen zerbrach, und ihn kein Leÿt gschah, also soll dir N: N: auch geschehen, das dich kein Büchs nicht krült, kein Baum nicht schnellt, kein schwerd oder bogen nicht schneid, davor behüt dich Gott heut und allezeit, bis ich dich wider sehe. 3 H[öchsten]. N[amen]. Amen

> N.N. Go forth into the battle. As the Lord God hath broken the doors of hell, and no injury befell him, therefore shall it also happen unto thee, N. N., that no gun shall fire, no tree shall overturn, no blade nor bow shall cut, therefore protect thee God, today and all time, until I see thee once again, in the Three Highest Names, Amen.

Manuscripts like Henninger's text, ranging from notations on slips of paper to lengthy collections of ritual procedures, can present significant challenges for those who find them among family papers, ledgers, or tucked into Bibles. The majority of these writings were not produced for posterity, but instead for private reference. Unless these powwow documents are used or found within a family, provenance can be difficult to establish without personalized inscriptions such as dates, names, or locations. Furthermore, even if such information is available, the majority of these texts were not written in English and instead were penned in non-standardized forms of early German. Even for those who are well-versed in modern Standard German, the task of translating these documents can be extremely difficult as there is substantial variability in early language for spelling, vocabulary, and grammar.

A dated sample from Northampton County provides some insight into the variability of German-language blessings recorded by speakers of English:

> 1837 The property of John Shively his paper a cure for sick cows when they have the blood:

> Buge und strige Blude Wige in Dos Say Ouse Dem Say in Den Rine Ouse Dem Rine in ine Stine Cum Nimer Mare Mit Meinem fe Do Hime.

While this text might be easily mistaken for a Pennsylvania Dutch language sample, the text is actually a High German sample written from memory by person who could not read or write German. The rendering of this German text with English phonetics maintained many of the original inflections and incorporated a few errors, but the English vowels are perhaps the biggest obstacle to identifying the German words in order to arrive at a satisfactory translation.

> [Bugger und Streiche, Blut weich in den See, aus der See in den Rhein, aus dem Rhein in einen Stein. Kumm nimmer mehr mit meinem Vieh daheim.]

> Buggers and tricks! Blood yield into the lake, from the lake into the Rhine, from the Rhine into a stone. Come no more with my cattle home.

Only rarely are powwow materials actually written in Pennsylvania Dutch, even though the language still plays an important role in learning to powwow. Occasionally memorized portions of the oral tradition were written down by speakers of Pennsylvania Dutch who could not read Standard German, or even sometimes by those who only spoke English, which results in phonetic renditions of powwow prayers. This was especially true around the turn of the twentieth century, coinciding with the gradual decline of literacy in Standard German following the American Civil War and the disappearance of German-language schools in Pennsylvania.

Sophia Bailer's manuscripts for instance show signs of a native speaker of Pennsylvania Dutch who was never taught to read or write standard German. Thus her writing of the language was heavily influenced by English approximations. Another practitioner, Kate Merkel,

Buge und strige Blude wige in Dos Say Cuse Dem Say in Den Rine Cuse Dem Rine in ine stine Cum Nimer Mare Mit Minem fe Do hime

1837 — The property of John Shively his paper a Cure for Sick Cows if They have The Blood

Front and back of John Shively's cures for sick cows, written in a phonetic rendering of German, dated 1837 from Northampton County, Pennsylvania. *Heilman Collection.*

interviewed in the 1950s wrote down only her English powwowing content, and memorized all the materials in Pennsylvania Dutch.[10] When asked why, she stated that she only spoke Dutch but couldn't read or write it, otherwise, she would have written everything down. Such anecdotes reveal that not all practitioners, past or present, feel strongly in favor of the admonition against writing down the oral tradition, and have more flexible notions about their level of discretion concerning the practice.

Pennsylvania Dutch is primarily a spoken language and has only become a written means of communication since the late nineteenth century. For much of the history of the Pennsylvania Dutch community, Standard German was the official written language, and was taught in schools and used in church for hymns, catechism, and sermons, as well as in legal documents such as deeds and wills, and for popular publications, such as almanacs and newspapers.

The Pennsylvania Dutch vernacular language, however, was the predominant language in everyday use in the home and in the community, and mirrors the use of oral forms in relation to written forms of language all over the world. Unlike standard languages, which are usually subject to explicit norms of usage, oral vernaculars such as Pennsylvania Dutch, by their very nature, are subject to greater variation and change over time. Ironically, it is commonly presumed that dialects (regionally defined vernacular languages) develop as a deviation or departure of standard language, but the opposite is true. Dialects predate their standard official counterparts. Pennsylvania Dutch is descended from the Rhenish-Franconian German dialects of the eleventh Century historically spoken in western central Germany. Yiddish, which also has its origins in Rhenish-Franconian German, is a close linguistic cousin to Pennsylvania Dutch. Modern Standard German is most closely related to written varieties in use in fifteenth and sixteenth-century Saxony in the eastern region of central Germany.[11]

Cypher Script

In addition to challenges resulting from Pennsylvania's variable language structure, some practitioners keeping private manuscripts created complex cypher scripts in order to obscure their texts from prying eyes. Some cyphers are merely numerical, with a number substituted for each letter,[12] while others are based in a series of symbols known only to the practitioner. An extensive manuscript written by Johann Kauffmann of Lancaster features a cypher that is peppered throughout the text.[13] Kauffmann introduces the title page of his cleanly bound journal with an inscription reading in translation: "This book belongs to me, John Kauffman, and I bought it for 2 Shillings and 10 Pence from the bookprinter in Lancaster on the 10th of September, 1789." Only the first portion of Kauffmann's book features the cypher that obscures just certain words rather than whole passages. This means that, given a little time and effort, I was able to crack the cypher by process of elimination. Again, variable spelling common to the time period only added to the challenge, but context

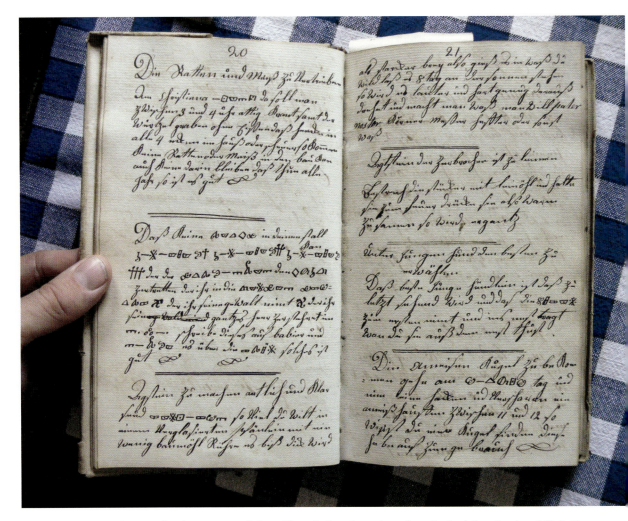

Lancaster practitioner Johann Kauffman's 1789 powwow ledger, with entries in cypher script, and a cypher key below. Courtesy of Clarke Hess.

from the surrounding words provided significant clues for completing the translation.

A seemingly unique entry in Kauffman's cypher describes a written blessing to be placed above the stable door to protect from a *Hex*. The inscription invokes an avenging angel Paraeuel, and the inscription that follows is derived from the Book of Genesis when God curses the snake:

"And I will put enmity between thee and the woman, and between thy seed and her seed; it shall bruise thy head, and thou shalt bruise his heel."[14]

> Paraeuel + Paraeuel ++ Paraeuel+++
> She shalt tread upon the serpent's head
> and he will strike her heel.
> She will take his power,
> but he shall destroy her entire army.
> In the Name of the Father, Son, and Holy Spirit. Amen[15]

In this case, Kauffmann's entry assumes that the *Hex* is female, and it is the serpent (the devil) who is striking her down, as well as her entourage of spirits.

```
S A T O R
A R E T O
T E S E T
O T E R A
N D T A S
```

Dieses sind ietzt die 25 Buchstaben und ist das Gesang welche die 3 männer Sadrach Mesach und Abedurgo gesungen haben die der König Nebucadnezer in den feurigen ofen hat werfen lassen denen hat gott einen heiligen engel geschickt der sie in der grausamen feuers gluth bewahret hat zu lesen im Propheten Daniel am 3 Capitel wer nun ein solches Lied bey sich trächgt oder im hause hat dem wird nicht leicht ein unglück über sein haus kommen sein hauß wird ihm auch nicht verbrennen auch wird ihm kein Donner oder wildes feuer einschlagen wenn auch kleine Kinder die gichter haben so schreibe die 25 Buchstaben auf einen Zettel lege es den Kindern unter den Rücken 2 stunden so ist das Kind frey und wird es sein lebtag nicht mehr bekomen ist an vilen proBirt worden wann iemand von einem wütenden hund gebissen und man gibt ihm diese worte zu essen so wirds ihm nicht schaden

An early manuscript variation of the SATOR square and an explanation of the "25 Letters" copied from the early powwow manual entitled *Various Sympathetic and Secret Ritual Arts (Verschiedene Sympathetische und Geheime Kunst-Stücke)*, ca. 1800. The manuscript was owned by the descendants of a Berks County healer. *Gift of Tammy Mitgang. Pennsylvania German Cultural Heritage Center Kutztown University.*

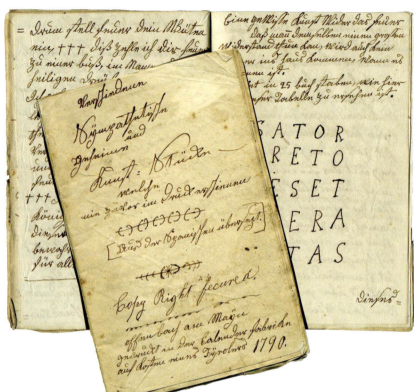

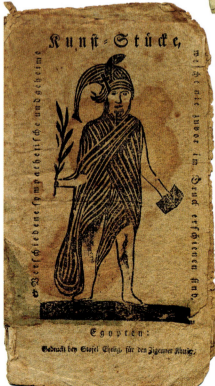

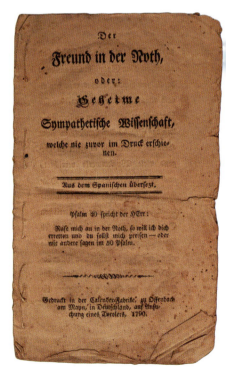

Clockwise from the top:
Isaac N. Kilmer's manuscript copy of the 1805 Reading imprint by Jungman & Bruckman of *Verschiedene Sympathetische und Geheime Kunst-Stücke* (*Various Sympathetic and Secret Ritual Arts*) ca. 1828, Stouchsburg, Berks County. Note the misspelled "Copy Right fecured" on the front of Kilmer's pirated transcription. *Heilman Collection.*

Der Freund in der Noth (*The Friend in Need*) 1813, printed by Johann Ritter, Reading, Pennsylvania. A lesser-known collection of cures and rituals, compiled by Johann Georg Hohman in 1813. Contents are identical to the *Kunst-Stücke. Heilman Collection.*

Verschiedene sympathetische und geheime Kunst-Stücke (Various Sympathetic and Secret Ritual Arts) ca. 1800, containing the false imprint "Egypt: Printed for the Gypsy King," with a woodcut of the Gypsy King, complete with book and stylus. *Pennsylvania German Cultural Heritage Center Kutztown University.*

An Early Healing Manual

Most of Johann Kauffmann's contents were also included in one of the earliest known printed powwow manuals in Pennsylvania, issued under several variations of the title, *Die Kunst-Stücke* roughly translated as "Ritual Arts."[16] This collection of remedies and rituals purports to have been discovered in the dwelling of a hermit who lived in a cave for over a century in a remote valley in the Swiss canton of Graubünden, where the hermit was famous for having driven away a dragon from the mountains of Unterwalden. The introduction alleges that the miraculous deeds of this wise and legendary hermit were recorded in 1752 in Freiburg in Üechtland, Switzerland, and printed by Hans von Leixner, but the existence of such a work has yet to be substantiated.[17]

The *Kunst-Stücke* appeared whole and in part in manuscript and printed form between the years of 1780 and 1830, with four separate editions printed after 1800 in Reading, Pennsylvania,[18] not to mention other editions in western Pennsylvania[19] and an English edition printed at Boonsboro, Maryland.[20] Usually consisting of about 36 entries, the work contained instructions for healing fevers, benedictions for protection from criminal violence, how to compel thieves to return stolen property, and instructions to extinguish fire without water, as well as a short section on "Omens and Their Meanings." Two separate entries in the printed versions of the *Kunst-Stücke* contain passages in numerical cypher, suggesting that the text was published from an earlier manuscript without deciphering the original text.[21]

One of the more unusual portions of the text includes a unique interpretation and spelling of the ancient SATOR square palindrome, and ties it to the biblical story in the Book of Daniel of the three holy Hebrew men, Hananiah, Mishael, and Azariah, (or Shadrach, Meshach and Abednego), who were condemned to death in a fiery furnace for their piety during the Babylonian captivity. According to the story, a miracle occurred when an angel of the Lord delivered them, and they emerged from the furnace unscathed.

```
S A T O R
A R E T O
T E S E T
O T E R A
R O T A S
```

These here are the 25 letters, and it is the song sung by the three men Schadrach, Meschack and Abednego, whom King Nebuchadnezaar threw into the fiery furnace. God sent a holy angel to them, who protected them in the cruel inferno, as can be read in the Prophet Daniel, in the 3rd chapter. Whoever now carrieth such a song with him, or hath it in his house, misfortune will not come easily unto him. His house will also not burn, likewise no thunder nor wildfire will strike him. Also when small children have convulsions, then write the 25 letters on a slip of paper, and lay it under the back of the child for 24 hours. Thus will the child be free from the convulsions, and will suffer it not a day more in its life.[22]

This story and the ritual application of the SATOR square highlights the once popular interest among the Pennsylvania Dutch in extra-biblical revelations found in the Apocrypha, a non-canonical portion of scriptural writings commonly included in Catholic and Protestant German family Bibles well into the twentieth century.[23] While these works are considered historically significant, they are no longer part of mainstream Protestant religious traditions. The Apocrypha included a book entitled, *The Song of the Holy Children*, which provides a transcription of the long, chanted prayer of Azariah, Hananiah and Mishael, allegedly excised from the Book of Daniel. While this litany is rich in cosmological imagery — calling upon the sun and moon, stars and heavens, light and darkness, night and day, heat and cold, etc., to praise the name of the Lord — there is little indication of why and how the SATOR square, called "*Die 25 Buchstaben*" (25 Letters), was presented as a codified version of Azariah's Song. Nevertheless, this version of the palindrome square, with and without its accompanying explanation of Azariah's Song, appeared in several subsequent powwow manuals, including one by the celebrated author Johann Georg Hohman, as well as in several works of midwifery.

Midwifery Manuals

Among the earliest known printed books of ritual instructions in Pennsylvania are works of midwifery, attributed to the Swabian bishop, St. Albert the Great and the Greek philosopher Aristotle, entitled *Kurzgefasstes Weiber-Büchlein. Enthaelt Aristoteli und A. Magni Hebammen-Kunst* (*Concise Women's Booklet, Containing the Midwifery of Aristotle and Albertus Magnus*), printed in four editions in the 1790s by Benjamin Mayer (1762-1824) from the brotherhood at the Ephrata Cloister, and by a related printer Salomon Mayer (d. 1811) at York. Although the bulk of this material includes conventional medicine of the times for fertility, prenatal care, child birth, and postpartum care, an addendum includes a series of useful rituals for domestic use, including the earliest known American publication of the celebrated, ancient SATOR square palindrome.[24]

The midwifery manual opens with the biblical verse "*Den wehmüttern die Gott fürchten, bauet Er Häuser.*" (And it came to pass, because the midwives feared God, that he made them houses).[25] Interesting typographical pieces are featured on the title page borrowed from the printing of the farmer's almanac, such as the image of the crescent moon and the signs of Gemini and Virgo, depicting twins and the virgin — all symbols suggestive of the health of women and children. Some later editions are also bound in wraps made from recycled almanac pages bearing the same type.[26]

While the bulk of materials contained in these midwifery books is not specifically powwowing, but rather basic herbal and clinical care of the times, such distinctions mattered little to the readers, who applied herbal medicine in an equally ritualized manner. Herbs and botanicals were not merely the vectors of healing compounds, but part of a symbolic world. This association with powwowing and herbal medicine is further corroborated by the fact that herbals contain manuscript entries of powwowing in the fly leaves.

One such example is found in the pages of a later edition of the *Concise Women's Booklet* including a supplement on dyeing printed by Gottlob Jungman and Carl Andreas Bruckman of Reading in 1802. The manuscript entries are for side stitches in a young man who is not only named in the text, but his father's name and location in Lehigh County is included in the words of the blessing:[27]

> *Vor daß stechen: Achen und stechen und Drogen gingen mit einander den berg hin auf begegnet im unser lieber Herr Jesus Christ. Achen und stechen wo wilt du hie? In Heidelberg Daunschip in des Görg Römölÿ sein Haus und will den Henerich Remelÿ sein fleisch und blut auf saugen Drohen das solt du nicht thun. Du solt gehen in einen wilden Wald, da ist ein Brinlein kühl und kalt, Da solt du drinken und essen und solt dem Henerich Römölÿ sein fleisch und blut vergessen das zehl ich im zuhr buss im X X X Du must aber hinaus under den freÿen Himmel gehen und gegen einen Wald wenden mit dein Angesicht abens und morgens unberuffen.*
>
> For side stiches: Aches, stitches, and pressing pains went together up the mountain, there they came upon our dear Lord Jesus Christ. "Aches and Stitches, whither goest thou?" "In Heidelberg Township, into the house of George Remeli, to devour the flesh and blood of Henry Remeli." "This you shall not do. You shall go into the wild wood, where there is a well, cool and cold. There you shall eat and drink, and forget the flesh and blood of Henry Remeli, this I render to him as penance in [the Name of the Father, Son, and Holy Spirit, Amen] X X X Thou must go outside under the open sky and [say the following words] with thy face turned towards the woods, evening and morning before speaking to anyone.

Side stitches, which are understood as relatively harmless today, were once considered to be part of a class of unexplained phantom pains that ranged from mild to severe and were occasionally debilitating. In cases such as these, illnesses were grouped with similar symptoms, based on location in the body and subjective, experiential descriptions, without regard to the cause of such disorders. Thus the idea of "stitches" could be applied to any and all abdominal pains including pleurisy, spleen disorders, and cramps, especially those resulting from physical activity.

Inscriptions in powwow manuals such as these are highly significant sources of biographical and genealogical data, reflecting not only the beliefs and practices of the family, but also the distribution of printed works throughout the region. This inscription for healing Henry Remeli(1777-1836) suggests that this midwifery book is likely to have belonged to his mother Maria Magdalena (Kocher) Remeli, who never inscribed the book with her own name. Even the handwriting of the inscription appears to be that of her husband George Remeli (1751-1827).[28] His name appears on the 1780 rolls of the Northampton County Militia under the command of Capt. Conrad Reader, and he owned a farm (*Plantasche*) in Heidelberg Township with additional lands in East Penn Township, and appears in the Census records of 1790-1820. In a time when documentation of the lives of women was largely defined by the writings created and left behind by men, Maria's engagement with the literature of midwifery and ancillary ritual practices is tacitly confirmed by the evidence in her midwifery manual.

Powwow Manual Inscriptions

As with prayer books, Bibles, and other significant works in Pennsylvania Dutch households, manuals of ritual instructions often bear the marks of ownership. In some cases inscriptions are as simple as a name, or as detailed as Henry Remeli's cure for side stitches. Others are formulaic, like the inscription of Samuel Leith found in an English-language collection of remedies printed in Schellsburg, Bedford County, for compiler Daniel Ballmer of Chambersburg:

> Samuel Leith is my name Heaven is my station in Lower Saucon Township Northampton County is my dwelling place and Christ is my Savior When I am Dead and in my Grave, and All my Bones are Rotten this Book will tell my Name When others have forgotten the Rose is Dear the leaves are grene an, look at this End think at me. When I am quite forgotten But now. if I Should Chance to lent this Book to any Friend of mine I Pray they may take great Care to Send it home in Time, So Much from me Samuel Leith January 12th A.. D.. 1837.[29]

While some took the time to inscribe and personalize their powwowing manuals, rarely are such works illuminated in the same manner as treasured religious texts. One particularly elaborate Pennsylvania document from 1892-93, decorated with stars and inscribed to a Lillie A. Moyer by an unnamed "friend," describes another cure for wildfire:

> For the Wildfire to Powwow:
>
> *Weldas.Faear.Weldar Brand.Fluck.and.Schmarz.Gerunnen. Blut.and.Kaldar.Brand Eech.um.faha.Dech.gott.der.harr. Ba.wara.Dech.gott.der.Est.Dar.allar.hachsta.man.Dar.Dech. Weldasfire.Weldar.Bran.Fluck.and.Schmarz.garunnen.Blut. And.Kaldan.Brand.and.Allan.Schadan.Wedar fon. Der:n Fardraeban.kan.+ + +*

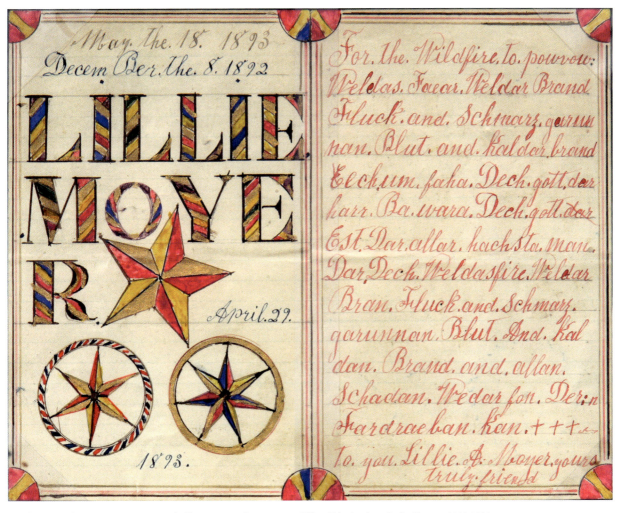

The illuminated powwow instructions of Lillie A. Moyer for treating wildfire, Tulpehocken, Berks County, 1892-1893. Formerly of the Lester P. Breininger Collection. *Heilman Collection.*

Wildfire and inflammation, rash and pain, running blood and gangrene, I circle thee. The Lord God protect thee. God is the highest one that can cast thee out, wildfire, inflammation, rash and pain, running blood and gangrene, and direct all harm, away from [baptismal name].+ + +

This document includes three separate dates between 1892 and 1893, and is signed "To you Lillie A. Moyer, yours truly, Friend," suggesting the possibility that the creator of the piece may have taught Lillie to powwow on the dates provided in on the document. Although the words of the cure were clearly transcribed from an oral source committed to memory, the text finds its origin in one of the most widely circulated books on both sides of the Atlantic: *The Egyptian Secrets of Albertus Magnus.*

Albertus Magnus

Like the early Pennsylvania works of midwifery, this work was also ascribed to St. Albert the Great, entitled *Albertus Magnus bewährte und approbirte sympathetische und natürliche Aegyptische Geheimnisse für Menschen und Vieh* (*Albertus Magnus' Tried and Approved Sympathetic and Natural Egyptian Secrets for Man and Beast*). European editions bearing imprints from the early eighteenth century appear to have made their way across the Atlantic with immigrant families, and later editions were imported by book sellers and reprinted in Pennsylvania throughout the nineteenth century.

Egyptians Secrets provides remedies and rituals for the purpose of healing, as well as a lengthy introduction describing the use of ritual among the righteous to

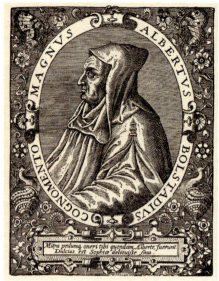 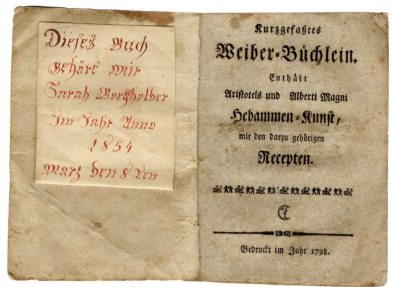

Left to Right: Portrait of St. Albert the Great, alleged author of several works of medicine, midwifery, and magic; *Kurzgefaßtes Weiber-Büchlein. Enthält Aristotels und Alberti Magni Hebammen Kunst* (*Concise Little Book for Women, Containing the Midwifery of Aristotle and St. Albert the Great*), Ephrata, Pennsylvania, 1791. Formerly of the Lester P. Breininger Collection. *Heilman Collection.*

counteract the works of the devil and his servants. An example of one classic ritual of exorcism included in the work aims to heal and protect one who is assailed by sorcery:

> Thou arch-sorcerer spirit, thou hast assailed N.N., so withdraw away from her, back into thy marrow, and into thy bone, as it was spoken to thee, I dismiss thee, by the five wounds of Jesus, thou evil spirit, and I dismiss thee, by the five wounds of Jesus, thou evil spirit, and I dismiss thee by the five wounds of Jesus from this flesh, marrow and bone, I dismiss thee, by the 5 wounds of Jesus at this very hour, let N.N. become well again, in the name of God the Father, of God the Son, and of God the Holy Spirit, Amen.[30]

It is clear from both the subject matter and the tone of the work that it was not actually written by the Swabian-born St. Albert the Great, who was distinguished for his philosophical and academic contributions to Europe as a Doctor of the Roman Catholic Church. Nevertheless, a whole body of pseudo-epigraphical, esoteric literature developed around this influential saint, such as *Secretis Muleorum* (Women's Secrets), another popular work of midwifery, and his alleged collected works *Book of Aggregations* (*Liber Aggregationis*) describing the virtues of herbs, minerals, and animals for ritual purposes. These latter works were printed in many editions in the seventeenth and eighteenth centuries, while the precise date of the first edition of *Egyptian Secrets* has been surrounded with some doubt. Many editions of the work claim to have been printed in 1725 in Brabant, and reprinted in Cologne, while some have suggested that the work is as late as 1816.[31] The language of the text favors vocabulary and idioms that point to a possible European origin within the region where Swabian-Allemanic dialects are spoken.[32]

Egyptian Secrets consists of several hundred entries in three consecutive volumes bound together as one book. A number of entries appear more than once with slight variations throughout the text, and there is no overall organization for the order of the entries in the work aside from an index. Healing remedies range from formulaic blessings, to concoctions of herbs and substances, both common and obscure, as well as sympathetic procedures for everything from opening locks to divination with bird songs. Many parallel entries can be found from the *Romanus-Büchlein,* which appears to be the predecessor to *Egyptian Secrets*, and other cures are attributed to the oral traditions employed by practitioners from a variety of locations in Europe, whence they came:

> A Mecklenburg farmer's formula to prevent any dog from becoming rabid:
> Dogs should have scraped silver filings given to them upon a piece of bread and butter, on Christmas Eve, New Year's Eve, and on the Eve of Epiphany. Dogs thus treated will never become rabid.[33]

> How a Midwife in Nürnberg Stops Blood:
> Jesus was born at Bethlehem, Jesus was crucified at Jerusalem, as true as these words are, so truly understand N. N. that thy blood shall also stand still, in the name of God the Father, the Son, and the Holy Spirit.[34]

Unlike other works of ritual procedures which assume prior knowledge, the compiler provides an explanation for the basic format of a powwow blessing:

> Wherever the two "N. N." occur, both the baptismal name and all other names of him whom you intend to help, aid or assist, will have to be added, while the † † † signify the highest name of God, which should always be added in conclusion. Every sympathetic formula should be repeated three times.

A number of entries involve cryptic alphanumeric abbreviations and inscriptions in garbled Latin, Greek, Hebrew, and other languages. Some of the passages appear to contain at least portions of legitimate phrases that have been mis-transcribed by the compiler. A protective inscription against "poisonous air and pestilence" is to be hung on a person or animal on a Friday in an uneven hour before sunrise:

> Sator Arepo Tenet Opera Rotas
> + J + C + S + H + H S b y l S a n n e t
> U S M m a t e r o n n y + S b a b e 2 S +[35]

The first four letters, following the SATOR palindrome are a variation of a common Latin abbreviation for "Jesus Christus Salvator Hominorum" (Savior of Humanity), as well as the names of three female saints "*H[eilige] S[i]byl*" (St. Sibylla), "*San[c]t U[r]s[ula]*" (St. Ursula), and "*M[aria] Mater*" (Mother Mary), while the third line may also contain misspellings of the Hebrew names of God "*Adonai*" (Lord) and "*Sabaoth*" (Lord of Hosts). Not all inscriptions in *Egyptian Secrets* provide enough context to infer meaning, and the intentions of some passages are either so well-encrypted as to appear random, or their meanings have been lost to time, or were possibly never abbreviating anything in the first place.

As the introduction proudly proclaims, a large portion of the work is devoted to anti-witchcraft rituals, some of which are protective prayers for humans and animals, such as one for curing a bewitched child:

> Stand with the child toward the morning sun, and say: Thou art welcome to me and God, sunshine, from whence thou hath come, bring aid to me and my dear child. God the Heavenly Father, I bid thee, to aid me in receiving the Holy Spirit, that he may restore the flesh and blood of my child. † † †[36]

Other anti-witchcraft measures include the the use of plants or specially prepared objects:

> Fetch alder buckthorn wood on a Good-Friday, cut the same while calling the highest names, and make chips from the wood, one to two inches in length. Carve upon them, in the three holiest names, three crosses, † † † Wherever one of the chips is placed, all sorcery will driven away.[37]

The compiler of *Egyptian Secrets* made no attempt to follow the biographical life of St. Albert the Great. Instead the compiler uses the saint's name as a platform for attempts to establish credibility and commercial gain despite statements to the contrary, which are too numerous and insistent to be taken seriously. The introductions to the chapters are signed "Albertus Magnus," and proudly claim that "for the purpose of rendering a great service to mankind, this book was issued, in order to bridle and check the doings of the devil." But elsewhere in an argumentative and defensive tone, the work claims that it was produced to help subsidize a needy family, and that the archangel Michael himself would protect the copyrights of the work from one who would "rob the real and legal owner of the means of deriving his daily bread from the sale of this publication." In no uncertain terms, the compiler suggests that copying the contents of the book would "incur the eternal curse," and that one who uses the book rightly would secure salvation:

> I, therefore, beseech every one, into whose hands this book may come, not to treat the same lightly or to destroy the same, because, by such action, he will defy the will of God, and God will, in return therefore destroy him, and cause him to suffer eternal punishment and grim damnation. But to him who properly esteems and values this book, and never abuses its teachings, will not only be granted the usefulness of its contents, but he will also attain everlasting joy and blessing.[38]

This awkward and theologically problematic introduction provides a perfect example of the type of controversy that powwow practitioners aim to avoid by recommending that the oral traditions not be submitted to public scrutiny through publication. The commodification of the tradition would appear to inspire these types of unnecessary digressions into defensive theological rants, as "Albertus Magnus" is but one of many published works to tread these murky waters throughout the centuries. At the same time, it is also clear that the compiler was unlikely to have been the original creator of the contents of the work – large portions of which were directly borrowed from *Romanus* and a variety of written, oral, and printed sources.

At least one source identified by name within the pages of *Egyptian Secrets* is that of a legendary doctor named Pleni Horati (or Pelin Horeb), allegedly a court physician from Cairo, Egypt of Romani background. Like pseudo-Albertus Magnus *Egyptian Secrets,* Pleni Horeb's association with Egyptian culture is due to the mistaken belief that the Romani came from Egypt (thus the term "Gypsy"), and were descended from a race of people possessing supernatural abilities. Thus the title "Egyptian" has less to do with the geographical location, and more to do with legendary ritual powers.[39]

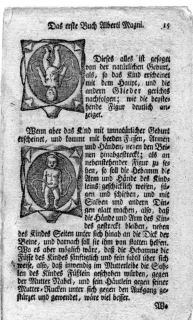

A Pennsylvania Dutch powwow doctor owned this fragmented eighteenth-century, European copy of the works of *Book of Aggregations* attributed to St. Albert the Great. The work includes a chapter on midwifery and the birthing process, and extols the virtues of plants, minerals, stones and animals. Elaborately illustrated diagrams such as the classic image of the cosmic man (see Chapter IV) explain celestial notions of healing from the early modern era. Illustrations below show the European *Wiedhopf* (Hoopoe), often cited in American healing manuscripts, and a legendary depiction of the Pelican feeding its young with its own blood - a symbol of Christ's Passion and sacrifice for humanity. *Pennsylvania German Cultural Heritage Center, Kutztown University of Pennsylvania.*

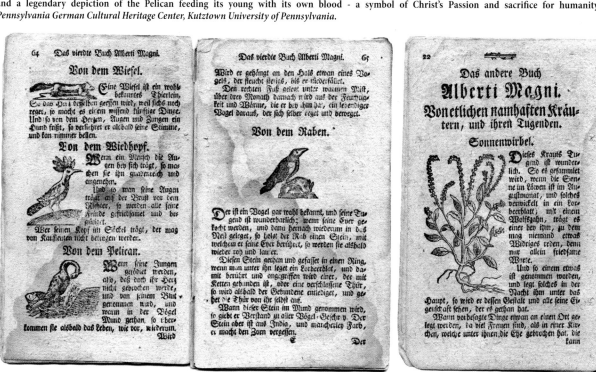

Pleni Horati's prognostication table of 42 unlucky days of the year appears in *Egyptian Secrets* to warn which days are ill-fated for childbirth, marriage, journeys, or construction of a building. The three unluckiest days were April 1st, the day that Judas the Betrayer was born; August 1st, the day that the devil was thrown out of heaven; and September 1st, the day Sodom and Gomorrah was destroyed. This table was originally printed in Pleni Horati's *Ein Schön neu-erfundenes Kunst-Büchlein, darinnen hundert fünff und zwantzig Stück vor Menschen un Vieh* (*A Fine, Newly-Compiled Book of Ritual Arts, Comprising One Hundred and Twenty-Five Entries for Humans and Animals*) printed in 1781 at an undisclosed location. Pelin Horati is also the source for copious other remedies found in *Egyptian Secrets* like fox-fat used to treat hernia in children, the use of black snails for removing warts, or the use of alder buckthorn to keep away witches.

The compiler of *Egyptian Secrets of Albertus Magnus* was by no means the only one to assume the legendary persona of a religiously influential figure in order to lend credence to a publication of ritual instructions. Nevertheless, not all such anonymous compilers were of the same ilk regarding their motivations for publishing.

Dr. Helfenstein's Secrets of Sympathy

One of the earliest and most unusual collections of powwow cures was from the nom-de-plume of an alleged European medical doctor, Dr. Georg Friedrich Helfenstein, entitled *Soli Deo Gloria (Glory to God Alone)*, consisting of seventy unbound broadsides, each printed with a cure on only one side of the page. A lengthy introduction tells the story of Dr. Helfenstein, a pious medical doctor educated in the Netherlands, who became a practitioner of spiritual healing methods after an enigmatic, supernatural being, identified only as a "gray man," appeared to him and taught him the "secrets of sympathy":

> And when this strange and mysterious man made known to me all that is included in this book, he vanished before my very eyes, and I never saw him again. Thus I, the author and a friend of mankind, became aware of this healing art, which is here newly reproduced and dedicated to the alleviation of the sufferings of my fellow men and neighbors, and to the glory of the Holy Trinity. Glory to God alone.[41]

Helfenstein's collection comprises three parts, each beginning with a short introductory paragraph, offering insight into the chapter. The first contains religious blessings to be used in healing the sick; the second, rituals for assistance in times of need, protection from witchcraft and criminal violence, as well as the stopping of thieves; and the third contains blessings for animals and livestock.

Strangely, although the work is attributed to Georg Friedrich Helfenstein, the introductory broadsheet is signed "J. H. Helfenstein" and is sealed with two wax seals depicting a fox and a lion. The unbound collection is a unique form of publication, as each broadside can be removed from the collection and used as a talisman or applied in healing rituals. The broadsides are printed very plainly, with only one cure on each page. Only about a dozen copies are known in Pennsylvania, most of which are cradled in decorative paper or tin boxes for safekeeping. Most copies of Helfenstein are incomplete as a result of the individual broadsides being separated from the collection for use and applied to the person for healing or protection. Leaves from my copies show evidence of having been folded and used as talismans.

Helfenstein's work was later released in bound book form as an undated chapbook printed at an unknown location and entitled *Georg F. Helfenstein's Sympathie; Eine Sammlung verzüglicher Heilmittel und Rezepte Für verschiedene Krankheiten der Menschen und des Viehes und andere Fälle, Gedruckt für den Herausgeber* (*Georg F. Helfenstein's Sympathy; A Collection of Reputable Healing Remedies and Recipes for Various Illnesses of Humans and Animals and Other Circumstances*).[42] This work was extensively overhauled and subsequently reprinted in 1853 by Scheffer & Beck of Harrisburg, Pennsylvania, in a dual edition with Johann Georg Hohman's celebrated powwow manual *Der lange Verborgene Freund (The Long Lost Friend)*. Helfenstein's broadsides were given a new title *Dr. Helfenstein's Vielfaeltig Erprobter Hausschatz der Sympathie* (*Dr. Helfenstein's Diverse Proven House-Treasury of Sympathy*). Three later English editions appeared in 1901, 1928 and 1938 from printers in Northumberland County. Circumstantial evidence suggests that Helfenstein's original broadside collection originates from above the Blue Mountain, perhaps at Shamokin or Sunbury — both early locations for German-language printing.

The persona of Dr. Helfenstein is an undisguised reference to one of the most celebrated lines of German Reformed ministers in Pennsylvania. Rev. Dr. Johann Conrad Albertus Helfenstein, was a famous pastor in Germantown, who served as the clerk of the Reformed Coetus in Pennsylvania in 1779 and 1787 and was president in 1781 and 1788.[43] He was also the progenitor of several generations of important Reformed (and a few Lutheran) clergymen, spreading from Philadelphia to Northumberland County, and even south into Frederick, Maryland[44] – although Georg Friedrich, compiler of the powwowing broadsides, was likely fictional.

A number of elements in the Helfenstein introduction, however, suggest intentional allusions to the actual line of Helfensteins. Georg Friedrich was supposedly raised by an uncle and patron Carl Augustus Helfenstein, whose initials match the celebrated Johann Conrad Albertus Helfenstein, a doctor of theology, who was ordained by the Reformed

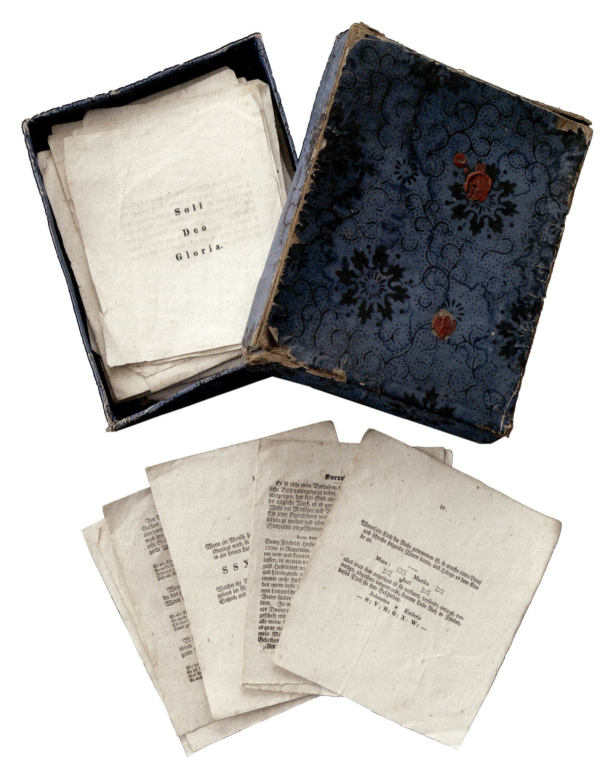

A rare unbound collection of broadside cures entitled *Glory to God Alone*, attributed to Dr. Georg Friedrich Helfenstein. ca. 1810, Northumberland County, later retitled *Secrets of Sympathy*. Formerly of the Lester Breininger Collection. *Heilman Collection*.

Synods in Holland. Thus even a careful reader could easily confound the fictionalized story of a Dr. Helfenstein from Holland and his uncle C. A. Helfenstein with that of the real Helfenstein family. Furthermore, a small hamlet named Helfenstein is located in Northumberland County, a mere 10 miles from Shamokin and 15 from Klingerstown, Schuylkill County, where the later English editions of *Secrets of Sympathy* were published.[45]

Although the name Helfenstein certainly carried with it a sense of religious authority, the name was also a German translation of the biblical place name of Ebenezer — literally meaning, "stone of help."[46] When the prophet Samuel brought all of Israel together, and they were attacked by the Philistines, Samuel made burnt offerings and prayed to the Lord for assistance. A great storm terrified the Philistines who were then defeated by the Israelites. "Then Samuel took a stone, and set it between Mizpeh and Shen, and called the name of it Ebenezer, saying, Hitherto hath the LORD helped us." Thus Ebenezer was a symbol of divine assistance rendered in a time of need, and a fitting parallel for Dr. Helfenstein's book, aiming to be "a deliverer in times of danger, a relief in pain and suffering, and a comforter of body and soul."[47]

Helfenstein's first chapter of cures for human illnesses is expressed in poetic biblical narratives drawing upon the imagery of the passion, and the miraculous healings of Christ and the Apostles, including the healing of the lame, the lepers, and the blind. For each ailment, a corresponding biblical healing encounter unfolds:

> And the bleeding ceased and he healed her at that very hour. Now, cease to flow in the name of Jesus Christ. So truly as Jesus hath turned water into wine, shall this flow take its proper course. The Lord hath made everything well, and considered humankind good, in the name of the Father, and of the Son, and of the Holy Spirit.[48]

This particular cure for menstrual complications mirrors the story of the woman suffering from hemorrhaging for twelve years, described in the Gospel of Mark:

> [She] had suffered many things of many physicians, and had spent all that she had, and was nothing bettered, but rather grew worse. When she had heard of Jesus, she came in the press behind, and touched his garment. For she said, If I may touch but his clothes, I shall be whole. And straightway the fountain of her blood was dried up; and she felt in her body that she was healed of that plague. And Jesus, immediately knowing in himself that virtue had gone out of him, turned him about in the press, and said, 'Who touched my clothes?' And his disciples said unto him, 'Thou seest the multitude thronging thee, and sayest thou, Who touched me?' And he looked round about to see her that had done this thing. But the woman fearing and trembling, knowing what was done in her, came and fell down before him, and told him all the truth. And he said unto her, 'Daughter, thy faith hath made thee whole; go in peace, and be whole of thy plague.'[49]

While Helfenstein's cure aims to quell bleeding, "when a woman has too much of her monthly cycle, so that the flow will not cease," just like the woman healed in the Gospel, a counterpart to this ritual makes use of the same biblical story but for the opposite purpose: when a period is delayed:

> And she touched his garment, and was healed. Thus I command thee blood, by the precious blood of Christ, to take thy regular course. I command thee congested blood, by the flowing wounds of Christ, to take thy regular course. So truly as Paul was bound, this sickness shall be overcome, in the name of the Father, of the Son, and of the Holy Spirit.[50]

The act of touching as a means to receive healing from the divine is echoed in other cures throughout the text in a variety of ways. Some suggest that the practitioner must pass (*fahre*) the hand or fingers over the suffering person, or, when appropriate, stroke (*streiche*), or rub (*reibe*) the afflicted part of the body, as an intermediary between the patient and God. In a cure for a whitlow, an infection of the finger, Helfenstein invokes the healing finger of God, and of the Apostle Paul to overcome the illness: "Thus shall this felon be slain, and this finger mend, through the finger of God, and the Lord worked great wonders through the finger of Paul…" Helfenstein instructs that the practitioner must stand outside under the open sky while the patient stands inside the house, pointing the infected finger out the window. This symbolism of liminal placement is similar to other rituals where the patient stands at the threshold of the house, suggesting that the illness is taken not only away from the person, but also away from the home and family.

The role of the hands and fingers in the symbolism of healing suggest acts of will and are not limited to the touch of eminently sacred people or God, but also apply to the hands of the practitioner, serving as the intermediary. Helfenstein's cure for a burn likewise makes use of the hand in narrative form: "There went a man over land, and found a hand, and the hand extinguished the brand." These words were to be spoken three times, while waiting ten minutes between each recitation, and blowing three times over the burn with each round.[51]

One unusual feature in Helfenstein's cures is that there are variations for certain cures according to the patient's gender. "For a burn received by a woman" the previous cure is reframed with a female protagonist seeking the healing hand. The same is true for two variations of a cure for erysipelas:

> Three women from the east went out to seek the Erysipelas-Stone: They search, they find, they come, they go, they run, they jump. Erysipelas, withdraw, and nevermore return. Fly out into the deep sea, be as a stone. In the name of Jesus, it shall be.

In the case of the cure for a man, the "three men from the east" suggests the Three Kings, Caspar, Melchior, and Balthasar, but for the three women, the Apocryphal accounts of Sts. Elizabeth, Brigid, and Matilda included in the *Gospel of Nicodemus* are likely candidates for the seekers of the healing stone – again a codified reference to Helfenstein and Ebenezer.

The idea of the healing stone appears numerous times throughout the Helfenstein broadsides, even in cures for animals such as one to drive out parasites:

> When a horse has botflies, lead him to a stone, and say the following words nine times, and between each three times thou must strike the horse on the belly with the stone. Each of the three times thou must wait one quarter-hour, and then lay the stone back at the same spot where it once laid:
>
> Peter plowed an acre with his golden plow, and under the plow lie three stones. The first is white, the second black, and the third red - thus I seize them, and strike the worms dead.[53]

Aside from Helfenstein's signature use of the stone, other ritual objects feature strongly as intermediaries to draw out, abate, or destroy illness.

> For mortification, take dead wood-coals, seven in number and tap with each one on the wound, and speak to each the following words: As this coal was once ablaze, and now burns no more, so shall this mortification be extinguished. Body and soul stand in the hand of God, therefore all evil be banished. The Blood of Christ atones for all. All flesh will perish, and the mortification cannot endure the stars so far, blue as heaven, as clear as the sun, in the name of John the Baptist. Afterwards, thou must grind them to powder, and strew them over flowing water.[54]

Just as the coals are deposited in flowing water, other objects are destroyed by fire:

> For wounds, bruises, punctures, and lacerations, take four pieces of pine-wood of equal length, and tap with each upon the wound and say to each one, the following words five times and then burn the wood: Upon Golgatha, upon Golgatha, upon Cyprus, upon Cyprus, upon Arrorat, upon Arrorat thy pains shall flee, into the deep sea thy pain shall descend, and by the wounds of Christ I lay thine. As this wood doth burn, So thy pains be drowned.[55]

The banishing of the illness to three mountains (Golgatha, where Christ was crucified; Cyprus where Paul and Barnabas introduced Christianity; and Arrorat, where Noah's ark settled after the flood), as well as to the depths of the sea, parallels a number of Helfenstein's cures whereby an illness is banished to a remote location:

> For fever, call the baptismal name of the sick person three times and say the following words:
>
> Heaven and Earth were created, and everything was good. Everything made by God is good, and only the fever is a plague. Therefore, yield from me, depart from me, remove yourself and vanish from me, fly to the highest mountains and thou shalt withdraw into the depths, withdraw from me in the name of John the Holy Apostle, and Jesus Christ the Son of God.[56]

In each of these instances, the source of affliction is called by name animistically and commanded to depart to locations of extreme height and depth, representing the extremes of the earthly kingdom. Banishing illness or evil spirits to geographic locations was not merely a metaphor, but an actual practice at locations such as Hexenkopf Hill in Williams Township, Northampton County, the site of the ritual operations of the notorious Johann Peter Saylor (1721-1803) and his son Peter (1770-1862).[57] However literal the interpretation of some practitioners may have been in regards to banishing illness into physical locations, Helfenstein explains the reference to the mountain and the depths in his introduction through the words of Christ in the Gospel of Mark:

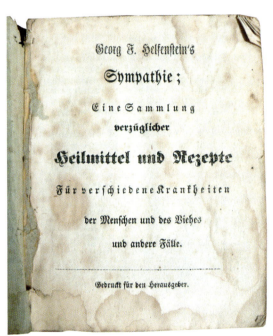

Georg F. Helfenstein's Sympathy; A Collection of Reputable Healing Remedies and Recipes for Various Illnesses of Humans and Animals and Other Circumstances, printed at an unknown location sometime in the early nineteenth Century north of the Blue Mountain. *Heilman Collection.*

> Have faith in God. For verily I say unto thee, that whosoever shall say unto this mountain, be thou removed, and be thou cast into the sea; and shall not doubt in his heart, but shall believe that those things which he saith shall come to pass; and he shall have whatsoever he saith.[58]

Within the context of the biblical story, these words of Christ are not merely meant as an inspirational passage, but as an explanation of the subordination of creation to the will of God, demonstrated in the preceding verses when Christ cursed the fig tree in Jerusalem and it withered the following morning.[59] This passage is the crux of Helfenstein's experience with the "gray man" and his new-found adoption of ritual healing methods to reveal the heights and depths of the power of the divine.

Helfenstein's second book is markedly different in tone, preceded with an admonition to avoid using its contents except when absolutely necessary – by the grace of God (*Gratia Deo*). Such instructions include how to ritually punish thieves and compel them to return stolen property,[60] how to render gunpowder ineffective, and how to take the vitality from one who wishes you harm. Other instructions include how to restore the milk of a cow that has gone dry because of witchcraft, as well as how to ritually punish a witch by creating a witch-bottle,[61] and as well as how to stop a conflagration by means of a ritual employed by a Romani in Prussia in the year 1714.[62] These methods stand in contrast to the religious piety exhibited in the first book of Helfenstein, and blend adversarial rituals with religious language:

> To take the power from a man, so that he cannot harm thee, say the following words:
>
> In the name of Jesus of Nazareth! I take from thee three drops of blood: one from thine heart, one from thine head, and one from thy virility. In the name of the Seven Angels that guard Christ, shalt thou be powerless, stand still, and harm me not. This I command thee by the power of God, who orchestrates and creates all.[63]

Although this set of instructions has appeared in numerous early Pennsylvania variations in works such as the *Kunst-Stücke*,[64] *Egyptian Secrets*,[65] and manuscripts throughout the region, Helfenstein's variation is unique in the sense that it invokes Jesus of Nazareth, the seven guardian angels, and the imagery of the creation. Although the particulars vary considerably, such as the source of the drops of blood from the lung, liver, and "manhood," or the tongue, lung, and heart,[66] this common ritual, and other contents of Helfenstein's second chapter, walk a delicate line between rituals for assistance and protection, and rituals of harm and aggression. This accounts for Helfenstein's admonition to make no misuse of the contents, and to employ them only when absolutely necessary.

The third book is for veterinary powwow rituals, especially for cows and horses. While Helfenstein's human and veterinary cures are very similar, one notable difference between his treatment of animals and treatments in other manuals such as *Romanus* or *Egyptian Secrets* is that Helfenstein suggests that the invocation of the Three Highest Names is not to be used for animals at the conclusion of a ritual. That no explanation is offered for such a distinction is puzzling and out of sync with other powwowing sources, but its implications could be theological, based in the fact that animals are not able to engage in belief-oriented discourse like humans, or the belief held by some that animals have no souls.[67] This latter belief, while certainly held by some, appears at odds with Helfenstein's omitting the Trinity while allowing other holy names. Helfenstein still suggests that rituals for animals are to conclude "in the name of Jesus," or Saints Matthew, John, Paul, and Peter:

> If a horse has collar boils, then take a bone from a dead horse that was found by accident, and rub the boil with the underside of the bone seven times, and each time say the following words: In six days the heavens and the earth were created, and it was good. Therefore all that has been created good shall be well maintained. Jesus hath banished all evil, and the good shall remain. So shalt thou be healed in Jesus' Name.[68]

Some of these entries make use of the names of the apostles and saints in a manner that suggests that each saint's invocation functions in a certain way:

> If a horse is constipated, then rub him with the hand seven times over the ribs, and say each time the following words:
>
> The disciples of Christ have healed all diseases by man and beast. In the name of John thou shalt be opened, in the name of Peter all things shall take their proper course. I bespeek thee in faith: thou shalt recover thine health. In the name of Paul shall thy pains abate.[69]

Thus St. John is responsible for opening, Peter for regimenting, and Paul for relieving. This is consistent with other uses of the saints' prayers, such as those to stop thieves, where St. Peter has the responsibility of binding while St. John is invoked to give the thief permission to depart.[70] Peter's role in the ritual is confirmed by his role in the Gospel of Matthew as the bearer of the keys:

An 1847 Pennsylvania Dutch illustration of St. Peter, depicted with the Keys to the Kingdom, as well as a stylus and book. Heilman Collection.

And I will give unto thee the keys of the kingdom of heaven: and whatsoever thou shalt bind on earth shall be bound in heaven: and whatsoever thou shalt loose on earth shall be loosed in heaven.[71]

The role of John the Evangelist in "opening" or "releasing" is less obvious in its biblical underpinnings: however Luther's German New Testament provides some clues. In the original German, The Revelation of John is titled *Die Offenbarung Sanct Johannis,* implying the revealing or "opening" of the heavens in John's visions, giving rise to his title as John the Revelator (*Offenbarer*). A less literal association that may be equally important to the idea of unbinding or releasing is in the depiction of John in many artists' renderings of the deposition of Christ, where in some versions of the story, John assists Joseph of Arimathea with the removal of Christ from the Cross.[72]

Paul as the reliever of illness is more straightforward, highlighting the healing miracles attributed to the apostle in his ministry, but also as one who suffered illness himself.[73] Several of Helfenstein's cures, especially in the third veterinary chapter appeal to Paul as a healer:

> If a cow or a horse has dysentery, then speak the following words softly in the morning to the animal, three days in succession:
>
> He who hath created and made all things, hath considered all things good. But take this illness from this animal, or as it is said: Paul's crown will persist, but this disease shall vanish. Dysentery I adjure thee by the power of faith, withdraw from this animal, the sufferings of Christ are enough.[74]

Paul's "Crown" appears in several biblical passages as a metaphor for his brethren in Christ: "Therefore, my brethren dearly beloved and longed for, my joy and crown, so stand fast in the Lord, my dearly beloved,"[75] and "For what is our hope, or joy, or crown of rejoicing? Are not even ye in the presence of our Lord Jesus Christ at his coming?"[76] Accordingly, in Helfenstein's conditional prose, the illness will abate, but the community of Christ and the blessings of heaven will persist. Moreover, regardless of the theological question of the existence of animal souls, Helfenstein's cure for dysentery nevertheless conveys the importance of animals as part of the order of creation.

Helfenstein concludes his work with an admission that the publication was underwritten by an anonymous benefactor, and suggests that, unlike other similar works, it was not a work intended for personal aggrandizement or profit, but for the glory of God (*Soli Deo Gloria*).[77]

> My dear reader and friend, male or female, this work was not revealed out of the desire for profit, but instead out of compassion alone, because it was intended only for the wellbeing of man and beast. It was compiled for the use of everyone and will be considered a treasury of the most useful writings ever to see the light of day. Also wilt thou, my dear reader, consider this collection a precious treasure, a gem, better than silver or gold, however one that is not expensive to obtain. It happened that a benefactor underwrote the first edition for one thousand dollars, so that it has been made available to the dear reader at half the cost it would have been otherwise. I am completely confident that thou wilt not regret the purchase of it, but instead, that it will bring thee great joy. Thou wilt consider it a friend to thine house, a deliverer in times of danger, a relief in pain and suffering, and a comforter of body and soul. Thus, I bid thee, dear reader, farewell, and commend thee to the protection and assistance of Holy Trinity.

Johann Georg Hohman

In 1820, a book that was later to become the most celebrated of all powwow manuals was printed in Reading, Pennsylvania, entitled *Der lange Verborgene Freund* (The Long-Hidden Friend) by Johann Georg Hohman, and commonly reprinted under the English title *The Long Lost Friend*.[78] This work has been released in dozens of editions, and has never been out of print in nearly 200 years. The collection was reissued in English for the first time in 1846 and spread rapidly outside of the German-speaking region, finding its way into the hands of healers, practitioners, and common folk throughout the Shenandoah Valley, the Midwestern states, and the Deep South.[79] The work also followed waves of German-speaking communities into Ontario, Canada, and copies were purported to have been found as far away as the Philippines.[80] *The Long Lost Friend* has come to both dominate and epitomize the American genre of powwow literature, winning Hohman legendary (albeit posthumous) fame.

Unlike other works of its kind, *The Long Lost Friend*, claimed no legendary authorship from saints, illustrious hermits, or celebrated physicians, but instead was penned by an ambitious and controversial compiler of popular printed works. Hohman was a Roman Catholic immigrant who arrived in Pennsylvania in October 1802 with his wife Anna Catharina and son Phillip, aboard the ship *Tom,* which departed from Hamburg, Germany.[81] Although Hohman's hometown was never recorded, another Hohman, named Johann Friedrich Hohman of Halberstadt in the Harz Mountains, emigrated in 1800.[82] If these two Hohmans were related, there is a possibility that Hohman would likewise have been of Prussian origin.[83]

George (as he was likely known) and Catharina departed from Europe as a family of redemptioners, who were immediately placed in servitude after their arrival in Pennsylvania to reimburse the costs of the family's passage across the Atlantic.[84] During his indenture, Hohman supplemented his repayment as a peddler of broadsides including birth and baptismal certificates (*Taufscheine*) and the earliest known American printing of a *Himmelsbrief*. This broadside printing included a contentious inscription that credited Hohman as the source of the one true *Himmelsbrief* in early Pennsylvania:

The heavenly letter from Magdeburg is a reprint of this one and it was not sent to Magdeburg but to Gredoria, which Georg Hohmann witnesses. It is caused to be printed by Georg Hohmann of Hellertown (Hellerstädel) in Northampton County. Yet no one can prove that this heavenly letter is false and concocted by human beings. For on the last Judgement Day many signs and miracles will happen, by which we will note that the time is very close and many miracles have already happened. Georg Hohmann brought this letter in the year 1802 from Germany to America, which it had until then been unknown; but a German brought a handwritten one forty-five years before from Germany to America.[85]

This inscription characterizes the type of controversy that Hohman inspired, aiming to simultaneously establish his credibility as well as to project his millenarian anxiety about the coming of the end times. In his customary fashion, he inserts his name in the credentials not once, but three times in the short paragraph – an unfortunate habit that is later echoed in *The Long Lost Friend*.[86] In the years following the release of this early broadside, Hohman became a prolific, entrepreneurial compiler and huckster of books and broadsides, ranging from the religious to the mundane – everything from a Roman Catholic Catechism to a children's book about a poodle.[87]

Although, *The Long Lost Friend* would later become his most influential work, he commissioned several works of a similar nature including an 1812 edition of one thousand copies of the *Kunst-Stücke* (*Ritual Arts*) printed by Johann Ritter of Reading.[88] This was the second of three editions of the *Kunst-Stücke* to be printed in Reading, as Gottlob Jungman & Carl A. Bruckman had released an 1805 edition Hohman's rival, Heinrich B. Sage, printed one in 1815.[89] Not to be outdone, just over two weeks after commissioning the *Kunst-Sücke*, Hohman ordered another thousand copies from Ritter; only he retitled the work, *Der Freund in der Noth* (*The Friend in Need*).

This new edition differed from others in name only, containing just twenty-four pages of thirty-six blessings for healing and protection, as well as a section on the use of omens for divination. Hohman borrowed the title from the catchy, popular aphorism: "*Ein Freund in der Not, getreu bis in den Tod*" (A friend in need is true unto death).[90] Not only an entrepreneurial decision aimed to set his work apart from his competition, *The Friend in Need* was also an opportunity for him to reassert his religious values, by echoing the title with the 50th Psalm directly on the title page: "*Rufe mich an in der Noth, so will ich dich erretten, und du sollst mich preisen*," – "Call upon me when in need, so will I deliver thee and thou shalt praise me." This biblical passage would later appear once again in *The Long Lost Friend*.

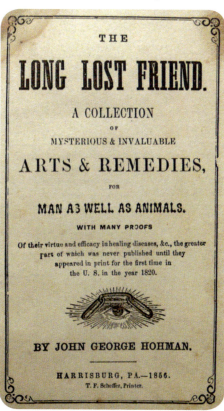

An English edition of Hohman's *Long Lost Friend*, by Harrisburg printer, Theodore F. Scheffer, 1856. Heilman Collection.

But for all of Hohman's enthusiasm, he remained impoverished for the duration of his life, and was unable to pay the costs of printing, so that Ritter officially cancelled his debts in 1826, after they were well-beyond a decade overdue.[91] Hohman alludes to a long-standing bout with financial and health troubles in an advertisement for *The Friend in Need* in Ritter's *Readinger Adler* (*Reading Eagle*) newspaper, where he introduces himself as a poor man suffering from chronic illness, hoping to earn money from the publication:

FINE BOOKS for purchase: A poor man, namely the subscriber, who has long been sick and is not yet rightly well, and for this reason has come into need, offers the following valuable book for purchase. It reads: "The Friend in Need, or Sympathetic Knowledge." It includes: to stop thieves, to have stolen property returned, for fever, for the evil thing, to disable a gun, also a sure remedy for convulsions in children and the bite of a mad dog, with 25 letters to render, that children will nevermore receive convulsions again. To describe everything in this book will take too much room; it includes 24 pages. – Price: ¼ Dollar. They are to be had: by Ritter and Company, in Reading; by Mr. Nehlo Beihl in Dums Tavern and Mr. DeJung, in Richmond; Heinrich Borkhalter and Heinrich Elias, in Rockland; Mr. Levan, in Kutztown; Mr. Price, in Pricetown; Mr. John Weiser, Abraham Ritter, Jacob Griesemer and Mr. Knabb, in Oley. Joh. Geo. Homan. The 9th of February, 1813.

The above aforesigned J. G. Homan, from Nockamixon Township, Bucks County, recommends this book, that it contains no lies, and should not be used with wicked intent. – Also the same is true with the 25 letters, that when they are in one's house, the house is free from thunder and fire.[92]

This period of illness and financial difficulty must have lasted for several years, as his prolific stream of publishing took a brief hiatus. His next three major works were released in succession beginning five years later in 1818. By this time, Hohman permanently relocated from where he was indentured in Nockamixon, Bucks County, to Rosedale, Alsace Township, Berks County, just outside of the City of Reading. Unlike *The Friend in Need*, Hohman's next major excursion into medical publishing did not consist of healing with words, prayer and benedictions, but contained ritual instructions nonetheless, as well as conventional domestic and agricultural remedies. *Die Land- und Haus-Apotheke, oder, Getreuer und gründlicher Unterricht für den Bauer und Stadtmann* (*The Agricultural and Domestic Apothecary, or True and Sound Instruction for Farmer and Urbanite*) outlined treatments and preventative measures for the health of humans and livestock, with an emphasis on horses. The work also contained a chapter devoted to the creation of dyes for domestic use.

In his typical fashion, Hohman begins his foreword with an affirmation of his authorship, "I, the author, Johann Georg Ho[h]man, wish with my whole heart that the following book shall be a blessing unto all who use it and an honor unto me." He later digresses into a mixture of entrepreneurial and religious tones, suggesting that subscribers who helped to underwrite the cost of production would be rewarded by God for doing so: "To all my subscribers, I thank you all one thousand times for the favor; the Lord in his heavenly kingdom will repay you when you die."[93]

While some of the contents of Hohman's medical advice appears consistent with trained physicians of his era, e.g. opening with statements regarding hygiene, the cleanliness of a bed-chamber devoted to recovery, and the documentation of treatment, most of his text is decidedly oriented towards sympathy and ritual. One remedy for healing degenerating eyesight as a result of a film on the eye suggests digging the roots of five or eight dandelions before dawn on St. Bartholomew's day, and hanging them on the neck in a bundle.[94] Borrowing from the works of Dr. Pleni Horati, he cites the use of black snails to cure warts and corns, and the treatment of atrophy with earthworm oil.[95]

Hohman provides a few clues about his activities in Europe through anecdotal descriptions of the treatment of disease. In a section dealing with venereal diseases of four types, amid the author's commentary that he wished he did not have to write about such things, Hohman admits that he saw many cases of such illness when he was a medic in the military (*Feldarzt*). While little is known of Hohman's life in Europe, this detail would suggest that he was involved in defending German territories during the French Revolutionary Wars (1792-1802), and was befitting of his description of syphilis as "*Franzosen*" – literally the "French disease."[96]

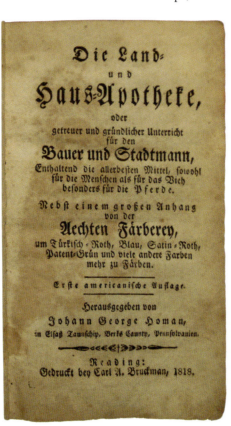

Hohman's Gospel of Nicodemus, a work of extra-biblical revelations printed in 1819 by Carl Andreas Bruckman of Reading. *Heilman Collection.*

This work raises a number of significant questions about Hohman and his publications. First, it is a lengthy and ambitious work – even for Hohman, who tended to edit and append, rather than create purely new materials for publication. The title page clearly states "*Erste Americanische Auflage*" (First American Edition) – but does this simply imply that it is the very first edition, or the first edition printed in America? Were there other editions of the same work? - and if so, was Hohman responsible for their publication in Europe? One possible source of inspiration was a work entitled *The Charitable Domestic and Agricultural Apothecary* (*Gemeinnutzige Haus und Land Apotheke*), printed in a dual edition with the *Kunst-Stücke,*. The titles are remarkably similar to Hohman's works, but the contents are markedly different.[97] Hohman would however, use copious entries from his own *Apothecary* to later populate his powwow manual, *The Long Lost Friend*.

In 1819, Hohman issued two religious works that were both on the fringe of the Pennsylvania Dutch spectrum of religious expression. The first was *The Small Roman Catholic Catechism* (*Die kleine Catholische Cathechismus*), with an aim to serve the Catholic congregation of the Most Blessed Sacrament in Bally, Berks County. Catholics comprised only 1% of the original Pennsylvania Dutch population, and such a work was not in high demand. Hohman claimed to have received official sanctioning to commission the catechism, and this was reflected on the title page: "*Mit erlaubnis Geistlicher Obrigkeit*" (With permission of the Ecclesiastical Authorities).[98] Whether or not such a license was actually granted to Hohman, this publication would appear to confirm his affiliation with the Catholic faith. In his later years, he lived near Fleetwood, Berks County, 2 miles north of Pricetown, where he may have attended St. Henry's Catholic Church, which was founded in 1823 but was disbanded by 1865. The church was later torn down, and the graveyard stands in the middle of farm fields today, where bricks from the church are occasionally plowed to the surface from the original building. This is a possible burial site for Hohman, whose precise date and location of death is unknown.

In 1819 Hohman also issued the most comprehensive edition of *The Gospel of Nicodemus, or A True Account of the Life, Suffering and Death of Our Savior Jesus Christ* (*Das Evangelium Nicodemus, oder Gewisser bericht von dem leben, Leiden und Sterben, unsers Heilands Jesu Christi*). This popular work of non-canonical books of the New Testament, featured the accounts of the events of Christ's crucifixion from the perspective of the Pharisee Nicodemus, a member of the Jewish religious authorities.[99] The work includes not only the *Gospel of Nicodemus*, but also the Testaments of the Twelve Patriarchs and numerous other Apocryphal letters and writings, as well as the popular legends of the late-medieval saints Genoveva and Helena.[100]

Two of the most notable pieces, nearly hidden in the midst of the volume, are two short texts devoted to the origin *Of the Wood of Chist's Cross, Where It went, and From Whence It Came (Von Christi Creuz-Holz. Woher es kommen, und wovon es genommen*), as well the *Revelation of Christ to the Three Holy Women, Saints Elizabeth, Brigid, and Matilda*.

The first piece tells how Adam was on his deathbed, and he sent his son Seth to the gates of the Garden of Eden to beg a fruit from the Tree of Life for healing. The Angel gave him three seeds, telling him to plant them so that they intertwine to create one tree, which would bear fruit to heal Adam and all of humankind. When Seth returned, his father had already died, but he planted the seeds as the angel instructed. The tree matured and was later cut down for Solomon's Temple. The strong trunk was used as a step to cross the stream of Kidron to the temple, but when the kings of Arabia visited Solomon's temple, they refused to step over the trunk because of a premonition that it would be used in the future to crucify a king. Solomon had the wood removed, and sunk into the pool of Bethesda. The 3000 year old log later surfaced and was set aside as salvage. It was put to use when wood was sought to build Christ's cross, and the angel's words were fulfilled: that the three seeds would make one tree, and a fruit that would heal all humankind would hang upon it.[101] This healing legend not only supports the connective narratives of biblical chronology, but also the notion that healing and salvation, like the three seedlings of the cross-wood tree, are thoroughly intertwined.

Although the narrative of Christ's Cross-Wood is decidedly legendary in nature, Hohman's presentation of Christ's Revelation to the three Saints Elizabeth, Brigid, and Matilda takes the notion of apocryphal accounts and chronology to a new level. According to the Revelation, these three Saints received a message directly from the mouth of Christ, detailing the numerology of his wounds:

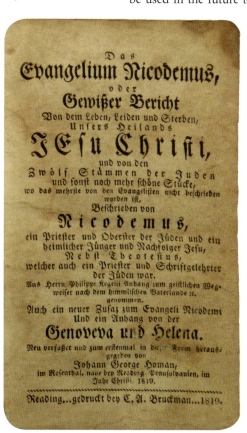

Hohman's Gospel of Nicodemus, a work of extra-biblical revelations printed in 1819 by Carl Andreas Bruckman of Reading. *Heilman Collection*.

Know, dear daughters, that I received 102 strikes on the mouth …30 strikes on the head, arms and breast… 30 strikes on the shoulders, body and legs… was pulled by the hair 30 times… I sighed 129 times from the depths of my heart… was pulled by the beard 73 times… a heavy blow caused me to fall to the ground while carrying the cross… I was whipped 6666 times… received 1000 pricks from the crown of thorns… 3 thorns punctured my head… was spat upon 73 times… received a total of 5476 wounds… there were 3,430 drops of blood…

These words were allegedly found at the Holy Grave in Jerusalem, and passed by word of mouth, until they were recorded in print. While Hohman does not precisely say that he authored the Revelation, he does assert credit for placing it in his compilation, listing his name in the by-line. However, the *Revelation* was certainly not penned by Hohman, as it appears in numerous compilations of European blessings such as *The True Spiritual Shield* dating to the eighteenth century, that claim the very text of the *Revelation* would serve as a protective blessing from evil and harm.[102]

Despite the fact that the Revelation is fraught with numerous anachronisms, these seemingly contradictory elements do not appear to have affected the desirability of the text as a work of contemplative religious literature. The three female saints, for instance, Elizabeth, Brigid, and Matilda, did not live contemporaneously, but were each about three centuries removed from the others in succession from the first to the tenth centuries. Elizabeth, mother of John the Baptist is the only saint that lived at the time of Christ, suggesting that Christ's revelation to the three women took place in an extra-chronological space, outside the bounds of history, and imagined in a heavenly, supernal realm.

Like the *Himmelsbrief* and *Our Dear Lady's Dream*, this Revelation would certainly be rejected by church authorities because of textual, doctrinal, and chronological inconsistencies. Nevertheless, these types of apocryphal narratives describe an important aspect of religious belief in an eternal space occupied by a cast of sacred personalities emanating their divine attributes through poetic dialogue. This conception of the heavenly sphere undergirds the wide range of creative expression found in the language of ritual blessings used for healing, protection, and assistance in times of need.

THE LONG LOST FRIEND

In 1819, Hohman completed his masterpiece in ritual literature, *Der lange Verborgene Freund*, or *The Long Lost Friend*, which has become the most widely distributed work of its kind in North America, used not only for powwow practice, but among healing practitioners of hoodoo in the south.[103] *The Long Lost Friend* contains prayers and rituals for healing, protection, and assistance, as well as herbal and botanical cures, and some miscellaneous household recipes. Although Hohman proudly claims credit for the publication of the compilation, he merely copied the majority of the text from classic eighteenth and nineteenth-century European collections of cures, such as the *Romanus-Büchlein*, or *The Little Book of Romanus*,[104] which had appeared a decade earlier than Hohman's edition under the title *Das Vortreffliche Zigeuner Büchlein*, or *The Splendid Little Book of the Gypsies* printed by Heinrich B. Sage in Reading, Pennsylvania around 1810.[105]

Hohman openly admits in his introduction to the use of a book written by a "gypsy" (*Zigeuner*) in developing *The Long Lost Friend*, but this has puzzled European scholars, who attribute *Romanus* to the saint, rather than the Romani people.[106] Thus it is possible that Hohman derived the contents of *Romanus* from Sage's edition, which claimed gypsy authorship. It is also possible that Hohman was not referring to *Romanus* at all, but to the works of the legendary Romani Doctor Pleni Horati, or to *Egyptian Secrets*. Several of Hohman's entries can be found in both works, such as Horati's prognostication table of "Unlucky Days" which appears at the end of *The Long Lost Friend*. A series of entries on the uses of certain herbs are likewise derived verbatim from pseudo-Albertus Magnus' *Book of Aggregations (Liber Aggregationis)*, expounding the secrets of

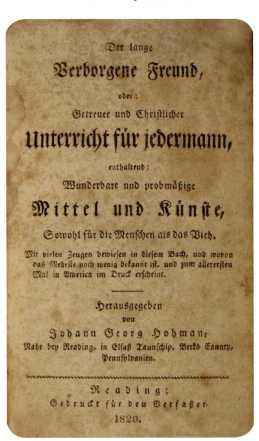

The first edition of Johann Georg Hohman's *Der lange Verborgene Freund* or *The Long Lost Friend*, printed by Carl A. Bruckman of Reading in 1820. Heilman Collection.

childbirth and the virtues of animals, birds, botanicals, and minerals.[107]

At least some of the materials included in *The Long Lost Friend* were derived from the oral tradition, which caused a stir among his contemporaries. Hohman alludes to the controversy in his foreword:

> I had not wanted to allow it to be printed, and my wife also opposed it, but my compassion for my fellow man was too great…Besides that I am a poor man in needy circumstances, and it is a help to me if I can make a little money with the sale of my books.[108]

However altruistic Hohman's desire may have initially been to help others through the publication of sensitive ritual material, Catharina Hohman's criticism of printing the work speaks volumes about *The Long Lost Friend*'s departure from tradition. In Hohman's introduction, among a series of testimonials on the efficacy of ritual process dated 1812-1819, Hohman's wife Catharina is mentioned as the practitioner in the earliest instances of healing that Hohman witnessed.[109] One could therefore justifiably wonder whether or not Catharina could have been the individual responsible for teaching Hohman in the first place, adding a personal dimension to her concerns over his publication. Catharina was also a first generation immigrant, and clearly a *Braucherin*, but her important story has been largely eclipsed by her husband's authorship. If Hohman learned to powwow from his wife, and then published certain materials against her wishes, one would sense that the author's struggles with controversy were not merely with the public, but also in his own home.

It is undeniable that Hohman's collected works, and those that both preceded him and followed in his footsteps, have enabled generations of the curious to purchase portions of *Braucherei* tradition, and essentially bypass the customary method of learning the oral tradition by word of mouth directly from another person. Perhaps of greatest concern is the way in which this literary method of learning has the potential to erode the sense of gender-neutrality that has so characterized the practice when a man learns from a woman, and vice versa. Without this human element, the literature of powwow can appear as a disembodied corpus of ritual procedures, stripped of its place within a larger system of traditional beliefs.

Notably, Hohman could have merely ignored the controversy his book created, but instead he anticipated the attacks from critics, and defended his work in advance in his foreword. In the midst of his long list of testimonials from local people, Hohman threatens to take legal action against any person listed in the book who would deny that Hohman and his wife were responsible for the cure of their infirmities:

> If any one of the above-named witnesses, who have been cured by me and my wife through the help of God, dares to call me a liar, and deny having been relieved by us, although they have confessed that they have been cured by us—I shall, if it is at all possible, compel them to repeat their confession before a Justice of the Peace.[110]

Although the anonymous author of *Egyptian Secrets* published portions of the oral tradition alongside equally problematic theological postulates and threats of legal action, what truly set Hohman apart from his predecessors was not only his lack of anonymity, but his level of unabashed self-promotion. Rather than hide from controversy, Hohman appeared to revel in the possibility of credibility through increased exposure. As in his previous works, Hohman was fond of asserting his authorial privilege by stating "I, Hohman…" before sanctioning portions of the work – listing his own name as many as five times on a single spread of two pages. His desire was not only for recognition from his readers, but from his creator:

The earliest known edition of Romanus printed in America, under the title Das Vortreffliche Zigeuner-Büchlein (The The Splendid Little Book of the Gypsies), ca. 1810 by Heinrich B. Sage of Reading, Pennsylvania. Courtesy of the Library Company of Philadelphia.

> I ask thee once again, friend, male or female, is it not at present an eternal praise for me that I have permitted such books to be printed? Do I deserve no reward from God on account of it?[111]

Not only does this statement appear to imply that Hohman believes that his publication has earned him salvation, he also states that any person who knowingly avoids the use of his book while their neighbor suffers from an illness "commits a sin, by which he may forfeit to himself all hope of salvation."[112] To Hohman, his book is a corollary to the biblical imperative cited in *The Friend in Need* from Psalm 50, "Call upon me when in need, so will I deliver thee and thou shalt praise me."[113] Thus to suppress or ignore his work was not only regarded as negligence, but as direct defiance of divine will.

On the other hand, Hohman praises the recovery of patients treated by ritual means as evidence of divine intervention, citing that such miracles serve as proof of a dualistic afterlife:

> There are many in America who believe neither in a hell nor in a heaven; but in Germany there are not so many of these persons found. I, Hohman, ask: Who can immediately banish the wheal, or mortification? I reply, and I, Hohman, say: All this is done by the Lord. Therefore, a hell and a heaven must exist; and I think very little of any one who dares deny it.[114]

While Hohman's self-aggrandizement, and threats of both legal action and eternal damnation, as well as hopes for monetary remuneration, are hardly desirable traits in a powwow practitioner, his aggressive statements of faith may have strongly appealed to some of his readers who sympathized with his millenarian and fundamentalist views. Hohman even expressed a tendency towards nationalism in his foreword to *The Long Lost Friend*, invoking "the freedom of the press and freedom of conscience" in the United States for justification of his publication, as opposed to "the kings and despots who rule with tyranny over the people in other nations."[115]

Hohman is correct that most works in Europe of a similar variety were banned by both secular and religious authorities and were, therefore, printed anonymously. His rhetoric, however, also subtly equates his contemporaries' criticism of *The Long Lost Friend* with the political suppression of similar works abroad – a bold misrepresentation of the cultural norms that discouraged powwow publications. Thus Hohman painted a picture of his critics as both anti-Christian and anti-American.

Despite Hohman's tendency towards publicizing his internal and interpersonal conflicts, it is clear that his statements were indeed reflections of his religious and social values. Although he admits in his introduction that he intends to profit from the sale of his books, he was neither successful in accruing nor maintaining a fortune. On the contrary, on Christmas Eve in 1826, Hohman's home and personal belongings were auctioned at a public sale to repay debts he owed for the purchase of a property near Reading.[116] For all intents and purposes, *The Long Lost Friend* was not a successful venture for Hohman, yet decades later, it became one of the best sellers from large commercial presses in Harrisburg. This was perhaps due to the fact that Hohman's greatest selling point for the book was not merely its healing instructions, but a short blessing that claimed:

> Whoever carries this book with him, is safe from all his enemies, visible or invisible; and whoever has this book with him, cannot die without the holy corpse of Jesus Christ, nor drowned in any water, nor burn up in any fire, nor can any unjust sentence be passed upon him. So help me. +++ [117]

When Hohman released his first edition, he included this passage nearly hidden at the end of the book. Editors of later editions moved this inscription to the front, where it increased the desirability of the book as a talisman, rather than only an instructional work. This may account for why so many copies of the book found among families in Pennsylvania show little evidence of having been read.

Aside from this missed opportunity in Hohman's first edition, his text was one of the first to provide a wide range of typographically impressive inscriptions, such as the SATOR square, and his own version of the *Abracadabra*, reading "AbaxaCatabax."

One of the most popular entries used for the blessing of homes and individuals "Against Evil Spirits and All Manner of Witchcraft (*Hexerei*)" features an arrangement of the Latin words for the Holy Spirit, and the abbreviation I.N.R.I.:

I.
N. I. R.
I.
SANCTUS SPIRITUS
I.
N. I. R.
I.

All this be guarded, here in time, and there in eternity. Amen.

Another typographical entry unique to *The Long Lost Friend* is Hohman's "Talisman." Popular among hunters and allegedly traced to a hermit in Europe, this inscription was supposedly given to a distressed, lame huntsman who feared punishment from he nobleman he served for the state of his hunter's pouch, empty of wild game. The hunter later, by means of carrying the Talisman, became one of the best hunters in the country:

Ut nemo in sese tentat, descendere nemo.

At praecedenti spectatur mantica tergo.

Hohman closes the entry with the advice "*Man thut am besten, un probirt es*" – "at best one should try it."[118]

The Latin in this talisman has proven, however, to proceed from an unlikely and ironic source. Scholar of esoteric studies, Daniel Harms identified Hohman's inscription in the writings of the first-century satirist Aulus Persius Flaccus (34-62), whose words originally decried the lack of introspection in his contemporaries:

> Not a soul is there—no, not one— who seeks to get down into his own self; all watch the wallet on the back that walks before! [119]

The irony is that either Hohman was totally ignorant of the inscription's true meaning, or he was well-aware, and included (or created?) the talisman with a sense of humor that would only be recognized centuries later.

Aside from the select few visually engaging typographical elements, Hohman's work runs the full gamut, from lengthy blessings invoking divine protection to concise ritual operations involving the use of an object and no words. Of the latter variety are cures for warts using fried chicken feet, or a bone like Helfenstein.[120]

Hohman also includes a variation of the classic lunar wart cure, with words to be spoken three times in one breath in the waxing moon: "*Was zunimmt, nimmt zu; was abnimmt, nimmt ab*" -"Whatever grows, does grow; whatever diminishes, does diminish," or "Whatever waxes takes on, and whatever wanes takes off," again echoing the dual meaning of the German words.[121]

Hohman is perhaps best known for his wide range of classic poetic blessings, featuring rounds of three: three holy men; three roses on Christ's grave; three wells; three worms:

> Three holy men go over the land;
> They did bless the heat and the brand;
> They blessed it so it burned not in,
> They blessed it so it burned out.[122]
>
> On Christ's grave grow three roses:
> The first is kind,
> The second is destined over many to rule,
> Blood stay still, and wound heal![123]
>
> I go through a green wood,
> There were three wells, cool and cold.
> The first is called courage,
> The second is called good,
> And the third is called stop the blood. + + + [124]
>
> Mary, Mother of God, went over the land;
> She had three worms in her hand;
> The first was white, the second was black, the third was red.[125]

For this last blessing, Hohman adds:

> Rub the person (or the animal), whom you serve. With each treatment, strike the person on the back; specifically, strike the person once for the first treatment; twice for the second treatment, and thrice for the third treatment; then determine a time for the worms, but no less than three minutes.

Hohman's suggestion of "determining a time" (*setze den Würmer ihre Zeit*) is to be an indication of how long the worms have to live until they are destroyed. Another version of this blessing included later in the text is more explicit, indicating that Hohman may have forgotten the last line of the former blessing, which would have completed the rhyme: "The one was white, the other was black, and the third one was red. Now all the worms are dead, in the name † † †."[126]

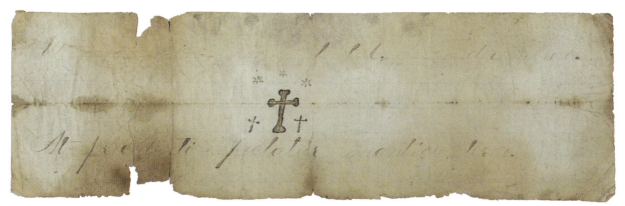

A faded copy of Hohman's Hunters' Talisman carried in the shooting bag of a late nineteenth-century Lehigh County hunter. *Heilman Collection.*

Hohman's collection is far from being organized in any coherent way. Like others of its kind, such as *Egyptian Secrets*, Hohman includes a table of contents at the end of the book, but the list includes all of the entries in narrative form. This means that the lengthy title of each entry is listed, such as "*Wieder ein Mittel, wenn jemand krank ist, so kann man es thun; den es hat schon Vielen geholfen, wo kein Doctor helfen konnte*" (Another remedy, when anyone is sick, so that one can cure it; it has already helped many, when no doctor could help). This title, like many others, does not explicitly state its use, but instead provides commentary on its effectiveness, so that looking for a particular illness in the table of contents is difficult.[127]

As in the case of Hohman's worm-cure, the original edition provides many useful hints and general rules for how *Braucherei* rituals were intended to be used, but these are located randomly throughout the text, or as commentary on a particular cure. Some of these are useful in getting an overall picture of how Hohman believed that ritual healing was to be performed:

> Make three crosses over the afflicted part with the thumb. All healing with words must be repeated three times, and wait a few hours between each time when you treat a person. For the third time, treat on the following day. The single N. indicates the person's first name; two, N. N., indicates the first and last name of the person one treats. This is the meaning of the N. N. throughout the entire book. One should bear this in mind.[128]
>
> Everything in this book that can be used to treat humans, can also be used for animals.
>
> The hand must be put upon bare skin in at the time of using sympathetic words.[129]
>
> When anyone writes a blessing for another, it must contain their name. [130]

Hohman also provides necessary commentary at the end of an entry describing one of many methods for blessing three sticks used for healing wounds and removing pain:

> With this rod and Christ's blood, I take your pain and poison out! Mark it well: you must cut one young shoot (a sapling) towards the rise of the sun in just one cut, and then cut three rods from it. Then you must roll them across the wound, one after another. When you take them in your hand, you must hold them by the right side first. – All rituals in this book must be used three times, even when the three crosses are not included [at the end of the entry]. All that is treated with words must be repeated in intervals of one-half hour, and the last repetition should wait over night [until the following day]. The wooden rods described above should be wrapped in white paper, and hidden in a warm location. [131]

The very same entry is listed elsewhere in the text without the additional commentary, and minus the words used to bless the rod. It is entirely possible that Hohman believed that the cure could be rendered with or without the use of a verbal component, as this procedure for curing wounds on humans and animals was widespread by the time of Hohman's release of *The Long Lost Friend*.

In 1810, the German-born Lutheran minister Frederick Henry Quitman (1760-1832) recorded the same procedure among the German-speaking inhabitants of the Hudson Valley in New York:

> When a horse has received a wound, three little sticks of a certain growth, and mysteriously cut must be applied to it in a certain direction, and the bark of them preserved in a very dry place…

Rev. Quitman derides the Trinitarian application of three sticks as superstition, "in favor with ignorant people," but states that the use of a stick in lancing the wound "to vent purulent matter" does indeed effect a cure.[132] Another Lutheran Clergyman of the time, James Patterson, suggested that such rituals were beneficial only because they prevented further treatment of the wound with "injudicious" applications of salves that could cause the wound to become infected.[133]

Some variations of the cure suggest using sticks or shoots of a particular variety. The manuscript account book of Frederick Sheeder, Jr., stage coach driver from Kimberton to Morgantown for the Philadelphia & Lancaster Mail Stage, records a similar procedure in 1831 for curing horses, using three stalks of "*Flöhkraut*,"[134] cut on St. John's Day. The stalks were to be cut into three pieces, and arranged in bundles like crosses tied in red flannel, which are to be tied onto the animal's mane if the wound is near the front of the horse, and on the tail if near the back.[135]

While these alternate forms of the wound-wood cure were certainly not derived from Hohman, they are powerful testimony of the breadth and variety of similar rituals in Hohman's day and age. In fact, forms of this ritual were still in use at the turn of the twentieth century, when a powwower named "Dr." John Rhodes from Rockland Township, Berks County made small bundles of three stalks of a certain herb tied with red flannel, and sold them to a wide range of clients across Eastern Pennsylvania. He recommended rubbing the tips of the stalks into a wound, and then hiding them "where neither sun nor moon can shine upon them." One was then to burn the bundle after the wound had healed.[136] Although Rhodes sold the bundles with which, he claimed, anyone could cure themselves, he refused to charge for powwowing beyond what anyone could afford or give willingly.

When compared to the prevalence of related cures used in the Eastern United States, Hohman's works appear far less vital to actually introducing ritual practices and were more important perhaps for the documentation and lending of credence to already well-established practices.

Despite the apparent lack of support that Hohman received for his initial publication of *The Long Lost Friend*, this important aspect of documenting regional and imported ritual practices would later contribute to Hohman's rise to popularity in the late nineteenth century.

Margaretha Croll's Healing Remedies

Although Hohman's work would later dominate the publication of ritual literature in Pennsylvania, other lesser known authors were popular in their day, and not all of them were men. In 1826, a collection of cures and rituals entitled *A Collection of Diverse Receipts of Healing Remedies to Use for Sicknesses among Humans and Animals* (*Eine Sammlung Auserlesener Rezepte heilsamer Mittel bey krankheiten der Menschen und des Vieh zu gebrauchen*) was published and attributed to the author M. Margaretha Croll. This is to date the only known powwow book written by a woman. The imprint merely states "*gedruckt in Pennsylvanien*" (Printed in Pennsylvania), but typographical evidence suggests that it was printed in Reading by Heinrich B. Sage. This work brings together a total of fifty-seven remedies of both botanical cures and ritual blessings, and opens with the suggestion: "May all that we do be toward the teaching and use of our community" (*Was wir thun, sey zu Belehrung und zum Nuzen des Nächsten*).

Croll's collection is purely instructional and offers no indication of biographical details of the author's life. It is possible that this is Maria Margaret (Geiger) Croll (1763 - 1832) buried at St. John's Lutheran, formerly a Union Church in Hamburg, Berks County,[137] however, this would mean that her collection of remedies was printed posthumously. If the author was indeed the same person, the book may have been based upon a collection of manuscript cures, and published by a relative in her honor.

Although quite a number of "Ladies' Books" (*Weiber-Büchlein*) were printed at Ephrata, York, and Reading, all of these works claimed spurious male authorship in Albertus Magnus and Aristotle. These works share at least one commonality with Croll, and that is an adapted version of the celebrated SATOR square palindrome. Croll includes the very same version of the SATOR square, as a means to protect the house and premises from fire, as well as to cure infant convulsions when written on a paper and placed in the cradle. This cure appears to have been popular, especially in works written for a predominantly female audience.

Croll's collection combines more than remedies for conditions, including a number of suggestions for preventative measures against illness. The last entry in the book suggests improving one's constitution and resistance to seasonal varieties of illness, by drinking a cup of the juice from sauerkraut. This type of remedy is being explored even today in probiotic therapies for a variety of illnesses.[138]

With a heavy emphasis on herbal and botanical cures, Croll's repertoire consists of domestic applications of plants common to Pennsylvania gardens and meadows made into teas, salves, decoctions, and compresses. Many of Croll's cures are practical in nature, and a number of them appear tried and true, such as the oral administration of molasses and lard to cure constipation in horses, the topical use of tar from a wagon wheel to dry out a wart or corn, and the use of red chalk dipped in honey as a lozenge for ulcers of the mouth.[139] Others feature compelling sympathetic cures such as one described for pain in the soles of the feet (*Weh' an den Fussohlen*):

Man schneide in der Grösse des Fusses einen Rasen in der Wiese aus, lege denselben umgekehrt wieder in sein Loch, das Gras hinunterwärts wie der Fuss darauf gestanden hat.

One must cut out the shape of the foot from the sod in the wheat, remove it, and place it back in the opening upside-down, with the grass facing downwards where the foot had stood upon it.[140]

M. Margaretha Croll's Berks County Collection of Diverse Receipts of Healing Remedies to Use for Sickness among Humans and Animals, 1826. Courtesy of Clarke Hess.

The idea here, as with other cures involving measuring parts of an ill person, is that an image of the person is captured in the measurement, and by manipulating or reversing the image, the person will become well. Thus when the image of the foot in the sod is flipped over, the illness will likewise be reversed and resolve itself. Croll indicates that this method is applicable for a wide range of ailments, including kidney stones, whitlow (an inflamed cuticle of the finger), and *Kazenspur* (a sore spot on the foot).[141]

A number of Croll's cures for both humans and animals are based in the well-established tradition of *Dreckapotheke*, or the use of excrement for healing. One such remedy for curing bloating of the digestive tract in horses (*Rehe*, or foundering from overeating) in horses involved the use of human hair trimmed from under the right and left arms, as well as the genitals (*wo es verborgene ist*, where it is hidden), tied into a bundle with human feces onto a horse's bit. The recipe calls for a woman's hair to treat a mare, and a man's hair to treat a stallion.[142] Such cures, while seemingly cruel and unusual to a modern audience, were aimed at suppressing the appetite of a horse that indulges too much in fresh, green grass, causing digestive issues.

For banishing toothache among humans, Croll suggests cutting the nails of the fingers and feet on a Friday in the waning moon, putting them in a piece of paper, and digging a hole on the north side of the house (*Winter Seite eines Gebäutes*) under the eaves. One was then to place the bundle into the hole and defecate (*verrichte deine Nothdurft*) upon on the bundle, and cover it over with earth.[143] The classic means of showing disdain to an illness is echoed in other cures recommended by Croll, who suggests that passing gas over a sore finger will prevent infection. Croll was modest about such suggestions, and even the verb for flatulation "*F-rtz*" is abbreviated in the text.[144]

For the toothache cure, however, Croll suggests performing the ritual three times each year to keep away the toothache, but that it is particularly effective when enacted on Good Friday in the waning of the moon. This latter piece of advice utilizes not only lunar forces to drive the illness into the ground, as the waning moon exerts a force towards the earth. Good Friday also reflects the symbolism of an opening of the earth to receive the body of Christ after the crucifixion and Christ's descent to the dead, as described in the Apostles' Creed - a time of cosmic significance for the removal of sin and infirmity, echoed in other ritual procedures.[145]

Such actions of burying in the ground play an essential role in many of Croll's cures, including one for itching of the skin, where a pig bladder is to be filled with lard rendered from a castrated boar, and buried under the eaves for three days. Twice, between each of the three days, the bladder should be exhumed and the lard squeezed around inside the bladder and reburied. After the third day, the itching part is to be anointed with the lard for five consecutive evenings, and then washed clean, at which time the itching will be gone.[146]

Two cures for erysipelas (*wilde Feuer*) sympathetically employ the tools used to make fire in order to banish the inflammation, one for humans and one for animals. The animal cure involves striking flint and steel to shower sparks over the length of the animal, starting at the top of the head, and proceeding down the back to the tail. This process is to be repeated nine times, and each round separated by three hours, and over again the following day. This progression employs the action of "chasing" described in other wildfire cures, used by Rev. Mennig and Sophia Bailer.

Croll describes three forms of "wildfire" for humans: that which is a rash-like topical poisoning (*Gift*), that which occurs in blisters (*Blasen*) like a burn, and patches (*Placken*)[147] on the skin. For treating humans, a woman who has borne twin sons must perform the ritual, and she must strike the flint and steel onto the head of the suffering person twice in two hours, two days in a row. This emphasis on two is echoed in some European sources,[148] but unlike the numbers, three, nine, seven, or five, there is no agreement about its symbolism. It is possible that the symbolic nature of the twins, being mirror images of one another, suggests a similar notion to the creation of an image or measurement for the purpose of healing.

Croll also makes use of herbal remedies to accompany rituals employed with words, timing, and manipulations of the hands. These types of rituals accompanied by words play only a minor role in Croll's work, however, with much more emphasis placed on symbolic ritual exchanges and transformations involving *materia medica*. Almost as if to satisfy the demands of her anticipated audience, she includes a cure for sweeny (muscular atrophy) towards the end of the book, entitled "*Eines mit Worten*" – One with words:

Man sagt: Guten Morgen Schwinden,
Bein, ich streich dich mit einem schiefen Stein,
Ich streich dir Haut, Fleish und Bein, Mark und Blut,
Das ist für 77gerley Schwinden Gut.

Den Stein, mit welchen man reibt, muss man im Keller holen wo keine Sonne hinscheint, dreymal den Athem über das Glied blasen, und im alten Mond drey Freytage hinter einander Morgens früh ohnbeschrauen, dieses brauchen; jedesmal aber den Stein wieder an seinen Ort thun.

One says: Good Morning Sweeny,
Bone, I stroke thee with a crooked stone,
I stroke thee skin, flesh and bone, marrow and blood,
This is good for 77 varieties of Sweeny.

The stone used to rub the affected limb, must be concealed in the cellar where no light shines upon it. One must blow three times over the limb in the waxing moon on three successive Fridays early in the morning without speaking to anyone, and each time replace the stone back in its place.[149]

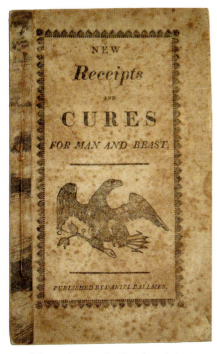 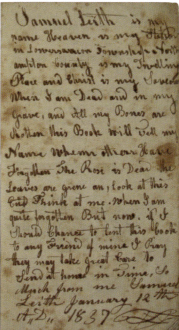 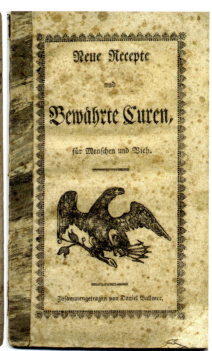

From left to right: Daniel Ballmer's English edition of *New Receipts and Cures for Man and Beast,* printed by Friedrich Goeb in Shellsburg, 1826, containing the inscription of ownership of Samuel Leith, Lower Saucon, Northampton County, 1837. *Pennsylvania German Cultural Heritage Center, Kutztown University*; Daniel Ballmer's German edition of *Neue Recepte und Bewährte Curen, 1826. Heilman Collection.*

Daniel Ballmer's Receipts

Also in 1826, at the time that Margaretha Croll's work was probably published in Reading, Daniel Ballmer of Chambersburg compiled the most influential powwow manual printed in western Pennsylvania. Entitled *A Collection of New Receipts and Approved Cures for Man and Beast* or *Eine Sammlung von Neuen Recepten und Bewährten Curen für Menschen und Vieh*, Ballmer's collection was printed by the former Lutheran minister and master printer Friedrich Goeb (1782-1829) in Schellsburg, Bedford County in 1827. This book was immediately issued in separate editions in both English and German, and distributed widely throughout Pennsylvania. It contained fifty-six cures for both humans and animals, as well as copious reflections on folk beliefs regarding medicine and domestic life.

The most common English and German editions feature an image on the cover of the patriotic symbol of the Golden Eagle, bearing an olive branch and a bundle of arrows in its talons - woodcut also featured on Geob's Schellsburg farmers' almanac *der Westlicher Menschenfreund* (*The Western Friend of Mankind*). A rare German edition of the same year features the image of a cherub draped with a laurel garland, blowing a horn, and carrying a sealed envelope. Variations of these two woodcuts are also found on birth and baptismal certificates printed by Goeb and and others in central Pennsylvania.[150]

While Ballmer's collection of cures focuses on detailed recipes for making and administering salves, his work includes a wide range of ritual procedures timed with the phases of the moon and saints' days, as well as just one written and three spoken blessings for blowing burns, curing warts and another to stop bleeding. The most striking of these cures is an inscription used to cure a felon or whitlow of the finger or toe.

Ḷ·A·V·S·V·S·R·A:

Now I rely on the name of God, that this word will destroy the seed of the felon.

The instructions state that this inscription is to be written on a piece of paper, with the letters and dots first, followed by the sentence, and tied on the finger or toe for 24 hours. Ballmer states that the inflamed digit will hurt terribly for the first twelve hours, but after, it will abate – but only if the inscription is applied at the very onset of the illness. This particular inscription has been found in manuscript form in Kutztown, Berks County, as well as in the Adams County manuscript of Levi Laydom.[151] In a German copy of Ballmer's Receipts from the collection of the author, the inscription was cut out of the book, rather than copied, and likely to have been used.

Ballmer also promotes a variation of the ritual wound-wood cures cited in Hohman; however, his procedure was used to stop blood rather than heal the wound. One was to take three small wedges of wood, and smear them with blood and drive them into a block of wood with a crack.[152] This very same procedure was documented in Morgantown, Berks County, by an Episcopalian storekeeper, James L. Morris, who described it in his ledger on November 13, 1844.[153] While this example could help to define the geographic spread of Ballmer's publication, like the inscribed copy owned by Samuel Leith of Lower Saucon, Northampton County, it is also possible that Balmer drew upon rituals and procedures already well-known in his day, just like Hohman.

A unique aspect of Ballmer's work is that the English and German editions were issued at the same time, unlike Hohman, whose work was translated decades later and by multiple people at different times.[154] Ballmer's contemporaneous editions allow for a comparison of his work in both languages, knowing that the author's intentions and mistakes are preserved in both editions. This is especially helpful in his entries for the ubiquitous lunar wart cure, previously described in Levi Laydom's manuscript. Ballmer's English edition includes the seemingly contradictory instructions to perform the ritual in the "increase of the moon" as well as to look at "the New moon" – an apparent astronomical impossibility that is echoed throughout his English edition.

This apparent contradiction, however, is a literal and accurate translation of the original German, which states that the ritual is to be performed on the third day in the "*Neulicht*" – literally, "the new light," meaning the earliest phases of the moon, i.e. waxing, as opposed to "*Altlicht*," indicating the waning moon.[155] Thus the author intended the ritual to be timed three days after the New moon, when the moon would technically be waxing once again.

Nevertheless, in the German directions, one is to look at the New moon (*Neumond*) and say, "*was ich sehe, das nimmt zu, und was ich greife, das nimmt ab*" or "What I look upon is increasing, and what I now touch is decreasing." Both the German and English words accompanying the ritual indicate that the moon is increasing or waxing, thus the potential for confusion lies with the suggestion that the New moon is to be three days old at the time of the ritual - an astronomical impossibility. Ballmer's language is not incorrect – it is just heavily nuanced. Levi Laydom's manuscript maintains this ambiguity in his transcription.

Many of Ballmer's entries involve applications of healing compounds administered at similarly ambiguous phases of the moon such as a salve used to prevent hollow horns in cattle applied "on the third day in the New moon in May," and the cutting of one's nails and plugging of the nail clippings into a tree in the "first Friday of the New moon" to cure toothache.[156] Unlike the wart cure, neither of these latter renderings in the English edition follow the German, which state, respectively "*auf den dritten Tag des Neuen Lichts im Monat May*," and "*im Neuen Licht*," both describing the "waxing moon" rather than the "New moon" as a specific phase.

Due to the difficulty in translating and distinguishing between the subtleties of *Neulicht* (waxing moon) versus *Neumond (new moon)*, it is no wonder that this ambiguity carries over into other oral traditions regarding health and healing, where it is not uncommon to find expression of differing and sometimes contradictory sets of beliefs regarding the moon and its effects. For example, two old adages in Pennsylvania Dutch suggest when the fingernails should be cut: "*Im Neimund schneit mer die Fingerneggel ab fer gut Glick*" (In the New moon, cut fingernails for good luck), and "*Im neie Licht soll mer die Fingerneggel abschneide, Zahweh zu verhiede*" (Cut fingernails in the waxing moon to avoid toothache).[157] These two attitudes may appear at first glance in Pennsylvania Dutch to suggest a similar timing, and even Fogel's original translation gives "new moon" for both the phases of the moon in both entries. This is incorrect, however, as Fogel's two entries specify two different states of the moon. The latter belief of cutting nails "*im neie Licht*" resonates with Ballmer's aforementioned toothache cure, which also suggests cutting fingernails in the waxing moon (*Neulicht*).

Interestingly enough, Ballmer's work also draws heavily upon common domestic beliefs of the times, including the use of lard in which Fasnachts were fried to keep away vermin and pests, timed according to the phase of the moon. Ballmer's instructions for driving weavils [sic] and mice from the barn in the waxing moon offer the following suggestion:

> Sweep your barn right clean on the third day in the New-moon before harvest (*Heuerndte*), then take a handful of hops and three handfuls of hoarhound, an equal quantity of chamomile & a full quart of fresh sheeps dung, put it all into a kettle full of water and boil it well, lastly pour it into a sprinkling pot (*Giesskanne,* watering can) and sprinkle your barn all over, as also the cracks, in which the weavils are. Besides this let your wife bake some cakes in hogs lard on shrove Tuesday, keep the lard till harvest when the grain is to be hauled in, and grease the wagon and the grain fork with it. By so doing you will not be troubled with mice or weavils.[158]

Similar to the warts, the toothache, and the hollow horn disease, the rats and weevils are unseated from their inhabitations in the barn by the waxing moon, which exerts a force up and away from the earth. Although Ballmer's language is not always easy to understand it is consistent in terms of orchestrating activities with lunar tradition.

A Paul Bolmer, possibly a son or other relative of Daniel, produced two later editions, one undated which bore a close resemblance to Daniel Ballmer's 1827 editions, with the image of a mortar and pestle on the cover, and another from 1831, claiming to have been printed in "Deutschland."[159] Although Daniel Ballmer's 1827 editions were widespread, his popularity faded as no new editions of his work were issued beyond the 1830's. Some of his recipes however, were described from memory over a century later by Sophia Bailer of Schuylkill County, where her father and brothers "washed" (emulsified) Venice turpentine in a stream towards the rise of the sun for the creation of a salve in the very same manner described by Daniel Ballmer. She also described the use of rattlesnake fat for curing earaches and deafness – but only if the animal has not bitten itself, as Ballmer advised.[160] Such accounts help to further describe the fluidity by which oral and written material are exchanged.

HOHMAN'S LATER EDITIONS

In 1837, a new German edition of Johann Georg Hohman's *Long Lost Friend* was printed in Skippacksville, Montgomery County, under the extended title *Der lange Verborgene Schatz und Haus-Freund* (*The Long Hidden Treasury and House-Friend*). This newly expanded edition plagiarized Ballmer's *Receipts* without so much as an acknowledgement, adding them at the end of the book as if they were the work of Hohman.[161] Although it is possible that this edition was commissioned by Hohman, the book shows several tell-tale signs of being an unlicensed, pirated edition. First, it only includes an abbreviation of Hohman's name on the title page as "J. H……..s" and nowhere else in the work. Hohman was never sparing with the use of his name. Secondly, the title page attributes portions of the work to an Arab named "Omar Arey, Emir Chemir Tschasmir," and given Hohman's propensity for seeking credit, it is highly unlikely that he would have deliberately attributed his work to another author. Hohman rarely cites other authors by name, except for example St. Albert the Great.[162] Third, the book contains a new foreword, which

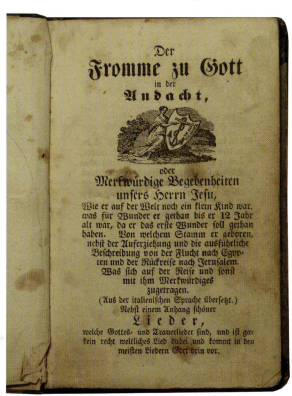

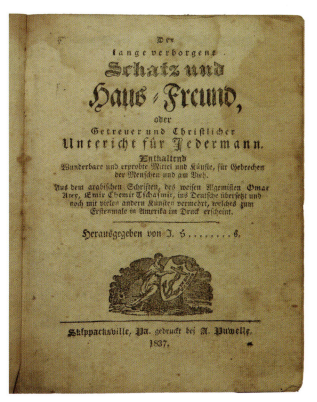

Left to Right: Hohman's 1846 book of popular and inspirational songs, *The Pious to God in Devotion*, featuring the frontis engraving with the motto "In God We Hope." The same engraving appears on the 1837 Skippacksville edition of *The Long Lost Friend* by A. Puwelle, which reprinted an appendix of Daniel Ballmer's *Receipts*. Formerly of the Lester P. Breininger Collection. *Heilman Collection*.

attempts to explain that the use of the Three Highest Names in ritual medicine was not to be confused with the commandment against taking the Lord's name in vain – but the foreword is only signed "*Der Verfasser*" (the compiler),[163] and Hohman would likely have used his full name as in his previous works, such as *The Long Lost Friend*, and *Gospel of Nicodemus*.

Nevertheless, Puwelle's Skippacksville edition bears the very same frontis illustration as Hohman's last known licensed work, *Der Fromme zu Gott in der Andacht* (*The Pious to God in Devotion*), printed in Reading in 1846. It depicts an emblem of a woman holding a shield with the motto "In God We Hope." This work begins with an infancy gospel of Jesus Christ, a narrative account of his early life and deeds as a child, and continues with a long series of religious and popular songs, including everything from murder ballads to devotional texts.

The 1837 edition of *The Long Lost Friend* was neither the first nor the last edition of Hohman to be pirated. Several later editions may have actually been commissioned by Hohman himself, such as one claiming to be the second edition printed at Ephrata in 1828, a third edition in Harrisburg in 1840,[164] and the first English edition also from Harrisburg in 1846.[165] over twenty different editions in German and English were printed before 1900 in various locations, including Chambersburg (1829), Skippacksville (1837, 1839, 1847), New Berlin (1843), Harrisburg (1843, 1846, 1850, 1853, 1856), Reading (1820, 1840), Carlisle (1863), Lancaster (1856, 1877), Kutztown (1872), and Philadelphia (1899). Two truncated, retitled editions were printed by Dreisbach in Bath, Northampton County (1847, 1857), and yet another by Ossman & Steel in Wiconisco, Dauphin County (1894).

The earliest known English translation of Hohman's collection bore the awkwardly translated title "*The Long Secreted Friend: or A True and Christian Information for Everybody*" and was printed in Harrisburg in 1846, claiming to have been "The First English Edition, translated from the German" by none other than "John G. Hohman, Publisher" himself. Although a few copies of the book were handsome, with a decorative stamped leather title cartouche on the clothbound cover,[166] the language was horrendous, and clearly the work of an amateur translator. An important example from this work contains Hohman's declaration that the work itself would function as a talisman for anyone who carried it with them, but the quality of the translation speaks for itself:

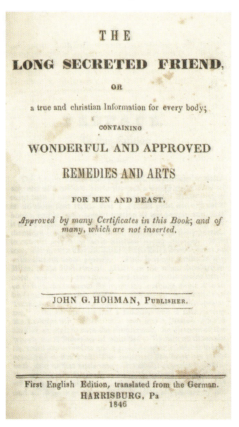

The first english edition of Hohman's Long Lost Friend, published at Harrisburg in 1846, possibly by Hohman himself. *Courtesy of Wright University Library, Archives and Special Collections.*

Direction to keep off balls: The sacred and heavenly Trompunes blow away all Balls from me. I flee under the tree of life which bears twelve kinds of fruit. I stand behind the holy Altar in the church. I recommend myself to the holy Trinity and the holy wounds of Jesus Christ. I N. N. hide myself behind the Corpus Christi that no mans hand shall take me, bind cut, shoot, stab or whip and conquer. This help me N. N. Whoever keep this little book with himself will be protected against all danger, and without the Corpus Christi he cannot die, drown or burn and none can say ought about it. To this help me + + +. [167]

This blessing, invoking powerful religious imagery, was intended for protection from bullets, but the meaning is eclipsed by the translator's lack of proficiency in English. Nevertheless, some portions of this English edition were true to the original 1820 edition, such as the spelling of the Latin in the hunter's Talisman. If this edition was truly authorized by Hohman himself as the title page states – could this have been Hohman's own translation?

Two other, more successful English translations were produced independently of one another at Harrisburg in 1850 and Carlisle in 1863. The latter translator used the literally correct, translated title *The Long Hidden Friend,* while the Harrisburg translator chose a title that was catchy, and built upon an already well-known English idiom: *The Long Lost Friend*. This would be the translation that would continue to be published for well over a century and a half up to the present day.[168]

It is telling that Hohman's work experienced a boost in popularity in the years immediately before and

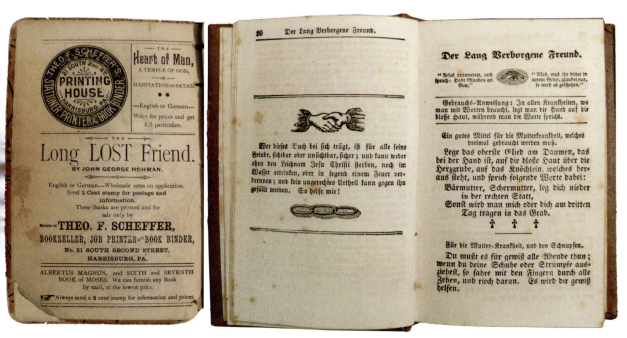

Left: Advertisement for Theodore Friedrich Scheffer's English editions of Hohman's *Long Lost Friend, Albertus Magnus,* and *The Sixth and Seventh Books of Moses,* produced in Harrisburg, Pennsylvania. Right: T. F. Scheffer's *Kunst-Buch,* a pocket-sized edition entitled *Hohmann's Lang Verborgene Freund,* complete with typographical emblems from the Fraternal Order of Oddfellows, printed ca. 1850. Heilman Collection.

shortly after the American Civil War, fueling the demand for the editions mass-produced in Harrisburg. This time period ushered in a number of significant changes in cultural awareness among the Pennsylvania Dutch, who not only were exposed to a broader cross-section of American culture through deployment in the national conflict, but were also undergoing a major shift towards the use of English only in local institutions of education, medicine, and religion. As a counter-response to these social pressures, Pennsylvania Dutch culture became increasingly nostalgic.[169] Powwowing practices resonated with these sentiments and appealed to a large portion of the Pennsylvania Dutch population seeking culturally-specific ways to assert their identities in a changing world.

Harrisburg would later come to dominate the printing of Hohman's book through printers such as Theodore F. Scheffer (1813-1883), successor to Gustav S. Peters (1793-1847), who is considered to be the first successful American commercial color printer.[170] In the 1850s and 60s, Scheffer printed *The Long Lost Friend* by the tens of thousands in English and German, and issued the very first pocket-sized editions bearing the title "*Kunst-Buch*" (*Book of Ritual Arts*) stamped on the cover. A member of the Masonic Lodge and the Fraternal Order of Oddfellows,[171] Scheffer frequently enhanced *The Long Lost Friend* with printing plates borrowed from the iconography of the Oddfellows, including the symbolism of clasped hands, three links of chain, and the All-Seeing-Eye, the latter of which were thought to evoke the Trinitarian contents of the book.

In addition, Scheffer recognized that the salability of Hohman's book was at least partially based in its promise of protection to the bearer, so he moved this passage from the haphazard location near the end of Hohman's original edition. Scheffer highlighted this inscription with printed embellishments, and placed it on the facing page of Hohman's first page of cures. At the beginning of these entries, Scheffer also repeated the title of the book, and inserted the image of the All-Seeing-Eye, along with verses of scripture from the eleventh chapter of the Gospel of Mark: "And Jesus answering saith unto them, Have faith in God... Therefore I say unto you, What things so ever ye desire, when ye pray, believe that ye receive them, and ye shall have them."[172]

HOHMAN & HELFENSTEIN

These very same words of scripture appeared on the title page of one of the most widespread German editions of Hohman, printed as a dual edition of Hohman and Helfenstein in 1853 by Theodore F. Scheffer and his early printing partner, Jacob M. Beck.[173] Although the German text of Hohman is unremarkable in this format, Helfenstein's collection underwent a series of substantial revisions and additions– everything from the title to the contents. Instead of the original title *Soli Deo Gloria* (*Glory to God Alone*), a totally new title was assigned,

Vielfältig erprobter Hausschatz der Sympathie (*Diverse and Proven Home Treasury of Sympathy*), with the addition of an anachronistic, and ill-fitting subtitle: *...oder, Enthüllte Zauberkräfte und Geheimnisse der Natur* (*...or, Unveiled Magic Powers and Secrets of Nature*). Helfenstein used the word *Zauberei* (magic or sorcery) only three times in his original work,[174] and each time, it appeared in the description of rituals designed to protect one from harmful acts of sorcery. Thus to Helfenstein, *Zauberei* was not a desirable experience, and certainly not one related to his particular brand of rituals aiming to heal and protect. Thus, Scheffer & Beck's efforts to increase the salability of Helfenstein's work by associating it with sorcery was incongruent with values presented in the original publication.

Unlike previous editions, Scheffer & Beck's new edition of Helfenstein was expanded with a long addendum that increased its size nearly by two fold, incorporating the contents from an earlier work by Sheffer's predecessor, G. S. Peters, entitled *Egyptische Geheimnisse oder das Zigeuner Buch gennant* (*Egyptian Secrets, or the So-Called Gypsy Book*). Although the title would ostensibly suggest a connection with the *Egyptian Secrets* of pseudo-Albert the Great, the contents are entirely different. The contents of G. S. Peters' *So-Called Gypsy Book* of 1844 shares a number of entries in common with an addendum entitled *Kunstreiche Stüche von Mancherley Art* (*Artful Formulae of Many Sorts*), found in the work of Daniel Schmidt printed in Carlisle in 1826, entitled *Das Gemeinnützige Haus-Arzeneybuch* (*The Domestic Doctor Book for the Common Use*).

Although Peters' work is comparatively late, the contents of Peter's and Schmidt's work are part of an early, distinctive collection of cures and instructions that was recorded in a late-eighteenth century manuscript

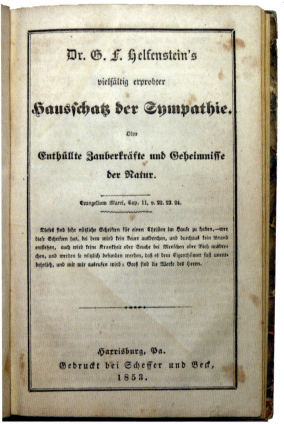

Dr. G. F. Helfenstein's *Vielfältig erprobter Hausschatz der Sympathie* (*Diverse and Proven Home Treasury of Sympathy*), published as a dual edition with the German text of Hohman's *Long Lost Friend* in 1853, by Scheffer & Beck of Harrisburg. Heilman Collection.

by the son of the Moravian Clerk at Bethlehem, Johann Christoph Pyrlaeus, Jr. (1748-1808). While Pyrlaeus was certainly not the author of this material, his collection is the earliest known American copy of this rare collection. An Allentown imprint from 1819 *Das Nützliche Haus und Kunst-Buch*, or *The Useful Domestic and Formula Book*, contains a total of thirty-three identical entries, and three others that are similar. Allentown's close proximity to Bethlehem suggests a related provenance in the Lehigh Valley.[175]

Interestingly enough, Hohman's *The Friend in Need* of 1813 contains three entries in common with Pyrlaeus, as well as the 1819 Allentown imprint. That Hohman and Pyrlaeus were able to access and record identical materials is no coincidence given their close geographical and chronological ties in the early nineteenth century at the border region of Northampton and Bucks counties. Beginning in 1802, Hohman lived in Nockamixon Township, a mere 15 miles from Bethlehem and also printed broadsides in Easton in 1811,[176] before eventually settling in Reading. Perhaps even more telling of the region's ties to ritual literature, is that one of the earliest known copies of *Romanus* produced in Pennsylvania is inscribed by Jacob Finsi in 1818, to a Tobias Schick (1782-1848) born in Springfield Township, Bucks County, a neighboring township to Nockamixon.[177] Schick later moved to Armstrong County in 1827, close to Pittsburgh following his service in the War of 1812, bringing his manuscript with him.[178] All of these early and interrelated works suggest that the Moravian settlement at Bethlehem, known for its early printing, binding, and importing of books, was a hotbed for esoteric publishing in the eighteenth and early nineteenth centuries that spread throughout the surrounding region, and eventually influenced other parts of Pennsylvania and North America.

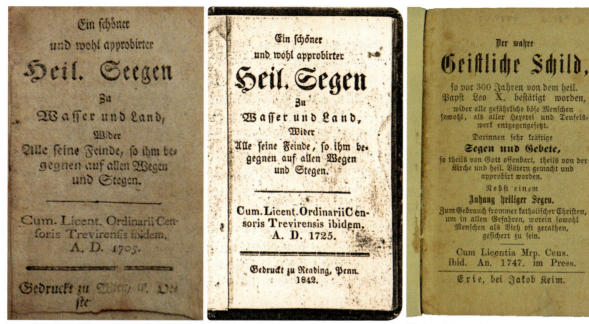

Three American editions of the *Heiliger Segen un Geistlicher Schild (Holy Blessing and Spiritual Shield)*, from left to right: An edition owned by Georg Henninger of Albany Township, Berks County, with a false imprint of Vienna; An 1842 "Reading, Pennsylvania" imprint of the *Holy Blessing*; Jacob Keim's edition of *The Spiritual Shield, Holy Blessing, and the Spiritual Shield Vigil*, with images of the saints. *Heilman Collection.*

THE MIDWEST & THE SPIRITUAL SHIELD

Similar books of sympathetic instructions were printed in Ohio and parts of western Pennsylvania, but few of these have survived to the present day, and more research is needed in these communities to determine their use and distribution. In Canton, Ohio, a work entitled *Die Wunder der Sympathie, zum zwecke für Heilungen an menschen, thieren, und pflanzen* (*The Miracle of Sympathy, for the Purpose of Healing Humans, Animals, and Plants*) appeared in 1855, printed by John Saxton and Son, for Daniel Prützmann(1813-1893).[179] Although powwowing manuals are a rarity in Ohio, there was apparently a demand for such works, encouraging Cincinnati printer Benjamin Boffinger to reprint the *True Spiritual Shield* in 1837. A Catholic minister publically shamed him for "disseminating lies and superstition among simple creatures."[180] Despite criticism from the clergy, the publication maintained relative popularity and later appeared in other communities of Roman Catholics, such as in Erie, Pennsylvania, where a Catholic German Family Bible was also printed in the 1870s.[181]

Evidence suggests that Reading printers were also responsible for earlier dual-editions of the *Spiritual Shield* and *Heiliger Seegen (Holy Blessing)* such as one claiming to have been printed in "Vienna in Austria" and owned by the son of Georg Henninger (1737 -1815) in Albany Township, Berks County, also named Georg (b. 1765) who inscribed it with his name.[182] Some of these American imprints do not include the images of the saints so common in the European editions, suggesting a Protestant appropriation of this Roman Catholic book of blessings. Many of those bearing a Reading imprint were from the press of Enßlin of Reutlingen,[183] who exported books to the United States, where they were distributed through the publishing houses of Wilhelm Radde of New York to meet the needs of American audiences for popular manuals of ritual healing.

OSSMAN & STEEL'S GUIDE TO HEALTH

As works by Hohman, Helfenstein, and Ballmer continued to evolve, a number of local publishers sought to cash in on the growing demand for powwow manuals in the late nineteenth and early twentieth centuries. One of the most unusual byproducts of Hohman's legacy is a compendium with the seemingly-unimpressive title *Ossman & Steel's Guide to Health or Household Instructor*, published in 1894 in Wiconisco, northeast of Harrisburg in Dauphin County.

Described as a manual for "Pow Wowing," Ossman and Steel's *Guide to Health* is an abridgement of *The Long Lost Friend*, with additional household remedies as well as recipes for the creation of salves, teas, and liniments.

The work aims, however, to impress the reader with large typographical reproductions of Hohman's Trinitarian formulas, featuring three crosses up to an inch in height that visually dominate the pages.

Although the first names of the authors are not listed, one entry, "I. D. Steel's Army Liniment," describes a recipe obtained during "the late war," and provides the necessary clues to determine the reluctant compiler's identity. Issac D. Steel of the Lykens Valley in Dauphin County (1835-1895) was a tanner by trade, and veteran of the Civil War, who enlisted in Company G of the Pennsylvania 7th Cavalry in winter of 1864, and served as a private for a year and a half.[184] A number of other remedies are attributed to "Mr. Steel" or "one of the authors,"[185] but never in first person – suggesting the possibility that Ossman did the writing.

Although it is unknown precisely who Steel's counterpart in the business was, there is at least one good guess. In the Federal Census of 1880, Isaac D. Steel is listed as living in Wiconisco with his wife Catherine, his four daughters Marrietta, Hannah, Maggie, and Amelia, and his widowed mother, named Ann Ossman. Just ten years prior, Steel is listed in the neighboring village of Lykens, having a housekeeper named Anne Ossman (b.1815), and a child of ten years named William C. Steel. William was later married and lived with his wife Susan in Lykens by 1880. In 1860, Isaac D. Steel is listed in Lykens as living only with a spouse named Sarah, who seems to have vanished from the scene within a decade. In 1850, at the age of fifteen, Isaac Steel lived in Lykens with Ann Ossman, aged forty. A somewhat complicated family narrative is suggested by this scant public documentation. Did Ann Ossman and Isaac Steel really publish the book at the respective ages of 59 and 79 – only for Isaac to pass away suddenly from heart disease one year later?[186]

As unlikely as it seems, these individuals, living under the same roof, are the only two people with the last names of the authors in the small village of Wiconisco at the time of the publication. The title page of the book suggests the possibility of sending mail to the authors, at "Ossman & Steel, Wiconisco, PA… To whom all communications should be addressed." The encouragement of the reader to contact the authors by mail plays an important role throughout the text of the book.

> In introducing our little book, entitled, *Ossman and Steel's Guide to Health*, we believe we have made something known that will be of much value to our readers. Our aim has been to present in as concise a form as is possible such information which will be useful, and to suggest many hints which, if followed according to our directions, will do a great deal of good. We have carefully arranged and condensed all the matter so that you may readily find almost any particular information in regard to Pow Wowing, &c., in a very short time. We hope and believe that this book will prove itself so full of information relating to everyday life, that after being thoroughly read, it will be carefully placed in a handy place for reference, and make for itself an indispensable household companion…

As with many powwow manuals, Ossman and Steel appeal to the reader's desire for proof of usefulness and benefit to others. Almost in anticipation of comparison to other less organized works of the same genre, the authors claim to have taken great pains to make the work more accessible, but offer little explanation for how the work is organized. Loosely, one can see that first part of the book contains selections from *The Long Lost Friend*, and the second half consists of additional powwow rituals as well as recipes for salves, plasters, and household remedies. The last and final section describes the creation of polishes, inks, adhesives, cosmetics, and cleaners. It is notable that the authors regard the total contents of the work – recipes, rituals, and remedies - as useful information for daily life, rather than the substance of legends peppered with the occasional domestic hint.

> …One feature of this book we wish especially to impress upon the mind of our readers, and that is, that every word, and every line, and every page, is true. Few books or pamphlets now published are strictly true. There is a thread of truth in them, but so much romance and fancy are woven around, that the single thread of truth is lost sight of. We give you the facts, not embellished, not enlarged upon, not exaggerated, but the plain unvarnished truth…

Here the introduction begins to exercise its rhetorical strategy, appealing to the reader with the promise of certainty, rather than lofty religious hyperbole. The authors may be taking a jab at Helfenstein's collection, which was likely to have been originally published somewhere within the tri-county area of Dauphin, Schuylkill, and Northumberland, and was known to have been distributed in multiple editions throughout the region. Helfenstein claims supernatural origins for the "secrets of sympathy" like Hohman's *Freund in der Noth*, the introduction of which included legendary tales of mystical hermits and dragons, copies of which also found its way into the Lykens Valley.[187] The indirect criticism of Hohman continues, by dodging the use of lengthy testimonials:

> We hardly deem it necessary to give the names and addresses of those who have been cured by our remedies, but should any one have the least doubt as to the veracity of our statement, we will take pleasure to convince such ones that every work we say is true, upon receipt of stamped envelope for reply. It is not necessary to commit anything to memory (although it is the better plan), as any intelligent person who has sufficient faith in it (as well as the patient), and who believes there is a Heaven and Hell, can Pow Wow with the greatest success simply reading from the book, and by following our instructions. Another point we wish to impress upon the mind of our many readers, and that is,

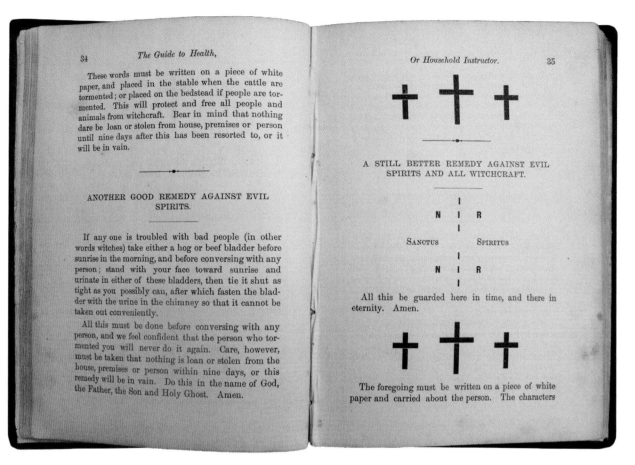

Ossman & Steel's Guide to Health, a rare collection of powwowing rituals and domestic recipes, published and distributed by mail order through two residents of Wiconisco, Dauphin County. *Heilman Collection.*

that every word we mention in regard to Pow Wowing is taken from the Scripture, and those who have no faith in the Scripture, had better keep their hands off our book, as they cannot be cured by this method.

You will note we consider some of our secrets worth ONE HUNDRED DOLLARS. We mean just what we say about this matter. ONE HUNDRED DOLLARS is a mere song for some of them, to say nothing of the many other valuable secrets that can be found in our book. WE WANT AGENTS EVERYWHERE, of either sex, and we don't hesitate to say that any intelligent person who devotes a little time to the study of this book, and who is not afraid to go from house to house and push the business, will make more money in one day that could be made in one week or more at any other employment. All that is necessary is to show the book, from beginning to end, setting forth each subject, &c., and we feel confident that no trouble will be experienced in effecting a sale, as nearly every person will see at a glance that the book is very valuable, and consequently subscribe for one, notwithstanding the fact that it will be necessary to economize elsewhere in order to obtain one. Write for circulars and terms to agents, enclosing stamps for reply. Ossman & Steel.[188]

The concluding portion of the introduction speaks volumes about the authors' intentions to capitalize on interest in powwowing throughout the region by not only suggesting a bloated monetary value, but also by shamelessly encouraging door-to-door sales of the work for personal gain. Indeed, the price of "ONE HUNDRED DOLLARS" and the suggested value "worth the cost of the entire book" is echoed throughout the text for diverse ritual and herbal entries – everything from how to compel thieves to return stolen goods, to snake bite rituals, to remedies for "Miner's Asthma" – black lung, a common complaint among anthracite miners in the region. Several of Ossman and Steel's cures conclude with the statement: "we don't hesitate to say that a great deal of money could be made by the sale of this preparation."[189]

These assertions of monetary value and projected income from powwowing are coupled with invitations to visit the authors in Wiconisco:

> Those who are inclined to doubt our word had better write, or come to see us personally, and be convinced that every word we say is true…Let good doctors and quacks talk about our assertions and book as much as they please. To those we can prove that we have permanently cured cases where some of the best physicians failed to affect a cure…Anyone desiring further information …call on us, or will write us, we will be glad to give further explanation. You will note that we can treat patients as successfully a thousand miles away as if under treatment personally, and that we conduct our own correspondence, which is strictly confidential.[190]

These statements seem to indicate that Ossman and Steel run their own entrepreneurial practice, treating patients from their home in Wiconisco, as well as remotely through the mail.

Other entries in Ossman and Steel's compendium are non-ritual in orientation, some of which are likely to cause direct physical harm through toxic applications of improvised chemical medicines or imprecise dosage. These include "neuralgia pills" made from strychnine, licorice, and gum arabic; medicinal "horse powder" containing large doses of gun powder, saltpeter, sulfur, and jimsonweed;[191] and chocolate coated pills made of camphor and opium claiming to cure both cholera and diarrhea.[192] While Ossman and Steel claim that these particular recipes originate from military cures used for humans and animals in the Civil War, a number of others claim to be "obtained from an old Indian doctor," "an old Indian remedy," "an Indian pain killer," and a "Gypsy remedy."[193]

Of all of the alleged sources that Ossman and Steel claim in their *Guide to Health*, the reference to George Washington is most prominent. The first entry in the book claims to be a copy of a blessing "carried in the Army as a protection by George Washington," containing the full text of Psalm 91 from the King James Bible. This blessing is followed by 44 pages of selections from Hohman's *Long Lost Friend*.

Beyond Ossman and Steel's entries from Hohman and the section of chemically-oriented remedies, a wide variety of basic sympathetic cures are outlined. These involve the ritual use of common everyday objects such as urinating into a hollowed out carrot that is to be concealed in the home to cure jaundice – stating that this "will cause the jaundice to disappear as the Urine absorbs," stemming from the belief that the yellow color of the skin from jaundice is healed through the absorption of yellow body fluids into a similarly colored vegetable.[194]

Other sympathetic cures featured in Ossman and Steel outline ritual practices associated with the dead such as the treatment of epilepsy by sewing into the sufferer's clothing small portions of rope with which a condemned criminal was hanged, a common nineteenth-century practice in Pennsylvania.[195] Along these lines, the *Guide to Health* also provides a wart cure, employing as many stones as there are warts, each rubbed on a single wart and deposited into a fresh grave where one has not yet been buried during the waning moon.[196]

A number of cures feature more complex dynamics in ritual structure such the notion that certain diseases must be healed by a member of the opposite sex. One cure for retention of urine features the abdominal application of a red band of flannel cloth that has been doubled over and urinated upon by a member of the opposite sex.[197] In other cases, it is not the gender of the person that matters, but only that the constitution of the healer is stronger than that of the patient.[198]

Like Hohman, Ossman and Steel do not provide much in the way of overarching recommendations for powwowing, but instead, instructions are situational and provided as addenda at the conclusion of each ritual. For example, a cure for erysipelas concludes by passing the hands three times over the naked body of the patient with bare hands from head to foot:

> **Pow-wow for patient three times a day, thus making nine applications. We have cured the worst kind of cases in a few days' time, and are still doing so from time to time. We are glad to say we have entirely cured cases that have been under the best physician's treatment, and whose remedies only aggravated the disease instead of giving relief.**[199]

In some cases, the passing of the hands over the body have to be timed with the moon. Unlike the previous wart cure involving the use of stones in the cemetery, the lunar aspects of the wart cure are further expounded in a cure for "wasting away of flesh on children" for which Ossman and Steel suggest powwowing on the first three Fridays of the waning moon, as well as on the first tree Fridays of the waxing moon, and the words must be altered to suit the occasion:

> When powwowing in the increase of the moon, say, what I look at shall increase, instead of saying what I look at shall decrease." Another similar cure for wasting among adults states: " Remember a cure cannot be affected by this method, unless it is done in either the increase or decrease of the moon.[200]

Aside from procedures that specify the passing of the hands over the body, some rituals become much more physically engaging through the act of anointing the patient and the use of massage. A remedy for individuals who are "heart bound" or "liver grown," requires the "greasing" of the supine patient with warm lard "from the shoulders to the pit of the heart, also along both sides of the ribs to the spine of the back."[201] One must then trace the same directional motions of the application of the lard with the thumbs, while reciting a variation of one of the usual cures for colic.[202] This must be repeated three times, and then the patient must be turned over onto their stomach, and the back is anointed and rubbed in a similar manner, along with the hands and feet. The patient's feet must face east toward the rise of the sun. They assert: "This remedy has never been known to fail."[203]

In other situations, Ossman and Steel offer advice when a ritual does not effect a cure:

> If this remedy does not cure (or any other of our pow-wowing remedies), there is no use in resorting to others, as any one who has faith in the Holy Bible will agree with us when we say that our dear Savior's medicine is above all others.[204]

Thus, if a ritual does not work, Ossman and Steel claim that it is not the fault of the remedy, but rather, that the illness is incurable. Most of the remedies found in *Guide to Health* are described as panaceas. Building upon the introduction's assertions of absolute truth, the work is interspersed with "never failing" remedies, as well as a few suggestions for the readers to engage in testing the remedies and rituals on their own. Perhaps the most audacious of these, is an addendum to the "*True Benediction Against Fire…*" suggesting:

> Anyone who has sufficient faith in this sentence, can check the largest fire by simply walking around it three times, each time repeating these words, and making a ring around it on the ground three times also. We don't pretend to say that the fire can be entirely extinguished by this method, but we do pretend to say that the fire won't and cannot possibly get over the rings made on the ground. We invite anyone to build a fire on some wooden floor, at the same time following our directions (the outskirts of the ring made on the wooden floor may be well soaked with kerosene if desired), and be convinced that every word we say is true.[205]

These types of dangerous suggestions are coupled with unusually-phrased, cautionary statements warning readers that certain rituals have the power to either heal or kill a patient. An entry explaining the use of the diminishing *Abaxacatabax* triangle inscription concludes with the advice:

> If this remedy does not effect a cure there is no use of trying others. It is mostly intended for children, and we would not advise any one to use it where there is but little hope of the patient's recovery, unless you either desire to effect a permanent cure or kill.[206]

These instructions not only suggest that ritual has the power to kill, they are also particularly reckless, because they appear to recommend to parents of sick children that if a powwowing ritual does not work, that no other course of action should be taken. This dangerous advice could threaten the life of a child.

In one similarly distasteful entry, a ritual for compelling thieves to return stolen goods appears to suggest that killing the thieves is not only possible by ritual means, but conceivably preferable: "we would advise you to release them within twenty-four hours, unless you desire to kill them."[207]

It is possible that the authors may have been employing some level of hyperbole, or even sarcasm, in their instructions to enhance the appearance of the text's power. Overall, the tone of their writing is decidedly cavalier, and gives no indication of whether or not they condone the use of ritual to harm. Despite Ossman and Steel's brazen approach to powwowing, it is clear that Hohman and

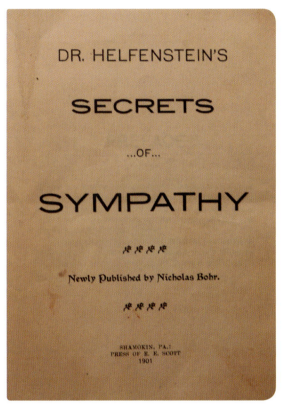

A twentieth-century edition of *Secrets of Sympathy*, an English version of the cures of Dr. Helfenstein, by Nicholas Bohr of Shamokin, 1901. *Heilman Collection.*

others like pseudo-Albert the Great had set the precedent generations prior for such an ethically complicated approach to the use of ritual, especially the publishing of sensitive material as a profitable commercial venture. Both Hohman's *Long Lost Friend*, and *Egyptian Secrets* warn against the misuse of their instructions – yet never actually defined any boundaries, aside from those of a philosophical and religious nature. This air of controversy would follow the genre of ritual literature into the twentieth century, when it would gain a wider popular audience and lose much of its original cultural context.

TWENTIETH-CENTURY RITUAL LITERATURE

By the turn of the twentieth century, two parallel trends of powwowing literature had developed, one of which experienced a wider acceptance throughout the United States, and the other of which remained local and rooted in religious healing. While the translation of Hohman's work into English allowed it to spread outside of Pennsylvania, and pulp editions become a favorite in both rural and urban populations in the manner of occult works of curiosity and magic, the works of Helfenstein were translated in to English but only retained a marginal reception among new generations of powwowers in North Central Pennsylvania.

Dr. Helfenstein's works appeared in three new additions after 1900 both of which bore the title *Secrets of Sympathy* – a phrase borrowed from Helfenstein's introduction. The first of these appears to be a direct translation from Helfenstein's original broadsides, produced by Nicholas Bohr of Shamokin in 1901. This is likely to be Nicholas R. Bohr (1852-1901) a Roman Catholic immigrant who arrived in the United States in 1872, having come from Detzem, in the Rhineland-Palatinate.[208] Bohr settled in the core region where Helfenstein was distributed and likely to have been originally published as broadsides. His translation demonstrates the acceptance of powwowing among later waves of German-speaking immigrants in the region, who used and even created English-language works as they adapted to the region. Alfred Shoemaker documented another English translation by William C. Kline of Shamokin, by the press of Shamokin Daily News in 1928. No copies are known to exist.[209]

An abridged version of *Secrets of Sympathy* was later reissued in 1938 in Klingerstown, Schuylkill County by William Irvin Beissel(1875-1949) of Leck Kill, Northumberland County. Beissel was a clerk for a lumber operation associated with a colliery near Shamokin, where he spent the rest of his days.[210] Both Bohr's and Beissel's editions referred to the contents as "sympathies" and were decidedly religious in their orientation, with no emphasis or exaggeration of exotic or legendary elements.

Bohr's edition maintains only a small portion of Helfenstein's introduction, but Beissel's edition includes no trace of it. Instead he offers advice out of his own experiences as a powwow healer:

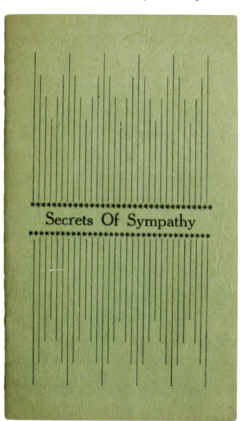

A third, abridged edition of the English collection of Dr. Helfenstein's *Secrets of Sympahty* by William Beissel at Klingerstown in 1938. *Heilman Collection.*

> I have used the sympathies in this booklet for the past forty years with great success. I, therefore, recommend this work and hope that its resulting blessings may be carried to many people everywhere. Anyone interested in helping others with physical, mental, and spiritual disorders may be fully assured with success if but a few simple rules are truthfully and faithfully obeyed.
>
> (1) Have faith and no doubt in your heart. Mark 11:22-23; Matthew 17:20. Also believe in the Holy Trinity. You cannot get success from God by using these sympathies if you are not a Christian or by using these words and not living a Christian life.
>
> (2) Use the Christian name for each sympathy in this booklet. If for example, the directions of the sympathy call for the use of the name and other actions three times [when] the name is said, the action performed (if any), and followed by the words of sympathy. This order must be followed three times (or whatever the number of times the directions of the sympathy call for). This is very important.
>
> (3) If the patient is very sick or has severe pain the sympathy may be repeated every 15 or 30 minutes for three times, or oftener as the case and condition may demand. If the suffering be great and the relief and success of the sympathy slow, the same procedure as just outlined above may be repeated every 3 days, or daily until fully relieved or recovered. If there is less suffering and the patient is weak every 7 or 9 days as experience may teach and call for or according to the effect the sympathy has and the strength of the patient. Experience will be a good guide.
>
> In way of general remarks remember that a sympathy may take hold at times and cause the patient to become very weak. At such times the repeatings of the sympathies must be regulated according to the strength of the patient. It is also true that at times when the one who administers the sympathy may receive a slight pain of suffering for a short period identical at the place in his body as the patient had for whom the sympathy was given. In severe cases of suffering a

number of sympathies may be given together or at one time. The beginner may not always be sure which one is needed and therefore can use several as the wrong ones will do no harm. It will be noticed that two sympathies are given at some places for the same thing. Either or both may be used according to the success received therefrom.

It is also important to remember that no one can be helped if they do not have a Christian name received through baptism. The full name including the middle name must be used. The patient may be absent if conditions of presence prove inconvenient or impossible for the one who is to administer the sympathy. The sympathy may be repeated verbally or silently. Success is also assured if any sympathy is used for yourself if you have faith and no doubt in your heart. The patient can only successfully be helped if he or she have faith in the Trinity and believe these sympathies. The one to administer the sympathy must be healthy and have a strong constitution. Certain severe diseases may be cured. Sometimes much patients [sic] and preserverence [sic] is required. The author knows of people that were helped that were given up as hopeless by doctors.

The author considers The Holy Fire and Pestilence Letter as found on the last pages the most important part of this entire booklet. He personally believes it should be in every home.

As a last word, my friend, if interested follow the directions closely and experience will teach you many things. You will be able to do wonders in years to come. As a beginner, have patience and keep trying until you get results and success. No success means that conditions have not been met and just as soon as they are met as herein described success is sure to follow. Remember, what you will do to help suffering humanity is to be TO THE GLORY OF GOD and not for personal gain, pride, or money. Use common sense at all times and be sure to follow directions exactly as given and success will be yours.[211]

Both of these later English editions stress those aspects of the powwowing experience that share the most in common with faith healing traditions, as opposed to magic. This is perhaps part of the reason that Helfenstein remains largely unknown in the present day, and was not appropriated by popular publishing companies to the degree that Hohman was. While Helfenstein drew a considerably smaller audience, Hohman continued to gain wider acceptance outside of Pennsylvania, and was adapted for use by vernacular healing traditions throughout North America.

In the twentieth century, Hohman's work was a favorite of esoteric publishing firms in Chicago such as Lewis de Claremont, Egyptian Publishing Co., and the DeLawrence Co., to name but a few. These companies specialized in a broad spectrum of popular occult works, and marketed *The Long Lost Friend* to a national audience. This was not without substantial restructuring of the image and presentation of the tradition. In de Claremont's late 1930s edition, Hohman is immortalized in comic-book illustrations, depicting him in nearly Dickensian attire amidst Egyptian pyramids and Turkish palaces. Instead of emphasizing the healing aspects of the tradition, advertisements for the de Claremont edition proudly boast that use of Hohman's book would help one obtain success, good fortune, and prosperity – and worse, a description of the book's contents promises ritual procedures that could be used to retaliate against enemies, gain advantage over others, prevent slander, manipulate the legal system, and gain invincibility.[212] This egomaniacal presentation of Hohman was further exaggerated by the fact that thousands of turn-of-the-century copies of *The Long Lost Friend* were printed in a dual edition with tracts against women's right to vote (*Woman: Her Duties, Relations, and Position*, 1899)![213]

Some have argued positively that, despite Hohman's distinctive personality, *The Long Lost Friend* has served to perpetuate and preserve traditional healing, which is perceived by some to be in a state of decline. While the act of recording this kind of material is certain to prevent it from being entirely forgotten, at the same time this contradictory approach to "cultural preservation," has attempted to prematurely embalm the body of ritual folk culture, long before any actual demise of the tradition has occurred. The role of Hohman's work, and other powwow manuals of a similar genre, have historically been overemphasized in the study of folk culture, when in the eyes of the folk, dependence on literature in ritual process is generally not looked upon favorably. The scholarly reliance on printed literature for folk-cultural analysis is understandable, however, as it is symptomatic of the challenges inherent in the acquisition of primary sources. It is far easier for some to study a book than to establish the trust of a community.

In some cases, publications of ritual instructions have also exposed the tradition to the ridicule and sensationalism by journalists, who through scathing editorials have done considerable damage to the image of the culture in the public imagination of America.[214] This disembodied literature has also revealed itself as the source of much abuse and fetishization of the tradition such as in the case of the tragic murder of Nelson Rehmeyer in York County in 1928, when an attempt to steal his copy of Hohman's book to break the power of a curse resulted in Rehmeyer's death.[215] The media's fixation on this tragic incident drew national attention to the region, and often grossly misrepresented the culture's traditions.

What is obvious in the marketing of the highly commercialized editions of Hohman is that the tradition was being forcibly removed from its cultural and community context in everyday life, and promoted as a self-centered practice used for personal gain. This loss of the original purpose of powwowing not only corrupts the practice and sullies its image in the public eye, but it also has the potential to compromise the survival of the tradition, by undermining the integration of ritual into everyday life.

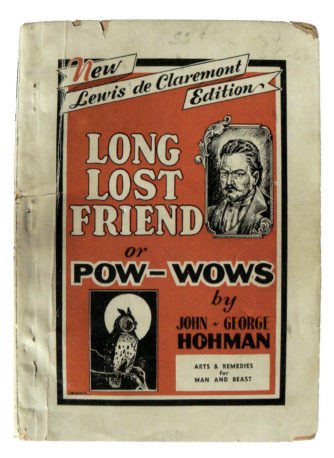
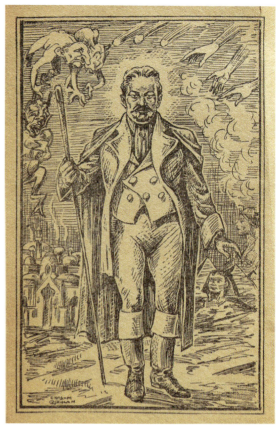

Above: Lewis de Claremont's *Long Lost Friend or Pow-Wows*, a 1930s edition of John George Hohman's classic work, featuring illustrations from the comic artist Charles M. Quinlain, who also illustrated golden-age titles such as *Lone Eagle, Masked Rider, Hopalong Cassidy, Super-Sleuths,* and *Cat-man & Kitten.* Heilman Collection.

Below: A newspaper advertisement for the Louis de Claremont edition of Hohman's *Long Lost Friend*, featured in the *Pittsburgh Courier* in 1939.

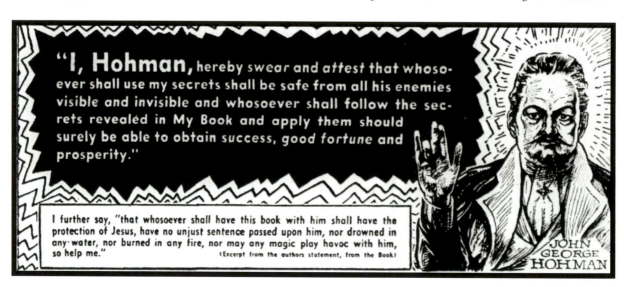

Sixth and Seventh Books of Moses

One of the more unusual books to be associated with powwowing that lacks any semblance of connection to daily life is the *Sixth and Seventh Books of Moses (Das 6te und 7te Buch Moses)*. This work alleges be the extra-biblical writings of the ancient Hebrews and Christian cabalists, claiming authorship from the most influential writer of the Old Testament. However, it is by no means a work of healing. Instead, the book held a sinister connotation, both in Pennsylvania and abroad, because its contents include seals and inscriptions of power allegedly used by Moses to visit the seven plagues upon Egypt, as well as instructions for the conjuration and command of evil spirits for a variety of purposes.

The book is visually complex, with illustrations of diagrams and sigils written in corrupted Latin, Hebrew, and Greek characters. The only aspects comparable to powwowing are two additional sections devoted to the ritual use of the Biblical Psalms and the Hebrew names of God for healing, protection, and beneficial purposes. Nevertheless, among the Pennsylvania Dutch this highly controversial book was believed to inform the practice of *Hexerei* (witchcraft), and it was from this book that the servants of the devil were thought to have derived their power. Although the *Sixth and Seventh Books of Moses* appeared in Pennsylvania relatively late in the development of powwowing, the book was feared for having the power to spell-bind a curious reader, causing them to be "read fast" – i.e. spellbound by the contents of the book. The remedy was to have a powwower read the text backwards to undo the effect.[216] On the other hand, many powwow practitioners saw *The Sixth and Seventh Books of Moses* as a work used to counteract *Hexerei*, and the book was owned by a wide variety of practitioners – some for use, and some merely for reference.

A European edition of the *The Sixth and Seventh Books of Moses*, complete with linen enclosures and waxed paper seals of a skull and crossed bones with a cross. The work claims to have been printed in Philadelphia, ca. 1880. *Heilman Collection.*

The earliest versions of the *Sixth and Seventh Books of Moses* appear to have been circulated in in manuscript form, as the earliest known reference to the work is from a bookseller's catalog from 1797 wherein a Latin text entitled *VI et VII Liber Mosis* was offered for sale among other ceremonial manuscripts and books.[217] Manuscripts formed the basis for the earliest and most authoritative edition compiled and first released in print in the 1840s by German antiquarian Johann Scheible (1809-1866). He included a standardized version in the 6th volume of his academic series on ceremonial magic, entitled *Bibliothek der Zauber-Geheimniss- und Offenbarungs-Bücher* (*Library of Magic, Secret, and Revelatory Books*) published in Stuttgart in 1849.[218] Shortly thereafter it became one of the most widely circulated works to inspire folk ritual practice on both sides of the Atlantic.

In the United States, early editions of Scheible's *Sixth and Seventh Books of Moses* were commissioned by American publishers and distributors across the Atlantic. The first and largest distributor was the book dealer Wilhelm Radde of New York in the 1850s. Radde carried a wide range of other works of ritual literature, including *The Spiritual Shield* and *Egyptian Secrets*.[219] In 1880, the English language edition appeared for the first time from Radde and was reprinted often throughout the late nineteenth and early twentieth centuries. These New York editions, in both English and German were the most readily available to Pennsylvanians, printed in both red and black text with copious plates and illustrations, and bound in black leather.

In Europe, *the Sixth and Seventh Books of Moses* rapidly rose to popularity as an underground banned book, and eventually the very title became a catch-all for many different works of ritual literature printed in Germany. Just like the popular presses in the Midwestern United States, German publishers such as E. Bartels, of Weissensee, Berlin, and Max Emil Fischer of Dresden published popular editions from the

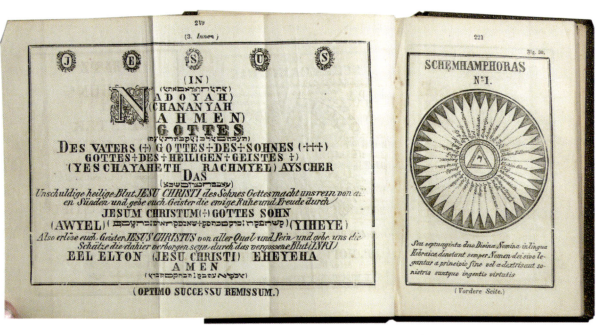

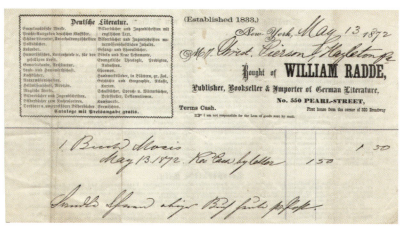

Above: A fold-out print from the Shemhamphoras - or the 72 Names of God, an addendum included in the *Sixth and Seventh Books of Moses*, with Latin, Hebrew, and German inscriptions. *Heilman Collection.*

Left: Order form from book distributor Wilhelm Radde of New York, who dealt in imported popular and religious books including *The Sixth and Seventh Books of Moses*, *Albertus Magnus*, and *The True Spiritual Shield*. This order form indicates that Christopher Peterson of Hazelton, Pennsylvania ordered one copy of *The Sixth and Seventh Books of Moses* for $1.50. *Heilman Collection.*

Opposite Page: 1931 German edition of *The Sixth and Seventh Books of Moses*, printed in Dresden, but bearing a "Philadelphia" imprint on the title page. This work was not only a new edition of the work, but it also includes commentary on the work, as its full title suggests "...Its Worth, and What People Seek in It." This particular edition appeared on the 1938 Nazi propaganda bureau's *List of Harmful and Undesirable Writings*, that urged the burning of the work and punnishment for those who possess, print, or distribute it. *Heilman Collection.*

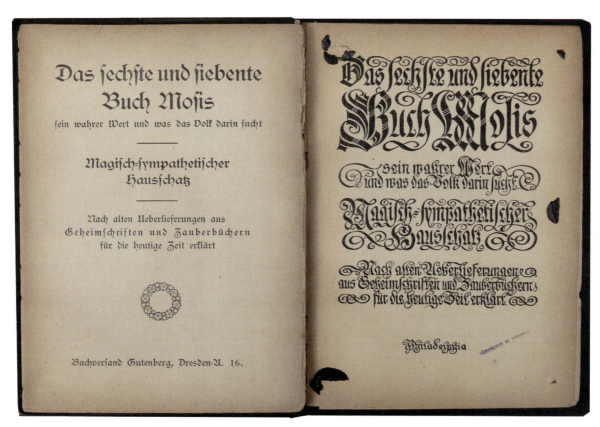

1880s through the 1920s. These contained a compilation (*Sammelband*) of many classic works banned by the Roman Catholic authorities, including *The Spiritual Shield*, *Our Lady's Dream*, and *The Seven Heavenly Bolts*. Bartels' compilations were often printed with black covers, sealed with wax emblems bearing skulls and crossed bones and bound with black linen wrappings over the pages that had to be cut open by the buyer.[220]

Some of these later editions, claiming to have been printed in Philadelphia, did not actually contain Scheible's text at all, but were sold as collections of occult curiosities. Additional collections, such as *The Eighth and Ninth Books of Moses* were of a similar nature, and tended to include a wide range of texts, such as *Romanus*, and *Egyptian Secrets*.[221] The Sixth and Seventh Books of Moses were later suppressed in Germany under the Third Reich, when a 1931 edition released in Dresden, complete with pentagram wax seals and claiming the false imprint of Philadelphia, was listed on the *1938 List of Harmful and Undesirable Writings* (*Liste des schädlichen und unerwünschten Schrifttums*) issued by Propaganda Minister Joseph Goebbels on December 31st, 1938.[222] This work was targeted and burned because of its alleged association with Jewish mysticism .Goebbels' list was mostly composed of works by Jewish authors and other intellectuals whose message opposed the fascist government. Presumably, punishment for owning books found on the banned list would have resulted in confiscation, and possibly deportation or incarceration in concentration camps.

Although no such extremist institutional censorship of the work ever took place in North America, *The Sixth and Seventh Books of Moses* was frequently burned in Pennsylvania if discovered among the belongings of a deceased person.[223] Although the work was certainly owned by both powwow doctors and sorcerers alike, fear of the contents of *the Sixth and Seventh Books of Moses* gave rise to the widespread notion that powwowing books in general were suggestive of sinister practices. Such perceptions, however, make no distinction between common domestic and agricultural rituals used for the health and well-being of others (*Braucherei*) and ritual used for harm (*Hexerei*). The boundaries and ethics that differentiate between these two forms of ritual practices are deserving of further exploration to better understand the dynamics of healing – especially the treatment of diseases that are perceived to be spiritual and linked to cultural attitudes surrounding the holding of a grudge or a *Hex*.

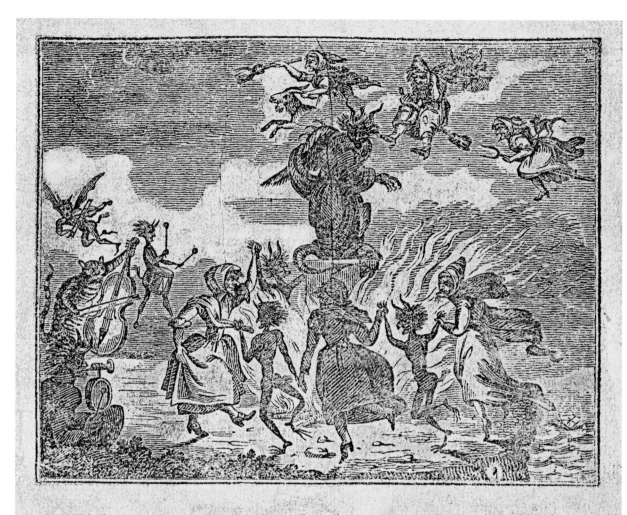

Engraving of the *Hexedanz* (witches' dance) on the Brocken Mountain in Germany, also known as Blocksberg. This detailed depiction appeared in the 1793 Philadelphia almanac entitled *Amerikanischer Stadt- und Land-Calendar* and is evidence of the persistance of European folk legend in Pennsylvania. The Eve of May Day (*Walpurgisnacht* or the evening of April 30) is significant in European tradition as the night that the witches gather on hilltops to dance for the "Witches Sabbath," and similar legends have been found in several counties of Pennsylvania, such as Hexenkopf (Witch's Head) in Williams Township, Northampton County, and *Hexebarrich* (Witches' Hill) in Virginville, Windsor Township, Berks County. Don Yoder Collection, Pennsylvania German Cultural Heritage Center.

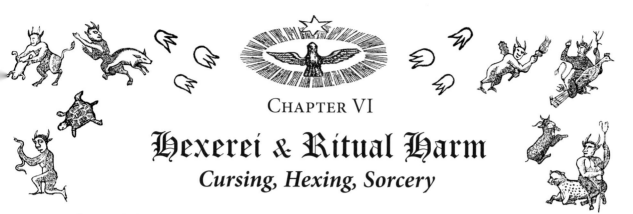

Chapter VI
Hexerei & Ritual Harm
Cursing, Hexing, Sorcery

Somewhere on the broad spectrum of Pennsylvania's powwowing practices is a line that marks a transition in orientation and intention from the honorable pursuits of ritual healing into a murky realm of predatory ritual behavior. Although this delineation is by no means unanimous, it is generally accepted among the Pennsylvania Dutch that *Hexerei* describes mercenary ritual practices, used for harm, revenge, monetary remuneration, personal gain, or control of another person. In this sense, *Hexerei* is diametrically opposed to *Braucherei*, which aims to bring about a state of well-being, and to heal, bless, and protect. Nevertheless, these boundaries, even up to the present day, are not always clear and have been defined in a number of ways over the centuries.

In its original connotation, *Hexerei* means witchcraft[1] and is unanimously regarded as a sinister practice within the context of Pennsylvania Dutch language because it is associated with ritual violence and harm. Those who are subjected to ritual antagonism of this sort may lose their health to disease, their family to disaster, their crops to failure, and their minds to insanity. It is the role of the powwower to identify the effects of this negative influence, and to ritually dispel it before it can do permanent harm.

A *Hex* is the word for both a curse laid under the auspices of *Hexerei*, as well as the term for a person who uses ritual to harm another person. The latter use of the word *Hex* is synonymous with a "witch" in the medieval sense of the word – one who is believed to have made a pact with the devil or other infernal spirits in exchange for power, or at the very least, has sacrificed their good nature to satisfy their desire for power over others. It is believed that such people do not act alone, but are assisted by spirit entities that can be sent to bring about harm or sickness in their victims.

There is, however, some ambiguity about the terms *Hex* and *Hexerei*, which have been absorbed into the English language and are considered by some to be synonymous with the role of the powwower in communities outside of the core cultural region of Southeastern Pennsylvania. This tends to be the case especially among monolingual speakers of English, who have adopted the term from Pennsylvania Dutch.

This neutral notion of a *Hex* is further compounded by the role of the hex-doctor, a practitioner akin to a folk exorcist, whose role is in curing a person of a curse or *Hex*, and in punishing the culprit who placed the *Hex*. Although this type of practitioner is called a *Hexedokter* in Pennsylvania Dutch, which implies the use of anti-witchcraft measures,[2] the term is often confused in English usage to imply that the *Dokter* is a *Hex* (witch), as opposed to one who cures a *Hex* (a curse). This dual definition of the word *Hex*, as both a negative state of being and a negative practitioner, has been the cause of much confusion and varying use of the word.[3]

This confusion is taken a step further through the modern adoption of the word *Hex* in myriad movements existing in the present day throughout Europe and the United States where the term "witchcraft" is used as a neutral and even positive term to describe contemporary reconstructions of a wide range of ritual traditions rooted in both Christian and pagan paradigms. Although these reconstructionist, religious movements are composed of well-intentioned people, there is no precedent among the Pennsylvania Dutch for using the word *Hex* in this manner, and no evidence to suggest that *Hexerei* was ever considered a positive facet of life in Pennsylvania Dutch culture, or in the Middle Ages, from whence the modern notion of a *Hex* proceeds.

Historically among the Pennsylvania Dutch tales of *Hexerei* are essentially continuations of medieval attitudes towards the nature of witchcraft, sickness, and calamity and include afflictions such as the ritual stealing of milk from cows, the prevention of sleep among people and animals, the striking down of infants and children with disease, or the driving of a wedge between married partners (see Chapter III). Often the perceived victims of this type of ritual violence are those who were once in a state of abundance and health and are forced to endure scarcity and disease, or those whose happiness or prosperity may be the object of envy.

Similar suspicions of malicious ritual activity formed the basis for witchcraft trials throughout Europe from the late Middle Ages to the Early Modern Era, and such offenses were punishable by death or imprisonment. These prosecutions were still the norm well into the time that German-speaking people arrived by the tens of thousands at ports in Philadelphia in the 18th Century, fleeing areas where these persecutions were quite severe. Coincidentally, the very same year that the first ship arrived in Pennsylvania carrying the German-speaking families who founded Germantown, Governor and Proprietor William Penn presided over Pennsylvania's very first and most famous witch trial.

In February of 1683, two Swedish women named Margaret Mattson and Yeshro (Getro) Hendrickson were brought before a grand jury in Philadelphia based on accusations of harming the health of their neighbors' livestock through witchcraft. Rumors and hearsay went so far that even Mattson's own daughter accused her of appearing as an apparition in the dark of night at the foot of her bed to demand the souls of a neighbor's cattle. As a Quaker who was well acquainted with religious and social persecution, Penn set an important precedent for the settlements under his administration. The jury found the women "Guilty of haveing the Comon fame of a witch, but not guilty in manner and forme as Shee stands Indicted" - thus Penn did not directly confirm or deny the reality of witchcraft, but instead challenged the manner in which such accusations were made on the basis of heresay.[4]

Penn's verdict set an important precedent in Pennsylvania nine years prior to the Salem witch trials in which the colonial government required the posting of 50 pounds each against the families of the accused to ensure their good behavior for six months, but declined to participate in any sentence of imprisonment or death. Inadvertently, this precedent diminished the role of legal authorities in settling disputes over perceived acts of ritual violence and witchcraft in Pennsylvania, fostering a culture whereby such conflicts were addressed not through legal recourse, but privately by counter-witchcraft rituals.

In classic cases, when the cause of the damage was understood to be coming from a human source, counter-witchcraft rituals were widely performed to punish the perceived culprit in order to force them to lift the curse or risk being destroyed by the reversal of the *Hex* upon its source. In some narratives, the aggressor is identified by ritual means, and other times a cure is performed without the discovery of the source of suffering. In the former instances such stories can be likened to lessons in morality, as the characters wrestle with issues of human emotions, like jealousy, hatred, and betrayal as motivations for ritual forms of revenge.

Powwowing is the means by which such situations of suffering are taken out of the realm of the personal, and placed within a cosmic and spiritual drama of good and evil – an equation where good always has the power to prevail. In one sense, this equation provides the much-needed answers to the age-old question of why bad things happen to good people, and what they can do about it.

THE ARCHETYPAL *HEX*

My distant relative by marriage, Elizabeth "Betz" Heilman (1820-1897), of Millmont, Union County, is the central character in a series of classic and perhaps legendary stories of *Hexerei* in central Pennsylvania in the late nineteenth century. Although Betz was in all respects a real person, her persona in the imagination of her community was tightly interwoven with a centuries-old stereotype for the petty, but highly dangerous, neighborhood *Hex*.[5]

All manner of wiles were associated with Betz, who was believed to have the power to strike fear into the hearts of anyone, or even kill with her stare; to ritually steal milk from cows at a great distance; to cause hunters to have bad luck shooting game; to leave her body and visit her enemies in their sleep; and to create all manner of illusions just to torment her neighbors. Betz's story is a tale of jealousy, and her first supposed act of *Hexerei* was to kill a former sweetheart who married another, by cursing him to death.

Betz had worked as a servant girl in the Buffalo Valley, in the village of Glen Iron and courted a young miner by the name of William Keinard. William spurned Betz and married another local woman named Sally. The couple took in the child of a local widower, Frederick William "Fritz" Heilman. Shortly thereafter, William was kicked by a mule at the mine, and Betz paid him a visit while he was recuperating. Allegedly, Betz sat alone with her former sweetheart for hours, speaking softly to him, and looking intently into his eyes. No sooner had she left the house than William took a turn for the worse and died within just a few hours of her visit. Everyone in Glen Iron assumed that Betz had taken her revenge against William by ritual means, and she became a persona non grata known as "old Betz," although she was not yet even middle aged.

Betz went on to marry Fritz Heilman, and the two lived in a log house near Penns Creek in Millmont, where the people of their neighborhood feared her and her sinister reputation. When a local couple had a baby, the wife frequently reported waking up in the night to the sight of Betz standing over her at the foot of her bed, even when the doors of the house were locked. As there was no ordinary means of entry, the couple assumed that she had entered through the keyhole. This notion of spiritual projection, the ritual act of leaving one's body and visiting remote locations to do harm, is a quintessential, supernatural power associated with *Hexerei*. Likewise, the idea that retaliation against such a spiritual projection could cause actual, physical harm to the *Hex* is a central motif of many accounts of *Hexerei*. The husband also was visited in his sleep by Betz, and one night he threw a tumbler from his nightstand at her specter, and found the next day that Betz had suffered an injury corresponding to the blow of the tumbler.

Moreover, at least two of her neighbors claimed to have actually witnessed Betz steal milk by means of a dish towel hung in the corner of her kitchen. Tugging the ends of the rag like an udder, she produced a pail of fresh milk from a cow some distance away. According to popular belief of the time, this legendary act of *Hexerei* was believed to have been derived from a pact with the devil and corroborated by popular Pennsylvania Dutch folktales of *der Deiwel im Budderfass* – the Devil in the Butter churn.

George Hartman of Hamburg shared the following story with Dr. Alfred Shoemaker in 1949. A farmer living in Windsor Township, Berks County, home of the legendary *Hexebarrich* or "Witches Hill," noticed that his neighbor produced an abundance of butter from only two cows. Eager to discover her secret he hid himself in the loft of her milkhouse on the day she did her churning. He spied her throwing a red dishcloth into her tiny churn, from which she drew a seemingly endless supply of butter. After discovering the woman's secret, the farmer tried the ritual himself at his own churn, hoping to produce a similar result. Instead, the devil emerged from the churn holding an infernal book, and prompted the farmer to sign his name, saying "It won't do you no good, my friend. Your name ain't in my book yet."[6]

Although this tale has been retold in a number of ways over many generations, it builds upon the basic notion that *Hexerei* could be used not only to steal milk, but to interfere with the butter-making process of others. As the legend suggests, the success of such seemingly impossible ritual feats depended entirely upon a pact with the devil. If butter did not come, it was assumed that the milk, the cow, or both were bewitched. The significance of this act is probably lost for most modern audiences who don't know that butter was more than a symbol of a farm's prosperity, it was the most profitable product from the farm. Although milk had a relatively short serviceable life, butter was more stable allowing for transport and sale, and was essential to the livelihood of rural families.

Butter was not the only thing that was "stolen" by witches. In addition, fertility of the fields or one's own vitality could be stolen by means of collecting dew at certain times of the year, especially on the first of May before sunrise. Mrs. Meta Immerman of Allentown was accused of cursing her neighbors by walking barefoot in the morning dew and was brought to court in 1911.[7] In 1887, Earl J. Wakeman of Mechanicsburg in Cumberland County describes the activities of the *Thaustriker* (Dew-Gatherer), a practitioner of *Hexerei* that steals the morning dew by riding over the fields to collect the dew with a linen cloth.[8] This cloth could be wrung out into the butter churn. This belief can be compared to old European practices in Altmark, Germany, where the first village boy to take his horse to pasture on May Day was called the "Thau-Schlepper" (Dew-Sweeper). He was adorned with wild flowers, and led from farm to farm to pronounce rhyming blessings for the year's growing season.[9] This nineteenth century fertility rite is clearly related to our Pennsylvania *Dew-Gatherer,* and suggests that rituals surrounding the May dew could be used for good or ill, to threaten production with scarcity or ensure abundance.

BLESSINGS AGAINST A *HEX*

For those who believed they had been preyed upon by a witch in this manner, a number of options were available to "restore" the butter, and punish the witch responsible for the incursion. The same was true if the milk was bloody, stringy, or watery. The simplest and least confrontational way to protect the cattle and ensure the production of butter was to place protective objects or written blessings in proximity to the stable doors. Protective objects could include forged iron such as horseshoes fastened to the stable door, or protective plants such as hazel, asafetida, elder, or ramps.[10] By far the most popular of anti-witchcraft measure, was the creation of written blessings, which were not only concealed within domestic and agricultural structures for protecting animals, but were also popularly carried in one's personal effects.[11]

Although many examples of written blessings have been discovered in buildings, one particular example directly addresses some of the nuanced agricultural beliefs concerning the effects of witchcraft on the health of livestock. An original barn blessing in the collection the Pennsylvania Folklife Society was reprinted by Dr. Alfred L. Shoemaker in 1953. The blessing was folded and concealed inside of the cow stalls of a barn in 1827, and was found in the twentieth century. The German language inscription was written and crossed out, an action aligned with the ritual sacrifice of the words themselves in order to release the essence of the inscription into the spiritual world.[12]

> V[ater].x.S[ohn].x.H[eilige Geist].x.
> Gott helffe diesen vor sei rind Vieh vor allen shaden und besen .x.x.x. amen in jesu namen amen Das Fierett seÿ diesen Vieh ist hat der Erbodin ist thut das nichts boses diesen Vieh fleisch oder blut keinen shaden dut. V.x.S.x.H.x. Amen dem Vater sein namen soll stehen von 1827 bis 1831 under 7 Planeten und under 12 himmlishe Zeichen.
>
> F[ather]. x. S[on]. x. H[oly Ghost].x.
> God help this person for his livestock from all harm und evil. x.x.x amen in the name of Jesus amen. May these cows be led, this undertaking is done, that nothing evil should be able to harm the flesh and blood of these cows. F. x. S. x. H .x. amen. In the name of the Father, this shall stand from 1827 until 1831 under the 7 planets and under the 12 heavenly signs.[13]

A series of celestial markings conclude the blessing, in addition to the biblical inscription I.N.R.I (*Iesus Nazarenus Rex Iudeorum* – Jesus of Nazareth King of the Jews). These concluding inscriptions are nearly identical to other blessings carried by humans for protection, presumably penned by the same practitioner.[14]

Perhaps most notable in this particular blessing is the fact that it is dated, and apparently only effective for a span of four years. Although one could surmise that a practitioner could have been paid to produce such a document (somewhat of a taboo in Pennsylvania Dutch culture), and therefore would profit from its renewal every four years, it is also equally possible that the number four had some form of sacred or calendric significance to the practitioner. Unlike some barn blessings, which are concealed in the structure at the time of construction,[15] this particular blessing was intended to address an illness in the cattle, believed to reside in the flesh and blood and described at the time of the blessing's creation as proceeding from an evil source – a common way to indirectly describe the work of a practitioner of *Hexerei*.

The most celebrated of all written blessings used to protect house and home from the influence of *Hexerei* is one addressed to an entity known as the *Trotterkopf* – a name that is not easily translated into English, but has sometimes been called "Trotterhead."[16] The name of this spiritual entity comes from the notion that it was believed to be a nighttime rider of humans and animals, which appeared in the form of a woman who would run horses to exhaustion, or would sit astride the body of a sleeping person and prevent their sleep.[17] Recent studies have shown that these beliefs about being subjected to the "nightmare," a "succubus," or being "hag-ridden" are not only mythical, but experiential, and part of a broad phenomenon across many cultures that attribute symptoms of sleep paralysis and insomnia to a spiritual entity.[18] Among the Pennsylvania Dutch, it was perceived that the *Trotterkopf* was either the spiritual form of a witch, or a spirit sent by a witch to cause harm. Johann Georg Hohman prescribes the following written blessing to deter the spirit by commanding it to complete a series of impossible tasks:

> To prevent witches from bewitching cattle, to be written and placed in the stable; and against wicked people and evil spirits, which nightly torment old and young people, to be written and placed on the bedstead: Trotter Head, I forbid thee my house and premises, I forbid thee my horse and cow stable, I forbid thee my bedstead, that thou mayest not breathe upon me: breathe into some other house, until thou hast ascended every hill, until thou hast counted every fence post, and until thou hast crossed every water - And thus dear day may come again into my house, in the name of God the Father, the Son, and the Holy Spirit. Amen.[19]

Barn blessing discovered by Alfred Shoemaker, written to be effective from 1827 to 1831, invoking the stars and planets. *The Pennsylvania Dutchman*, February 5, 1952.

178

The prefix *Trotter-* also stems from *Trude* or *Drude*, an archaic German word implying a feminine, nocturnal spirit, demon, or elf[20] – the latter giving rise the English use of the word "Bed-Goblin" in the English translation of *Egyptian Secrets*,[21] where pseudo-Albert the Great states that he has seen many humans and livestock, even whole towns, brought to ruin by the *Bettzaierle* (Bed-Goblin). This word *Trude* also appears in the form of a European protective emblem used to ward off the influence of a *Drude*, known as a *Drudenfuss* which is composed of a star of five sides or pentagram.[22] The use of the *Drudenfuss* for this purpose was immortalized in the work of Johann Wolfgang von Goethe (1749-1832) in his classic play *Faust*, where the devilish Mephistopheles is detained by this magical emblem.

While there is no use of the word *Drudenfuss* among the Pennsylvania Dutch, many of whom emigrated long before the play was penned by Goethe in 1808, allied words such as the *Groddefuss* (Toadfoot), *Gensefuuss* (Goosefoot), and *Hexefuuss* (Witchfoot) have been documented in oral tradition by Pennsylvania folklorists,[23] but the actual forms of these emblems are ambiguous.

Folklorist Edwin Miller Fogel recorded several variations of this ritual procedure in Berks, Carbon, Dauphin, Lehigh, Lancaster, Northampton, and Snyder counties: "*En Gensefuuss uff die Schtalldier mache, halt die Hexe draus*" (Put the foot of a goose on the stable door to keep the witches out).[24] While Fogel speculates that "putting" the goosefoot on the door may imply the drawing of a pentagram, it is equally likely that the actual foot was nailed over the door, as in another statement documented in all of the same counties, as well as in Lebanon: "*Wann die Kieh verhext sin, naggelt mer'n Groddefuuss an die Dier, no gehn die Hexe Weck un's halt sie aa draus*" (Nail a toad's foot over the stable door to drive away the witches and keep them out of the stable). However another statement suggests that the same emblem can also be drawn. "*Mach Groddefiess mit Greid an die Bettlaad, sell halt die Hexe weck, odder innewennich owwich's Fenschder odder Dier*" (Draw toads' feet with chalk on the bedstead, this keeps the witches away, or in the room above window or door).

Interestingly enough, toads have five toes on their hind feet - as many toes as the points of a pentagram - thus it is possible that the word *Groddefuuss* may have applied to both an actual foot and a geometric five-toed star. The goosefoot on the other hand, has only three toes, and when drawn as an emblem, has been called a "*Hexefuss*" (Witch-foot)[25] In some cases, this word was not only used to designate a ritual mark placed on a doorway, window, or bedstead, as suggested by Fogel, but it was also believed to be the mark or footprint left behind by a witch who took the form of a bird or animal. This dual nature of the *Hexefuuss* as both protective emblem and as supernatural indicator is reflected also in the European counterpart, the *Drudenfuss*.[26] which is also the word for footprint of a demon. As in Martin Luther's accounts of witchcraft, a footprint could be used ritually to ensnare a person or spirit.[27] Thus, the folklore of the *Trudenfuss* and *Hexefuss* suggests that placing the image of a demon's footprint in a circle allows for the coercion or repulsion of the spirit.

A Berks County barn blessing used to ward off the influence of an evil entity called Trotterkopf, *rendered here in English as "Trotter head." This blessing was created in the late nineteenth century by the reknowned powwow practitioner, Dr. Joseph Hageman, whose specialized in creating written blessings. Courtesy of the Henry Janssen Library, Berks History Center.*

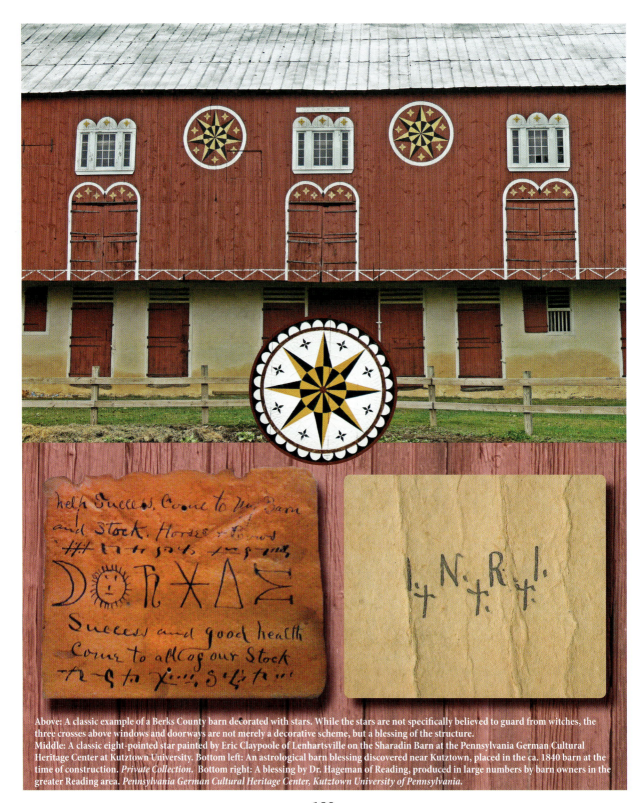

Above: A classic example of a Berks County barn decorated with stars. While the stars are not specifically believed to guard from witches, the three crosses above windows and doorways are not merely a decorative scheme, but a blessing of the structure.
Middle: A classic eight-pointed star painted by Eric Claypoole of Lenhartsville on the Sharadin Barn at the Pennsylvania German Cultural Heritage Center at Kutztown University. Bottom left: An astrological barn blessing discovered near Kutztown, placed in the ca. 1840 barn at the time of construction. *Private Collection.* Bottom right: A blessing by Dr. Hageman of Reading, produced in large numbers by barn owners in the greater Reading area. *Pennsylvania German Cultural Heritage Center, Kutztown University of Pennsylvania.*

So-Called "Hex Signs"

This idea of the *Hexefuuss* would have remained relatively obscure had it not appeared in the popular accounts of a retired congregational minister, celebrated photographer, travel journalist, and antiquarian from New England, Wallace Nutting (1861-1941). In 1924, Nutting wrote *Pennsylvania Beautiful*, featuring a fanciful explanation of Pennsylvania barns and the decorations featured on their facades. It is because of Nutting's account that these designs are called "hex signs" today.[28]

According to Wallace Nutting, a single source from Bethlehem told him that such a "decorative mark" was called a "hexafoos" and regarded as protective from witches and devils.[29] Nutting's summary states:

> They are a decoration sometimes applied on the door heads or on or about the door. They are supposed to be a continuance of a very ancient tradition, according to which these decorative marks were potent to protect the barn, or more particularly the cattle, from the influence of witches. It is understood by those who are acquainted with witches that those ladies are particularly likely to harm cattle. As the wealth of the farmer was in his stock, contained in his remarkably substantial barn, the hexafoos was added to its decoration as a kind of spiritual or demoniac lightning-rod![30]

There is no doubt that Nutting learned from his unnamed informant about the powwowing practice of creating ritual marks on doorways, as echoed in the work of other folklorists in the early twentieth century. The problem with Nutting's account lies in his application of this story to all decorations on Pennsylvania barns. Furthermore, as a collector of early American furniture, Nutting should have recognized that the motifs on barns extend all across early American culture in other artistic traditions – from New England to the Shenandoah. While the subtle, hidden "marks" in chalk or otherwise were certainly ritual in nature, the large-scale exterior public displays of color and artistry were commonly called "*Schtanne*" (stars) and "*Blumme*" (flowers) by speakers of the dialect,[31] and were not regarded as "hex signs" until after Wallace Nutting's accounts were widely distributed.[32] Furthermore, the stories of the artists and craftsmen who painted "various star patterns" on Pennsylvania barns are well-documented at the time of Wallace Nutting's travels in Pennsylvania, and no supernatural meanings were originally attributed to these celestial designs.[33]

While there are a wide variety of ritual practices associated with protecting barns including written blessings and some carved or painted graffiti, in the core geographic region of the "hex sign" in Berks and Lehigh counties, there is absolutely no evidence to suggest that powwowers actively painted barns, and to this day there are no barn painters actively powwowing.[34]

Instead, the traditions of powwowing and barn star painting are at best parallel expressions of the folk-culture, sharing in common a cosmological orientation. Occasionally, these traditions have cross-pollinated and shared motifs, as there are many examples of powwow blessings that incorporate stars. Usually these expressions are not nearly so artistically developed as the barn murals produced in Berks and Lehigh counties. There are a few barns that feature painted crosses, or even protective inscriptions like I.N.R.I, but these are extremely rare, and totally unlike the bulk of the tradition. In a few rare cases, it has been documented that barn stars were painted over prayers written in pencil or chalk on the barn siding. While I personally know of three examples in Berks and Lehigh counties, these were contemporary requests by barn owners and not the decision of the artists.

Historically and presently, vocational barn painters themselves were commercial painters with varying opinions about the symbolism, numerology, and religious significance of the designs that they painted, but with no direct experience of powwowing.

Ironically, those painters, like the legendary Johnny Ott, or the silk screen printer Jacob Zook, who styled themselves "hexologists" and feigned magical power in their work, never actually painted on barns, but instead produced a new line of tourist commodities based in images that are entirely distinct from the designs originally painted on barns. These twentieth-century designs were purported to have historical ritual significance, but were largely invented in the 1950s. Ott, a Roman Catholic, furthermore expressed contempt for powwowing to the press of the Allentown *Morning Call* newspaper in 1962, when asked about the spiritual content of his work:

> "I tell them to have faith and never mind the tobacco-chewing pow-wow doctors…A lot of people think I am a hoodoo man. They think I just have to wave my wand and get them out of trouble…I tell people over and over to go to church and have faith and everything will come out all right – even if it takes a little while. But they ask where is a good pow-wow doctor. What good can they get out of a pow-wow doctor that is just a tinsmith or a railroad worker?"[35]

Beyond the attitudes of artists like Ott, who both publically railed against powwowing while at the same time capitalizing on and promoting public misperception of "hex signs," it is clear that the brightly colored, intricate patterns espoused by commercial painters are distinct in every way from the ritual "marks" described by farmers. While Fogel suggests the pentagram as an explanation for these marks, that are comparable to the German *Drudenfuss*, the fact remains that five-pointed stars are statistically found on less than 2% of decorated barns

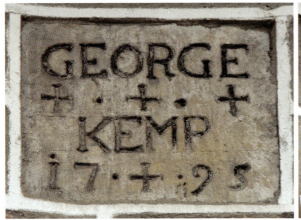 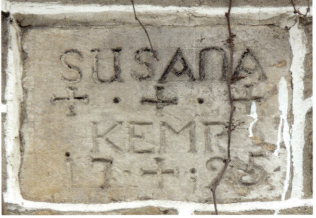

Blessing stones from the 1795 Kemp Hotel in Maxatawny, just outside of Kutztown, show the use of three crosses as articulations between the owner's names, blending both the religious and secular, public and private aspects of house blessing stones.

in Berks County, and all of these are twentieth-century paintings.[36] Overall, designs with eight points are the most numerous, followed closely by six – thus the narratives concerning actual content and context of use for the ritual marks do not match the Pennsylvania evidence. Nevertheless, these two distinctive traditions have been compounded in the cultural imagination, and have led to the contemporary use of twentieth- and twenty-first-century, commercially produced "hex signs" as protective blessings throughout the United States.

The ritual nature of graffiti can be especially difficult to discern on historic structures, as geometric patterns are placed on wooden surfaces for a variety of different purposes aside from protection. These include decoration, amusement, demonstration of skill, or in some cases are part of a timber-framer's layout. Six pointed stars, for instance, commonly created with hayforks by farmhands, are far too ubiquitous to have ritual intentions attributed to them in all cases.[37]

Out of hundreds of samples of graffiti that I have documented in homes, barns, mills, and outbuildings, only a handful of markings have been positively identified as ritual in nature. These include seven crosses carved in series on the stone quoins of a barn near Kutztown, the word "Spiritus" painted in blood on the door-jamb of a stable in Pike Township, Berks County, and on the same property, the stamping of three crosses on each iron strap hinge of the master bedroom and the ancillary workshop. In all of these cases, the carved or painted images are subtle and not likely to be seen by anyone but the property owners.

However, some public examples are visible in the form of three consecutive crosses carved into date-stones near Kutztown such as the 1795 house of George and Susana Kemp or three crosses painted on barns above doorways, in nearby Maxatawny and Albany townships in Berks County. Such public expressions of protection are part of broader traditions of the blessing of barns and homes with the use of formal blessing inscriptions, some of which blend inspirational and protective text such as a pair of stones from the border of Berks and Lebanon counties:

GOTT GESEGNE DIESES HAUS UND WAS DA GET EIN UND AUS GOT ALEIN DIE EHR UND SONST DEN KEINEM MER J770 AU 14 WER GOTT VERTRAUT HAT WOL GEBAUT IN HIMMEL UND AUF ERDEN WER SICH VERLEST AUF IESUM CHRIST JACOB A. WERT J770 MARGREDA L. WERDIN.

The use of three painted crosses above the windows and doorways of barns finds its origins in protective traditions, rather than mere decoration. Maxatawny Township, Berks County.

God Bless this house, and all that go in and out. Glory to God alone, and none to anyone else. 1770 August, 14. He who trusts in God has built well in heaven and on earth, and who relies on Jesus Christ. Jacob A. Wert. 1770 Margareta L. Wert.

Such formal religious blessings aim not only to bless, but to counteract a wide range of calamities, sickness, and misfortune. They do so without ever identifying oppositional forces. Thus formal house-blessings are part

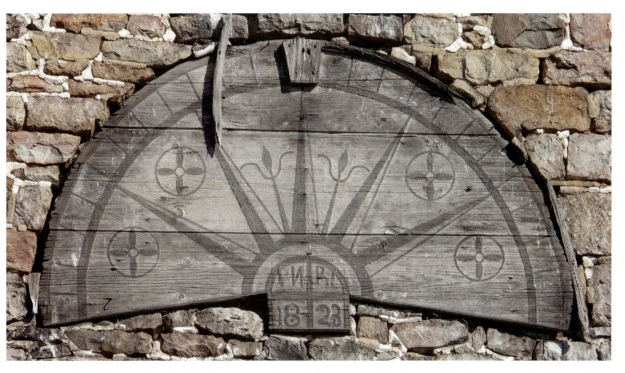

A highly unusual Lehigh County barn blessing plaque that combines the iconography of the barn star with religious symbolism. The use of the inscription I.N.R.I above the date 1823 and placed within the four quadrants of a central cross is unique and atypical for barn decorations.

of a broad spectrum of acceptable apotropaic measures to ensure safety from natural disasters and the forces of evil, including witchcraft and the influence of a *Hex*. Only one house blessing in Pennsylvania specifically addresses the barring out of evil spirits. It is from the 1731 house of Hiram C. Anders in Worcester Township, Montgomery County:

> *Ihr höllen Geister, packet euch,*
> *Ihr habt hier nichts zu schaffen,*
> *Dies Haus gehört in Jesu reich,*
> *Lasst es nur sicher schlaten. 1731*
>
> Ye spirits of hell, be gone,
> Ye have naught here to do,
> This House belongs in Jesus' realm,
> Let it abide in peace.[38]

Ritual Retaliation Against a *Hex*

Other far less savory techniques were also once employed to counteract the effects of a *Hex* on the health of cattle and the production of butter. Many of these techniques involve ritually showing disdain or violence to the source of the perceived *Hex* by means of secondary, sympathetic objects. One might whip the churn full of milk with a hazelwood rod, stab the milk with a scythe blade,[39] burn, fumigate, or otherwise destroy the milk in order to not only cure the cow, but to wreak vengeance upon the witch by proxy.

Although such acts are in themselves deliberate enactments of curses placed by ritual means upon the perceived culprit, this form of retaliation was not uncommon. One example from the early nineteenth century of such a procedure for punishing a witch describes the process of sympathetically inflicting an injury to a person by means of shooting at a cookie baked in the image of a human form.

> *Wie man Hexen und Zaubern dott, oder ein Glied, oder ein bein, oder ein auge ab schießen kan – „Man macht ein Deig von Mell und dan macht man ein Bild dar von; ja, ein Bild, wie ein Weib wann man weiß das ein Weib ist, ist es aber ein Man, so muß auch ein Bild seÿn, wie ein man; ist daß Bild gemacht von Deich. Dan dhutt man es backen im Ofen, und den mensch sein namen muß abends auf dem Bild ein Sterrn geschrieben seÿn, un die flind muß abens mit einer Silber Kugel gelatten seÿn, morgens frie ohne beschrauen vor sonnen auf gang nimmt man selbes Bild und flind: steld selbes Bild auf ein Fens Eck man gehet 9 schritt zurick spand den Hanen und zielt aufs Bild wo man es schießen will -Und sagt du Georg oder Mallÿ, wie er heist – ich schiesse dir verfluchte sehle dein linken Arm – al + + +*

> How one can kill a witch or sorcerer or to shoot an arm, or a leg, or an eye out - One must make a dough of meal, and then he must make an image out of it, indeed, an

Folio Manuscript of Instructions to Kill a Witch, ca. 1820, Georg Börstler of Schwartzwald, Berks County. Heilman Collection.

image, like a woman if one knows that it is a woman, but if it is a man, the image must be of a man, and the image must be of dough. Then it must be baked in the oven, and in the evening the name of the person must be written upon the brow of the image, and the gun must be loaded in the evening with a silver bullet, early next morning, without speaking, before the rise of the sun, one must take the image and gun, place the image in a fence corner. Then one must go 9 paces back, cock the gun and aim it at the image where he wants to shoot it. And you must say "George or Molly," whatever he is called, "I shoot you, accursed be your left arm," etc. + + + [40]

These instructions were penned by the hand of Georg Börstler, a resident of Schwartzwald, Exeter Township, Berks County from around the turn of the nineteenth century.

This method of shooting the image of a witch with a silver bullet was widespread, and the same manner of death of an eighteenth century "witch of great repute" from Valley Hill, Chester County, was memorialized in a poem by James B. Everhart of Philadelphia in 1868:

Kate Spider was yclep'd (called) a witch,
And filled the folks with dread:
For she gave the cows the murrain,
And made the milk turn red!
And had a sort of mummy look,
As if she had been dead!

And she dwelt upon the hillside,
Within a natural cave;
And when she went abroad they said
She issued from the grave -
And she could ride upon the air,
Or walk upon the wave.

Now some witches may be tender,
And beautiful withal,
As they paint the witch of Endor,
Who told the fate of Saul;
But in Kate, her best defender
Could see no charms at all.

She was dark, and deeply wrinkled,
Her nose was hook'd and thin,
And her eyes were like a devil's,
That gloated over sin;
And when she tried to smile, she made
A very horrid grin.

And then, too, she carried with her
Her kittens and her cat,
Who, often, on her head and arms,
In antic postures sat;
And would walk upon their hind legs,
And do such tricks as that.

'Twas said they were her messengers,
And brought infernal news,
For their early race o'er meadows
Dried up the morning dews;
And when the cowboy crossed their trail,
He trembled in his shoes.

And forsooth! she read the secrets
Of fortunes at a glance,
And announced the times and places,
And surnames of gallants,
When young damsels dropp'd their money
Amongst her simm'ring plants.

But the public ban was on her,
Her patrons gazed, with awe,
Upon one who seemed unfettered
By any kind of law,
And into the world of spirits
And misty future saw.

Some nail'd a horse-shoe o'er the sill,
To bar the entrance way;
Or stuck a fork beneath her chair,
Near fire to make her stay;
Yet these were rather meager plans
To keep a witch at bay.

So they got a clever artist,
Who sketched her on a door,
Which they shot with silver bullet,
That made it ooze with gore—
And Kate Spider, in that region,
Was seen not any more.[41]

Betz Heilman of Buffalo Valley was also allegedly subjected to a wide variety of such acts of ritual vengeance, such as shooting with silver bullets and the stabbing and burning of effigies made in her image. Although some claimed to have succeeded in injuring her, she lived to be over 70 years old and died of natural causes.[42] Betz is buried in the cemetery at Buffalo Valley Church of the Brethren.

Another particularly salient account of haunting and a subsequent ritual punishment of a witch made it into local newspapers in 1875 from Rossville, York County, when an unidentified old woman arrived unannounced and asked to stay the night at the residence of the Nesbit Family on the William Ross farm. Mrs. Nesbit declined, but the woman unsuccessfully persisted in her requests until she angrily asked Mrs. Nesbit how she would like it, if she were unable to rest. Mrs. Nesbit, unsure of the woman's intent, said she did not know, and sent the woman away.[43]

Shortly after this incident, Mrs. Nesbit was bedridden with an acute attack of rheumatism during which time she was unable to sleep. Shortly thereafter, she began to receive nightly visits from a shadowy specter of a naked human being with flaming eyes that would roam the house and one of the outbuildings on the property as if looking for her. The Nesbit family described that the figure would appear at the foot of her bed and then drag Mrs. Nesbit along with her blankets to the floor, where she was subject to fainting and fits of convulsions. News of the haunting of Mrs. Nesbit soon spread throughout Rossville, and one evening nearly the whole neighborhood gathered at the home to see if there was any truth to the story.

According to the *Lebanon Courier* of November eighteenth, 1875, reprinting the story from the *Mechanicsburg Journal*, the house was so crowded, that many stood outside of the home, waiting for a chance to witness the haunting. The lights were all extinguished, and Mrs. Nesbit went to bed, putting her baby in the cradle next to her. At ten o'clock, the spirit appeared to the group of townspeople waiting in Mrs. Nesbit's room.

Instead of a figure, they only saw a pair of flaming orbs, which appeared to advance upon the woman's bed. Seven of the men sought to intervene, but as Mrs. Nesbit fainted, the fiery orbs instead seized the infant in the cradle. The bystanders were able to wrest the child from the clutches of the spirit, which suddenly vanished. The spectacle confirmed the Nesbit's story to numerous witnesses, and the community responded with deep concern.

A local man, a *Braucher* by the name of Dr. Gusler,[44] offered to assist the Nesbits with the haunting, claiming that it was caused by witchcraft. He told Mrs. Nesbit that on a certain day at a certain hour, she was to heat a sickle red-hot, and pass it along her arm as close as possible without burning herself. The family was instructed that if anyone came to the house, they were not to give anything to anyone who might ask. The following day, the very same old woman, who had inquired about lodging several weeks prior, came to the door with a burn running the length of her arm. She asked if she could have some lard to grease her burn. Mrs. Nesbit refused, whereupon the woman asked if they had a strip of cloth to cover the wound. When she was refused again, she asked for a pin. When Mrs. Nesbit told her in no uncertain terms that she would receive nothing from the household, she left them alone. Apparently, the haunting ceased after the ritual was performed, and the culprit's request was denied.[45]

Unlike the Nesbit's terrifying experience, some stories of hauntings and curses were told in humorous form and have become a sub-genre of oral folktales recorded among the Pennsylvania Dutch. Such is the tale of "Aunt Sybilla," written by her niece Elsie Gehris Creswell[46] much to the chagrin of the whole family.[47]

Aunt Catherine Sybilla Gehris Miller (1862-1952) of Washington Township, Berks County, owned a farm with her husband Henry, where she attributed many troubling events to predations from a *Hex*. When valuable meat spoiled, the setting of eggs failed to produce chicks, cream would curdle in the crock before it could be churned into milk, and cows gave stringy or bloody milk, Sybilla visited a woman "hex-doctor" who lived in a shack near the farm.

This woman was described as eccentric, according to Sybilla's daughter, Birdy Miller, who said that the woman frequently went about with her hair and eye brows singed from working rituals over a cauldron in her hearth. She told Sybilla to rise early in the morning, take some fresh cow dung from a young sick cow, place it in a stoneware crock in the cold oven of her wood-fired cook stove, and light the firebox under the range. The woman indicated that when this ritual was completed, the person responsible for laying the *Hex* on the cows would be burned.

Sybilla dutifully performed the ritual, which caused the methane gas from the fresh dung to accidentally ignite and blow the door off the oven, burst the stove pipe of the flu, and send the burners flying. Although her husband Hen was known for his stinginess, he was forced to buy a much-needed, new cook stove, and he forbid Sybilla from ever "laying a *Hex*" again. Coincidentally, the same day, the woman hex-doctor with whom Sybilla had consulted was badly burned on her face and hands.

Aunt Sybilla's story, although purported to be entirely true, was originally written as a humorous and critical account of beliefs held within Berks County families. At the same time, the humorous nature of the conflicts in such a *Hex* story need not eclipse the fact that these scenarios are not merely literary constructions or moral lessons, but actual experiences interpreted through a set of cultural expectations and norms.

Furthermore, Aunt Sybilla's encounter with *Hex* reversal provides some detailed insight into the nature of such ritual transactions. The woman with whom she consulted was a "hex-doctor," typically understood as one who specializes in the removal of curses, but whose motives and intentions are often suspected to be mercenary in nature. A hex-doctor typically has no qualms about returning a *Hex* back from whence it came, often with dramatic consequences that either ritually injure or even kill the one suspected of being responsible for the curse. It is also not uncommon for such methods to backfire, and occasionally implicate the hex-doctor as a manipulator, and the original author of the curse, which is suggested by this story.

However, Henry suggests that Sybilla had herself "laid a *Hex*" by performing the ritual with the cow dung, furthering the notion that ritual retaliation is in and of itself considered an act of *Hexerei*. This perception is based in the notion that fighting sorcery with sorcery has historically been forbidden in Christian communities in Pennsylvania, as well as in Europe since the middle ages.[48]

Powwow healers on the other hand, both historically and presently, tend to steer clear of dealings of this type, and focus instead on restoring health and prosperity without participation in rituals to identify the source of a *Hex*. There are taboos against a powwow doctor participating in revenge against a perceived adversary for the very reason that one could be wrong about an accusation and multiply suffering. As an alternative to rituals aimed at vicarious violence, blessings are employed to counteract the effects of the curse, and such procedures place the patient in the care of the divine. It is this capacity to make sense of suffering and integrate it into a broader network of spiritual and communal relationships that produces conditions favorable to a powwow cure.

This ethic of curing spiritual ills by means of blessing rather than by ritual retaliation is characteristic of the very same ethics put forth in the manuals of exorcism compiled in the late medieval and early modern eras, such as the *Flagellum Demonium*, as well as in advice for secular courts in prosecuting witchcraft such as the *Malleus Maleficarum*.[49]

Despite these strict codes of conduct, the early modern era provides numerous examples of how notions of *Hexerei,* the historical term for witchcraft in German-speaking lands, could be dangerous if taken to the extreme, and many innocent people suffered from false accusations of culpability in the era of witchcraft trials.[50] Historically, it is no coincidence that the executions of supposed witches in Europe were at their height during times of religious and social upheaval, as well as widespread crop failure and famine, as a result of a cooler European climate. Thus those accused of witchcraft became scapegoats for a Europe plagued by fears and actual economic insecurities.

As a result of critical perspectives on this traditional framework, the equation of *Hexerei* has expanded and become more complex over the centuries, with the breakdown of the dualism that once characterized so much of western thinking. In the present day, a *Hex* could also be the result of holding a grudge, misplaced aggression or envy, or the harboring of ill-will against another until it negatively affects one's own well-being. A contemporary powwower in Berks County once confided to me that in her experience most cases of the placing of a *Hex* upon another is unintentional, and the result of careless projecting of negative emotions.[51]

The Unintended *Hex*

A retired public school teacher from Berks County once related a story to me that reflects this form of unintended *Hex,* retold from her parents' experiences in dealing with an unexplained developmental disorder that she had endured in early childhood:

The woman explained that through nearly the first two years of her life, she had suffered from a rare, unidentified developmental disorder that terrified her parents and baffled doctors, who were unable to identify its cause or even recommend a treatment. As a newborn, the little girl appeared perfectly healthy, but as she grew older, she simply didn't progress as other children did. Although at first she was just considered a "late bloomer," eventually doctors began to visit the home regularly to monitor her progress, recommending that the parents be patient and wait to see if the little girl improved on her own. By nearly two years of age, she remained silent, showing no inclination towards speech whatsoever, and her motor skills were so entirely impaired that she was unable to even crawl like normal children less than half her age. Instead she would inch her way across the floor sideways using one arm for leverage. The doctors continued to observe that the child was physically healthy in every way, and that there were no clues as the cause of her delayed development. The parents, tired of waiting, decided to take matters into their own hands. They consulted a female powwow doctor living in the neighborhood, who specialized in childhood ailments.

The powwow woman paid a visit, and after briefly examining the child and the home, concluded the child had fallen victim to a *Hex* or curse. The parents were beside themselves and asked the woman how this could be. The woman explained that this was not a simple equation, and asked family if there was an item that the little girl treasured, something she held close as a means to comfort herself. The parents volunteered that the little girl had always been very close to a stuffed rabbit that had been given to her as a present shortly after she was born. Despite her immobility, the child was able to cling to the stuffed rabbit, and carry it with her wherever she was. The powwow doctor inquired who had given the rabbit to the child, and the parents reluctantly began to tell a tale of family jealousy:

They admitted that the rabbit had been a present from a neighbor who lived just down the street. This woman was the mother of a man who had been, in his younger years, an old sweetheart of the mother of the child. It was well known that the neighbor begrudged the family, wishing that her son had been the one to marry the child's mother and that she wished the child was her own grandchild. The powwow doctor immediately understood that the gift, although perhaps well intentioned, had been poisoned by the woman's envy and that her unbridled jealousy was the cause of the child's disorder. She immediately ordered that the rabbit be burned, and despite the family's dismay, they did as the powwow woman ordered. The child cried and wailed at the loss of her favorite toy, but much to the surprise of the parents and the family's physician, the child immediately began to show signs of recovery. Within just one year's time, the little girl had caught up to her peers and was able to walk and talk like the others. She went on to be a very intelligent and productive person, despite the difficulties of her first two years.[51]

One important aspect of this story is that a cure was produced without multiplying ill-will. The rabbit was burned and the case was closed. There was no need or desire to punish the woman who had given the gift and the issue was pursued no further. This is typical of the ethics of powwowers who identify as healers, as opposed to the ethics of those who identify as "hex-doctors," who often suggest means to harm the one perceived to be ritually responsible for a *Hex*. Although the neighbor was indeed jealous of the child, the family wished no ill-will against the woman, and hoped only for the child's recovery. This serves to highlight the reason why many powwowers refused to participate in ritual retaliation, because of the repercussions of such actions within the community.

It was believed that a *Hex* could be transmitted by means of an ill-intended gift, food, or even a child's toy, like this stuffed rabbit.

A Child and a *Hex*

Infants and young children are featured prominently in *Hex* stories, and generally are believed to be the most susceptible and vulnerable to the power of a curse. It is easy to see that these cultural attitudes correspond to one of the most challenging phases of life for parents, when so many aspects of a child's health and development can be cause for anxiety and concern. Colic, insomnia, teething, night-terrors, and unusual behavior were once considered to be supernatural in origin, rather than purely physical and psychological concerns.

One contact from the coal town of Macadoo, Schuylkill County, recounted a story from the 1940s when her parents believed that her sister had been subjected to supernatural torment from a strange old woman who appeared in the neighborhood.[53] The family owned and operated a general store in the village, and when her sister was born, the baby was frequently kept in the store with her parents. The baby's bassinet was along the edge of the counter, and many customers would stop to admire the healthy little girl. One day, an old, unfamiliar woman came to the store, explaining that she had heard that there was a new baby in the family, and asked if she could hold the child. The parents, who knew their community of customers very well, had never seen the woman before, and were uneasy about the request. But, without wishing to offend her, they acquiesced and allowed her to stand over the bassinet to admire the child and to hold her. The baby cried, and carried on, seemingly upset by the woman's touch. The woman held her for only a short while, and inquired "How well does the baby sleep?" The parents explained that she was sleeping quite well, and they took the child back from the woman, who left the store without buying anything.

The truth was that the baby had been sleeping very well – that is, until the incident with the old woman. From that day forward, the child was inconsolable as soon as the sun went down. She cried constantly for hours, and refused to sleep in her cradle, permitting her parents little to no sleep. Throughout the night, they would take turns pushing her in a carriage up and down the streets until the early hours of the morning. Eventually, the baby would fall asleep and each night the parents would expend great energy to gently lift the carriage up the stairs and onto the landing by the bedroom so that they could be near her and still catch a few hours of sleep.

During this time, the old woman would occasionally visit the store, and smile knowingly, while inquiring about how the baby was sleeping. This greatly disturbed the parents, and led them to believe that the old woman was somehow the cause of their torment. The child continued to get worse, and the insomnia persisted well beyond the normal duration of a case of infant colic. The couple endured miserable months of this routine, until the mother, nearly at her wits end, went to speak with their minister.

The local Lutheran pastor agreed to meet with the mother, who brought the child along. The mother told her story, of the healthy child and of the abrupt turn of events. She admitted that she didn't wish to be superstitious, but she explained to the minister about the strange old woman in the store, and her concerns that the woman may have caused the child's insomnia. Although the mother respected the pastor, she was concerned that he would think she was crazy. The pastor surprised her by saying that he understood her concerns, and agreed, despite the unpopularity of such beliefs, that there are indeed wicked people in the world who are capable of causing illness and calamity for others. The pastor asked the mother if he could pray with her and the baby, to which she agreed. Together they prayed for the child's recovery, and for the dark cloud to be lifted from over the home of the family.

That evening, when the mother was giving the baby her bath, she noticed something she had not seen before – a long, thick, white hair had been tied in a series of intricate and intentional knots, again and again, around the baby's toe. The hair was so obvious that the mother

The discovery of mysterious objects hidden in one's personal effects, like the red mitten above, is a common feature of stories of *Hexerei*, and stories of witchcraft from the Middle Ages. Because such objects appear in seemingly impossible circumstances, the belief was that these objects were placed by spiritual entities and were the source of illness and misfortune.

knew this was not something she could have missed. She believed that the prayers of the minister had worked to reveal this material manifestation of the curse, which had been invisible to her up until this point, and she carefully removed the hair. From then on, the child slept peacefully.

The next day, the woman appeared in the store, asking about the child, but the parents were adamant, and refused to allow her to see the child. Greatly incensed, the woman left the store, and never returned.

Although my contact suggested that her parents had believed that the curse had been placed by the woman who had stealthily tied the hair around the baby's toe when she first admired the child in the store, and that the invisibility of the hair was supernatural, other *Hex* narratives indicate that such devices could be attached to a person or their personal effects remotely by supernatural means. This notion is identical to the medieval notion of *ligaturae* (ligatures or bindings) and other objects that were placed in a person's bedstead or even inside their body by spirits conjured by a sorcerer or witch.[54]

One of the most elaborate of such cases proceeds from the memory of Dora Mae Edwards (1875-1926) of Ebensburg in the Allegheny Mountains of Cambria County. Mrs. Edward's daughter Irene (1902-1975), who lived in Johnstown, and worked in a silk mill in Hornersville, was betrothed to a Harry Mishler (1895-1951), also of Johnstown. Prior to their wedding in the 1920s, Irene became incredibly ill and went to her parent's farm to recuperate. While she was there, she complained that she was sleeping terribly and that her pillow hurt her head. Although her pillow appeared normal, Irene continued to lose sleep and her illness grew more severe. In the height of her distress she exclaimed that she thought she would die before she ever married Harry.

Mrs. Edwards decided to take Irene to a powwower named Mr. Myers in Ferndale, just south of Hornersville. He listened to their story and to their surprise, immediately suggested the following course of action: "Go home, and take the pillow away from the house; cut it open. You will find a red mitten and two objects woven in the feathers that look like wings that you could use for hat decorations. They will be woven so tight you cannot pull them apart. In the center of each is a rosette. One is finished, the other is not but don't wait. If it gets finished, Irene will die. Burn the contents. Also, the person who is doing this to your daughter will be the first person not of your family who comes through your door after the pillow is burned."[55]

The Edwards' went immediately home. Mr. Edwards, who would not have approved of the consultation with Mr. Myers, was not informed of the outcome of their visit. When they were alone, and Mr. Edwards was out in the barn, they took the pillow outside and cut it open. Inside, just as Mr. Myers had said, they found a red mitten and two intricate wings woven from the feathers. Only a very small section of one of the weavings was unfinished. Irene recalled saying that she would die before marrying Harry, and now she believed that she most certainly would have died, had she not visited Mr. Myers and revealed the source of her illness.

They burned the pillow and its eerie contents, and went back into the house. Suddenly and without any prior notice, Mrs. Mary Miller Mishler (1873-1948), the mother of Irene's fiancé Harry, arrived at the farm for a visit and appeared at the door. The Mishlers lived in Johnstown, about 20 miles away, and Mary's unannounced arrival at the farm was highly unusual. The family suspected that Mary was responsible for the curse, but never addressed it with Mary.

Following the ritual burning of the contents and revealing of the source of the curse, Irene recovered her health, the couple went on to get married, and Irene was no more subject to supernatural harassment. Her mother, Mrs. Dora Mae Edwards, characterized by her family as a woman of strong religious convictions, felt so strongly about this experience that she recorded it in entirety for posterity.

First-hand accounts of *Hexerei* are by nature one-sided. Whether in the case of Mary Mishler or the old woman in Macadoo, rarely do those who are suspected of harming another by means of ritual have the chance to explain the happenings from their own perspective. Furthermore, such stories always beg a number of questions: If according to such beliefs, a *Hex* can be placed upon another simply by means of a grudge, was Mary aware of the effect she had on her daughter-in-law-to-be? Was it intentional? Did the wings have significance, as a foreshadowing of Irene's near-death? Did the mitten represent the subtle hand that wove the feathers?

Such narratives are often recorded by the people who endure the tribulations of *Hexerei*, but rarely are such victims willing or able to interpret these experiences beyond the level of innuendo and gossip. Although not every person considered a *Hex* is female, historically, there tends to be a strong bias towards relegating women to the role of a *Hex* within Pennsylvania Dutch culture especially those who are independent, powerful, non-conformists, or those who are elderly, vulnerable, disfigured, or solitary. Mother-in-laws, "old maids," and widows are often cast in this role, and it is not always clear what those suspected of *Hexerei* would stand to gain from terrorizing others. Nevertheless, such women became the targets of anti-witchcraft rituals. Some forms of ritual retaliation were also essentially, acts of *Hexerei,* as they were intended for inflicting harm upon those perceived to be responsible for misfortune and illness.

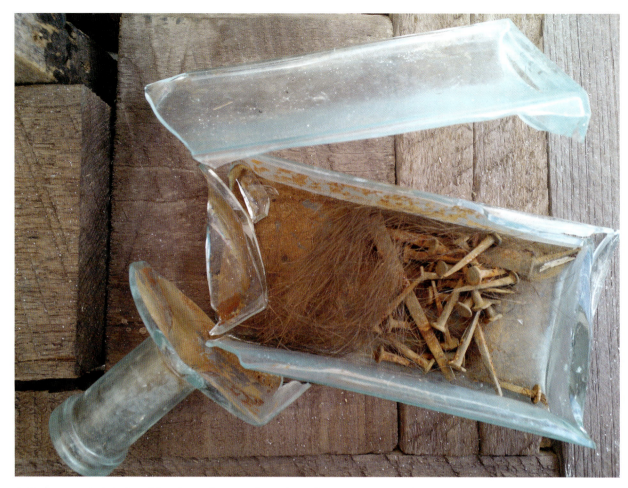

A ubiquitous practice in both English and Pennsylvania Dutch populations for overcoming the ritual predations of wicked people is the use of a witch bottle. The afflicted person would place a sample of their own hair as well as pins, needles, or nails into the bottle, and then urinate into it, and stop it up. Then the bottle was buried or locked away. The belief was that the witch would be unable to urinate and have to beg their victim for forgiveness.

Borrowing, Lending & Witch Bottles

This overarching sense of suspicion of others carried over especially into domestic forms of reciprocity, where borrowing, lending, or the giving of gifts plays a central role in the notion of *Hexerei* as a form of cultural transaction. One who expresses undue generosity to a family may be suspected of cursing them, and on the other extreme, one whose generosity or request is refused may curse out of revenge.

A mid-twentieth century story from Mohnton, Berks County, describes a woman who stopped by the house of a mother and a small baby to give them a gift of some food she had prepared for them. After her visit, when the baby's temperament abruptly changed, and the child cried incessantly for extended periods of time, the mother arrived at the conclusion that they had been cursed. She took a pail of hot water to the middle of the parlor, and drove a red-hot poker into the water, while speaking the words of a prayer. The next day, she found out that the woman who had visited the home had been scalded to death. This confirmed the mother's perception that the woman who had brought them food was actually trying to curse them.[56]

No matter how good one's intentions may be, the outcomes of these narratives of ritual retaliation are cruel and violent. However one form of ritual retaliation was favored for its ability to summon a person responsible for a curse without killing them using an item called a *Hexeboddle* (witchbottle). Each time the culprit is given the option to lift the curse and avoid harm, or suffer devastating consequences.

Sophia Bailer described a classic formula to punish a *Hex*, which she advised in a variety of cases of illness or calamity believed to have proceeded from a malicious ritual source. She advised that one obtain a new bottle that had never been used before, and have the plagued person urinate into the bottle without speaking to anyone. Then nine new pins and nine new needles were to be carefully placed into the bottle, all pointed upwards, and the bottle was to be placed under lock and key. The keyhole was to be puttied shut and the key carried by the afflicted person. Sophia said that this method worked every time, and that the person guilty of placing the *Hex* would soon arrive at the house of the afflicted and ask to borrow something. If the afflicted person wishes to end the curse, they must refuse the request, even if the person begs. Thus anyone who appears at the home under such circumstances is believed to be the culprit.[57]

According to Sophia, the guilty person is compelled to appear at the home of the victim not only to borrow something in order to regain power over them. The belief is also that, in actuality, the ritual locking up of the *Hexeboddel* (witch-bottle) makes the culprit painfully incapable of urinating, unless the bottle is destroyed, or the culprit reverses and removes the *Hex*. Sophia Bailer warned that keeping the bottle locked up will eventually kill the person. She claimed that under her own direction, such a bottle was created that resulted in a woman's death,[58] and later remarked, "She must let that patient go or she'll die. Now that is true, and I say, God is with me when I do it."[59]

This practice is also well documented in Anglo-American communities, as well as in Britain, especially Suffolk, where a large number of bottles from the seventeenth century have been unearthed.[60] This period of time also corresponds to the publication of a manual of *Astrological Practice of Physick*, by Joseph Blagrave of Reading, England in 1671, where directions for creating the witch bottle are provided:

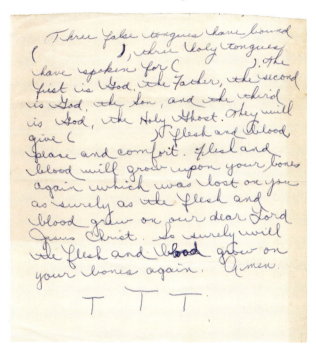

A "Ruhkbrief" (sleep-blessing), written by the hand of Sophia (Leininger) Eberly, namesake and apprentice to "Aunt" Sophia Bailer of Schuylkill County. *Heilman Collection.*

…Stop the urine of the patient, close up in a bottle, and put into it three nails, pins or needles, with a little white salt, keeping the urine always warm: if you let it remain long in the bottle, it will endanger the witches life: for I have found by experience that they will be grievously tormented making their water with great difficulty, if any at all, and the more if the Moon be in Scorpio in Square or Opposition to his Significator, when it is done…the reason… is because there is part of the vital spirit of the Witch in it, for such is the subtlety of the Devil, that he will not suffer the Witch to infuse any poisonous matter into the body of man or beast, without some of the Witches blood mingled with it…"[61]

Puritan minister Cotton Mather of New England, best known for his role in the Salem Witch Trials, condemned the practice of counteracting witchcraft with bottled urine in communities in Massachusetts, saying that "this may be to heal a body, but it is to destroy a soul."

I shall relate something that do not approve; and that it is, the urinary experiment. I suppose the urine must be bottled with nails and pins and such instruments in it as carry a shew of torture with them, if it attain its end…. [62]

Hohman describes a similar means to punish a witch:

Another remedy to be applied when any one is sick; which has effected many a cure where doctors could not help. Let the sick person, without having conversed with any one, make water in a bottle before sun-rise, close it up tight, and put it immediately in some box or chest, lock it and stop up the key-hole; the key must be carried in one of the pockets for three days, as nobody dare have it except the person who puts the bottle with urine in the chest or box.[63]

Although Hohman does not describe how the cure is supposed to operate, one can assume that his audience of readers implicitly knew what to do with such instructions.

Another variation of these instructions suggests: "Someone will come to loan, but be careful so as not to loan anything from the house, premises or person, within nine days, or this remedy will be in vain. Care must also be taken that nothing is stolen from either of these places."[64]

Helfenstein includes an incantation to be used with the *Hexeboddel*:

> Just as Paul was bound, so be thou defeated. In Jesus' name, thou shalt burn, in the name of Peter thou shalt burst. Make good what thou hast harmed, or else the bonds of hell will rest upon thee. Thine heart shall burn in thy body, thy blood shall run away like water. Thou shalt grow lame and crooked, deaf, and dumb. Thy bladder shall burst. In the air thou shalt be scorched, in the name of the Holy Spirit, and the Holy Guardian Angels.[65]

As a counterpoise to these methods, Sophia Bailer also employed a softer way to provide relief to one who was subject to the predations of a *Hex*, and whose rest was "stolen" by means of witchcraft. A *Ruhkbrief* (Letter of Rest) was composed and placed under one's pillow, containing the following text derived from Hohman's rendering of a prayer found in *Romanus*:

> Three false tongues have bound N. N. Three Holy Tongues have spoken for N. N. The first is God, the Father, the second is God, the Son, and the third is God, the Holy Spirit. They will give N. N. flesh and blood, peace and comfort. Flesh and blood will grow upon your bones again which was lost on you as surely as the flesh and blood grew on our dear Lord Jesus Christ. So surely will the flesh and blood grow on your bones again, Amen. + + +[66]

This prayer addresses the notion that a person has not only lost their rest, but they have become withered in body and spirit. The act of growing flesh and blood on one's bones is likened to the incarnation of Christ, and the prayer restores balance in the person through Christ's perfected human form. The "Three Holy Tongues" counteract the "Three False Tongues" without harming the one perceived to be responsible for the loss of rest.

Sophia Bailer's perceptions of witches, both male and female, were more complex than the one-dimensional characters so common in tales of Pennsylvania witchcraft. She claimed to have known several people personally who practiced *Hexerei*, and not all of them were exclusively predatory in nature. One even used his power for good, although he admitted that the source of his power came directly from the Devil himself.

THE SORCERER OF TREMONT

Sophia's family had a boarder, a hired man, who was married to their maid, and he displayed supernatural knowledge and abilities on numerous occasions. One incident involving a stolen cow made him famous among his neighbors. The morning that the family discovered the theft, the hired man used a deck of cards to determine the location of the cow. He warned the family that the cow would be slaughtered in one half hour, if they did not immediately bring three hairs from the cow's stall to him. Sophia's brother John retrieved the hairs, and the hired man went out into the field to perform a silent ritual. The family watched from a distance, and to their great surprise when he was finished, the cow came running. The heifer jumped over the fence, went right up to hired man, and let out a bellow that was loud enough to be heard by everyone.

Word spread, and soon, members of the local congregation, assuming that he was a powwower, sought to engage his services. They offered him money to discover the identity of an arsonist who attempted to burn the church on two occasions. The hired man explained that he could summon the culprit, but he couldn't accept the money, or "the devil would tear him to pieces."[67] This frightened the church members, who began to speak ill of him, calling him a liar and saying that he had no such abilities. Instead he offered to show a small group

The devil's role as temptor is featured in many Pennsylvania stories of witchcraft and sorcery as both the instigator of evil deeds, and the tormentor of those under his power. Engraving from the *Temptation of Christ*, 1704 Merian Bible, Frankfurt am Mayn. *Courtesy of the Evangelical and Reformed Archive, Lancaster, Pennsylvania.*

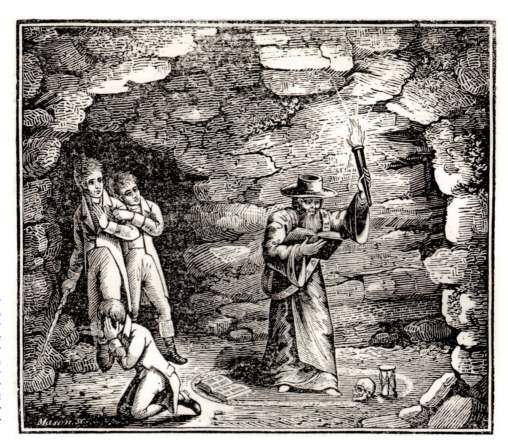

The clandestine discovery and defeat of a sorcerer is a motif common to many European legends. Some of these stories made their way to Pennsylvania, such as in this engraving by Pennsylvania printmaker Mason, featured in Conrad Zentler's *Americanischer Stadt und Land Calendar 1843*.

of the men something out in the woods. He took them to a clearing near a spring and made sure they were alone. Then, to everyone's surprise, a dark, dandy gentleman appeared by the spring, who had a horse's hoof for a foot, and he dug at the earth with his hoof.

The men from the congregation returned from the woods, dumbstruck and terrified, vowing never to ask the hired man for assistance ever again. One of them said "*Mit sellem, Dunnerwedder, will ich nix meh zu duh hawwe*" (With that man, [expletive] I will have no further association).

Eventually, the hired man and the maid moved away from the area, but one day they stopped by to visit. Sophia overheard him speaking to her mother, describing his plight that the devil would appear to him where he worked in the mines, and torment him by making the coal so hard that he could not pick it loose. For a coal miner who was paid by the load, this meant personal ruin. Finally, the man renounced the devil, and began attending a church in order to make "peace with God."

THE SORCERER NEAR GREEN POINT

Unlike the sorcerer of Tremont (in Sophia Bailer's recollections), whose proximity to the community certainly played a role in his story of redemption, others were regarded as social outcasts, living in remote areas on the fringe of society, with little hope for reintegration.

A friend from Lebanon County spent his childhood in the 1940s near Green Point at the base of the Blue Mountain. Bill Unger's family lived in the last house on Gold Mine Road just at the base of the steep rocky ascent over the mountain, and they shared the duplex with a reputed sorcerer named Mr. K and his wife.[68] Because of the remote location, the sorcerer had very few people upon which to impress his ritual abilities, aside from his wife and the family next door. His relationship with his wife was described as tumultuous by my friend Bill and his sister, who witnessed the hostile environment as children. The family was well-aware that Mr. K would use *Hexerei* in petty ways to aggravate his wife.

On one occasion in the midst of a heated argument, Mrs. K went out to the back porch to wash clothes. She pumped the water and heated it on the coal stove. After pouring it into her wash bucket, she grated the soap by hand. It was no sooner that she immersed the clothing in the hot water, that the children heard her scream and overturn the wash-bucket in frustration. Watching from the window, Bill and his sister saw Mrs. K run back into the house to confront her husband. There lay the wash bucket on the porch in the heat of the summer - frozen solid with the wash still in it. There was no satisfactory explanation for the freezing of the water, except that Mr. K had frozen the bucket by ritual means in revenge.

The whole family was frightened of Mr. K, who appeared to operate unencumbered by the laws of nature. One winter evening, after a heavy snow fell, Mr. K approached the Unger family outside about where they had parked their truck, saying he wished them to move it on account of accessibility to the driveway. Bill's father had been unable to move the truck because of the snow, and told Mr. K that he would move it the next morning. Just after Mr. K returned to his side of the house, the family noted that he had left no footprints whatsoever, despite the fact that everyone else's footprints from playing in the snow were clearly visible. To the family's surprise the following morning, the truck had been mysteriously moved according to Mr. K's wishes, without his access to the truck keys. Furthermore there was not a single mark or tire track in the snow, while the marks from the family's activities were still clearly visible, and there had been no drifting. Such puzzling events with no explanation only added to the mysteries surrounding Mr. K's reputation as a *Hex*.

According to my contact, Mr. K was not only perceived to be responsible for unexplainable events, he was also beyond eccentric. He tamed snakes and had one particularly large black snake that he kept as a companion and used in his ritual work. Mr. K would leave the house before dawn and go up the mountain with his snake. One day while Bill was walking outside by the stream that flowed across the road from his house, he saw movement on the hillside. To his surprise, the rocks began to shimmer with movement, as dozens of snakes of all sizes emerged from their lairs among the rocks. Bill climbed onto the dam-breast at the edge of the stream to get a better look, and saw that Mr. K. was standing above on the road wrapped in his big black snake with his arms outstretched. The snakes on the hillside all crawled toward Mr. K, as if drawn by an invisible force, but they did not bite him. Bill remained hidden, and from his perspective, Mr. K appeared to become semi-translucent, and he cast no shadow as the sun's rays appeared to shine directly through him.

This event, a form of sinister transfiguration that revealed the true nature of the sorcerer, affected Bill so strongly that he decided to seek retribution for all the disruption that Mr. K had caused for the two families. One day, while Mr. K was away, Bill clubbed his snake to death. When Mr. K discovered the body of the snake, he angrily confronted the boy. Bill openly admitted to killing the snake, and Mr. K shook with rage, but was seemingly unable to do anything overtly to retaliate against the boy in front of his family. The Ungers later moved from the property. Thus, a determined young boy with a precocious sense of justice had out-played the passive-aggressive sorcerer near Green Point.

Not all sorcerers were so easily overcome as Mr. K, yet petty quarrels were a common feature in many tales of witchcraft. Stories of grudges and competition between neighbors, centering on issues of revenge and the control of others, suggest that *Hexerei* was not merely relegated to the actions of skilled practitioners, but, like powwowing, was often employed by common people in the hopes of securing some advantage in everyday affairs.

Hexerei Shooters

Second only in popularity to witchcraft stories associated with dairy farming, are those associated with hunting and fishing – perhaps because the outcomes of both activities are subject to forces beyond individual control. Because hunting and fishing stories are often told among men as evidence of masculinity, such stories also highlight gender tensions, as women were often associated with bad luck, curses, or *Hexerei* used to obstruct a hunter's success, or even to "take the power" from gunpowder so that a shot does not properly fire.

Betz Heilman of Union County was reviled by hunters who would pass by her mountain dwelling on their way to the game lands, because from the comfort of her front porch she would sagely predict their inability to shoot game.[69] Naturally, when hunters returned from the mountains in their unsuccessful expeditions, Betz was to blame; and hunters assumed that she had emasculated them by ritual means.

While it is easy to see that women like Betz became scapegoats for the failure of men to return home with game, there are numerous documented rituals to prevent poaching, and most of them are geared towards women. While some rituals merely suggest that a woman need only to take off her apron and hang it over her shoulder in disgust to make the shot of a hunter miss its target,[70] Helfenstein offers an accompanying incantation to use "when thou wishest to take the power from the gunpowder of another, so that he can hit nothing, say the following":

Christ's fire was dear,
Thy fire is severe,
Vexation marks thy shot,
So shall it miss, and reach thy target not.
I invoke you by the Wind, Lead, iron, and powder,
that ye shall go astray without power, and reach not your aim, dispersed and commanded by the wind.[71]

While one can imagine that such rituals may have been popular among women who may have had few alternate forms of recourse if men with guns were spotted on their property, it is apparent that such rituals can be used to both protect and to harm – a tell-tale indicator of *Hexerei*. While most *Braucherei* rituals have no alternate uses beyond healing and protection, those rituals which are used for assuring positive outcomes can also be used for personal gain at the expense of another.

For those hunters, however, who were not to be dissuaded by the wiles of empowered women, there were other ritual options that invoked infernal forces to assure the accuracy of a shot. Casting bullets at a crossroads was one sure way to achieve this goal, typically at the liminal occasion of New Year's Eve or Christmas, but one should expect the arrival of the Devil,[72] seeking either a signature in his Book of the Damned, or merely to discourage the completion of the ritual. Bullets created in this manner are believed to have the power to strike an enemy no matter how far away the shooter may be.[73] Such deadly rituals were occasionally enacted in diverse and unexpected ways.

In 1915, two young Berks County men decided to attempt a ritual assassination of Kaiser Wilhelm in order to put an end to Germany's aggression in World War I. They took branches of elderwood and formed a circle at the crossroads of Lobachsville Road, Bertolet Mill Road, and Long Lane by the bridge over Pine Creek on New Year's Eve, and stood within the circle. Although elder is a wood that is considered unlucky to burn, the boys lit the circle of branches and made a fire to cast a silver bullet. One of them had successfully unearthed the skull of a criminal for the occasion, which was to serve as a stand-in for the Kaiser. They placed the skull in the center of the circle and loaded a flintlock pistol with the silver bullet – but something went wrong. A dark figure appeared at the intersection, his cloven hooves kicking up dust from the unpaved road. One of the youths panicked and sprang out of the circle, and ran in the opposite direction. As the devil approached the circle of elder wood, the remaining young man fired the gun into the skull. But the spell had been broken by his companion's exit, and as the devil vanished, the shot rang out louder than any earthly gunshot, and could be heard as far away as Kutztown ten miles away.[74] Needless to say, the Kaiser remained unaffected by the attempt.

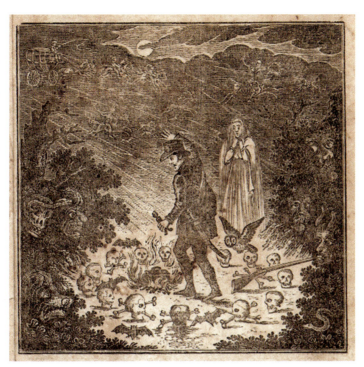

A hunter casts bullets at the crossroads in a circle of skulls while surrounded by apparitions, in an illustration from the German almanac *Amerikanischer Stadt- und Land-Calendar,* by Conrad Zentler of Philadelphia, 1833.

While such stories tend to function as cautionary tales, warning against making agreements with the devil, accounts of *Hexerei* also tend to serve as reinforcement of cultural norms and ethics forbidding the use of harmful ritual for even seemingly altruistic goals – like ending the war. When such overzealous and utilitarian desires result in the use of rituals enlisting help from sinister forces, the consequences are unpredictable and insufficient to justify the means.

In a broader sense, these conflicting motivations, desires for control, and tendency to assign blame, allow *Hexerei* narratives to provide the cultural context to assess and explore the darker side of the cosmic equation and its effect on the human experience.

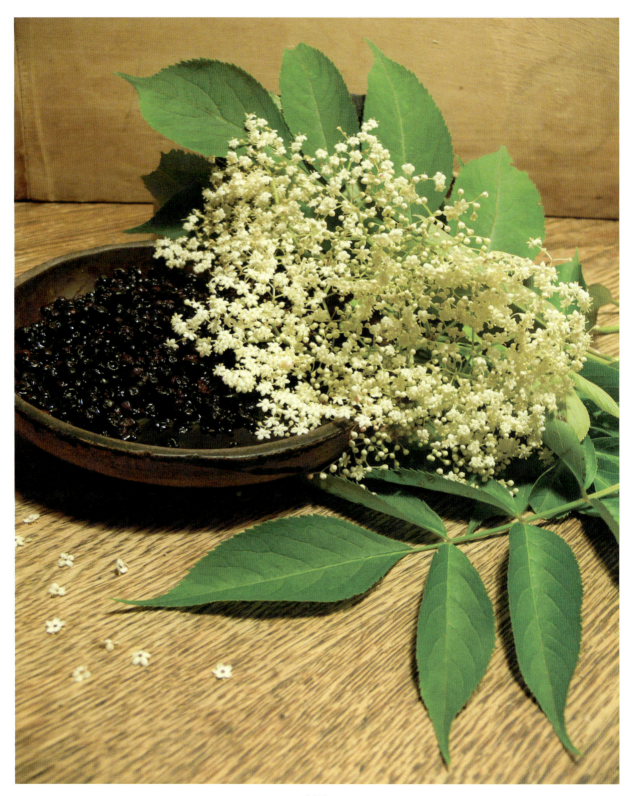

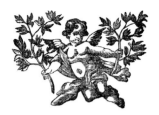  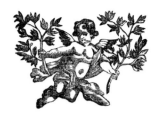

Chapter VII

Herbal Rituals
Trees, Shrubs, and Botanicals

The use of herbs and botanical cures is one of the oldest, most fundamental forms of medicine. Throughout the ages, plants have not only sustained humanity as an essential source of food and life, but the patterns of growth and the changing of the seasons have inspired conceptions of cosmic order for cultures across the globe. In Europe during the Middle Ages, the exploration of this botanical kingdom was an endeavor to reveal the will of the divine at work in the created world.[1] This notion was embraced by Protestants and Catholics alike, and the development of early botanical and natural science was perceived to be a fulfillment of the biblical promise in the sacred Garden of Eden at the dawn of creation: "Behold, I have given you every herb bearing seed, which is upon the face of all the earth, and every tree, in which is the fruit of a tree yielding seed; to you it shall be for food."[2] The use of herbs to nourish and heal the body, therefore, served not only practical purposes, but as reinforcements of humanity's place in a sacred world, seeded with divine order.

At the same time, herbal cures are a forerunner to modern biochemical medicine, and the efficacy of many herbal compounds in the treating of disease is supported by scientific investigation. Nevertheless, it is important to remember that the many uses of herbs in traditional healing systems cannot be easily reduced to the types of measurable techniques employed in the practice of conventional medicine. Instead the role of herbs and botanicals are defined by nuanced, cultural attitudes and part of a network of relationships interpenetrating agricultural, domestic, social, and religious spheres of life.

For the Pennsylvania Dutch, chemical and ritual cures are so generously interwoven in folk cultural expressions of herbal practices throughout the centuries that it is may be difficult to determine if a particular herbal remedy is more influenced by scientific or religious attitudes. More importantly, it is evident that no such distinction was recognized by the majority of Pennsylvania's early practitioners of traditional medicine. Mountain Mary, the legendary powwow healer of the Oley Valley, whose healing with herbs was inextricably linked to her religious piety, set the standard for the archetypal powwow practitioner, blending both worlds – botanical and religious medicine (see Chapter II).

The same was true of Christopher Sauer Jr., printer, apothecary, and Brethren activist in colonial Germantown, who compiled the first book of botanical medicine in North America.[3] Sauer's herbal was released between 1762 and 1778 as a serial publication in his *Hoch Deutsch Amerikanische Calendar,* a popular farmer's almanac distributed widely throughout the region. Sauer's work, based largely on the works 17th-century Swiss botanist Theodor Zwinger, contains a combination of both clinical and ritual medicine – a byproduct that, while academically outdated for the time, was not out of place with Sauer's religious orientation, nor that of his readership.[4]

In theory conventional medicine of the eighteenth and early nineteenth centuries was based on academic notions of medicine. In practice, most physicians also incorporated empirical knowledge acquired in the field from experiences within a traditional context. Undoubtedly the benefits derived from such mixed applications are at least in part due to an herb's chemical properties, but the methods of employing these herbs were often highly ritualized in terms of the symbolic timing and manner of their harvest, application, and frequency of use.

A classic example is the use of bark from the dogwood tree, which was believed to produce both emetic and purgative effects based upon the particular manner of harvesting of the bark. If the bark were peeled

Elderberry leaves, bark, blossoms, and berries are common *materia medica* in powwow cures. Illnesses were not only treated with elderberry compounds, but were also ritually transferred to the plant, suggesting a cultural relation to the elderberry beyond it's chemical properties.

from the tree in an upwards direction and in spring when the sap was rising, it would have an emetic effect to induce vomiting when decocted in boiling water. If the bark were to be stripped downwards, in autumn when the sap is flowing into the roots, it would have a purgative effect, following the direction of human evacuation.[5] The association of directional qualities with the effect on the human body is an example of sympathy – the notion that two bodies sharing subtle qualities of correspondence have the ability to act upon one another even without physical proximity. The movement and direction of the dogwood's sap corresponds to the action of peeling upward or downward, and importantly to the desired effect produced in humans from the bark. By consuming the bark, one is not only consuming the tree's qualities, one is also consuming the directional force of the practitioner's actions.

The same rule is applied to harvesting the leaves of the herb boneset (*Darrichwax*), when employed for a similar effect, and follows an identical pattern when stripped upwards or downwards: "*Wammer's Laab vun Darrichwax iwwerschich abschtrippt un macht en Tee davun, macht der Tee em breche; unnerschich, laxiert er.*"[6] (If one strips leaves upwards from boneset and makes tea from it, the tea will make him vomit; and downwards it is a laxative.)

Such overarching systems of thought are applied to a wide variety of plants and their interactions with human concerns. These attitudes were reflected in a substantial body of literature in early Pennsylvania and reinforced by the range of household apothecary books available to consumers. One such work printed in Harrisburg in 1841 by Gustav Peters suggests mugwort is reported to be valuable to women for regulating monthly periods. If the stem of the herb is cut downwards towards the earth it will encourage bleeding when a period is late, and end a heavy period if cut upwards, away from the earth.[7]

Borsdorf apple is harvested in a similar manner. It works like a laxative, when one shaves with a knife the bark from a branch towards the blossom and then eats it, but if one shaves toward the stem and eats it, they become constipated. Likewise, the same work suggests that the new, green inner bark of the elderberry bush, when harvested and boiled in milk has either an emetic or laxative effect according to the upward or downward motion of the harvest.[8]

Elderberry (*Sambucus negra* in Europe, *Sambucus Canadensis* in North America) has a long-standing role of providing a variety of medicinal compounds that are still widely marketed today. In Pennsylvania, elderflower tea was once widely used to combat inflammation, especially for erysipelas and other bacterial infections of the skin,[9] and even today the berries are still cooked and combined with brandy to make cordials as a remedy and preventative for colds. While these examples may be compatible with attitudes towards the use of herbs today, still other examples represent a broader spectrum of use, informed by the plant's role, not merely as the origin of a chemical compound, but as a veritable force of nature capable of delivering healing properties simply by virtue of proximity, and every bit as effective as when ingested.

A Berks County native from the Hamburg area described that up until fairly recently, Pennsylvania Dutch workmen in Berks County would carry elder leaves in their back pockets to prevent chafing on the job. The herb did not need to have any direct contact with the skin. Likewise, blossoms could be used in a similar manner to deter skin rashes, such as eczema.[10] Uses of elderberry bark varied considerably, including recipes for purging parasites, curing jaundice, as a skin wash for sores, and to reduce swelling. It was also useful to women to relieve cramping when a warm compress of the leaves or the bark made into a paste was applied warm to the abdomen.[11]

The elderberry among the Pennsylvania Dutch is a subject worthy of ethnobotanical study, for alongside these examples of medical rituals are personal rituals emphasizing a potentially sacred significance to the elder. Like many traditional cultures, the Pennsylvania Dutch have placenta burying rituals following the birth of a baby, and the most common location to bury the placenta was either under the shade of the elderberry bush, or under an apple tree. The shade of the elder bush in particular was also the site of healing rituals for chronic childhood ailments,[12] and apple trees were documented in the eastern United States for healing fevers.[13]

These attitudes of healing in Pennsylvania find their origins in European veneration of the saints where both elder and apple trees are associated in antiquity with female saints, and protectors of children and mothers. An old legend from Baden suggests that the Virgin Mary hung the Christ Child's diapers on the branches of the elderberry bush to dry.[14] St. Leopold founded the Abbey at Klosterneuberg after seeing a vision of the Virgin Mary under an elderberry bush, where he miraculously recovered his wife's wedding veil that had been missing for nine years.[15] Other legends suggest that the Holy Cross was made of elderberry wood or apple wood.[16]

Aside from its identification with the Tree of Knowledge of Good and Evil in the Book of Genesis, the apple plays other roles in legends of the saints. St. Dorothea is responsible for a miracle of making apples and roses appear in her bonnet following her martyrdom, which has been depicted in renaissance art,[17] and is the patron saint of midwives and apples.

Sources suggest that Christian legends surrounding these important trees were introduced to supplant earlier legends rooted in the worship of pre-Christian deities.[18] The Pennsylvania Dutch name for elderberry, *Hollebier,* is possibly derived from the name of the patron goddess Holle, associated in antiquity with mothers and childbirth, although others liken the etymology to that of Holland,[19] being "of the forest."[20] The association with Holle may also be the result of folk etymology that, while unconfirmed in an academic sense, reflects attitudes about the association of ideas with words that sound similar.[21]

Regardless of origin, these Christian and pagan attitudes, both support the widespread European German notion that one should tip their hat when passing by the elder tree.[22] An elder tree by the home was considered the resting place of protective spirits; whatever befell the tree would have repercussions in the family.[23] Out of respect for the bush, there were taboos associated with burning the wood.[24] The punishment for burning such wood was to contract Erysipelas (*Rotlaaf*) an inflammation and infection of the skin, likened to the fire. In this case, the elder is both the healer and the source of the illness, depending upon one's conduct around the plant.

As with many Christian symbols, a generous mixture of cultural forces are at work in the origins and significance of expressions of religious veneration, both in Europe and North America. For example, many herbs and plants were once associated with particular saints, and their patron's names are preserved in vernacular and botanical terminology such as St. John's wort (*Hannesgraut*) which was believed to drive away evil spirits, and currants (*Johannesbeer*) are named in honor of Saint John the Baptist, whose feast day on June 24th marks the day when the currants ripen. Red currants in particular are also called *Gichtbeer*, and the name implies their use in treating epilepsy. Hamburg parsley is associated with St. Peter (*Pederliliewatzel/Pederli/Pederslilienwurzel*), masterwort with St. Paul (*St. Pauls-Wurzel*), motherwort (*Muddergraut*) with the Virgin Mary, scallion with St. Jacob (*Jakob-Zwiebel, Allium Fistulosum*), to name but a few associations.[25]

Many herbs, although not associated by name with a particular saint, are best when gathered on particular days. The most popular of these practices in the Dutch Country, even to this day, is the gathering of dandelion greens on *Griener Dunnerschdaag* (Green or Maundy Thursday of Holy Week). Dandelion greens are picked and eaten as a spring tonic to prevent illnesses, lice and fevers; and to invigorate the liver and blood in the body. An old Pennsylvania Dutch proverb states that if you don't eat something green on Green Thursday, you'll be a dumb mule all year long; meaning you'll be sluggish and toilsome.[26] This notion of eating greens at this season may be informed by the Christian borrowing of the practice from the Jewish celebration of Passover during which bitter greens are eaten in commemoration of the hardship of slavery in Egypt. With typical Pennsylvania Dutch flair, however, the bitter dandelion greens are served with hot bacon dressing, and are a favorite at local church suppers in Berks, Lebanon, and Lehigh Counties.

Dandelion is still called *Biss-Bett* (Pee-the-Bed) in Pennsylvania Dutch because of its diuretic effect when decocted into a tea and also because of its yellow color. This notion is reflected in the once-common practice among children to take the yellow flower and hold it under another's chin – if the color is reflected onto the skin, it means that one is a bed-wetter. I recall this as being common even in my own childhood in the 1980s in Lebanon County. These beliefs and practices are indirectly related to the eating of dandelion greens on Green Thursday because the diuretic effect was an extreme form of the properties valued as a spring cleansing.

Ascension Day (*Himmelfahrt*) is still maintained as a holy day among the Old Order Mennonites and Amish, when shops are closed and everyone refrains from work. This observation used to be widely practiced among the Pennsylvania Dutch population, but is no longer entirely observed in the present day. In previous generations, Ascension Day is well documented as an important time for gathering medicinal herbs, which were believed to be most potent on this holiest of days. If one drank tea made from seven herbs gathered on Ascension Day, it was believed to prevent illness over the course of the year,[27] and as with many herbal traditions centered around the liturgical calendar, it was the holy day that was responsible for this power of prevention – not always the herbs in and of themselves, which is why the types of herbs are not usually specified in documentation of the tradition. This was not always the case, as one York County physician from the turn of the twentieth century described harvesting snakeroot and sarsaparilla on holy days as an activity every bit as charged with religious feeling as the act of prayer.[28] Teas were also gathered on the day when the celebration of reformer Jan Huss is observed on July 6, as well as *Maria Himmelfahrt* (The Assumption of Mary) on August 15.[29]

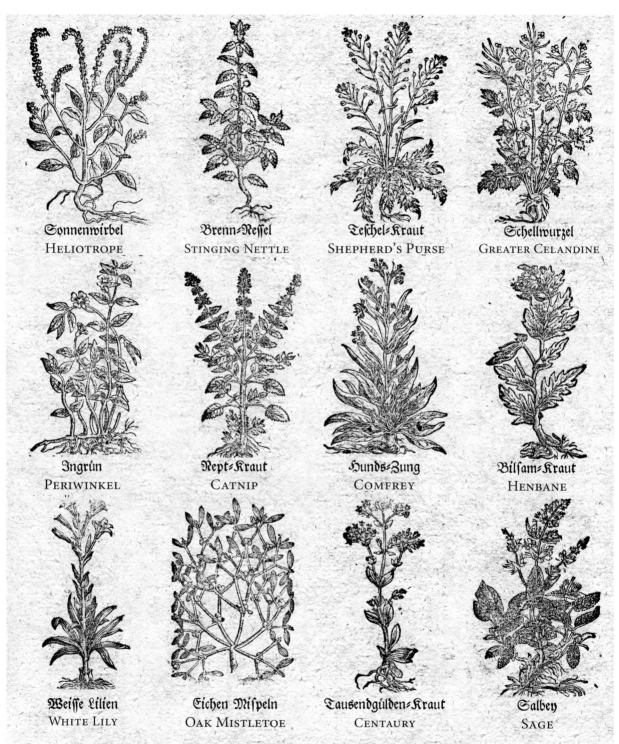

A wide range of herbs and their healing properties is expounded in the widely circulated *Book of Aggregations* attributed to St. Albert the Great. Each herb is illustrated and described for its virtues in healing and astrological correspondences. *Pennsylvania German Cultural Heritage Center, Kutztown Univeristy of Pennsylvania.*

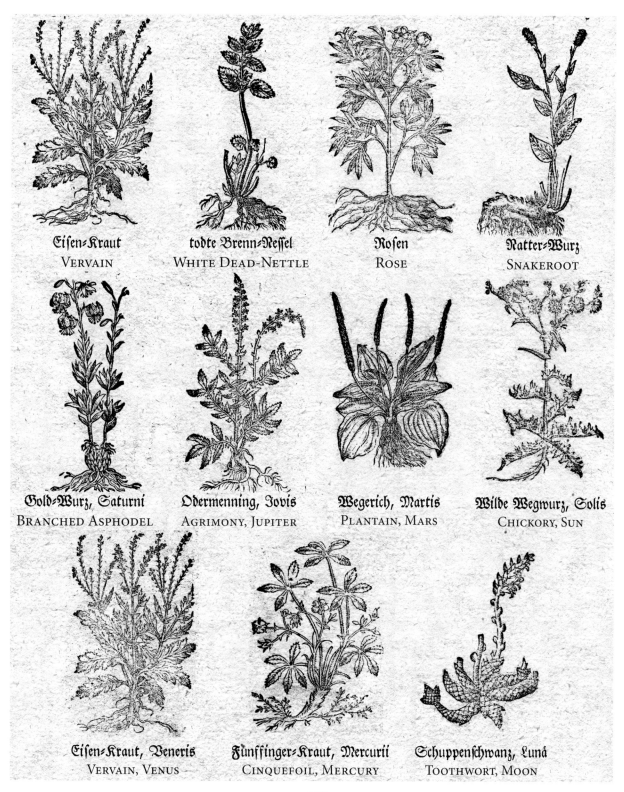

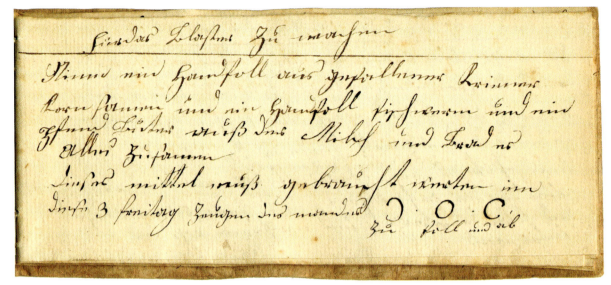

Recipe "To Make a Plaster," from *Conrad Raber his Docter book*, ca. 1800, Tulpehocken Township, Berks County. Note the diagram showing the progression of the moon. *Pennsylvania German Cultural Heritage Center, Kutztown University.*

The writings of Conrad Raber, *Braucher*, blacksmith and farrier in Tulpehocken suggests that the means of acquiring a plant determines its qualities and use, as cited in recipes for healing salves and plasters.[30] One such recipe that requires grain that has not been purchased, or even harvested, but that which has fallen on the ground of its own accord:

> Take a handful of fallen, clean grain seed and a handful of earthworms and a pound of butter and bake it all together. This recipe must be performed on the 3 Fridays in witness of the moon, as it waxes to full and wanes.).O.(

Just as the moon would affect the potency of herbs gathered on certain days, so too was the lunar effect equally important for ritually administering herbal compounds at certain times. Symbols at the end of Raber's inscription of the progression of the moon are illustrated directly above the words "*zu foll und ab*," (as it waxes to full and wanes), and each phase of the moon is reflected in the closing statement. Reflecting the notion of the moon exerting force on terrestrial bodies, this recipe may be intended as a drawing ointment in the waxing moon, and to release its healing properties in the waning moon. It is also possible that the sore or wound which was treated with the plaster was expected to wane along with the moon's decrease.

Salves were once extremely common in home remedies, and many of the recipes specify certain types of fats (goose, dog, bear,[31] groundhog, etc), each with properties distinct from the herbal compounds infused in the fats. The timing or manner of application was equally important, as reflected in an anecdote from the fieldwork of Anna Mae Gourley, who described a patient that received simultaneous treatment from a conventional doctor and a *Braucher* in the early twentieth century. The doctor was so impressed with the curative effect of the salve administered by the *Braucher* that he asked for the recipe. The *Braucher* willingly gave the recipe, but with the implication that the cure was necessarily in the composition, not of the salve but in the timing and manner of its application. Interestingly, the doctor compared the recipe to his own, and found little difference in the salve's ingredients.[32]

Although the notion of Conrad Raber's "plaster" is practically unheard of in the present day, salves, teas, decoctions, poultices, and tinctures are still popular means of administering healing herbs in modern herbalism. I know several modern clinical herbalists who still allow tinctures and other extracts to steep for the length of one moon cycle so that the mixture will achieve maximum potency.

The moon's effect is most easily discernible in the ritual use of potatoes and onions for the removal of warts. Although some claim that both of these plants contain trace amounts of salicylic acid, which is the active ingredient in modern wart removal medication, it is the ritual that receives the attention. Similarly, a recent Lehigh County contact described a neighbor carrying a potato in her blouse pocket to treat rheumatism, and among descendants of the Pennsylvania Dutch that

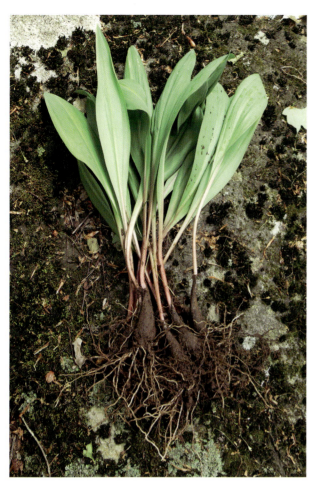

The wild leek, the closest Pennsylvania equivalent to the Alpine leek, *Victorialis*, *Allermansharnisch-Wurzel*.

Of the powers and virtues of the rightful *Victorialis*, which is endowed by God with miraculous functions, as follows: It is written that this root is to be a sure and proven remedy when hung over the door of the house or stable, so that no sorcerer (*Zauberer*) nor conjurer of the devil (*Teufels Bänner*) can enter into the house or stable. The root is a good remedy for inflammation in humans and animals. There is no better remedy for an over-ridden horse than hanging the root around its neck. The same serves well against cramps, when one hangs it on the afflicted limb. When one is lacerated, stabbed, or cut, take some of the outer layers of the root and lay it over the wound, and it will stop the bleeding. The root is good for cracked skin when working and for spasms of the limbs, when one hangs it on or lays it under the person. This root is good for pregnant women, so that that mother and child shall not die in childbirth when it is kept with them. One should clasp the root in the left hand, and the birth will proceed. No black magician (*Teufell Künstler*) or witches (*Hecksen*) can remain where this root is kept in one's house, or carried on one's person, and it is good for all obstacles when it is kept in your handkerchief. Such *Victorialis* is good to hang on all people, young and old, so that evil people cannot harm them. Terrible things can be done to those who are to be joined [in marriage], as some have experienced enough suffering, that they were made to be crippled, lame, or utterly blind, or a rift can be made between the bride and groom. For this reason, young women and men who are betrothed should seek out *Victorialis*. Also for livestock and horses, it should be hung on the stable door. *Victorialis* is also good to keep in the house or carry on one's person to protect from evil spirits, just as the mountain folk use it to drive away spirits that assail them. In total, *Victorialis* is highly prized, and the virtues exceed any description.[33]

These claims were refuted, however, by an academic medical encyclopedia popular among the intellectual elite in early Pennsylvania, *Gazophylackum Medico-Physicum oder Schatz-Kammer medicinisch- und natürlicher Dinge* (*Treasury of Medical-Physick or the Treasury of Medical and Natural Things*), by Johann Jacob Woyts, doctor of medicine in Königsberg, Prussia. Woyts cites all of the apotropaic uses of the herb against spirits (*Gespenstern*) and describes the common European practice of hanging the herb over a stable door, or burying it under the threshold. However, he attributes the practice to diverse superstitions endorsed by charlatans (*Quacksalbern und mancherlei Aberglauben*).[34] Although Woyts and his contemporaries condemned using *Victorialis* in this manner, the herb was valued more for its subtle virtues than for its medicinal and culinary role. *Victorialis* commanded high prices in the streets of Berlin even into the twentieth century,[35] and was commonly carried by soldiers as a remedy to stop bleeding from wounds.[36] In Pennsylvania, Woyts' work was advertised in the *Neue Unpartheyische Lancaster Zeitung* (*New Impartial Lancaster Newspaper*) on December nineteenth, 1792, and was available as far as the City of York, but his influence in Pennsylvania was minimal among the rural inhabitants

moved to Ontario, a horse-chestnut or buckeye is carried for the same purpose. A friend in Southern Appalachia related that a buckeye, polished with oil from one's nose, and carried in a pocket will protect a person from dying an untimely death while drunk.

Many botanicals and herbs are valued for both their protective and healing qualities, and in many cases no distinction is made between these two purposes in written descriptions of these plants in private household recipe books. The wild onion is a well-documented example of this notion. An early nineteenth-century collection of manuscript cures from Reading, Berks County, is attributed to a father and son, Peter and Samuel Hain, who cited *Victorialis*, the European Alpine leek (*Allermansharnisch-Wurzel* – literally 'everyone's armor') as a sure remedy for exorcising evil spirits and the damage done by witchcraft and sorcery.

of Pennsylvania, except perhaps among apothecaries such as Samuel Ensminger (1763-1840) of Manheim, who inscribed his personal copy.[37]

Although the Alpine leek, *Victorialis,* is not to be found in the hills of Berks County where Peter Hain penned his manuscript, the closest American equivalent is the ramp (*Allium tricoccum*), a type of wild leek, which is native to Pennsylvania. Growing in moist woodland clearings, Ramps are popular in many parts of the United States in regional cookery, but they are threatened as a species from overharvesting for commercial consumption. Although the Allium family is known for its medicinal qualities, the pungent smell of the wild leek is at least partially responsible for its reputation as a powerful herb.

Perhaps the most celebrated of all herbs for pungency in ritual applications is asafetida (*Ferula Assafoetida*) a powdered resin with a powerful stench. Asafetida is native to Asia and is common in Middle-Eastern and Indian cuisine, but has been exported to Europe since the Middle Ages. Commonly known as Devil's Dung (*Deiwelsdreck*), the herb has many regional names and pronunciations throughout Pennsylvania and southern Appalachia.

The resin of the plant was once widely available in drug stores and although it has biochemical uses, it was widely purchased in the Dutch country for ritual and pharmacological medicine. Typically granulated or powdered asafetida was placed in small linen bundles and worn around the neck to ward off disease. My grandfather, Kenneth Galbraith (1932-2009) of Lebanon, recalled his mother making him wear 'asperfidity' to ward off illness when he was sent to elementary school. The potent smell was certainly enough to keep his classmates at arm's length, thus potentially avoiding communicable illnesses. But he was not the only child in class to wear the herb; in fact it was once quite common in both rural and urban areas for adults and children.

The herb was also ingested to treat colic in cattle and horses, to stimulate digestion, and relieve gas in humans and animals.[38] Some even chewed the substance like tobacco.

But every tradition has its critics. An anonymous, entrepreneurial correspondent in the Readinger Adler Newspaper in 1893 suggests the following:

Deel Leit duhne alleweil Deiwelsdreck kaafe in der Apothek un duhne des Stoff tschabe fer Krankhete abhalte. De seem zeit laafe sie rum mit ausgeworne Schuh un Schtivel un hen nasse Fiesz. Ken Wunner dasz seller Deiwelsdreck sie nix batt. Sie deete besser grad geh an der Eagle Schuh Schtore uf Eck der 6te Penn Schtrosse, Reading fer en verstannige pore Shuh.

Some people frequently buy Devil's Dung in the drug store and chew the stuff to keep away illness. At the same time, they walk around with worn out shoes and boots, and have wet feet. It's no wonder that Devil's Dung doesn't work for them. They had better go straight to the Eagle Shoe store on the corner of 6th and Penn Streets, Reading, to buy an outstanding pair of shoes.

Asafetida was not only carried on one's person, but, like *Victorialis*, was included in many apotropaic applications for protecting horses and cattle from spiritual attacks of sorcery:

Take wormwood, black caraway, five-finger grass and asafetida, three cent's worth of each, fava bean straw, and together with some of the dust that collects behind the stable door and a little salt, make it into a little bundle and put it in a hole bored into the threshold where the cattle pass in and out, and plug it shut with a plug made of alder buckthorn wood.[39]

This can be compared to a parallel procedure suggested by Dr. Helfenstein:

So that no witch nor spirit may harm thy property: take rue, bread, salt, and oaken coals. Bore a hole in the door sill, where the cattle go in and out, and put the powder into a rag and stuff it into the hole with the tine of a harrow, thus will the cattle be safe.[40]

What is notable here is that the words for alder buckthorn (*Ezelbaum* or *Elsebaum*; *Rhamnus frangula*) and the harrow tine (*Eggen Zahn*) are so similar, that a transcription error is likely to have occurred at some point in Europe, whether in oral or written tradition, producing divergent ritual procedures. The harrow tine is a removable tooth from an agricultural implement with the role of tearing and dredging the soil, and is used in this case to force the bundle into the hole. As a possible

Two nineteenth-century, linen asafetida bags used in Lancaster County, actual size. *Courtesy of Clarke Hess.*

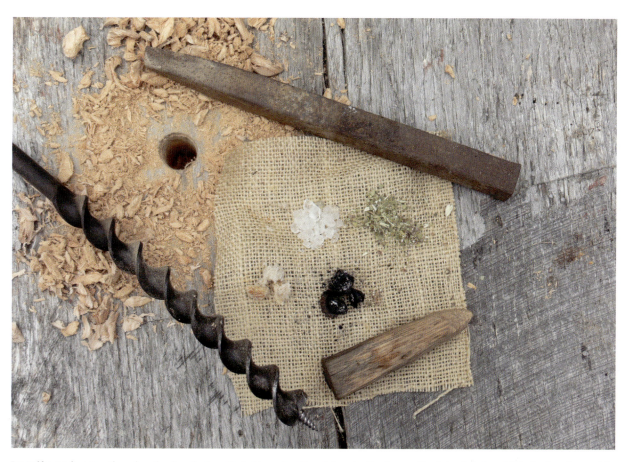

Dr. Helfenstein's recipe of rue, bread, salt and oak coals, tied ino a bundle and forced with a harrow tine into a hole bored into the door frame of the stables. Such recipes are a possible explanation for non-structural pegged holes found in historic Pennsylvania barns.

source of symbolism, this tool relates to the extra-biblical story of Christ's "harrowing of hell" to release the saints from captivity, featured in the non-canonical *Gospel of Nicodemus*, a favorite book of extra-biblical narratives among the Pennsylvania Dutch.[41] At the same time, alder buckthorn wood, also known as *Zapholz* (literally, "plug-wood") plays a role in many apotropaic procedures where a plug is necessary. One ritual outlined in *Egyptian Secrets* suggests that the buckthorn plug itself is what "keeps the witches out," rather that any herbal compound held in place by the plug.[42] Some have suggested that Christ's Crown of Thorns was woven of buckthorn,[43] adding a layer of biblical symbolism to a protective ritual otherwise lacking in any specificity, religiously or otherwise.

Whether pressed in place with a harrow tine, closed up with a plug, or worn on the person, discrete bundles of herbal mixtures are featured in many aspects of ritual practices, placed in architectural deposits in barns and stables, as well as in personal amulets for protection and talismans worn for short durations for their healing properties.

An early nineteenth century Berks County remedy for a fever suggests digging five broadleaf plantain roots (*Wegerich*) on a Friday morning before the sun comes up:

> **In an uneven hour, sew up the roots in an unbleached cloth with unbleached thread, and hang the bundle on the person in an uneven hour until the ninth day, when the bundle is to be cast into flowing water or buried in manure.**[44]

Broadleaf plantain was valued for its curative properties in the eighteenth century, and described at great length in Sauer's herbal as treatment for a wide variety of ailments including illnesses of the urinary tract and fevers as a decoction as well as topically in the form of poultices for sores and inflammation.[45] It is clear, however, that while the use of plantain roots in a bundle to be worn around the neck as a cure for fever is a departure from many of the more distinctly clinical methods endorsed by Sauer, some measure of the curative properties assigned to plantain are implicit in the selection of the herb as a ritual form of anti-inflammatory.

Sauer cites a similar ritual burying procedure using smartweed:

> Various surgeons have written that if this herb is drawn through fresh water, and then bound over an old, open wound, until it is well warmed, and the bandage then buried in a damp place [the manure pile], this will have the remarkable power to heal the wound as the herb rots in the ground.[46]

Sauer's remedy bears most of the earmarks of the former ritual involving plantain roots such as flowing water and the dung heap, except for the timing. The requirement of an uneven hour for the application of the herb, although seemingly arbitrary to the modern mind, is indicative of a state of change and instability, and intended to influence the abatement of the illness. Like the movement of the water, and the decomposition of the manure pile, the fever is to leave the person, enter into the bundle, and be carried away by a brook, or neutralized through decay.

Other traditions suggest burying the roots in soil, often after dark, or at a particular time following a ritual procedure. In this case, interring the disease evokes symbolism of the grave and the demise of the illness. If the herbs are tied up in white linen, it is suggestive of the funeral veil.

In the year 1889, a woman in Akron, Lancaster County was so frequently observed "stealthily" digging up roots after dark, bringing them into the house for a ritual behind closed doors, and then burying the roots wrapped up in white linen in the backyard that it caught the attention of neighbors who reported it to the local press. The story ran in newspapers as far away from Akron as Pittsburgh with descriptions of her procedure, and the explanation that "a lot of people have great faith in her treatment."[47] Although local readers could easily infer that the neighbors were being *Wunnerfitzich* (nosey) and equally "stealthy" in their observations, it is important to note that the woman was likely to have been operating under particular ritual conditions. In some cases, gathering materials for powwowing must be done silently and without being noticed (*unbeschraue*), and many rituals involve rising before the sun, while fasting (*nichtern*) and speaking to no one.

In other cases, speaking is an important part of the ritual – where prayers and invocations are spoken over the plants that are gathered, and in many cases, the ritual involves speaking to the plants. The plants are called by name, in much the same way that illnesses are addressed in powwowing cures, only instead of being invoked and dismissed like a sickness, the plants are blessed or asked to contribute to the cure.

A remedy for "restoring milk" is given in the collection of Dr. Helfenstein, describing a ritual procedure involving common ground-ivy (*Glechoma hederacea*). Milk was considered "stolen," "spoiled," or "bewitched" if its consistency was too thin, and lacked sufficient milk-fat to produce butter or cream. This was typically the result of poor nutrition, but was perceived to be the result of malicious witchcraft. Even still, the condition was frequently mitigated with herbal supplements of the ritual variety in the eighteenth and nineteenth centuries:

Gunt Reben, Christus hat dir Gnade geben, Der hat erschaffen die Wolken, und Bring mir die Milch wieder, mier das meine, und jeder das seine im Namen des Vaters, Sohn und Heiliger Geist + + +

Broadleaf plantain, used in rituals for reducing fever, inflammation, rash from poison-ivy, and bee stings.

Ground-ivy, Christ hath given thee grace. He hath created the clouds, and bringeth back the milk to me: he shall restore mine unto me, and to each his own in the name of the Father, Son, and Holy Spirit.

These words were to be spoken to the ground-ivy (*Gunt-Reben*) before it is harvested, while passing one's hand over the plant in a circular motion. Once the words are spoken, the plant can be plucked and given with a little salt to the cow to eat.[48] A European variety of the ritual suggests making three wreaths out of the ground-ivy and milking the cow through the wreaths before feeding them to the cow.[49]

An manuscript source from the convent of St. Blaise in Baden, penned in 1617 suggests plucking the ground-ivy in honor of the Virgin Mary and Christ, and throwing it into the air to bless it, saying "I throw thee up to the clouds, so that the Lord Jesus Christ, will return my milk and cheese to me."[50] This invocation echoes Helfenstein's dedication of the ground-ivy to "he who hath made the clouds," suggesting a common origin for the ritual. Likewise, the ground-ivy is sprinkled with a little salt and given to the animal to eat.

Another European invocation asks the ground-ivy a question:

Konrebel, du edle Saft, weiß du, was Christus Jesus sagt? Du sollst vertreiben die Mundfäul und die Bräun und was noch dabei möcht seyn.

Ground-ivy, thou of noble sap, do you know what Christ Jesus says? Thou shalt drive away the thrush and sore throat, and whatever else be with it.[51]

Another from Landstuhl in the Pfalz describes an apocryphal chance meeting between Christ and St. John in the fields:

*Sankt Johannes ging über das Land
Begegnet ihm Jesus Christus mit seinem Gesand.'
"Sankt Johannes warum bist du so traurig?"
"Warum soll ich nicht trauern?
Mein Mund muss mir verfaulen!"
"Sankt Johannes hol drei Gundelreben
Und lass sie durch deinen Mund schweben
So wird dein Mund gesund werden!"*

Saint John went over the land
He happened upon Jesus Christ with his envoy,
Saint John, why art thou so mournful?
"Why should I not mourn?
My mouth is rotting away!"
"Saint John fetch three ground-ivy sprigs
and sweep them through thy mouth,
so wilt thy mouth be made whole!"[52]

The accompanying ritual procedure for a similar invocation was documented in 1941 for a case of infant thrush in Witgenstein, Germany describing the use of the herb which was plucked by a woman from the edges of the path through the barnyard, and drawn three times through the mouth of the child to transfer the illness to the herb, and then hung in the chimney of the bakeoven where it was to be ritually smoked (*beräuchert*), so that the smoke would drive away the illness.[53]

This ritual is used for thrush, a throat infection often affecting infants, causing white lesions on the inside of the mouth and on the tonsils, known as *Mundfäule* or *Bräune*.

Historically, this use of the ground-ivy is the ritual counterpart of other medical applications of teas and infusions made of the herb to be used as a mouthwash.[54] Ground-ivy is somewhat mucilaginous when bruised or chewed (thus its derivation from old Gothic *"Gund"* meaning puss), and it can be likened to mallow, which is used to coat and sooth a sore throat. Although at first, this use of ground-ivy as a treatment for thrush and sore throat within the parameters of historical forms of conventional medicine may appear to inform the selection of the herb for ritual purposes, the reality is that the plant plays a dual role in both forms of medicine. The use of ground-ivy in ritual is no more derivative of conventional medicine of the past than the conventional use was derivative of the ritual use. Both treatments historically existed side by side, and occasionally, were used simultaneously, suggesting the likelihood that both forms of treatment were influenced by earlier traditional uses of the plant, which may have combined both ritual and conventional components without distinction.

A ringlet of ground-ivy used in rituals to ritually restore stolen milk from dry cows.

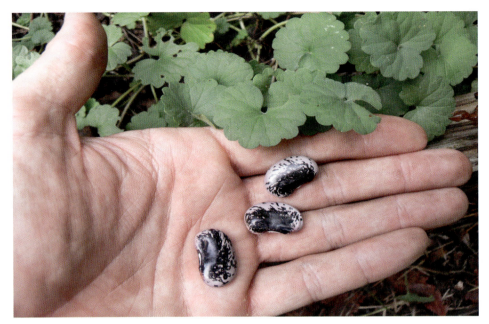

The ritual offering of three beans when harvesting herbs for ritual use is a practice that proceeds from practitioners living in the hills surrounding the Oley Valley of Berks County. Offerings like these are common to many cultures, as a symbolic observation of reciprocity.

The invocations of the ground-ivy and Christ's suggestion to St. John imply the perception that the virtues possessed by the ground-ivy were God-given, and part of the order of creation. The plant-invocations also grant the ground-ivy some level of agency in the ritual as a sentient being and adds additional meaning to some old European renderings of the herb's name in the dialect of the Pfalz as *"Gundermann"* – implying a form of animistic personhood. Some sources have suggested that the common proximity of ground-ivy to the paths of the house and farm led to this naming of the plant as a comparison to a beneficent house spirit, a *"guter Man"* (good man).[55]

This correlates to the shamanic practices of other cultures across the world, such as the Kuna of Panama, where not only are plants considered sentient spiritual beings, but a shaman must ask permission prior to harvesting plants for ritual purposes, and such plants are believed to be ineffective for cures if permission is not granted.[56] While the ground-ivy ritual makes no exact mention of permission, the fact that some rituals require invocations that must be spoken prior to harvest indicates some level of sanctioning of the harvest within a spiritual framework. Permission to harvest the *"Gunderman,"* was therefore at least partially dependent upon engaging the plant in a ritual dialogue.

When I learned to powwow in 2006, I was advised by my teacher to make an offering of three beans anytime that I gathered a plant for a healing purpose. Although I was never advised that the offering itself had any effect on curative or protective properties, it was described instead as a way to honor the sacrifice of the plant by conveying a sense of reciprocity.

Some invocations of sentient plants are far less honoring and consensual in certain samples of the ritual literature of the Pennsylvania Dutch. Johann Georg Hohman's borrowed a ritual from *Romanus* for compelling a thief to return stolen property:

> Walk out early in the morning, before sunrise, to a Juniper bush, and bend it with the left hand towards the rising sun while you are saying: Juniper tree, I shall bend and squeeze thee, until the thief has returned the stolen goods to the place from which he took them. Then you must take a stone and put it on the bush, and under the bush and the stone you must place the skull of a malefactor + + + [in the Three Highest Names]. Yet you must be careful in case the thief return the goods to unloose the bush and replace the stone where was before.[57]

Although the distribution of Hohman's book was extensive, there is no documentation of actual use of this particular ritual among Pennsylvanians, and the use of the skull certainly adds a sinister element to the juniper ritual. While there is a precedent for the use of cadaver bones in ritual procedures, usually these elements are considered to be part of the spectrum of *Hexerei*, and are not looked upon favorably. Furthermore, while skulls are occasionally featured in healing rituals, there are several in which skulls play a signature role where a theme of violence prevails, such as in several procedures related to casting enchanted bullets at a crossroads.[58]

The treatment of the juniper bush is likewise a ritual of coercion and force, and is not unlike conjurations described in the *Sixth and Seventh Books of Moses* that aim to detain spirits and compel them to perform tasks. Nevertheless, this juniper ritual substantiates the notion that trees and other plants are treated as simultaneously physical and spiritual entities, capable of assisting humans in a variety of ways. This same line of thinking undergirds the notion of plugging illness into trees which has been well-documented among many cultures — Pennsylvania Dutch, Lenape, and English. Early accounts provide details of this procedure, and evidence of "plugged" trees have been found up until the twentieth century.

An undated series of mid-nineteenth-century instructions, written in the hand of Dr. Johann Peter Saylor of Northampton County, describes the ritual procedure, but does not specify what type of illness was to be cured:

> Take a goose quill and cut it of[f] where it begins to be hollow then scrape off a little from each nail of the hands and feets [sic] put it into the quill & stop it up after bore a hole towards the rise of the sun into a tree that bears no fruit put the Quill with the scrapings of the nails into the Hole and with three strokes close up the Hole with a bung maid [sic] of pine wood It must be done on the first Friday in the New moon in the morning.

While no title or explanation accompanies this set of instructions, the process clearly illustrates the practice of removing illness by transferring it into a tree, and it is identical to an entry in Daniel Ballmer's *Receipts* used for removing toothache.[59] This practice is well documented in Pennsylvania as well as in the Ozarks,[60] and occasionally, such deposits are discovered when trees are cut down as evidenced by a cross-section of a tree displayed in the Thomas Brendle Museum at Historic Schaefferstown. The remnant of a plugged oak tree was discovered by a farmer chopping wood on a farm between Reistville and Schaefferstown, Lebanon County. According to the farmer's observations, the tree was believed to have been close to a century old when the peg and ritual deposit was placed for transferring illness into the tree. The ritual deposit took place over a century prior to having been cut down. One hundred twenty annual growth rings had grown over the peg.

Although some have related this practice to protective rites derived from the worship of trees in pre-Christian times, these instructions would appear to indicate instead that in this particular instance the tree is used as an object of transference rather than worship and that the illness is being sympathetically withdrawn from the person into the tree by means of the nails from the hands and feet. Perhaps the most important piece of evidence indicating that the tree becomes the vessel of the illness is the cryptic admonition the tree must bear no fruit – negating the possibility that a human being would accidentally contract the illness by eating a piece of fruit.

The scheduling of the ritual within these particular cosmological constraints serves to articulate a portion of the folk-cultural beliefs surrounding the effect of the moon upon earthly affairs. The moon was believed to exert a particular force on the Earth which varied according to its phase: as the moon waxed to full, it was believed to exert a force which pulled away from the Earth, and as it waned to the new moon, it exerted a force towards the Earth. This force was believed to be the strongest at either extreme.

The use of the influence of the new moon in the case of plugging trees is appropriate, because the force of the moon is directed towards the earth, fixing the illness within the tree. As a corollary to this, it was believed to be beneficial and of good luck to cut one's nails in the new moon, which would prevent nails from becoming ingrown.[61] In addition, a new moon falling on a Friday was considered universally among the Pennsylvania Dutch to be the best day for healing.[62] Ancient European folk processes concerning ritual deposits in bushes and trees also make use of Friday as the preferable day for the work to be done, as well as the use of the direction of the rising sun as a feature common to such rituals.[63] This combination of circumstances - the new moon, Friday, rising sun - was a deliberate choice on the part of the practitioner, to make use of the most beneficial arrangement of celestial forces.

In 1885, Charles W. Ash of West Caln, Chester County discovered a "wooden pin" deep within the growth of a white oak tree that was cut down on his property, and reported it in the *Daily Local News*. An anonymous reader responded by describing a memory of having witnessed a cure for sweeny (muscular atrophy) in a mare when he was just a boy, involving a tree-plugging ritual. Before dawn, he accompanied a neighbor, and together they led the horse to a woodlot located in Uwchlan Township about a quarter-mile south of the turnpike (along present-day PA Route 100), where a yellow poplar tree had been selected and a hole had been bored on the previous evening. The neighbor cut three tufts of hair from the top, middle, and bottom of the hollow of the atrophied shoulder of the mare, and stuffed the hair into the hole. He then slid a plug into the hole and waited silently, facing east for the sun to rise. When the sun began to crest the horizon, the neighbor used the butt of an axe to drive the peg into the tree with three strokes. Although the neighbor had not spoken to the boy throughout the procedure, when the

> Take a goose quill and cut it of where it begins to be hollow, then scrape off a little from each nail of the hands and feets put it into the quill & stop it up after bore a hole towards the rise of the sun into a Tree that bears no fruit put the Quill with the scrapings of the nails into the Hole and with three Strokes close up the Hole with a [hamm]er made of pine wood It must be done on the first Friday in New moon in the morning

Manuscript Directions for Transfering Illness Into a Tree, ca. 1860-1880
Heilman Collection.

These manuscript instructions provide a process for ritually transferring an illness into a tree, involving the use of a goosequill, into which nail clippings of the fingers and toes are placed. A hole must be bored in a tree that bears no fruit, into which the quill is to be placed, and sealed up with three strokes of the hammer on the first Friday of the new moon.

The timing of this ritual was crucial, for the new moon was believed to exert a force down and inward, driving the illness into the tree; it was believed that the movement of the sun westward would reinforce the same movement of the illness into the tree. Friday was considered a beneficial day to begin such an undertaking because of its association with the crucifixion of Christ on Good Friday, and the initiation of the salvation and healing of the world in Christian tradition.

Plugged Oak Tree Remnant, mid-nineteenth century, Schaefferstown, Lebanon County. Thomas R. Brendle Museum, Historic Schaefferstown.

Discovered by a farmer chopping wood on a farm between Reistville and Schaefferstown, Lebanon County. According to local interpretation, the tree was believed to have been close to a century old when the peg and ritual deposit was placed for transferring illness into the tree, over a century prior to having been cut down. One hundred twenty annual growth rings were counted from the bark to the peg.

The practice of "plugging" illness into trees is well-documented among many cultures — Pennsylvania Dutch, Lenape, and English. Early accounts provide details of this procedure, and evidence of "plugged" trees was still found in the twentieth century.

> Wer GOtt vertraut? Und dem Segen Jacob's glaubt; Und an Jesus Christus glaubt: Der werde weiters Macht haben, als Teufel, noch bösen Thieren, noch Wuth. Das in das Loch in ein Baum gethan, und ein Wasser hinein gemacht, und ein Zapfen darauf geschlagen.
>
> Baum, Gott segne mich.
>
> in fanto das ist Der
>
> farce, in, etina : afa : Wirba : farce, in, feba : refa : bnua : farce, in, naba : freba : etna :

"Baum-Segen" Broadside Prayer and Tree Plugging Instructions, ca. 1790-1810
Heilman Collection.

"Who trusts in God, and believes in the blessing of Jacob and in Jesus Christ, will have the power to overcome the Devil, wild animals, and danger. Put it into a hole in a tree, and urinate into it, and hammer a plug thereafter. Tree, God bless me." This broadside also has cryptic inscriptions that follow, which appear to be written in cypher.

process was complete the neighbor later explained "If it should not cure her, it will do her no harm" – echoing a Pennsylvania Dutch maxim: *Batz nix, schad's nix* (If it doesn't work, it won't hurt).[64] The writer concluded that the mare had improved rapidly and "soon became efficient in her place on the farm."[65]

The Medical and Surgical Reporter of 1885 describes common cures used for asthma, when a person would allow a lock of hair still attached to the head to be carefully plugged into the tree. The hair was then to be cut, freeing the person suffering from asthma, who was to walk away without ever looking at the tree again in order to be cured. The editor cited this procedure as an explanation for reports of mysterious bottles found lodged in trees in Beaver Township, (either Snyder or Columbia County). Some of the bottles were filled with unidentified fluid, and corked shut. These were used in much the same way as a wooden plug, and held cuttings of hair in place in the tree.[66]

An early, rare Pennsylvania broadside provides insight into the possibility that the bottles may have contained urine, as another means to transfer illness from the person by means of materials taken from the body. The broadside offers the following cryptic inscription:

> Wer Gott vertraut? Und dem Segen Jacob's glaubt; un an Jesus Christus glaubt: Der Werde weiters Macht haben, als Teufel, noch bösen Thieren, noch Wuth. Das in das Loch in ein Baum gethan, und sein Wasser hinein gemacht, uud[sic] ein Zapfen darauf geschlagen. Baum, Gott segne mich…
>
> Who trusts in God? And believes in the blessing of Jacob? And believes in Jesus Christ? He shall furthermore have power, over the Devil, against wild animals, and rabies. All this placed in a hole in a tree, and urine passed therein, and a plug driven over it. Tree, God bless me…[67]

In this case, the text seems to suggest that the tree plays the role not so much of a receptacle for illness or object of transference, but instead as a preventative and protective source of power.

A fever remedy, from *Egyptian Secrets* attributed to St. Albert the Great recommends using a nut tree, perhaps with the notion that anyone or anything to eat such a nut would assist with the cure and take on the illness, which in this case was fever:

> Nut tree, I come unto thee to take the seventy-seven-fold fever from me. I want it to remain therein. † † †

This must be written upon a slip of paper, and before the sun rises go to a nut tree. Cut out a plug from the tree and insert the paper. Recite the above inscription three times, and put the plug in its place again, so that it may grow together."[68]

A similar procedure is described as a remedy for a hernia. The text provides a number of different procedures for plugging illness into trees.

To transplant a hernia from a Young Man

Cut three tufts of hair from his cowlick and bind them together in a clean cloth. Carry it to another property. Cleave a young willow tree and place it within, so that it may grow over the spot. † † †[69]

Another cure, again addressing a willow tree, bears a number of similarities to the previous two descriptions of tree plugging, although instead of plugging the tree, knots are tied in strips of bark, which are deposited in flowing water.

> Willow tree, I propose to thee: I bid thee take away from me my seventy-seven-fold spasms. This must be spoken three times, three Fridays in succession, when the moon is waning. In the morning, before sunrise, go to a flowing stream, and turn thy face in the direction that the water runs, and tie three knots on each of three strips of willow bark, in the three highest names."[70]

The procedure of tying knots and disposing of them appears in cures for warts, only instead of tying three knots three times as a reference to the trinity, a knot is tied on a string for each wart and disposed of in flowing water.

The action of tying was not only employed with strips of bark, but string was used to bind illness to trees, either in a symbolic form, such as with scraps of fabric from a sick person's clothes or in written form. Such trees, with appended devices were known in Germany as *Lappenbäume* (rag-trees).[71] An example from Hesse cites biblical reasoning for the selection of the elderberry tree for tying fever into its branches:

> *O Fliederbaum, du lieber,*
> *Mich quält das kalte Fieber:*
> *Weil Judas sich an dir erhänkt,*
> *Sei das Fieber dir geschenkt!*
>
> O elderberry, thou dearest tree
> The cold fever tortures me,
> Because Judas hung himself upon thee,
> so shall the fever to thee given be.[72]

As indicated in this blessing, according to some regional folklore found across Northern Europe and the British Isles, the elderberry was the tree upon which Judas took his life after betraying Christ.

This idea of hanging a fever on a tree is reflected in an account from 1833. It describes a ritual of tying white and blue string together into a loop attached to an apple tree on one end, and encircling the wrist of a young girl who suffered from a fever. The girl was to slip her hand from the loop, and run into the house without looking back.[73]

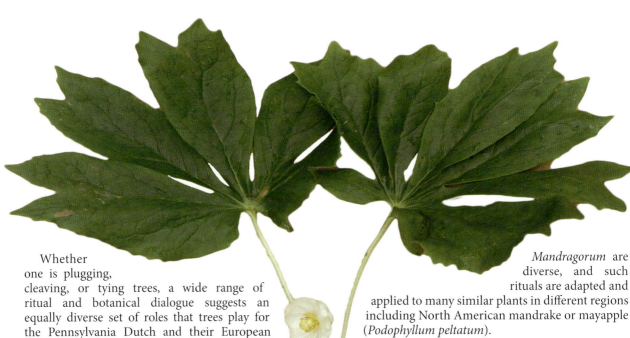

Whether one is plugging, cleaving, or tying trees, a wide range of ritual and botanical dialogue suggests an equally diverse set of roles that trees play for the Pennsylvania Dutch and their European predecessors: as sentient protectors, as dwelling places for spirits, or as receptive vessels for sequestering and neutralizing illness.

On the other hand, some ritual procedures imply that certain plants can be spiritually dangerous, but still capable of providing profound healing properties. Such is the case for European rituals surrounding the legendary mandrake (*Mandragora officinarum*) used for ritual purposes in the ancient world. Having a bifurcated root that appears like the form of a human's arms and legs, with two types of fruits distinguishing it as either male or female, the mandrake is believed to be a particularly powerful stand-in for a human being and is associated with love and fertility rituals, as indicated in the Vulgate translation of the Book of Genesis and Song of Solomon.

According to ancient sources, the mandrake will let out a powerful shriek when harvested for ritual purposes, a sound that has the power to kill or drive a human to insanity. The Jewish scholar Titus Flavius Josephus (37-100), whose works *The Jewish War,* and his 20 books of *Jewish Antiquities* were re-published by Pennsylvania Quakers Kimber & Sharpless in Philadelphia for Pennsylvania Dutch audiences in 1820, suggests a safe way to harvest the root without harm. One can tie a dog to the stem of the plant and bait the dog to pull forward and uproot the mandrake, so that the person can safely keep distance while the dog is killed by the herb.[74] The European varieties of mandrake from the family *Mandragorum* are diverse, and such rituals are adapted and applied to many similar plants in different regions including North American mandrake or mayapple (*Podophyllum peltatum*).

Although the more ornate rituals surrounding the use of mandrake are rare in Pennsylvania, the twentieth century herbalism and celebrated midwifery practices of Dora Dick Drumheller of *Hetricherschteddel*, now Mount Pleasant, Berks County, was documented at length by the botanist Walter Lewis Stevens, who verified the efficacy of some of her cures with chemical analysis at the turn of the last century.[75] Dora recommended the use of the fruit of the local variety of mayapple (*Moi-Abbel*) for expectant mothers, an unconscious parallel to its use in the ancient world in fertility rituals.[76] More interesting, however, is Dora's use of the root of the may-apple in the creation of "images" that were given to mothers suffering from post-partum, to ensure "prosperity." Dora used the Pennsylvania Dutch word *Bild-Watzel*, literally, "image root," suggesting that the root was likened to the "image" of the human form as it was in antiquity. Although very little information is given in Stevens' account of Dora's process for creating such images, such accounts are consistent with the use of the root in the Middle East for making dolls used for protection from demons and stimulation of sexual vitality.[77]

In these ancient accounts, the image of the human form is used as a distraction by proxy against demonic forces that would target the doll rather than the person. Although Dora's practice makes no mention of spiritual forces at work in the ritual, it is clear that the idea of transference of certain qualities to the image takes place. In her account, women with postpartum difficulties are politely described as "doting mothers," and the little image was intended to provide a relief from anxiety by periodically turning the mother's attention away from the new baby, and directing it towards the image as an amulet.

Such ritual dolls, which may have been widespread in use and diverse in function, are rarely documented, and even more rarely saved and preserved after their use is over. One such doll, possibly containing some form of herbal compound was discovered as a ritual deposit in an architectural void in the floor joists of an eighteenth-century log house in Lancaster County when the house was dismantled in the 1980s. Due to the complete inaccessibility of the void where the doll lay hidden, it is clear that the doll had been deliberately placed within the structure of the house at the time of its construction. It is uncertain whether the doll contained any *Bild-Watzel* or another herb in the tight spherical bundle that comprised the doll's homespun head, as opening the bundle would inevitably destroy the doll, which was miraculously intact after two centuries. Another such rag doll was found concealed in the return flue of an early *Kacheloffe* (tile stove) of the Friedrich Antes House in Montgomery County. The individuals that discovered the doll have avoided the possibility of a ritual interpretation, suggesting instead an elaborate and imaginative narrative of a child having "lost" the doll in the flue while playing.[78] For this reason, no attempts have been made to examine whether the doll contained any botanical substances beyond the tow stuffing that spilled from the head, or if there are any other indicators of ritual activity. Such enigmatic discoveries of ritual dolls, combined with Dora's use of the Pennsylvania Dutch word *Bild-Watzel*, suggest the possibility that evidence of a broader and more nuanced tradition may still exist in historic structures throughout the region.

What is interesting from Stevens' account of Dora Dick Drumheller is that although this notion of the doll is clearly an operation of sympathy in powwowing, Stevens, as a botanical chemist, seems to place the practice idea under the category of home-remedies rather than anything to do with ritual traditions or powwowing. Only later does he identify her somewhat indirectly as a powwower by suggesting that "necromancy" was not outside of the realm of services she rendered in her community. He relates two stories of Dora's activities not related to healing, but as functions of interpersonal ritual manipulation. In one instance, when a poorly organized, visiting country band played in her neighborhood, she ritually chewed a lemon to distract and intimidate the players into flubbing their performance so that they would not return. Another story involves her helping a young man to ritually retaliate against a young suitor who wanted to court his sweetheart. Dora instructed him to sprinkle saltpeter on the steps of his sweetheart's steps the night that the suitor appeared for courting. Allegedly the young man witnessed the humiliation of his rival later in the evening, when he slipped and fell on the way out the door. The rival became angry when the young woman laughed at his clumsiness, and subsequently he was never asked to return for another evening of courting. The rival, however, learned of the trick, and knowing that he was defeated in his pursuits of the young woman, sought revenge instead on Dora. He stole her prized egg-layers when they wandered from her chicken coop. Her remedy was to place sassafras roots in the coop to keep the hens from roving.

Narrative accounts from powwowers like Dora Dick Drumheller help to illustrate the broad range of interactions that have taken place over the centuries in Pennsylvania Dutch communities centering on the use of subtle qualities of herbs in healing, protective, and ancillary measures. As a highly significant part of everyday experience, the world of plants is yet another way that ritual can be seen as an integrative force in daily life, and that for every concern, need, or infirmity, a remedy could be derived from materials and botanicals that were immediately available and accessible to all. The role of the powwower in these situations is to serve as the community's repository for such culturally significant knowledge of the subtle relation of the spiritual and natural realms of life, and to provide access to possible solutions to life's difficulties.

An eighteenth-century ritual doll, no more than 4" in height, constructed of homespun linen dyed with calico from a Lancaster County log home. This doll was discovered intact in a structural void, where it was placed at the time of the building's construction. *Courtesy of Clarke Hess.*

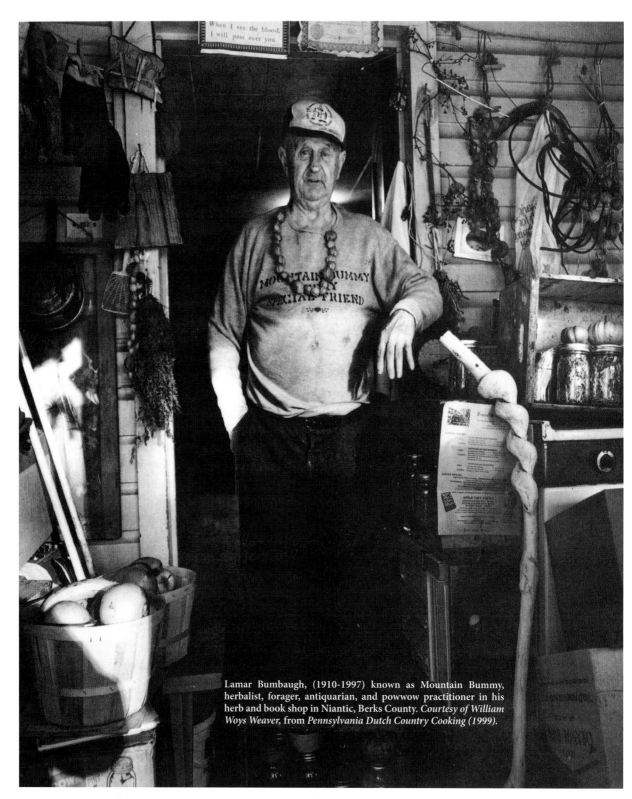

Lamar Bumbaugh, (1910-1997) known as Mountain Bummy, herbalist, forager, antiquarian, and powwow practitioner in his herb and book shop in Niantic, Berks County. *Courtesy of William Woys Weaver,* from *Pennsylvania Dutch Country Cooking (1999).*

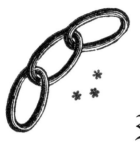
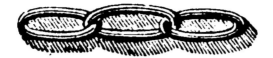

Chapter VIII
Ritual Objects of Power
Canes, Knives, Stones, Carvings

As a spiritual expression, powwowing can be a deeply personal practice, allowing room for the tailoring of ritual elements to one's individual tastes and aesthetics. This level of personal preference applies not only to the manner in which one employs ritual prayers and gestures, but also to the choice of setting and the use of ancillary ritual objects. These objects generally fall into two categories – mundane objects with a limited temporary role in ritual performance, and personalized objects of power created or adapted for a permanent role in ritual practice.

In most cases, objects employed in ritual process consist of common household or agricultural items and implements such as a piece of string, a dishcloth, a frying pan, a coal shovel, a dung fork, or a broom, which are all returned to their normal place in everyday life after their role in a ritual is finished. Some ritual elements are also perishable like eggs, potatoes, or a rind of bacon, and thus are limited to one-time use. For mundane objects, ritual power is symbolic and reflective of an object's role in daily life. A mundane object's virtues are the subtle result of repeated use in day to day circumstances.

On one hand, this relationship between ritual and the mundane can appear to normalize the power of ritual objects and diminish their apparent power; however, it is equally true that this mixing can serve to further describe the interrelationship of life and ritual – not as separate aspects of existence, but as intimately entwined facets of daily experience.

In contrast, the deliberate creation of specialized, ritual objects of power are a rarity in Pennsylvania Dutch practices. Such objects of power are either created or adapted for exclusive use in powwowing, and do not typically revert back to use in mundane affairs. Unlike everyday objects used in powwowing, ritual objects of power maintain their significance long after the performance of a particular ritual, and are used repeatedly for a specialized purpose, as part of a series of ritual events. These objects can be compared to consecrated items and substances used in traditional liturgical functions. They carry with them a sense of immanent sacredness and ritual power that is separate from life. The most common object used in this manner is the Bible, but a wide variety of other objects have also been used, created, or adapted for ritual purposes throughout the generations.

Examples of created ritual objects are canes, staves, or rods; carvings (either flat or dimensional in wood or stone); or worked iron. Other objects permanently adapted for ritual use are natural or found objects like stones, bones, or shells, but some adapted objects include those imbued with religious significance after many years of repeated use such as basins, cups, or chairs.

For some practitioners, especially those leaning in the direction of professional practice, personalized objects play an important role in shaping ritual procedures. Such objects are guarded as deeply personal and may be kept secret or stored in a special location as part of their ritual function. Because of this level of discretion, if objects become separated from their users, or if a practitioner dies without disclosing an item's provenance or purpose, the specifics of the object's use are often difficult to determine. Such objects are regarded as suspicious or enigmatic, and as a result they rarely survive. Local narratives indicate that families out of concern for their reputation often burn ritual objects, books, and papers when a healer dies – or occasionally, such burnings are, at the request of the practitioner. Other times, these objects of power are passed on to new generations of powwowers, or families maintain them as heirlooms.

Objects of power serve a fundamentally different purpose from items created for a specific, single healing event such as written blessings or materials used as amulets or talismans. Although these articles of healing or blessing are understood to be powerfully transformative to a sick or vulnerable person, objects of power are intended to create a temporary change in the state of being in both the patient and practitioner, bringing both people out of the realm of the ordinary and into a designated ritual space. To a patient, such objects can be visually impressive or conspicuous and are often incorporated into a ritual in a manner that reinforces the specialized role of the practitioner as an effective healer. At the same time, such objects of power are empowering for the practitioner as a means to focus the attention and serve as a symbol or extension of the practitioner's will.

Powwow Canes

As a common personal item, walking sticks and canes are nothing unusual to have in the home, especially among the aged or those with difficulty walking. Although in the present day, most canes used for assistance with walking conform to standards of the medical industry, this is not always the case, and many people of both genders use personalized canes in everyday life.

In the late nineteenth century, canes were also regarded as part of necessary formal wear among men, and many canes were tailored to a person's tastes. Although fashionable canes embellished with valuable materials like ivory handles or silver hardware were more common in urban or upper-class homes, such items were also not out of place in rural communities. A cane could communicate many things about a person's place in society, and frequently canes were embellished with symbolic content, especially among those who served in the military or were part of fraternal organizations such as the Freemasons or the Oddfellows. It is also not uncommon to find canes composed of exotic or unusual woods with unique features used by those who rely on them for mobility.

Canes known to have been used by powwowers share many common characteristics with personalized canes of the usual variety – the difference lies in how they are used, and scant documentation exists to fully describe their specific ritual functions for particular individuals. As with many aspects of ritual practice, these specifics are things that most practitioners would never write down, but instead are preserved in local narratives that leave much to the imagination.

One particular powwower and maker of canes was Lamar Bumbaugh (1910-1997) or "Mountain Bummy," a Berks County herbalist who harvested wild herbs for medicine and ritual purposes.[1] Bummy ran a unique antiquarian bookstore and herb shop once located in Lyon Station, just outside of Kutztown in Berks County, and later in Niantic on the border of Berks and Montgomery counties. Dr. Don Yoder purchased many rare and unusual powwow items from Mountain Bummy over the years, as Bummy, a powwower himself, was able to obtain such items because of his well-established connections with traditional practitioners in the area.

One item of interest was a late nineteenth-century cane carried and formerly used by a deceased powwower from Montgomery County, whose identity was known by Bummy but never shared with anyone else. Composed of an unknown species of wood, the cane appeared, for all intents and purposes, to be a normal cane – except that evidence showed that there were two places on the cane that once had three rings of brass, and each ring was held in place with three thin brads. As with many ritual objects, it remains unanswered if these were decorative embellishments or symbolic elements. In addition, the handle of the cane was naturally formed at a right angle, indicating that the plant from which the cane was fashioned grew out of the side of a hill or embankment. This right angle allowed the cane to be easily gripped loosely in the hand with the long shaft of the cane parallel to the ground, in a similar manner to one particular style of dowsing rod that is intended to sweep left and right to direct the user to the location of things that cannot be seen with the eye.

As with many ritual objects, this particular cane could easily have been discarded following the death of the original owner had Bummy not saved it. Nevertheless, the narrative that accompanied the object is lost to the sands of time. Interestingly enough, Bummy may have saved the cane because he was a maker of canes himself, although his work was totally unlike the nineteenth-century artifact. Bummy's canes were naturally formed, and he selected specially shaped saplings for the creation of his signature spiraled canes.

When young shoots of sassafras become entwined with the creeping honeysuckle vine the shoots' growth is constricted, and the result is a spiraled growth formation that is visually distinct and prized for making canes. Mountain Bummy was not alone in making these canes, as many traditional wood carvers such as Clarence L Griesemer (1913-1979) of Spies Church, Berks County, also harvested sassafras for the same purpose.[2] I have known many people possessing such canes across Pennsylvania, as this particular growth phenomenon is widespread. However, a number of documented canes suggest that this growth pattern was believed to possess particular qualities favorable for powwowing. One such naturally formed, spiral cane used by a powwower in southeastern Pennsylvania was preserved by Henry Chapman Mercer at the turn of the twentieth century, along with other more elaborately carved examples that link the spiral growth pattern to symbolic images of serpents[3] – universal symbols of healing in the ancient world.

Two of Mercer's serpent-canes were associated with powwowing practices in Pennsylvania, with spiraled snakes carved along the length of the canes. One cane in particular in the Mercer collection features three ascending snakes, and according to Mercer's notes, it was used in rituals for helping butter to properly churn – a reference to the notion of "stolen milk," ubiquitous in early rural Pennsylvania. The cane features snakes that ascend in a manner that bears much resemblance to the Rod of Asklepios – an ancient Greek symbol of medicine. The temples dedicated to the god Asklepios kept non-poisonous snakes that would slither over the sleeping bodies of the sick who visited the temples for healing.[4] The Rod of Asklepios is echoed in the Bible, when Moses is instructed by God to make a fiery serpent and place it upon a standard in the desert, so that anyone who looked upon it would be healed of the bites of vipers.[5]

Another cane in the Mercer Collection, purchased from Claude W. Unger of Pottsville, Schuylkill County, featuring two carved pairs of opposing snakes was used by a male powwower identified as a "hex-doctor" from Hamburg, Berks County sometime around the turn of the twentieth century. The cane is painted a reddish-brown, and one pair of snakes is green, and the other pair is black. A wooden knob handle at the top was heavily worn from use. The two pairs of facing, spiraling snakes are suggestive of the ancient Greek herald's staff known as the caduceus of Hermes, the messenger God associated with commerce and communication, and later with alchemy and esoteric practice.[6]

Left: A powwower's cane formerly owned by Mountain Bummy, used as a wand for healing and divination, Montgomery County. *Heilman Collection.*

Middle: A cane wrapped with four carved serpents, used by a powwower from Hamburg, Berks County. *Courtesy of the Mercer Museum, Doylestown, Pennsylvania.*

Right: A naturally formed spiral cane from vine, used as a powwow cane in Berks County. *Courtesy of the Mercer Museum, Doylestown, Pennsylvania.*

At least two other serpent canes were once owned by Unger who attributed them to Schuylkill County powwowers, one with a single spiraled rattle-snake ascending the cane, and another more elaborate cane with twin speckled serpents spiraling along its length, and myrtle leaves as embellishments at the upper handle of the cane. Both canes were depicted in illustrations and a photograph in the Allentown *Morning Call* in 1931, along with a compilation of legendary accounts of the life and activities of the original owner of the more ornate cane, Paul Heym (1715-1808) of Brunswick Township, Schuylkill County. The cane was passed down through direct descendants of Heym, who described his use of the cane in "drawing mystical figures on the ground of floor of buildings in the practice of his art."[7]

According to a highly romanticized narrative recorded by the Honorable Judge D. C. Henning of Schuylkill County,[8] Paul Heym emigrated to Pennsylvania and settled on the banks of the Schuylkill River near Fort Lebanon (later called Fort William), located directly between Deer Lake and Auburn. Heym lived there in 1755 during the period of intense conflict of the French and Indian War, but was never harmed, nor was his property attacked. Allegedly, this was because Heym was renowned for possessing supernatural powers of divination and shape shifting such that the Indians feared him. He used the cane in his ritual practice and never left home without it.

Judge Henning described a ritual performed by Heym that provided protection to him and his family, as well as his premises each time that he left his home:

He would write the words of the Holy Trinity on a square piece of paper about two inches square, thus:

Im Namen Gottes Geh Ich aus;
Der Vater wahr mir dieses Haus;
Der Sohn mit seiner Lieb dabei
Das Haus bewahr in alter true;
Und Heil'ger Geist, lass night heran,
Ein' Sach dass dies Haus Schaden Kann.

Henning provided a "free and liberal translation of the words:

> In God's name I do now go out;
> The Father shield this House about;
> The Son with all his love thereto,
> Defend the House with grace renewed;
> And Holy Spirit keep Thou alarm,
> Whatever might this house do harm."

Heym would hold the paper in his hand, and beginning at his entrance door, process clockwise three times around his house. With each round, he would recite a couplet from the prayer in succession. Finally, facing the front door, Heym would fold the paper into a triangle, repeat the fold three times, and place the paper into the left pocket of his trousers. Having completed this ritual, he would leave the house unlocked, and travel on his white mare, unafraid of harm. Henning described that no human or animal could approach the house within a radius of 100 feet without being "transfixed" to the ground, unable to move until Heym returned, at which time he was able to dispatch his enemies.[9]

Although Henning's lyrical account of Heym's narrative is characteristic of many turn-of-the-century romanticized retellings of legendary events from the colonial period, the story highlights the presence of highly developed ritual activities among the first generation of German-speaking immigrants in the region. This story also appears to suggest that the use of serpent canes is not unique to the United States, but was already an established part of the ritual traditions brought with the earliest immigrants to Pennsylvania.

Although Unger boldly asserts that Heym's ritual use of a serpent cane is modeled after the biblical rod of Aaron, there are no accounts of Heym having attributed this symbolism to his cane, and Henning makes no mention of the idea.[10] In the Bible, Aaron's staff was involved in two miraculous events in Exodus and Numbers. The incident in Exodus is directly related to the symbol of the serpent where Aaron is asked by God to cast his staff upon the floor in Pharoah's court, and it turns into a snake. Pharoah's court magicians do the same, but Aaron's serpent is larger and swallows the magicians' snakes, foreshadowing the seven plagues that would be visited upon Egypt.[11] The second miracle of Aaron's rod is that it miraculously sprouts, blossoms, and gives forth ripe almonds as a symbol of the priesthood of the tribe of Levi.[12]

Unger likewise applies the same symbolism to the Hamburg powwow cane in the Mercer collection. Unlike the almond-wood rod of Aaron, the practitioner and original owner of the Hamburg powwow cane indicated that it was carved from hazelwood, and had to be so in order to be effective for use.[13] Although no detailed documentation exists to describe how this cane was used in the healing process, the species of wood offers some possibilities for comparison with documented rituals in Pennsylvania Dutch literature. According to the works attributed to St. Albert the Great, hazel is a tree prized for creating divining rods,[14] and is a central feature in ritual practices involving divination and anti-witchcraft measures.

One ritual that highlights the role of the snake and hazelwood as symbols of wisdom involves locating a white adder accompanied by twelve young underneath a hazelnut tree, and consuming it with food in order "to see and discern all secret and otherwise hidden things."[15]

This role of hazel wood as a means to secure, understand, or affect things vicariously may undergird the Hamburg powwower's advice regarding the use of hazel for efficacy. As a "hex-doctor," his role would have been to intervene on behalf of those suffering from perceived curses or attacks from witches, and, possibly, to punish the witch by returning the curse.

Three entries attributed to St. Albert the Great suggest the use of a hazel rod to punish a witch,[16] and describe in detail how one is to harvest and bless such a rod:

> Observe when the moon is new on a Tuesday before sunrise, or on a Golden Sunday (Easter) or Good Friday, go to a hazelnut bush before sunrise, which you have selected in advance. Stand before the rod toward the rising of the sun, take hold of it with both hands in God's name, and speak: Rod, I grasp thee, in the name of God the Father, the Son, and the Holy Spirit, that thou shalt be obedient unto me, that I may surely hit him whom I intend to thrash." Then take your knife, and cut the rod in three cuts in the three highest names, and carry it home without speaking, and guard it well, so that no one steals it.

Two examples of ritual canes from Schuylkill County, attributed to Claude W. Unger of Pottsville. *Allentown Morning Call, all rights reserved.*

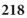

The instructions continue that if you wish to strike the person who laid the curse, call them by name, and walk around the afflicted person or animal backwards three times. Then take a hat or a jacket laid upon the threshold or a mole-hill,[17] and beat the hat or jacket as though you were beating the person.[18] The notion is that the blows of the hazelwood rod will reach the person vicariously, and they will receive the strikes, even if they are at a great distance.

Although it is uncertain whether the hazelwood cane from the Hamburg hex doctor was used in a similar manner, it is interesting to note that one of the entries in *Egyptian Secrets* employs hazelwood for vicariously thrashing a witch as a means to restore milk that has been stolen. By thrashing the milk in the churn, comparable to the documented purpose of the other powwow serpent cane in the Mercer Collection, as "causing butter to churn.[19]

Typically, the recommendations for creating such implements of punishment were not as heavy as a cane, but were switches, often indicated in various sources as being either just one or three year's growth.[20] One method for harvesting these young rods recommended using a "sympathetic weapon" to slice through the rod with three strokes. This would seem to indicate that, in some cases, one ritual object was used to beget another – a ritual switch was cut by means of a ritual knife.

The Ritual Knife

Among the rarest of all accounts of ritual implements used in powwowing practices in Pennsylvania are stories of the ritual knife. These knives were marked with three or nine crosses, and were used only in a ritual context, and not as tools for utilitarian purposes. These knives are mentioned briefly in a number of European sources,[21] indicating that, like the serpent-cane, the tradition arrived in North America with some of the earliest immigrants.

The 1775 private manuscript of Johann Georg Henninger (1737-1815), an Alsatian immigrant who settled in Albany Township, Berks County, describes a process for creating a knife marked with nine crosses in the time of the new moon, and an accompanying prayer to be used in conjunction with the knife for protection from enemies. This ritual is a survival of a well-documented process in the Tyrolean Alps, where folding pocket knives marked with nine moons and nine crosses were created between the seventeenth and nineteenth centuries in conjunction with the dialect phrases, "*Neun Stearn mit neun Mun Greifen alle Teufel un*" (Nine stars and nine moons assail all devils), and "*Neun Kreuz und Neun Mon Gwiagg alles Hexenwerk*" (Nine crosses and nine moons destroy all witchcraft).[22] Sometimes called Trudenmesser, such knives were kept on the bedstead, or driven into a doorframe to keep away demons that were believed to prey upon people in their sleep.[23]

Henninger's process for creating and using such a knife is specific:

Laß ein Messer machen mit 9. + im Neuen Mond, Trags beÿ dir, Wann dich einer mit einer Degen Stechen, oder erschiessen will, so sprich diese Wort, über die Waffen oder Büchs, Ich beschwöre dich, durch die allerheiligste Dreÿfaltigkeit, über sich ich dich, in der Mitten durch sich ich dich, und unter sich helff mir überwinden unser Herr Jesus Christ. Amen.

Let a knife to be made with 9 crosses in the new moon, carry it with you, when one with a sword wants to pierce you, or shoot you, thus speak these words over the weapon or gun, "I adjure thee, through the All-Holy Trinity, over thee, in the middle through thee, and under thee, help me to prevail, Our Lord Jesus Christ, Amen.[24]

The accompanying prayer invokes the Holy Trinity "above…middle…under" – verbally implying the equation of 3 x 3 = 9, although it is uncertain whether the knife itself is used to make the sign of the cross three times in each position.

A variation of this ritual was described in 1969 by Gerald Landis, whose family from Bechtelsville, Berks County, possessed a *Dreikreitzer Messer* (Three Cross Knife) handed down to him from his great-grandfather.[25] The process outlined by Landis for creating such a knife is extremely specific, citing that the iron was to be obtained honestly, but without paying for it, and without saying what it was for. The iron must be forged between midnight and one o'clock on New Year's night at a crossroads, with only three strokes of the hammer per year, over the course of three years. The ritual required two people to perform: one to forge the iron, and one to walk clockwise in a circle reciting the *Vater Unser* (Lord's Prayer) to repel the evil spirits which would inevitably be drawn to the process with the intention of preventing the knife's completion. According to his retelling of his great-grandfather's account, the pair were beset each year by "*feirdliche geschpenster, brillende leewe, und wiescht gashtige gediere, un der deiwel selwer*" - Ferocious apparitions, bellowing lions, and ugly horrid animals, and the devil himself.

The Three Cross Knife (*Dreikreitzer Messer*) of Gerald Landis of Bechtelsville. Present whereabouts unknown.

Gerald Landis' maternal grandfather, John Hoffman (1847-1917), was a farmer from Huffs Church, Berks County, but also a blacksmith, carpenter, blood-letter, and powwower on the side. Hoffman created the Three Cross Knife sometime in the late nineteenth century at the crossroads called Five Points, just above Fredericksville, where Five Points Road, Fredericksville Road, and a farm lane all intersect.[26]

The knife was used by the family primarily for anti-witchcraft measures such as placing the knife under one's pillow for relieving disturbed sleep, and under the butter-churn to ensure that the thickening of the butter would not be hindered by witchcraft. The knife was also handled by members of the family when an evil influence was perceived. Although the accounts of Henninger and Landis corroborate the continuation of European ritual process in Pennsylvania, documentation of this particular process is isolated and rare.

The use of the Three Cross Knife is well documented in Europe however, with a number of very specific uses that suggest several avenues of symbolic interpretation. In Swabia it was used for stopping blood from a wound, implying that a blessed knife can heal the harm done by another knife – suggesting the ancient notion that like cures like, or *similia similibus curantur*.[27] In Northern and Eastern Germany, a Three Cross Knife is thrust into the overhead beam in the stove-room (*Stube*) and left in situ to protect the house[28] – again, possibly echoing the idea that similar things take care of each other, so that a knife protects from violence, even when it is not used as an actual weapon. Likewise, in the Pfalz, the Three Cross Knife is simply placed underneath a butter churn when the milk will not yield butter.[29]

Unlike other methods used to punish a perceived supernatural butter thief where a knife, or a scythe is jabbed into the butter[30] – the Three Cross Knife is rarely used to actually cut anything physical. This also lends insight into the Hessian tradition of having a bride and groom step over a Three Cross Knife, perhaps in keeping with the medieval doctrine that witches create *ligaturae* or bindings to curse a marriage and cause impotence.[31] Thus the knife becomes a means to cut invisible fetters or obstructions.

Another early Pennsylvania manuscript from around 1810 by the hand of John Rohrer of Lebanon County describes the use of a three cross knife for divination and healing of consumption:

Vor die auszehrung zu curieren

Mache ein Messer darauf mache 3 Creutz darnach neme eine Brot Gruste so Groß daß du dieses Messer drein stecken kanst stecke das Messer in die Brot Gruste und wan du schlaffen gehest so lege die Brot Gruste daran das Messer gestecket ist under deinen Kobf mit der Grust Seite [x] gegen[x] von dem Kobf darnach das Morgens ziehe das Messer auf dem Brod wische es saubar an der Brot Gruste ab Darnach geb die Brot Gruste einem schwartzen hunt im namen x x x so wirst du gesunt werten ist das Messer rostig wan du es aus der Brot Grusten ziehest so ist es die Auszehrung ist es aber hell so ist es die Auszehring nicht.

To cure consumption

Make a knife with 3 crosses on it, and take a crust of bread big enough that you can stick the knife into it entirely. When you go to bed, place the crust with the knife in it underneath your head, with the crust side down, and in the morning pull out knife and wipe it clean on the bread, and feed the bread to a black dog in the name [of the Father, Son, and Holy Spirit] +++ thus will you be made healthy. If the knife is rusty when you pull it from the bread, the illness is certain to be consumption, and if it is bright, it isn't consumption.[32]

A similar set of instructions attributed to St. Albert the Great suggests the following procedure to cure a cursed child, prior to applying a plaster made of almond oil, deer tallow, rose-infused vinegar, and caraway seed:

Before applying the plaster, the mother, after eating supper, must take her knife and cut three thin pieces of bread with it. The knife must be thrust into the three pieces of bread, and placed under the child's back [in the cradle] during the night. If the child is cursed, the knife will be completely rusted the following morning. Then take the bread from the knife, spread butter on it, and feed it to a black dog. One must put an old shirt on the child, and after three days and three nights take it off, and bury it with the plaster before sunrise under an elderberry bush without speaking to anyone.[33]

In both cases, whether for curing the infant or the person suffering from consumption, the idea is that the knife is a symbolic collector of the illness, likening the curse or consumption of the body to the deterioration of the metal. The knife, which is polished smooth once again can be likened to the ideal, healed person, and the rust is transferred to the black dog, an entity widely identified in European and American folklore with the devil,[34] suggesting the return of an illness to its source.

This use of a knife to cut bread as a symbol for healing transformation is also featured in the ubiquitous powwow prayer used to cure inflammation from the topical infection erysipelas, recorded in *Egyptian Secrets* of Albertus Magnus:

Ich ging durch einen rothen Wald, und in dem rothen Wald da war eine rote Kirch, und in der rothen Kirch da war ein rother Altar, und auf dem rothen Altar da lag ein rothes Messer, nimm das rothe Messer und schneide rothes Brod. + + +

I went through a red wood, and in the red wood there was a red church, and in the red church there was a red altar, and on the red altar there lay a red knife, take the red knife and cut red bread. + + +[35]

Just as in other powwow prayers featuring poetic expressions of biblical and divine metaphors, this prayer describes a supernal reality and a progression into the innermost reaches of the human soul. With these words the healer descends into a symbolic wilderness to approach the patient's spiritual body or temple[36] in order to retrieve a transcendent instrument of healing from the altar at the inner sanctum of the Spirit. The color red is not only the color of the heart, but of the Holy Spirit's manifestation in fire.[37] It is unlikely that an actual red knife is being suggested as a means to affect a cure, as the knife is every bit as much a part of the progression of spiritual elements as is the wilderness, which is a non-literal, symbolic space.

Although the "bread" at the "altar" may at first appear to suggest the Holy Eucharist,[38] it is important to remember that the Body of Christ is typically broken, not sliced with a knife.[39] One possibility is that, while the temple corresponds to the spiritual body, the bread represents the patient's physical body undergoing a form of ritual surgery and the red knife is an allusion to sacrifice and renewal. Another possibility is that the bread represents the vector of the illness, since rye contaminated with ergot was responsible for St. Anthony's Fire or the infection caused by ergot poisoning, and the German word *Rothlaufe*[40] applies equally to both Erysipelas and ergotism.

It is also possible that this reference to bread relates to a common folk medical cure for erysipelas involving the use of bread as a poultice or compress, which was applied to the infected lesions as a carrier for other medicinal compounds.[41] It is entirely possible that this method occasionally proved effective because the procedure introduced yeast to compete with the streptococcus bacteria present in erysipelas. This notion is echoed in several other entries in St. Albert the Great, where a written blessing,[42] a scrap of red fabric,[43] or clary sage[44] is administered to an animal suffering from erysipelas by means of a piece of bread:

> To cure erysipelas in cattle:
>
> Write the following upon a piece of paper as follows, and feed it to the cattle: Three maidens went over the land. They carry a piece of bread in hand. The one said: we want to divide and cut it; the third said: we want to heal N. N.'s cow of erysipelas. † † † It must be spoken three times, written upon a piece of paper, and given to the cow in a piece of bread.[45]

What is notable in this variation of the "Three Maidens Prayer" is that again the three women are cutting the bread, and not breaking it, although no knife is explicitly mentioned.

Bread used in healing rituals occasionally involves cutting the sign of the cross three times in succession on the top of the dough with a knife before baking it.[46] This may have proceeded from the baking of bread on the Feast of Epiphany marked with Three Crosses,[47] an extension of the liturgical blessing of chalk on Epiphany used to mark homes and barns with three crosses and the initials of the three magi, Caspar, Melchior, and Balthasar, or C+M+B+.

It is likely that the Three Kings Crosses[48] are related to the practice of marking a knife with three crosses for ritual purposes. The creation of the knife on New Year's Eve in Landis' Berks County narrative is telling, as New Year's Day is directly between Christmas and Epiphany, one of many symbolic intersections featured in the creation of the Three Cross Knife.

It is also likely that this rare use of a consecrated, ritual object within powwowing tradition is at least partially informed by European practices in ceremonial magic such as those described in the classic grimoire, *The Key of Solomon*.[49] Two knives, one with a black handle and one with a white handle are consecrated, each in a very specific manner. The white knife is heated three times in the hour of Mercury, when Mars is in the sign of Aries or Scorpio, and the steel is quenched in the blood of a gosling and the juice of a pimpernel. The black knife is heated in the hour of Saturn and quenched in the blood of a black cat, and the juice of poison hemlock. The white knife is to be inscribed with one of many sacred Hebrew names of God, AGLA, an abbreviation for the phrase *Ateh Gibor Leolam Adonai* (Mighty art thou forever, Lord). Such knives occasionally turn up in a simplified form, having been adapted for use in ritual practices on the folk-cultural level. One marked with ALGA and three crosses from the sixteenth-century was documented by Ralph Merrifield in the British Isles as an architectural ritual deposit in the walls of a house to protect from witchcraft.[50]

Although some of these procedures may appear exotic for Pennsylvania's particular brand of ritual traditions, Johann Georg Hohman describes a process for empowering knives with ritual inscriptions in his classic powwow manual, *The Long Lost Friend*, borrowed from the *Romanus Büchlein*:

> Another still more certain way to stop Bleeding:
>
> If the bleeding will not stop or if a vein has been cut, then lay the following on it, and it will stop that hour. Yet if any one does not believe this, let him write the letters upon a knife and stab an irrational animal, and he will not be able to draw blood. And whosoever carries this about him, will be safe against all his enemies:

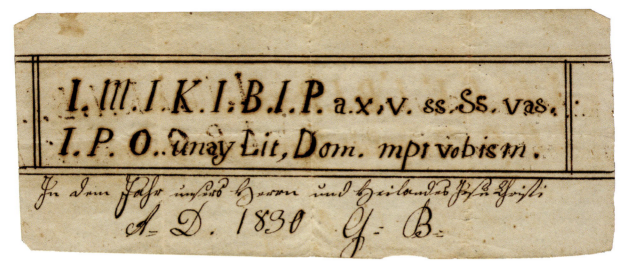

Cryptic abbreviations associated with protection from enemies and the stopping of blood from wounds, written and signed by Georg Börstler, Exeter Township, Berks County 1830. Börstler lived only just a few miles from Johann Georg Hohman's residence in Rosedale near Reading, and the inscription as likely copied from an original edition of *The Long Lost Friend. Heilman Collection.*

I. m. I. K. I. B. I. P. a. x. v. ss. Ss. vas I. P. O. unay Lit. Dom. mper vobism.

And whenever a woman is going to give birth to a child, or is otherwise afflicted, let her have this letter about her person; it will certainly be of avail.[51]

In this case, the use of the knife is framed within a procedure to test the efficacy of the inscription for stopping blood and is unlikely to have been actually used. The inscription itself was once popular in both Europe and the United States as a protective blessing. Soldiers in Europe carried the inscription into battle,[52] and numerous Pennsylvania copies have survived to the present day. This inscription however, was even more ephemeral when used to empower a knife, as it is written on the blade temporarily, and not forged permanently. No known knifes with such an inscription have survived to attest to the use of this method in stopping blood.

There is another inscription widely distributed in Pennsylvania for empowering a sickle or shovel used to ritually cure a cow whose milk has been stolen by supernatural means. Consisting of a jumbled series of moons, crosses, numbers and letters, the inscription was to be written on the blades of three common sickles or three shovels, and they were to be heated red hot and quenched in milk. This typographical version of the inscription, appears to be a corruption of the aforementioned Tyrolean nine crosses and nine moons theme. The printer probably reproduced the inscription by approximating it with available type, which may have only loosely resembled an original handwritten example or a printed plate from another edition.[53] There are three moons, five instances of the letter "c" and one "9" – nine in total, and all of which have a crescent shape. There are only 2 crosses, four cases of the lowercase letter "t" and one inverted "y" - a total that is 3 short of nine approximated crosses. In addition, there are "m" and "B" letters, indicating that the inscription may have included the initials of the Three Kings, CMB.

In contrast to an actual everyday knife or sickle in such procedures, if Gerald Landis' account is to be taken as the norm in Pennsylvania, the Three Cross Knife is not even sharpened. Furthermore, the most significant difference perhaps is that such a knife is not forged of tempered steel like those described in *The Key of*

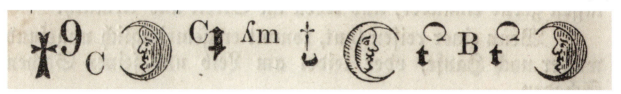

Characters to be written on a sickel or shovel used to ritually cure a cow whose milk has been stolen by supernatural means, from the *Egyptian Secrets of Albertus Magnus,* printed by Harlacher & Weiser, Allentown, 1869. *Heilman Collection.*

Solomon, but is fashioned of simple wrought iron. The relative softness of iron as opposed to steel reinforces the notion that the Three Cross Knife is not typically used to cut physical things, but to create and sever boundaries of a spiritual nature.

The iron composition of the knife is highly significant, as a substance associated with fire, purification, and protection.[54] In Pennsylvania, the act of heating and forging in fire is associated with neutralizing evil, giving blacksmiths and the objects they create special significance in powwowing. This is further substantiated by magnetism, suggesting that iron both "attracts" and neutralizes negative forces.

Iron objects such as horseshoes, nails, chains, and votive figures have been used historically in both Europe and the United States to protect buildings, bless livestock, and promote health and healing. In some rare circumstances, iron objects associated with blessing are stamped with symbols much like the Three Cross Knife such as the strap hinges used throughout the 1753 Jacob Keim Homestead of Pike Township, Berks County, where three crosses are stamped on each hinge. More commonly, iron objects associated with ritual practices are subtle, like the use of the horseshoe.

The Iron Horseshoe

The horseshoe is universal in the western world for its association with good luck and protection. Among the Pennsylvania Dutch, the horseshoe with the prongs facing downward above the barn door is a symbol of protection in keeping with Central European use.[55] The opposite is true in Anglo-American tradition, and when the horseshow points upward like a chalice, it is a vessel to hold luck. There is much disagreement about these two cultural perspectives, as those who believe the latter, generally question the Pennsylvania Dutch method of positioning the shoe, citing concerns that "the luck will spill out" – a statement I heard in my childhood in Lebanon County.[56]

In some areas such as Adams County, where both English and Pennsylvania Dutch influences are found equally, early examples of horseshoes are sometimes found nailed to the doorjambs of stables sideways,[57] with the tines of the arch facing inward. This is echoed in some parts of Europe, where it is stated that horseshoes should not be placed with the arch facing outwards, lest the horse take all the luck with it when passing out of the stable.[58] This two-fold logic present in the use of the horseshoe suggests that both English and German sources are equally significant in Pennsylvania, undergirding the horseshoe's dual use as both an apotropaic and beneficent object.

Unlike many objects with permanent ritual power, the horseshoe must be found, not purchased or created. However, specific actions are sometimes ritually associated with securing its curative and beneficial properties. In Europe, as in Pennsylvania, it is considered unlucky to drive past a horseshoe without picking it up. In Europe, if one cannot pick up the horseshoe, at least walking around it three times will secure its blessing.[59] Certain days such as St. Sylvester (New Year's Eve) or the Eve of St. John the Baptist (June 24) are powerful days for finding such objects, and only second to Holy Saturday (*Karsamstag*, between Good Friday and Easter), when one can pick up items from the ground without being hindered by spirits on account of Christ's descent and harrowing of Hell, according to Christian legend.[60] A rare ritual involves throwing the horseshoe

Top: A rare, eighteenth-century Swiss iron horse votive, used to bless livestock in the barn. While actual use of votives varied, this piece was intended as a stand-in for the actual horses, and was brought to church for blessing on appropriate days. The votive would then be placed in the barn as an annual tradition. Iron votives of horses and cattle were once common in Europe, and some have speculated that such practices may have migrated to Pennsylvania, however, this has never been substantiated. *Heilman Collection.*

Bottom: A studded draft horseshoe, for winter and muddy conditions. Berks County, Pennsylvania. *Heilman Collection.*

backwards into the air to secure its positive effect, but more commonly one can simply carry it home without directly touching it with the hands, and without speaking to anyone.[61] In all cases, the shoe must be found, and not bought or taken in mundane circumstances.

A horseshoe with some or all of the nails found intact was believed to be especially effective in powwowing. Such horseshoes were not only nailed above the barn door, but were also essential to certain ritual cures and procedures. A preventative for rabies documented in Berks, Schuylkill, Lehigh, and Montgomery counties, involved cauterizing a wound from the bite of a "mad" dog with a horseshoe "*mit all de Nagel drin*" (with all the nails intact).[62] Such horseshoes endowed with nails were also placed under or within the bedding of an infant's cradle to cure or prevent *die Gichdre* (infant convulsions).[63] The typical "regulation" number of nails used in a standard horseshoe was eight.[64]

Such nails could be removed from the horseshoe and suspended on a cord around the neck of a child suffering from convulsions (eclampsia infantum) an echo of the European *Fraisketten*, a chain upon which are suspended various amulets, *Brevia* (written blessings) and saints' relics, common in Roman Catholic communities in Austria.[65] A ring made from one of the horseshoe nails would keep away rheumatism,[66] and a nail from a coffin was used in much the same way but connected instead to the notion that the dead would take away illness from the living.[67] Horseshoe nails were also fashioned into rings, and worn for protection from both illness and storms.[68]

One of the most elaborate rituals involving a horseshoe is included in certain editions of Dr. Helfenstein's *Soli Deo Gloria*, for ritually binding thieves and forcing them to return stolen property:

If something is stolen from thee, then take a horseshoe with three nails in it, make it red hot, and sprinkle salt and pepper on it, and let it cool at the spot where the stolen item was located. Lay three black chicken feathers on it, cover it with a black rag, and make three white crosses on it, and say the following words three times:

Five evil angels shall pursue thee. Thy conscience shall despair. I adjure thee in the name of the Holy Trinity: Bring back what thou hast stolen at this very time. Thou shalt burn as fire, wander as a monstrosity. The Seventh Commandment condemns thee to hell and flames of fire. I command thee by the power of Heaven, bring back what thou hast taken away. The Earth shall devour thee, if thou dost not bring it back. Restlessness shall afflict thee, Lucifer shall chase after thee, and thou shalt become lame and immobile, until thou bringest what thou hast stolen. In the name of the Twelve Holy Apostles of Jesus Christ."

And after this, take a red onion, and stick the three nails which have been made red-hot by fire into the onion, and say the following three times:

As red as this onion is, so is thy corrupted heart. In the Name of the father, I drive a glowing nail into thine heart. In the name of the Son, I drive a glowing nail into thy lungs and liver. In the name of the Holy Spirit, I drive a glowing nail into thy virility, until thou returnest what thou hast stolen, by the will of Jesus Christ and in the names of the Twelve Apostles."

When a thief returns the stolen goods, then thou canst release him by the following means and retrieve all related things, by saying the following words three times:

I release thee from thine anguish and vexation in the name of the Father, Son, and Holy Spirit, and take all heavy bonds placed upon thee, and commend them to be sunken into the deep sea in the Name of the Power of Jesus Christ of Nazareth.[69]

The materials featured in Helfenstein's ritual to compel a thief to return stolen property: A horseshoe, a red onion, three nails, salt, pepper, a black handkerchief, and three black chicken feathers.

The ritual heating and cooling of the horseshoe is both literal and symbolic, and links the process of the blacksmith's craft both literally with the purging fires of hell, aiming to torment the conscience and body of the thief. The ritual concludes with a symbolic form of quenching the fire, as the bonds placed upon the thief are sunken into the sea.

This use of the horseshoe nail as a means to inflict pain upon the thief is also known in Central Europe and comparable to another European ritual use of a horseshoe heated red-hot to ritually "mark" a witch.[70]

While some have compared the ritual use of a horseshoe to ancient Germanic pre-Christian religious veneration of the god Wodan to whom the horse was sacred, others have also suggested that the horseshoe may have been a common means of supplication to the patron saint of horses, St. Leonard. This is corroborated by the fact that horseshoes were attached to the doors of churches sacred to St. Leonard,[71] and that iron figures of horses and cattle were also offered as votives to be blessed on the saint's feast day on November 6.[72] Such iron votives were common in the eighteenth and nineteenth centuries in Roman Catholic areas of Switzerland and Austria and were placed in stables for the protection and health of the cattle. As with many other aspects of European folk culture, both Christian and pre-Christian narratives undergird the historical origins of such practices, and add important layers of meaning to practices that are often puzzling to modern audiences.

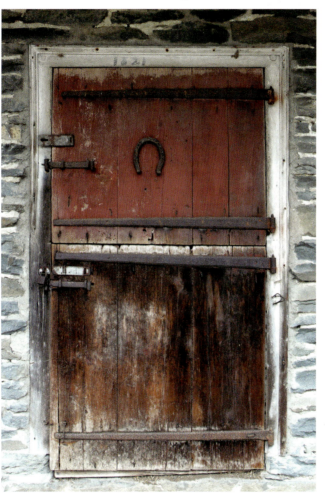

A horseshoe on the stable door of an 1826 stone Pennsylvania barn in Greenwich Township, Berks County, hung in the traditional orientation among the Pennsylvania Dutch, with the prongs down.

Ruhkschtee (The Stone of Rest)

One historic element of Pennsylvania's ritual tradition that can be directly traced to ancient European thought is the *Ruhkschtee* (the stone of rest). Since at least the beginning of the early Roman era when European farmers plowed their fields and found prehistoric pointed stone-age tools or oblong belemnite fossils, such remnants of bygone eras were regarded as highly mysterious in origin. Since the time of the Iron Age, Europeans were no longer making stone tools, and thus had little awareness of the technology of previous millennia. A once commonly accepted explanation was that these were the remnants of lightning strikes and attributed to the power of deities such as Jupiter among the Romans and Donner among the pre-Christian Germans. As evidence of sacred points of intersection – between the gods and earth – these artifacts assumed healing and protective properties, and were carried by Romans for ritual purposes,[73] and such practices continued well into the modern era. The Pennsylvania Dutch in North America continued this association with the "Stone of Rest" – believing that such stones would cure insomnia when placed under one's pillow.

Wammer sich en Ruhkschtee unnich's Koppekissli legt, kammer gut schloffe.

When one places a stone of rest under the pillow, one can sleep well.[74]

Dr. Edwin Miller Fogel of the University of Pennsylvania documented this Pennsylvania Dutch language cure for insomnia in Berks, Dauphin, Lebanon, Lancaster, Monroe, Northampton, Snyder, and York Counties in 1915. Fogel, who lacked any form of English equivalent for the *Ruhkschtee* never translated it as a stone of rest, but instead as a "small roundish stone found lying on fenceposts in the country districts. Probably an echo of the *Donarkeil*."[75]

At the turn of the twentieth century, as an American proponent of the romanticized notion of Germanic heathendom, Fogel described the stone of rest as one of many "survivals" of the veneration of the Germanic gods, and equated it with the Standard German *Donnerkeil,* (thunder-wedge), and the mythological Hammer of Thor, *mjölnir*.[76] Fogel does not explain why his narrative locates these stones on fenceposts, but presumably, being distinctively smooth and pointed, such Paleolithic relics were discovered by farmers while plowing and placed on top of fenceposts for temporary safe-keeping. It is unknown if the fencepost, marking a liminal space such as a property line, held any particular significance for this particular object, as it does in other rituals.

Folklorist Ezra Grumbine in his 1905 collection of Lebanon County folk beliefs, described a memory as a young boy, when a schoolmate showed him a "thunderstone," explaining that "it was believed that the lightening hurled stones, which, on striking, caused damage and death."[77] Grumbine's description is that of a "a smooth, roundish, flat stone" and clearly an inspiration for Fogel's later description as "roundish," except that he does not include "flat" as one of the descriptors. Grumbine's "flat" description closely matches one of two European varieties of the thunder-stone – those which were in fact Paleolithic axe-heads or strike-a-lights[78] as opposed to those which are cylindrical and pointed, and actually fossilized cranial structures of belemnites from the Jurassic age.[79]

The European *Donnerkeil* or *Donneraxt* (thunder-axe) was so-called because of the prevalence of early, wedge-shaped, Paleolithic axe-heads which were used in this manner, but the actual shape, size, and qualities that designated a thunderstone were incredibly diverse. Some thunderstones had holes in them, and were later known as a "*Lochstein*."[80] The belemnite fossil, on the other hand, comes from the Greek term for "dart," because of its conical shape. The Romans called them *ceraunia* (thunder-stone), and this became the later scientific term for the phenomenon throughout the Middle Ages and into the early modern era.[81] It is clear that despite the varieties in forms – everything from arrow-heads to fossils – Europeans likened the destructive power of lightning to weapons hurled by the gods, and later among Christians, by God himself. Such notions were seemingly confirmed by the occasional and terrifying landing of meteorites such as the Ensisheim meteorite of 1492, which landed in Alsace and captured the public imagination as an omen of the victory of King Maximilian I against the French. This event was publicized in a series of broadsheets by Sebastian Brant, whose poems about the "*Donnerstein*" were accompanied by images of a pointed stone falling from the sky towards Ensisheim.[82]

It was not until the 17th century that *ceraunia* were finally understood to be Paleolithic tools and differentiated from meteorites.[83] Even once natural scientists understood the origins of the thunderstone, the tradition of using them among the folk continued for generations, in widespread regions, including Britain, Ireland, Scandinavia, France, Germany, Holland, Portugal, Italy, and Greece. In the British Isles, where large geological deposits of Belemnites as well as Paleolithic tools have been unearthed, such objects continued to be called thunderstones, and were placed in the house to protect from lightning, as well as a wide variety of human and veterinary medical uses.[84]

Interestingly enough, despite detailed accounts of the European varieties of thunder-stones and their uses, it is rare to find mention of the stones as cures for sleep disorders in the same manner that the Pennsylvania *Ruhkschtee* is a remedy for insomnia. One such reference, in a poetic treatise on the virtues of precious stones by a 12th century Bishop of Rennes, Marbodaeus Gallus, suggests among many uses, including protection of one's person and home from lightning, safe passage at sea, success in warfare and legal matters, - *Et dulces somnos et dulcia somnia præstat* – and provides sweet sleep and pleasant dreams.[85] There are other clues, however to the possible origin of this notion in accounts of the stones being called "*Trudenstein*"[86] and "*Alpschoss*"[87] in Germany, and "Elf-Shot" in the British Isles and parts of Pennsylvania,[88] suggesting that their origin is perceived not so much to be from lightning, but instead as the creations of supernatural beings capable of using such stones to inflict illness. In order to combat such illness, the stones themselves are used or invoked as a cure, in a like-cures-like relationship.

Ruhkschtee, a "stone of rest," originally an ancient stone pestle used by Native Americans living in the region of what is today the Delaware Water Gap, Pennsylvania. *Heilman Collection.*

It should be no wonder then that in German-speaking lands, the *Trudenstein* and *Donnerstein* are used to ward off a wide variety of predatory entities identified as *Hexen* (witches), *Truden* (succubi), *Maren* (nightmares), *Alpe* (elves), and *Gschpenster* (spirits), all of which are believed to be responsible for stealing the rest from people and animals in their sleep by riding them to exhaustion. This phenomenon has been documented as a supernatural experience by many cultures, and has been described in North America as being "hag-ridden."[89] As a corollary to the "stone of rest," the use of a hagstone, or a stone with a hole in it, appears in traditions of the British Isles and Southern Appalachia as a remedy for being hag-ridden, and corresponds in form to one of the variations of the European thunderstone.[90]

The Pennsylvania Dutch tradition alternately refers to the entities responsible for stealing rest as "*Trotterkopf,*" (sometimes translated as trotter-head) or "*Bettzeierle*"[91] (see Chapter VI). It is likely to be implicit, although Fogel's informants did not specifically say so, that to "sleep well" meant to be free from supernatural harassment. Dialogue surrounding these perceptions of the supernatural origins of insomnia appears extensively in defense of Dr. Hageman's use of written blessings for children suffering from a loss of sleep in his 1903 civil suit against the *North American Newspaper* in Philadelphia (see Chapter IX). It is unlikely however, that the relation of the *Ruhkschtee* to the notion of the *Trudenstein* had any bearing on the thinking of rural Pennsylvanians.

Belief in the healing powers of the *Ruhkschtee* did not last much longer than the time that Fogel and Grumbine were collecting folklore in the early twentieth century. What is surprising, however, is that unlike the Europeans of the Middle Ages who were thousands of years removed from a time when stone tools were used, European settlers in the eastern United States had extensive contact with cultures still manufacturing stone tools, and yet the story of the *Ruhkschtee* as a thunder-bolt remained until fairly recently. Although interaction with the indigenous cultures of the Americas is cited as one of the most significant influences in the re-thinking of the mythology of the thunderstone in Europe,[92] the fact that North Americans continued to use the *Ruhkschtee* well into the twentieth century is evidence that the beliefs surrounding the "thunderstone" may have evolved into something more complex in order to withstand the test of time. Although Fogel associates the *Ruhkschtee* with the Thunderstone, this parallel may not have been uniform among the Pennsylvania Dutch, and thus the Stone of Rest may have been used independently of any idea that could have been contradicted by modern science – mainly, that such stones were dropped from the heavens. In rural Pennsylvania, where reminders of the presence of indigenous cultures are commonly turned up each year with plowing, the notion of the Stone of Rest persisted as a means to put such objects to use in a ritual context in the modern world.

Ritual Carvings

Carvings in wood, like personalized powwow canes, are well-documented, but extremely rare. Often such objects are difficult to interpret due to the level of discretion surrounding the use of the object. Some carvings for instance, play a role in the performance of a ritual which is witnessed by a client or patient while others are discrete and kept entirely private.

One particular type of rare carved object that is visible during the performance of a healing ritual is a unique, personalized plaque that is clutched or held against a Bible. One such piece was described by a Berks County resident, whose family from Albany Township, described an aunt who powwowed with a circular plaque made of wood or possibly ceramic that was held against her Bible. The plaque was carved with symbols including astrological images of a sun and moon and was small enough to fit within the parameters of the

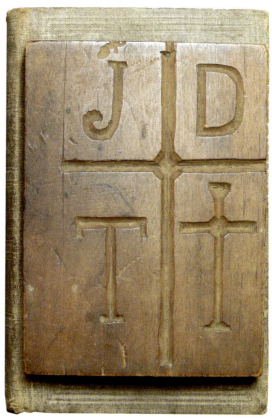

Wooden Bible-board with carved symbols, placed upon the cover of a pocket-sized New Testament, used by a powwow doctor near Emmaus, Lehigh County, and carried for protection. *Courtesy of Willard Martin. Heilman Collection.*

Bible's front cover and be held with one hand.⁹³ The plaque was destroyed following the death of the owner, whose activities were considered suspect to certain portions of her family that confused her powwowing with witchcraft.

Only one such plaque has survived to the present day from South Mountain, near Emmaus, Lehigh County, but the name of the original owner has been forgotten. The plaque measures approximately 3" x 4," and is carved into four quadrants by the form of an offset cross. In each quadrant around the cross is a carved symbol, with J D in the uppermost half, and a T and another cross in the lower portion. The offset cross leaves a blank margin along the left side of the plaque, an arrangement which echoes the use of the golden ratio throughout the geometric layout of the cross and the symbols in each quadrant. The plaque is small enough to fit on the cover of a pocket New Testament, and the blank edge on the plaque also suggests the front board of a bible, offset to accommodate the binding. This board was carried with a pocket New Testament for protection up until fairly recently by a previous owner.

Another form of plaque, in the shape of a paddle carved with symbols was owned by the antiques collector Earl F. Robacker, who presumed its alleged significance in powwowing, but was unable to substantiate his claims beyond the notion that it contained "cryptic inscriptions." The paddle was less than 1 foot long, with a circular plaque at the top, measuring approximately 5 inches in diameter. A six-pointed rosette divided the circle into equal areas, and on each of six lobes, was a symbol. The elements were both carved into the paddle, and highlighted with a coat of white paint. In each lobe of the rosette, appearing clockwise from the top was a cross, a diamond eye shape, a capital J, a W, an S, and the last lobe is divided in half, with the top portion painted white. In between each lobe was a triangle, and around the outermost edge was a border composed of triangles pointing into the center of the circle.

This paddle was associated by Robacker with a decorated wafer iron also of alleged powwow significance due to "cryptic inscriptions." The wafer iron likewise had a rosette and cross pattern, as well as unidentified writing around the edge of the circular shape. Both of these images appeared in a photograph by Robacker featured in *Pennsylvania Folklife*,⁹⁴ the journal of the Pennsylvania Folklife Society. Dr. Don Yoder, who edited the journal, told me that he was not convinced of the paddle and water iron's alleged significance for powwowing, but instead suggested that that the paddle was a butter or cheese mold, and that both items closely resembled European culinary items decorated to the particular taste of the owner.⁹⁵ Robacker had no record of the provenance of the paddle and wafer iron, as they were purchased on the antiques market and thus the items remain somewhat of a mystery. This tendency to assign meaning relating to powwowing with unusual items that turn up at public sales is inherently problematic, but unfortunately many ritual objects do get preserved by collectors, who lose sight of the narratives associated with such items.

Collector Richard S. Machmer owned a number of carved figures associated with powwowing, including three carvings associated with a "Doc Moyer" from the greater Kutztown area. These carvings were shaped from bedposts, carved into crude figures. Two of these carvings featured snakes climbing the height of the post and swallowing a human form. In the back of each figure was a plugged chamber used to insert a lock of hair or other subtle personal trimmings, much like the practice of plugging hair into a tree to remove illness. Richard Shaner discovered another carved human effigy used in this manner by a powwow doctor from Emmaus around the turn of the last century. The figure also included a hole in the back for inserting hair.⁹⁶

Richard Shaner of Kutztown also collected a story from a farmer from District Township, Berks County, explaining the possible use of such a figure. As a child the farmer had been taken to a powwow doctor in Emmaus for advice concerning a mysterious childhood illness. The powwow doctor suggested that the father of the child carve an effigy of the person responsible for placing the *Hex*, and then to hammer a nail into part of the body – any part but the heart, or the

A digital recreation of Earl F. Robacker's elaborately carved powwowing paddle, current whereabouts unknown.

person would die. The father then buried the figure under the eaves of the house to let it rot. Shortly, a woman down the road suffered an injury on the same location on the leg that the father had nailed, and the child recovered.[97]

Shaner also discovered a number of highly significant ritual objects in the 1960's at the home of his uncle Freddy H. Bieber's (1885-1978) farm at Ruppert's Eck in Rockland Township, Berks County, that related to his Aunt Annie J. (Buchert) Bieber's (1874-1960) powwowing activities. These including a small, flat, wooden board, measuring no more than a few inches, carved with three geometric shapes: a triangle, a square, and a circle.[98] Although it is unknown what the board was used for, another nearly identical board was purchased from a local book dealer known to have been associated with powwowing (probably Lamar Bumbaugh). Shaner suggested that the three shapes represented the elements earth, fire, and water.

Also among Freddie Bieber's belongings was a wooden chair marked with a Star of David in chalk under the seat. Although chairs are a common feature in many healing rituals, typically these chairs are ordinary objects that are used in ritual circumstances but hold no permanent significance. Such a chair might be a kitchen chair requisitioned for temporary use upon which a patient is to be seated.

One known exception to this rule is the "Powwow Chair," formerly used by a Manheim powwow doctor, and now in the collection of the Thomas Brendle Museum at Historic Schaefferstown. This chair was donated to the museum on the condition that the name of the powwow doctor and his family be kept secret; otherwise a curse would be visited upon the museum.[99] The story associated with the chair is that each of its features and carved embellishments was actually a codified set of symbols designed to evoke sacred concepts in both the healer and the patient who would sit on the chair throughout the ritual healing process.

Although appearing to be a normal chair in all respects, the explanation provided by the daughter of the original owner of the chair was quite detailed, elevating what might easily be seen as common decorative forms to symbols of biblical proportions.[100] The chair was painted red to symbolize the blood of Christ, and two arches in the cresting rail were to remind the patient of the Two Tablets of the Law given to Moses, upon which the Ten Commandments were inscribed. The two large vertical stiles of the chair's back were to represent the pillars of the church,[101] and the three vertical spindles were the apostle Paul, Jesus, and Peter, the Rock. The front lower stretcher was to symbolize Judas the betrayer, a rung upon which the patient should rest her right foot in disdain. The three rings on the legs were to invoke the Holy Trinity, and the low construction of the chair was to humble the patient to receive healing.

The chair itself is humble, and unassuming, begging the question: did the symbolism develop to match the chair's construction, or was the chair created to match these symbolic specifications? While the latter seems unlikely to some,[102] no details have been recorded regarding this important part of the chair's provenance. In fact, given the high level of detail present in the oral history about the chair, perhaps an even more important observation can be made: it may not have mattered whether the symbolism was adapted to the chair's features, or if the chair was symbolically constructed – what mattered most was the content of the narrative set into play by the practitioner who used the chair for acts of healing. It may well be that such questions reveal more about our modern expectations for objects imbued with ritual power, than about the nature of the chair itself. If such a seemingly ordinary piece is actually reflecting such extraordinary themes, perhaps the ritual power of the chair rests not in the chair itself, but in the relationships between the people who used the chair that make it spiritually significant.

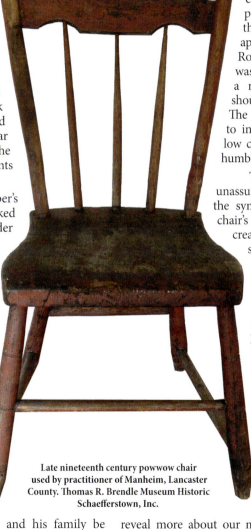

Late nineteenth century powwow chair used by practitioner of Manheim, Lancaster County. Thomas R. Brendle Museum Historic Schaefferstown, Inc.

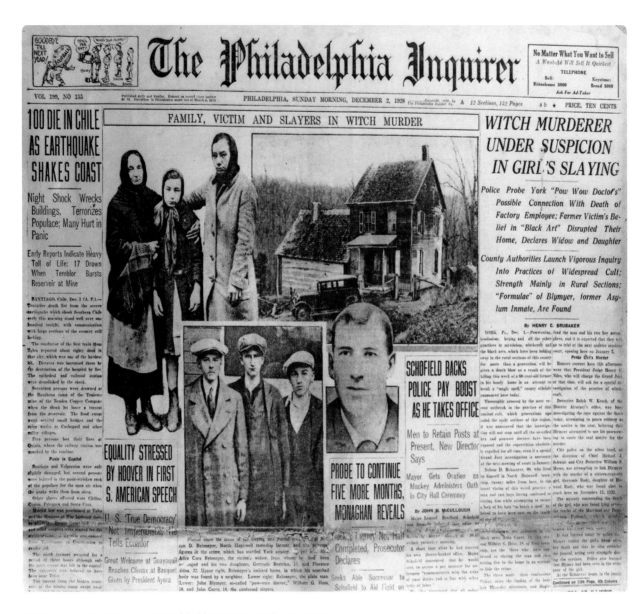

York Hex Murder Media Coverage 1928, *Philadelphia Inquirer*. Heilman Collection.

The murder of powwow doctor Nelson Rehmeyer in York County, dubbed the "Hex Murder," received national attention in 1928-1929. The murderer, John Blymire, an escapee from a mental asylum, was convinced that Rehmeyer had placed a curse upon him. In an attempt to break the "hex" by obtaining a lock of hair or Rehmeyer's copy of John George Hohman's *Long Lost Friend*, Blymire and two accomplices John Curry and Wilbur Hess, killed Rehmeyer two days before Thanksgiving in 1928. The trial drew national media attention to the persistence of beliefs associated with powwowing in Pennsylvania. However, this media attention was heavily biased, and promoted many negative, false, and culturally insensitive stereotypes about Pennsylvania Dutch people and the communities of York. The incident is often indicated as the single-most defining moment in Pennsylvania's anti-powwowing crusade, which swept across the state. Threats from lawmakers, physicians' councils, and civic organizations forced traditional healing to be conducted in secrecy for fear of prosecution for practicing medicine without a license.

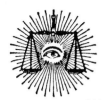

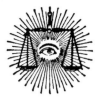

Chapter IX
Powwowing & The Authorities
Medical, Legal, Educational, Media

With the standardization of scientific medicine in the late nineteenth century and the consolidation of legal and educational authority for medical licensing, traditional practitioners of many varieties found themselves on the wrong side of the law. Although initially medical licensing was merely a formality, and even some powwow doctors were technically registered practitioners in the State of Pennsylvania, the organization of local, regional, and national medical societies initiated widespread efforts to eradicate traditional practices throughout the nation.

The media played an important role in this process, publicizing any form of controversy that centered on the activities of non-sanctioned medical practitioners – especially those practitioners whose clientele overlapped with licensed, conventional medical doctors. Rather than tolerating these alternative and complementary practices that existed side by side with conventional medical institutions of the time, doctors, journalists, police, lawyers, and citizen crusaders participated in efforts to "expose" traditional practices as inherently deceptive, predatory, and profit-driven.

Powwowing, with its close ties to the use of the German language, came under fire at precisely the same time that Pennsylvania's educational institutions began the gradual process of shifting to English-only schools in regions that were formerly bastions of German-speaking people. As children began to receive education in English, and many families gradually discontinued the everyday use of Pennsylvania Dutch in the home, this language rift highlighted the ever broadening gap between two parallel societies, defined by language, but characterized by distinctive traditions and practices.

Powwowing, like many other forms of traditional medicine across the nation, was targeted in southeastern and central Pennsylvania, but the majority of practitioners were impossible to prosecute. Typically powwow practitioners make no charge for services, administer no chemical compounds that are not essentially home remedies, perform no invasive procedures, and bar no one from visiting other medical professionals. These generally accepted norms tended to insulate powwow practitioners that offered their services to friends, family, and their immediate community. However, powwowers of the "professional" class, serving clients by the thousands, were regularly engaged in legal defense from a variety of charges and allegations. Some of these practitioners gained relative notoriety and prominence from media attention, while others received media attention only after devastating incidents left them disenfranchised or dead.

The following three accounts of prominent practitioners in Pennsylvania highlight significant narratives in three core regions of ritual activity in the commonwealth at the turn of the century: Dr. Joseph H. Hageman (1835-1905) of Reading, Berks County, D. Dennis Rex (1863-1944) from the Lehigh-Carbon border at the Blue Mountain, and Nelson D. Rehmeyer (1868-1928) of York in Central Pennsylvania. While reflecting sharply contrasting sources of controversy, their stories provide insight into broader conflicts that shaped the culture and contributed to the ebb and flow of powwowing in Pennsylvania.

READING CITY'S JOSEPH H. HAGEMAN

A century and a decade ago, the city of Reading lost the most prolific and influential folk healer of the nineteenth century among the Pennsylvania Dutch of Berks County. Dr. Joseph Heinrich Hageman (1832-1905) was a second-generation healer, having followed in the footsteps of his father Heinrich Herman Hageman (1801-1882), a well-known herb doctor in the city. Joseph Hageman (also spelled Hagenman, Hagaman, etc.) was not a medical doctor in the conventional sense, but a *Braucher* or powwow doctor by vocation, whose healing by means of prayers and written blessings was highly sought after by members of the Pennsylvania Dutch community. Despite the fact that his methods were far from conventional,

Hageman was described in 1898 as "one of Reading's leading and most successful practitioners of medicine, [who] possesses, in addition to a lucrative office practice, an extensive patronage in the surrounding territory."[1]

Dr. Hageman was best known for the creation of highly sophisticated German-language blessing inscriptions intended to be carried on one's person for the healing of physical ailments, or hidden in the house and barn for protection from malicious spiritual forces. Examples that have survived to the present day have been found inscribed in his beautiful German script with the names of people who were sick or troubled and needed his care. Others have been found concealed in furniture or on the lintels of barn doors in Berks County.[2] In addition, the blessings consisted of prayers asking for divine assistance, as well as sections written backwards that addressed the spiritual entities believed to cause illness and misfortune. These blessings were produced in scores beginning about 1850 until 1905, and were used in the greater Reading area by city and rural folk alike. The 1st floor of his brick Victorian row home, located at 836 Elm Street, was used as a waiting room and consultation space until the time of his death in 1905, and was identified by a tin sign bearing the name of his practice. Reports in 1900 indicated that his waiting room was rarely empty, and that clients visited him daily to receive his written blessings. Although it is unknown how many of his blessings have survived to the present day, hundreds of such inscriptions must have been made in the decades of his successful practice in Reading.

Despite Joseph Hageman's wide acceptance within the community of Reading, the Hageman family was distinct in a number of ways from their Pennsylvania Dutch neighbors. They were part of the later waves of German immigration taking place throughout the nineteenth century. German-American immigrants were typically part of urban and industrialized populations from Europe, rather than the rural, pre-industrial communities that earlier characterize the eighteenth century immigrants later known as the Pennsylvania Dutch. The Hageman family would blend these two distinct German-speaking populations, but even their dialect would set them apart from their neighbors for two generations.[3] Although far from the romantic notion of a "rags-to-riches" story of immigration and integration into the fabric of Pennsylvania's diverse society, the Hageman's family narrative provides considerable insight into the diversity of Pennsylvania's ritual practitioners, as well as the continental European practices of folk medicine.

Joseph Hageman's father, Heinrich Herman Hageman, was born in the mostly rural town of Lübbecke, Westphalia, in the Kingdom of Prussia to Anthony Wilhelm Hageman and his wife Catherine Mary in 1801.[4] As a young man he was trained as a baker, and at the age of twenty-five he emigrated on the ship *Agenora* to Philadelphia in 1827.[5] Upon his arrival in Philadelphia, Heinrich married first-generation immigrant Elisabeth Burke in 1828, and together they had a son, Joseph Heinrich Hageman, born December 12th, 1832, who was baptized into the German Reformed Church on January sixteenth, 1833.[6] His brother Abraham was born two years later in 1834. The family then relocated their home to Rockland Township, Berks County, in 1835,[7] where they appear on the US Federal Census in 1840, and later in Ruscombmanor in 1850, where Heinrich is listed, not as a doctor, but as a "Laborer." Joseph had three siblings, Abraham and the twins, William and Sarah. It is unclear what year Heinrich began to practice medicine, but sometime following Abraham's death in 1853, and Elisabeth's death in 1857,[8] Heinrich moved to Reading with Joseph, and remarried to Anna Maria Wünsch, another first-generation German immigrant.[9] By 1860, Heinrich Hageman is listed in the census as a doctor, living with his new wife and his son Joseph, who is listed as a laborer.[10] By the time of his death in 1882, Heinrich was described as "a well-known herb-doctor."[11] It would not be until 1890 that Joseph Hageman was listed as a physician in the Federal Census. This latter designation could be misleading, as practitioners of folk medicine among the

Above: Portrait of Reading powwow practitioner, Dr. Joseph H. Hageman, ca. 1890. Courtesy of Thomas Gable and Family.
Right: Family picture of Dr. Joseph H. Hageman, with his wife Emma (Hinnerschitz) Hageman, and five of their children in front of their home at 836 Elm Street, Reading. Dr. Hageman's subtle tin sign for his practice can be seen along the edge of the doorframe. Courtesy of Thomas Gable and Family.

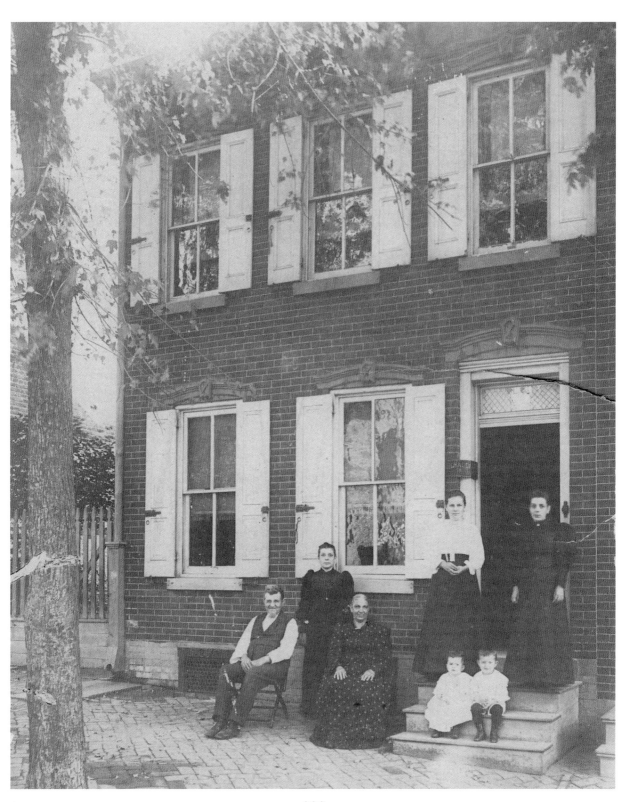

Pennsylvania Dutch rarely do so in a professional capacity, and are frequently tradesmen or farmers. Only rarely are individuals actually listed as a "powwow doctor" in the US Census.[12] *The Biographical Sketches of the Leading Citizens of Berks County*, states that Joseph began to practice in Reading around 1864,[13] but Reading City directories only list him alternately as a carpenter and laborer until 1891.[14] Towards the end of his life, he would recall the date 1858, but this disagrees with his obituary, which states 1846.[15] Despite this uncertainty, the Hageman family is exceptional for having been publically recognized with the title of "physicians," when they were in fact powwow doctors.

Another important exception for the Hageman family is that practitioners of folk medicine among the Pennsylvania Dutch typically pass their traditional knowledge across lines of gender – that is, a female must teach a male, and vice-versa. If Joseph learned from his father, this would be somewhat unusual, although occasionally, in some families, a father could teach his first-born son and a mother her first-born daughter, as the single-exception to the rule. Another famous line of powwowers in Reading was the Schmidt-Eberth family, where for three generations the women in the family were regionally renowned as healers, and the title *die Wascht-Fraa* (The Sausage Lady) was handed from one generation to the next. The women of *Wascht-Fraa* dynasty, however, passed their knowledge to their husbands, who in turn would train the next generation of women how to powwow.[16]

In addition to the possibility of having learned his practice from his father, the young Joseph Hageman worked mixing medicines in a pharmaceutical dispensary, Derringers of Reading.[17] It would later be revealed by his family that Joseph was presumed to have some connection with the celebrated Doctor Charles A. Gerasch of Kutztown, former treasurer for the Keystone State Normal School, known for his "high reputation among his brethren for skill in the art of healing."[18] In addition, a Samuel Winters was also listed as an influence to Hageman's practice,[19] although Winters is listed in the U.S. Federal Census as a farmer in West Donegal Township, Lancaster County in 1880.

Regardless of how knowledge was passed in the Hageman family, it would seem probable that Joseph inherited his father Heinrich's clientele following his death, as Joseph continued to operate from the same house as his father on Elm Street. Joseph would later describe his practice as having commenced in 1858,[20] but it is uncertain to what extent his particular practice had anything in common with his father's. Although Joseph's practice was extremely well documented at the turn of the century, only scant mention of his father's methods can be found. The title of "herb-doctor" can be ambiguous, referring alternately to botanical or clinical herbalism, or as a polite means of identifying a powwow practitioner who made ritualistic and magical uses of herbs. No documentation exists to classify Heinrich's methodology, but one important clue helps to differentiate his herbal practice from his son Joseph's use of written blessings: Heinrich was illiterate according to the 1880 US Census. If that Census is correct, this means that although Joseph could have learned a great deal from his father in terms of the creation of the tinctures he would later dispense, the written component of Joseph's blessings was not learned from his father. Despite his apparent lack of formal education, Dr. Heinrich Hageman's practice flourished, and so much so, that a Reading conventional physician located just down the street, Dr. S. B. Keckman, admitted in 1903 that his practice had been so threatened by Heinrich's presence that he had to move and relocate his clinic in favor of more business elsewhere in Reading.[21]

Although little is known of the specifics of Heinrich Hageman's herbal practice, a late nineteenth century German language newspaper account describes a visit to a local Reading herbalist (of the ritual variety) in great detail. *Der Readinger Hexendoktor* was known to continually brew herbal decoctions over an old stove in the corner of his office, praying incantations over his brew, and while stirring the pot with three ladles held only with three fingers three times every three hours from sunup to sundown, for three days, three nights, three hours and three minutes. Although one could wonder if the doctor in question were Dr. Heinrich Hageman, it is doubtful, as the author describes his dwelling place as a single story building of frame construction, on the edge of town – nowhere near Heinrich was known to have lived. Further, if Heinrich was unable to read, he could not have been the Doktor, who admitted that he had a book of cures for all illnesses bound in snake skin, which he stored buried under seven inches of ashes and would consult when he was fasting and the moon was full.[22]

This highly embellished account, whether based on actual events or not, is an early example of the wave of journalism that would later portray the city of Reading as "*Hexe-Schteddel*" (The Little City of Witches)[23] and all of Berks County as the single-most largest concentration of ritual activity in all of the United States. The Hagemans' influence played no small part in supplying a steady stream of anecdotal content to national newspapers, and by 1911, just four years after Joseph Hageman's death, the *New York Times* would declare him to be "the greatest powwow doctor who ever lived."[24]

It is therefore both ironic and unfortunate that the majority of what is known about the practice of Dr. Joseph Hageman is based on popular media rather than first-hand accounts. While the dramatic stories of his incantations, blessings, and laying-on-of-hands were often highly detailed and are valuable descriptions of ritual practice, it is hard to discern the thin veneer of truth which served to disguise what amounted to little more than extremely prejudiced, anti-German sensationalism on the part of the press. Although some of the earliest newspaper accounts of Pennsylvania Dutch folk medicine occur in the 1860s,[25] papers all over the country carried stories of Pennsylvania's powwow doctors by the 1880s, and this trend continued well into the twentieth century.

It is no wonder that the penultimate anti-powwow article of the turn of the century specifically targeted Dr. Joseph Hageman in 1900.[26] The exposé, entitled "The Reading Witch Doctor's Sway Over the Trusting and the Ignorant," written by Alice Rix of Philadelphia, is a full-page article, one-fourth of which is occupied by a caricature of Dr. Hageman clutching a bible, bearing the libelous caption:

> THIS MAN DEALS IN NECROMANCY: There is a Witch Doctor, a Brager [sic], a Pow-wow man, who has a thinly-disguised, remunerative practice under the very noses of the Reading authorities. His name and address are in the Reading Directory – Doctor Joseph B. Hageman of 839 Elm Street, and his waiting room is rarely empty. He sells powders, potions, forbiddings, blessings and charms. – A gross, grizzled, dirty old man, huge of head and face and jowl, and hanging chin, with the monstrous body, long, thick arms, and short, thick legs of the bear; with big, fat, greasy hands like suet puddings boiled in bags; with squat, square feet; with a mouth open over a single row of brown and broken teeth; with bright, blue, questioning, kindly, smiling eyes – two spots of innocent blue upon a field of filth, like forget-me-nots dropped on a dirt heap."

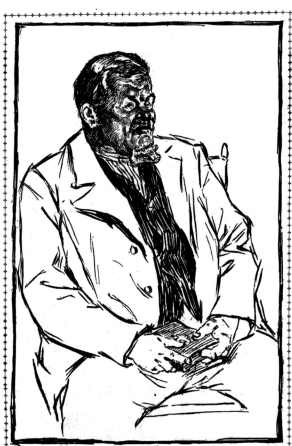

Illustration of Dr. Joseph H. Hageman, from Alice Rix's exposé in *the North American*, "The Reading Witch Doctor's Sway Over the Trusting and the Ignorant." May 22 1900.

Rix's crusade was inspired by the anti-powwow rhetoric of the medical doctor and member of the Berks County Medical Society, John M. Bertolet of Reading, who had delivered a lecture to his colleagues on the evils of powwowing in Reading City in the previous year, a transcript of which was later published in the December issue of the *Philadelphia Monthly Medical Journal* under the title "Witch Doctors and Their Deceptions."[27] This address called for the prosecution of all powwow doctors, according to 1861 Pennsylvania State Law P.L. 270: "Any person…who shall for gain or lucre pretend to affect any purpose by spells, charms, necromancy, or incantation, shall be guilty of a misdemeanor, punishable… with fine and imprisonment or both." It is interesting to note here that the law defines a "witch-doctor" as anyone "pretending to do something impossible to accomplish," ultimately resting on the premise that deception is involved, with no discussion of cultural practices and beliefs. Likewise, the Berks County Medical Society urged legislators to enforce these laws, saying that "many such in Reading do business on what might easily be called false pretense… [and] extort money from the public by imaginary cures of all sorts."[28] It is obvious that these accounts not only cast doubt upon the efficacy of the cures, but also the sincerity and ethics of the practitioners. This form of negative publicity would later inspire Hageman's patients to defend him from such accusations.[29]

Albert M. Burkholder, editor of the *Reading Eagle*, arranged a meeting with Dr. Bertolet, Alice Rix, and Gertrude Partington, the artist responsible for the illustration of Dr. Hageman. At the meeting, Dr. Bertolet provided the address of the Boyer family living on Cotton Street where Dr. Hageman had been treating their son

William. Together, Burkholder, Rix, and Partington interviewed the family, presumably without explaining their real purpose, as the family was decidedly sympathetic to Hageman and his method of healing. With an all-too-familiar anti-Pennsylvania Dutch sentiment, Rix used the Boyer family interviews as ammunition to depict the local people of Reading as tragically uneducated and feeble-minded. While the name of the family is intentionally omitted in the article, a life-sized photograph of a blessing obtained from the family is included. Although the portion of the booklet that was reprinted was written backwards, the name "Warren William Boyer" is clearly discernible in the inscription.

Finally, the three journalists planned a deceptive appointment with Dr. Hageman himself. Rix was able to receive a walk-in consultation, under the false pretense of seeking help for a sister in Harrisburg who was "strangely afflicted," and subject to "nervous spells at night," whereby she would awaken suddenly in the night to the vision of "black-robed figure of a woman," and the "forms of cats jumping across her bed, one after another." Entrapping him with her questions, she inquired if witches sometimes take the forms of cats, and apparently Dr. Hageman replied to the affirmative. Rix purchased a charm for five dollars, which she provides in translation at the conclusion of her exposé. None of the specifics of the deception were included in Rix's article, but were later relayed by Burkholder who remained in the hallway outside of the waiting room where Dr. Hageman would not recognize him as the editor of the Reading Eagle.

Although she mentions nothing of her secret collaborations with Dr. Bertolet or Mr. Burkholder in her article, Rix was the only member of the conspiracy who did not live in Reading, and therefore she could take much greater liberty in her writing – a freedom that Dr. Bertolet and Mr. Burkholder did not have as prominent citizens of Reading and neighbors of Dr. Hageman. This is further confirmed by the fact that Burkholder wrote as a correspondent on the subject for publications in New York City but would not do so in his own town.

Although Alice Rix's horrid depictions of Reading citizens raised no complaints against *The North American* newspaper, Dr. Joseph B. Hageman took particular offense to the article – not from a personal perspective, but rather as a response to the claim that his cures were created under false pretenses and thus, ineffective. In an attempt to re-establish his dignity as a doctor with the public, he filed a lawsuit which commenced, after several delays, on March 6th, 1903, in the city of Philadelphia. The plaintiff's lawyers based their case purely on the writings of Alice Rix, believing her work to be so inflammatory that the jury would decide in their favor; however, the defense lawyers for *The North American* were representing the interests of C.E.O. John Wanamaker, former U.S. Postmaster General and a very wealthy and powerful citizen of Philadelphia. Whether out of confidence in the outcome of the case or out of a sense of self-protection, *The North American* printed the entire transcript of the trial in the paper. (It is interesting to note that while The North American goes to great length to condemn the practice of folk medicine, the products advertised on the very same pages as the publicity of the trial are for various popular patent medicines, claiming to

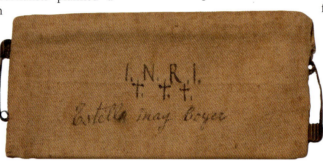

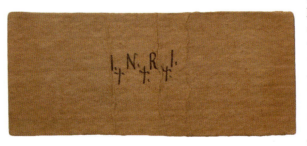

Left: Personal blessings for healing and protection, made by Dr. Joseph H. Hageman of Reading, Berks County, for Estella May Boyer, 1895. In 1911, the *New York Times* called him "the greatest powwow doctor who ever lived." Hageman's blessings were derived from a European book of blessings called *Der Geistliche Schild und Heiliger Segen (The Spiritual Shield and Holy Blessing)*. Pennsylvania German Cultural Heritage Center, Kutztown University.

cure everything from deafness, to kidney failure, and promising the "secret of long life and health" – essentially early-modern, commercial quackery.)

Although the full details of the week-long lawsuit are far too exhaustive to summarize in great length, several notable examinations took place of witnesses who testified not only to the efficacy of Dr. Hageman's charms, but also of the various ways in which his clients blended conventional medicine and folk medicine in a hierarchy of resort, where many clients turned to the help of Dr. Hageman when conventional doctors were unable to help, or in some cases they consulted a conventional doctor at the same time. In addition, linguistic specialists were brought in to analyze Hageman's blessings, calling them "a collection of words from different languages, either memorized and written down from memory, or else transcribed immediately from different books." These testimonies are a valuable resource in determining the particulars of folk medical practices in the beginning of the twentieth century, and the way in which the scandal pitted the forces of tradition and cultural identity against the waves of health care reform that were rapidly sweeping across America.

Over the course of trial, the majority of the witnesses called by the defense were women living in Reading, who had consulted with Dr. Hageman because of sick infants. The defense used these cases to prove that Hageman's methods were unconventional, and further, that his practice was based in the creation of charms and that public perception was that he was a "witch doctor." The mothers' testimonies were that typically they had already consulted with conventional doctors (sometimes several)

Above: Blessing made for Emma Jane Weidner, 1887, by Dr. Joseph H. Hageman of Reading, Pennsylvania. Hageman's blessings were derived verbatim from European collections of folk-religious blessings, such as the Geistlicher Schild (Spiritual Shield) and the works attributed to Saint Albertus Magnus. Heilman Collection.

for their sick children, and had turned to powwow based on the reputation of Hageman as a successful practitioner. Although many called him a "witch-doctor," (English for *Hexedoktor*), their testimonies demonstrated that in general Hageman's method were no more or less effective than many of the other conventional practitioners consulted, especially if the illnesses were particularly tenacious. In some cases, just like the conventional doctors, Hageman would also inform his patients of when he felt that the illness was beyond his abilities.

What made these reports difficult, however, for the court, were the diagnoses described by Hageman in the cases of illness among infants. The witnesses reported that Hageman described that their children's "rest was taken," (*Ruh genumme*) a common early nineteenth century perception among the Pennsylvania Dutch, which could apply to a wide variety of ailments including insomnia (*Unruh*), colicky babies or children who were "livergrown" (die *aagewaxne Kinner*), as well as marasmus (*Abnemme*), often referred to as the wasting disease.

Hageman also suggested that some of the sick children were "hypnotized," or "magnetized to the earth." While the defense lawyers attempted to pressure the mothers into describing who had taken the rest, most were unsure, and made no attempt to elaborate. In many instances, the witnesses expressed a lack of interest in how or why Hageman's methods were intended to function, and more concerned about the results.

Hageman was no stranger to infant illness, as he and his wife Emma buried six of their children, five of whom were two years or younger at the time of death, and the youngest of which was only four days. The high rates of child mortality in American families at the turn of the century is one of the most important, albeit unspoken, aspects of Hageman's trial. Most of the witnesses testifying in his defense were mothers who had turned to Dr. Hageman when there was no other recourse. His willingness to treat children that had been considered too far gone for conventional care was one of his signature services to his community.

The first witness called by the defense was Mrs. Maggie Hohl of Reading, who described that in 1899 her twelve-year-old daughter, Katie E. Hohl, was afflicted at night with bouts of screaming, "saw all different kinds of things in the wall," and wouldn't leave the house by day. Hageman's diagnosis was that the girl was hypnotized, and he gave her an unidentified 2oz bottle of medicine, and a few days later, a written blessing. By the end of the week, the screaming fits stopped. However, when the child's overall health did not improve, and Hageman felt as though he had done all he could, the mother sought another doctor. Despite this change in physicians, the child continued to wear the blessing for two months. Although the lawyer for the defense attempted to lead the witness in the direction of discussion of a curse, asking if the child had enemies or "any person who had looked into the eyes of the child," objections were raised and sustained.

Several other witnesses were of particular interest, especially two women, a mother and daughter named Lavina Babst, and Lizzie (Babst) Winter. Their testimonies may have represented a generational shift that occurred at the turn of the century, with Lavina as a firm believer in the efficacy of powwow, and her daughter Lizzie, a young mother who was uncertain about Hageman's folk medicine, but would try anything to restore the health of her infant. It was her parents and friends who suggested that Lizzie visit Dr. Hageman.

Unfortunately, her mother Lavina Babst was the laughingstock of the trial. She was a very animated witness, and one can discern a thick Pennsylvania Dutch accent from the manner in which her narrative was transcribed. Despite her sincerity, she became enraged when she perceived that she was being mocked. Lavina was also singled out, because although many witnesses had possessed copies of Hageman's blessings, Lavina was actually wearing hers, and she refused to turn it over, citing biblical scripture as the justification for her belief in the efficacy and appropriateness of Hageman's clinical methodology.

According to Lavina's daughter Lizzie Winter, in 1894 Lizzie's child, Nora Amelia Victoria Winter, was sick, and although she had taken her to several doctors, the child's condition did not improve. Dr. Hageman attended the child at their home, and his diagnosis was that she was "hypnotized." Lizzie reported that when she received one of Hageman's blessings, consisting of a multipage document written in German and enclosed in a canvas envelope, she pinned in to Nora's undergarments, and it was used over the course of five years. The blessing was only removed after the family was certain that the child had fully recovered and would never relapse.

This same procedure was followed for Lizzie's son Howard who was apparently more severely afflicted than his sister, as the right side of his body was the site of the illness as described by his mother. Hageman had Lizzie make a cross with salt at the foot of the child's bed, place the pillow over it, and have the child sleep opposite his usual posture. Lizzie was instructed to do this for nine days. When pressured by the cross-examination to be more specific about the objective of the rituals, Lizzie testified that Hageman had told her the ritual would "keep them off" – implying that the affliction was caused by "something that had come into the house."

While the witness was unable to be specific about what this meant, other witnesses reported Hageman telling them that they were not to borrow or lend anything during the duration of the nine days. Unbeknownst to the jury, composed of Philadelphia citizens, this was a classic process in the Pennsylvania Dutch community for avoiding a curse or hex, whereby common household objects that were borrowed and came into the home were perceived to potentially carry negative consequences, either by intention, if someone were actually attempting to place a curse, or more commonly, if a person was carrying a grudge and unintentionally brought misfortune upon the household they begrudged. The nuances of this cultural perception were lost on the members of the jury.

To Hageman's credit, throughout the course of the trial, it was apparent that Hageman was not engaged in assigning blame to other members of the community for causing illnesses or placing a hex. Out of hundreds of narratives, only in one instance did a witness, by the name of Ida Eckenroth describe that Hageman believed a person was responsible for a child's illness, admitting that he knew it was a lady, although he gave no indication of how he knew this. When Mrs. Eckenroth inquired about whether he would "bring the lady" – that is, to summon or ritually compel her to visit the house of the sick person to account for her curse – Hageman explained that this he was unwilling to do this, because it would put too much of a strain on him to perform such a ritual.

Instead Hageman gave her liquid medicine in bottles, as well as a written blessing, but he also instructed her to sprinkle salt across her front door, outline the child with salt in the bed, and burn one of the baby's diapers in the woodstove while invoking the "Three Highest Names" of the Father, Son and Holy Spirit, and to say the child's name and invoke the compassionate spirits of "all his

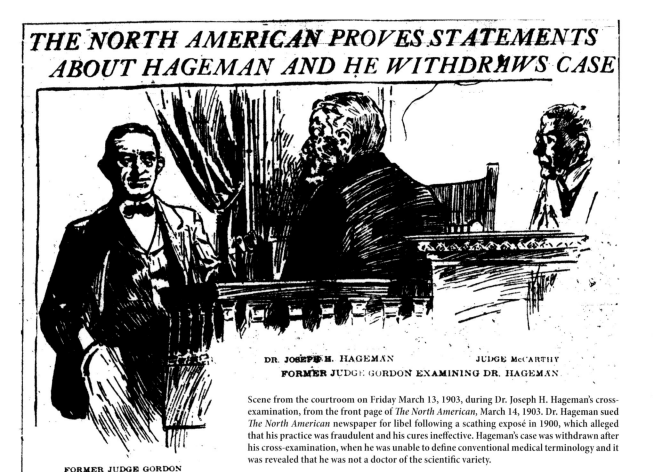

Scene from the courtroom on Friday March 13, 1903, during Dr. Joseph H. Hageman's cross-examination, from the front page of *The North American*, March 14, 1903. Dr. Hageman sued *The North American* newspaper for libel following a scathing exposé in 1900, which alleged that his practice was fraudulent and his cures ineffective. Hageman's case was withdrawn after his cross-examination, when he was unable to define conventional medical terminology and it was revealed that he was not a doctor of the scientific variety.

friends who are invisible" and conclude with the name of the Holy Trinity once again. Although Ida's son died from his advanced case of marasmus two weeks later, the child was also under the care of another physician at the time, who, likewise, was unable to affect a cure for the infant.

Many of the testimonies are tragic, like the story of twenty-year-old daughter of Elle Zimmerman, whose health was on a steady decline in 1895. She was sick for seven months prior to her death. Dr. Hageman had been called in after several unsuccessful physicians attended her, diagnosing it as a complication of diseases. Hageman administered medicine, and gave her a blessing to wear, saying that the poor girl was "magnetized to the earth." She was attended by several other physicians after that time, each saying that they didn't know what specifically ailed her. She was bedridden for three weeks, and in the absence of improvement, she refused to see anyone. In her final week, she asked her mother to remove Hageman's blessing, and three days later she died.

The final testimony was from Hageman himself, who was grilled with specific questions from the defense concerning the science of medicine, anatomy, chemistry and his credentials. When it was apparent that he was not even remotely versed in conventional medicine, was not familiar with the words pathology, or hygiene, and failed to accurately describe the concept of blood circulation, the civil suit was dismissed with "prejudice" so that no appeal could re-open the trial.

It is tragic that this final day of court proceedings constitutes the only source containing Hageman's own words, aside from the nonsensical quotations from Rix's article. The cross-examination is anything but a dialogue, with Hageman forced into a defensive position, never even having the opportunity to describe in any detail what type of medicine he actually practiced. His testimony, mostly consisting of admission that he did not know, or did not remember the correct answers to the defense's questions, fell upon deaf ears, and instead they gave him a proverbial shovel and somewhat reluctantly, he proceeded to dig a very deep hole.

Interestingly enough, it was Hageman's own lawyers that addressed the court, asking for the verdict to be delivered without any further questioning, as well as a pardon for them being aware of the extent of his ignorance of conventional medicine. What is unclear in the whirlwind of agendas and legal process, is whether Hageman's motivation for filing the complaint was actually consistent with his lawyer's interpretation. Was Hageman less concerned about his label of "hex doctor" and more concerned that his sincerity and ability to affect cures was questioned?

Accounts of Hageman's activities following the dismissal of the trial vary considerably. Some imply that he was forced to close his practice under close scrutiny of Reading officials, and while this is an easy assumption to make, it has never been confirmed that Hageman had any further brushes with the law. Other sources say that he went on as before, and his business never lapsed.[30] Without citing any sources whatsoever, one popular author claimed that Hageman had a protégé named "Gentzler" from Oley,[31] and furthermore asserted that Gentzler became entangled with other media sensations such as the York County murder of Nelson Rehmeyer in 1928. In a very real sense, these accounts of hearsay are evidence of the persistence of Dr. Hageman's influence in Pennsylvania. Without the closure of a neatly-packaged ending to Hageman's story, his narrative would continue nevertheless to inspire media coverage for decades to come.[32]

On June twentieth, 1905, Dr. Joseph H. Hageman passed away and the following obit was submitted to the *Reading Eagle*:

> Dr. Joseph H. Hagenman died of bilious fever, aged 73 years, Sunday evening at his residence, 836 Elm, after an illness of some time. He was bedfast since last Monday. He was a son of Henry and Elizabeth Hagenman (nee Burke), and was born in Philadelphia. He came to this city with his parents as a boy, and received a common school education. He studied medicine under Dr. Gerasch at Kutztown, and later with Dr. Samuel Winters of Lancaster. In 1846 he began the practice in this city, and he has been located here ever since. His wife, Emma E. (nee Hinnershitz), died four years ago. These children remain: Daniel C., Charles A., Annie H., Mary E., wife of Elias Phillips; Emma, wife of William Luppold, and Milton; also seven grandchildren. He was a member of St. Luke's Lutheran Church. Dr. Hageman was widely known in Eastern Penn'a, having been professionally called to attend a large number of cases of nervous prostration and a variety of nervous complaints, marasmus and mental afflictions, in which he achieved considerable reputation.

Just like many of the other conflicting documents surrounding Dr. Joseph Hageman, his life and practice, this conclusion to his life's narrative leaves more questions than answers, and opens up room for more speculation concerning the nature of his legacy of folk medicine in Reading.

The following blessing was written for Emma Jane Weidner of Kutztown in 1887. May these words tell the story of Dr. Hageman in a way that no public document or newspaper could ever convey: his worldview and sincerity, his belief and compassion, and his persistence in tradition despite an ever-changing world.

I. N. R. I.

+. +. +.

Jesus of Nazareth, King of the Jews, may this triumphant title of Jesus Christ the Crucified be between me, Emma Jane Weidner and all my visible and invisible enemies, that they can neither approach me, nor harm me, Emma Jane Weidner, neither in body or soul, Amen. Jesus + Maria   In the Name of God the + Father, and of the + Son, and of the Holy + Spirit, Amen. God Elohim, God Tetragrammaton, God Adonai, God Sabaoth, God Emmanuel, God Hagios, God O Theos, God Ishryos, God Jehova, God Messiah, God Alpha and Omega, together with all the names of God the Father, of the Son, and of the Holy Spirit, strengthen and preserve me, Emma Jane Weidner, today and for all time, against my corporeal and spiritual enemies, Amen. + The Uncreated Father, + The Uncreated Son, + The Uncreated Holy Spirit. + The Bornless Father, + The Innate Son, + from which proceeds the Spirit. God the Father + The Creator, God the Son + The Redeemer, God the Holy Spirit + The Sanctifier protect and preserve me, Emma Jane Weidner now and for all time against all violent storms, ghosts, and witchcraft, Amen. Christ Jesus Triumphs, Christ Jesus Reigns, Christ Commands, Christ Jesus expels all violent storms, sorcery, and devil's work, through the power of his divinity, through the power of his bitter suffering, through the power of his Holy Cross, through the power of his rose-colored blood, and through the power of his Holy Name, Jesus Christ, the Son of the Living God come down from Heaven, into the body of the most blessed Virgin Mary, through which he became holy human flesh: With it, he expels the devil and all evil spirits, and casts them into hell, these will he disperse, and me, Emma Jane Weidner, he will unbind from all those that the devil has bound, and through his damnable work has blinded, Amen. By the sign of the Holy Cross + release me, Emma Jane Weidner, O God, from all my enemies, Amen. The Word became flesh, and dwelled among us, born of the Virgin Mary, and will protect me, Emma Jane Weidner, through the witness of his mercy, in which he lifted us up from our highest affliction, and through the intercession of the most-blessed Virgin Mary, as well as the Four Evangelists, John, Matthew, Mark and Luke, against all spirits of Satan and his servants, and all acts of witchcraft, cursing, delusion, sorcery, spell-binding, and enchantment performed against me, Emma Jane Weidner, or could yet be performed against me, or could yet be performed against me, from all stalking by the Devil's evil will, from lightning, thunder, hail, violent storms, walking dead, and from all evil. He who reigns with the Father and the Holy Spirit from eternity to eternity,

Amen. In the Name of J. J. J. Amen. I, Emma Jane Weidner. Jesus Christ is the true salvation, Jesus Christ is the true salvation. Jesus Christ reigns, governs, and triumphs over all enemies, visible and invisible, Jesus be with me, Emma Jane Weidner, in all places, ever and always, on all paths and bridges, on water and land, on mountain and dale, at home and in the entire world, where I am, where I stand, walk, ride, or drive, where I sleep or wake, eat or drink, there be thou Lord Jesus, at all times, early and late, all hours and moments, when going in or out, the five wounds red of our Lord Jesus Christ protect me. Be they secret or public, may they avoid me, and their weapons cannot harm or wound me, so help me, Emma Jane Weidner. +. +. +. Jesus Christ, with his shelter and shield, protect me, Emma Jane Weidner, at all times from daily sin, earthly harm, and against injustice, against condemnation, against pestilence and other sickness, against fear, murder, and pain, against all evil enemies, against all false witness and slander, and that no gun may harm my body, so help me, Emma Jane Weidner +. +. +. That, yea, no thieving servants, nor gypsies or bandits, arsonists, witchcraft, or all types of demons can sneak into my house and yard, yea, much less break in. All this be protected by the dear Virgin Mary, and all her children, that by God in Heaven, are in eternal bliss, and may the glory of God the Father refresh me, Emma Jane Weidner, the wisdom of God the Son enlighten me, Emma Jane Weidner, and the virtue and grace of God the Holy Spirit strengthen me, Emma Jane Weidner, at this hour until eternity, Amen. In the Name of God, I cry out: God! I, Emma Jane Weidner, cry out: God the Father be above me, God the Son be before me, God the Holy Spirit be next to me, Emma Jane Weidner. Whosoever is stronger than these three men, shall approach me, Emma Jane Weidner. But whosoever is not stronger than these three men, shall leave me alone. J. J. J. So long as the Lord lives and reigns, therefore, so truly shall his Holy Angel protect me, Emma Jane Weidner, in all my comings and goings. God the Father is my might + God the Son is my power + God the Holy Spirit is my strength. May the angel of God smite all of my enemies away. Amen + + +

I. N. R. I.

+. +. +.

February 7 A.D. 1887[33]

Dennis Rex: Healer of Slatedale

With increased pressure on county courts to prosecute powwow doctors, just a decade after Dr. Hageman's debacle, another local healer took front and center of the local papers for allegations of "necromancy." Dennis Rex (1863-1944), farmer, beekeeper, and lumberman living just a few miles north of Slatedale, at the foot of the Blue Mountain was arrested by the Lehigh County Detective Bureau on charges of fraud and brought to trial in October of 1914.[34]

Like Dr. Hageman, Dennis Rex had a wide base of support in his community despite the allegations, and members of prominent families in Allentown appeared in court to show their support for him and his work in the community. Rex's story was typical of professional powwow practitioners, treating cases where doctors failed to

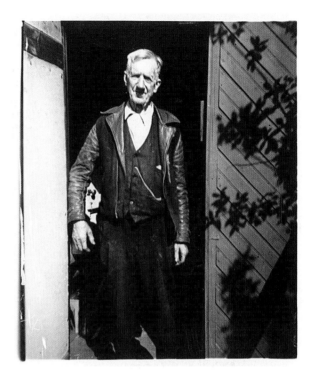

Powwow doctor Dennis Rex of Slatedale, standing in the doorway of his mule-drawn medicine wagon and wearing his driving jacket, ca. 1920. *Courtesy of the Rev. Brian Haas and Family.*

provide relief from nervous dyspepsia, sciatic rheumatism, insomnia, a wide range of reproductive issues for women, nervousness, and other ailments.[35] His procedures were traditional, and described as laying on of hands, while offering silent prayers, after which he would give written blessings in sealed envelopes that were to be worn on the patient against the skin, and burned three days later.[36] As a charismatic and well-respected healer, Rex's clientele ranged from all over the region, and as far away as New York. According to his family, cars would line the road for miles along the winding dirt road that led to Rex's home at the base of the mountain, and some would even pitch tents to wait overnight for the next available appointment. He specified no particular charge for his services, but his patients were generous - so generous in fact, that Rex's practice became too lucrative for it to go unnoticed by the authorities for long.

Rex was arrested once before in Carbon County for practicing medicine without a license, but it did not discourage his activities in Lehigh.[37] Aside from working out of an outbuilding in his back yard[38] as his primary office, Rex had also opened an office in Allentown, where he held regular hours,[39] and according to oral history in Slatedale,[40] he also made house calls from a horse-drawn medicine

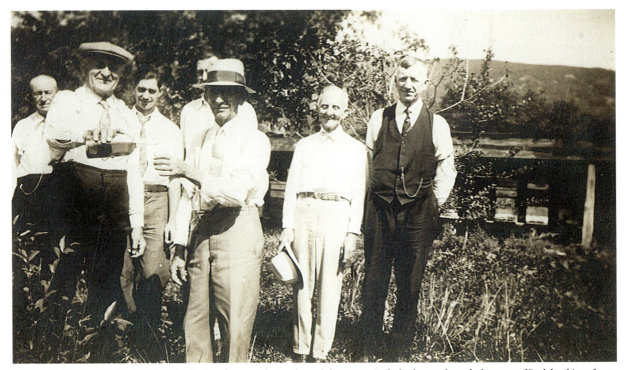

Left: Dennis Rex (far right) and his friends, sharing a beverage during the prohibition era. In the background stand a long row of Rex's bee hives, from which he derived some of his cures. *Courtesy of the Rev. Brian Haas and Family.*

Opposite, above: Mrs. Emma (Krum) Rex, ca. 1920. Below: Dennis Rex and his granddaughter Lillie Kerschner. standing by the porch of his house at the foot of the Blue Mountain in Slatedale. *Courtesy of the Rev. Brian Haas and Family.*

wagon. Both his wagon and his offices were quite private, and this sense of secrecy, as well as the fact that most of his clients were women, raised many concerns from jealous husbands who were suspicious of his practices.[41] Rumor had it that, in addition to occasionally supplying herbal compounds to induce abortions, Rex was also in high demand for his "honey treatments" sourced from his own bees, which he himself applied for women's reproductive issues.[42] It was because of this that Rex's activities were reported to the authorities, who were notified that he was breaking up homes. One local woman in particular vowed that she would rather leave her husband than stop seeing Rex for treatment.[43]

Despite these cases of marital issues, Rex was held in high esteem by both men and women alike in his community. Those who took the stand in his defense in 1914 were described as believing "religiously" in Rex's healing,[44] so that the District Attorney struggled to extract incriminating testimony.[45]

Rex's accusation of necromancy was not without precedent, as demonstrated by the case of Dr. Hageman of Reading, and was based in the Pennsylvania Legislation of 1861: "an act for suppression of fortune telling and similar purposes, and those who shall for gain or lucre pretend to affect any purpose by spells, charms necromancy, or incantations, shall be guilty of a misdemeanor."[46]

Dennis Rex was acquitted, however, on account of a highly convincing statement from his defense attorney, George A. Miller, who cleverly invoked the controversy of Christian Science to his advantage. At the time, Christian Science was the fasted growing religion in the United States,[47] and two of the members of the jury were Christian Scientists. Miller stated that if Rex were found guilty of a crime on the basis of powwowing, then it would set a precedent enabling the courts to likewise bring criminal charges against adherents of Christian Science for practicing their own brand of religious healing. Whether these two members of the jury were able to sway the outcome or whether it was because the heated debate took all night, in the end Rex was fined $107 in court costs and was sent on his way. Judge Groman apparently admonished the jury for their decision, calling Rex a "charlatan," warning him that if he were to turn up in court again, he would be sentenced without a jury.[48]

Rex nevertheless continued his practice virtually unhindered, and was somewhat of a celebrity personality because of his brush with the law. A Pennsylvania Dutch dialect columnist from the Allentown *Morning Call*, writing under the pseudonym Obediah Grouthomel (cabbage-head, dolt) featured Rex as the butt-end of a joke in a humorous tale about Hen Blose the farmer and "Schtuckey" Wannamacher the Tax collector:

> *Now der Hen Blose wase immer ebbes; er wase fiel sacha os net so sin ow'r er komt oft noch Allentown un do kon mer all arta sacha uf picka. Er hot kertzlich die rumatism kot, udder war's der gout? Er hot so grossa schmerza kot os ken doctor ihm ma helfa hot kenna, no het er for der Dr. Dennis Rex g'schickt un mit hond uf laga un mit schtondhafter glawva is es glei besser werra.*
>
> Now Hen Blose always knew something; he knew many things that weren't so, but he often came to Allentown and here one can pick up all sorts of stuff. He got rheumatism recently, that no doctor could help him, then he sent for the Doctor Dennis Rex, and with the laying on of hands and steadfast belief, it got better right away.[49]

The Humorist Obediah Grouthomel wasn't the only person who disapproved of Dennis Rex and doubted the sincerity and efficacy of his powwowing. In the years to follow his acquittal in 1914, he was subjected to repeated lawsuits, many of which were based in his relations to female clients and patients that took personal issue with him and alleged sexual misconduct.

In 1929, controversy struck yet again, as Dennis Rex was accused of being the father of a child with a 22-year-old woman named Carrie P. Ziegenfuss, whose mother was a regular patient of Rex for two years until her death

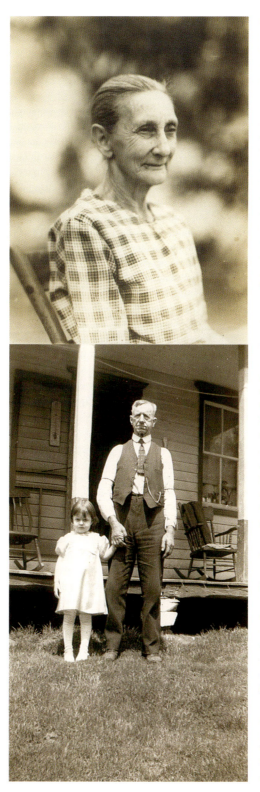

from cancer. Ziegenfuss claimed that Rex had told her that his treatment of her mother's cancer would only be effective if they had relations together, occurring twice a week at the time of her mother's cancer treatments, when he would visit their home in Little Gap, Carbon County. The child was born on April 9, 1929.[50] Although a jury was selected, and the trial was scheduled in Carbon County courts, a settlement was reached outside of court and the charges were subsequently dropped. No details of the settlement were disclosed and Dennis Rex's powwowing continued unaffected by the charges.[51]

Again in 1930, Rex was accused of assault and battery by a woman named Mrs. Charles Winters, who had consulted with Rex about a ritual means to secure her husband's bail from prison. Charles Winters had been arrested on charges of larceny and had been awaiting trial. Mrs. Winters claimed that on August 22, Rex had uttered mysterious words, and then took her to the backyard where she underwent "antics termed, in the least, undignified" and was taken to an outbuilding where she was allegedly assaulted, resulting in an injury to her back.[52]

Although coverage in the local papers appeared to favor Mrs. Winters' initial testimony, the charges were quickly dismissed on the grounds of insufficient evidence.[53] Dennis's wife, Mrs. Emma Rex testified that she and two young girls had hidden behind a shrubbery and had witnessed the whole incident. One of the girls was her granddaughter, Lillie Kerschner, who also testified in court that Dennis had done nothing to harm the woman. Mrs. Rex reported that Mrs. Winters had appeared two days prior the alleged assault, and that she had not looked kindly upon the manner of her visit, prompting her to keep watch when she visited a second time. Following the testimony of Rex, his wife, and granddaughter, the charges were dropped and the case was dismissed.[54]

Although Rex made no more appearances in court, and was not the subject of articles in the local papers thereafter until the time of his death in 1944, the latter portion of his career was by no means uneventful. At the same time that he fended off criticism and allegations from former clients, Dennis Rex was also in the middle of a feud with another local practitioner, a chiropractor and powwower named Joseph "Doc" Kuntz, who operated out of Allentown.

Doc Kuntz was not a licensed chiropractor by today's standards, but was a college educated practitioner of chiropractic medicine, who specialized in an eclectic array of alternative medical practices. He was known to perform "psychic surgery" and to powwow remotely using the telephone. Doc Kuntz' son Mark, who later became a licensed chiropractor himself, recalled traveling with his father to obtain a copy of a mysterious book from a minister in Philadelphia.[55]

In one account of his ritual surgeries, Kuntz recited verbal blessings while unfolding white towels over the abdomen of a man suffering from severe stomach ulcers. Although Kuntz used no surgical implements and made no incisions, the patient claimed that it felt as though Kuntz had entered his body cavity near his stomach and performed a procedure that resulted in a full recovery from his chronic symptoms.

Such dramatic and seemingly cutting-edge ritual practices were in direct competition with Rex, who also had a practice in Allentown. Allegedly, the rivalry grew so intense that Rex placed a *Hex* on Doc Kuntz by placing a series of stones in a large circle around the perimeter of the Kuntz property. Kuntz became aware of the stones and placed them all in a metal canister, punched with holes. He sank the canister in the dark waters of a nearby slate quarry, and rumor had it that Dennis Rex began to immediately suffer from edema and swelling in his legs.[56]

Dennis Rex died on February 15, 1944 without passing on his knowledge or practice to any relatives or associates in the vicinity. His medicine wagon, presumably auctioned with the rest of his movable property at his farm sale that April[57] stood parked at a property in Slatedale for decades after his passing, as an all but forgotten, local monument to his legacy as a healer.

Dennis Rex was one of many healers whose biography was defined by controversy documented by the media, rather than by any initiative of his own. The fact that powwowers did not often actively participate in the telling of their own stories is a central feature of these early twentieth century accounts. This lack of agency demonstrates that these narratives tell less about the healers and their patients and more about their critic's biases and beliefs.

The "Hex-Murder" of Nelson Rehmeyer

On Thanksgiving of 1928, the braying of an unfed mule led neighbors to the discovery of the body of a powwow practitioner, Nelson D. Rehmeyer (1868-1928), in his blood-spattered home in North Hopewell Township, York County. His body had been severely beaten, bound in ropes, and burned the evening two days prior by a trio of young men, seeking to end a curse that the victim had allegedly placed by means of obtaining a lock of his hair or his paperback copy of Hohman's *Long Lost Friend*.[58] This tragic event ignited not only one of the most infamous series of murder trials in the history of Pennsylvania, but also the most widely publicized attempt to eradicate the ritual healing traditions of the Pennsylvania Dutch.

The killers were charismatic powwow dabbler John H. Blymire (also spelled Blymyre) (1895-1972), and two youthful accomplices, John C. Curry (1904-1963) and Wilbert G. Hess (1910-1979), aged 14 and 18 at the time of the slaying. The thirty-three year old Blymire was the only one of the three who personally knew Nelson Rehmeyer in any capacity, and their personal connection was through powwowing. Rehmeyer was one of a long list of practitioners that had treated John for an acute adult case of *Abnemme* – literally wasting, or "pining away."[59] Blymire's difficulties had begun early in his life, and some sources indicate that Nelson had treated him for childhood illnesses as well and had later employed the boy to help on the farm with harvesting potatoes.[60] Little did he know that Blymire would later blame him for unexplained illness, and kill him in cold blood.

Descended from three generations of male powwow practitioners, Blymire had shown an aptitude for healing in his early years, but was later subject to severe emotional and mental collapse, so that he was unable to sleep, work, or lead a productive life. Blymire's older sister Helga had suffered a similar collapse after "seeing visions" and died in a county home for the mentally disabled.[61] Blymire sought help from numerous doctors, who diagnosed him with a nervous disorder called "hypochondriacal melancholia,"[62] characterized by depression, obsessive ideas, hallucinations and illusions.[63] At least one doctor treated Blymire with electroshock therapy, but he turned again to powwowing after conventional treatments proved ineffective. Believing that a curse was responsible for his condition, he gradually developed a paranoia that would later poison his familial relations and drive him to murder.[64]

Attempting to lead a normal life, Blymire married Lilly Belle Alloway (1900-1986), the daughter of one of his landlords but their marriage was marked by tragedy, and they lost two of their three children, Richard H. and Josephine L. Blymire.[65] Stricken with grief and suspecting that the death of his children was further evidence of his curse, his behavior became so unpredictable and verging on violence, that his father-in-law took him to the York County Almshouse for examination in 1923. The county's psychiatric doctor committed him to the Harrisburg State Hospital, where he stayed for four months but eventually escaped while attending a baseball game with the other patients.[66] No one pursued Blymire immediately following his escape. When he returned home, his fits of violence became so intense that his wife had him arrested and taken into custody. Authorities from the state asylum were allegedly still looking for him, but having little cooperation with police at the time, they were unable to locate him because he was in the county jail. A year after his disappearance from the asylum, his case was considered closed, and he was officially discharged by default.[67]

Upon his release from prison, Blymire kept his distance from his family, and his wife officially divorced him. Afterwards, he became a drifter, taking up residence in rented rooms in York City, and spending a significant portion of his time on the road. He traveled a circuit to the most renowned powwow doctors in the region including Andrew Lenhart of Reading and Dr. Genzler of Oley, Emma Knapp of Marietta, and Samuel Schmuck, Rufus Murray, Charles Dice, and Nelson Rehmeyer of York County.[68] He sought treatment for his persistent suffering from his perceived curse, which made him unable to consistently sleep, work, or eat, with a resulting loss of weight and overall agitation.

When he was able to work, he did piece-work for a local cigar factory in Red Lion and later in East York, and during this time began to powwow again for his coworkers in the factory as well as for friends and the general public. His landlords were used to the late-night traffic of powwow clients arriving for treatment at all hours, and some even reported that he powwowed under a pseudonym as John Albright.[69]

At the cigar factory in East York, Blymire made the acquaintance of fellow cigar-roller, John Curry, a strong and capable young man who struck out on his own at the age of thirteen with no more than an eighth-grade education. Curry had fled the home of his alcoholic step-father who physically abused him, and suffered tremendously from his estrangement from his family. He described symptoms similar to Blymire's – he had become thin and weak, and couldn't sleep or eat – until Blymire powwowed for him. Curry would later recall, "if it had not been for Dr. Blymire, I would be dead by this time."[70]

The summer of 1928 marked a turning point for Blymire and his mysterious disease. After a long series of visits to a powwower and fortune-teller in Marietta named Emma Knapp (1855-1933),[71] Blymire became convinced that Nelson D. Rehmeyer had cursed him. Knapp was able to provide traditional powwowing treatments, but Blymire consulted her instead for information regarding the origin of his disorder, and for this she turned to a repertoire of rituals for divination.

A sensational depiction of the slayers of Nelson Rehmeyer, John Blymire (center) Wilbert Hess (Right) and John Curry (Left), and images suggesting the occult from *The Sixth and Seventh Books of Moses*. Inset is a small illustration of the dollar-bill divination trick used to identify Rehmeyer as the source of Blymire's Hex. Clipping from *The Reaing Times, Wednesday, January 9, 1928.*

245

Although frequently a reader of cards, Knapp employed a common parlor trick for which she utilized a dollar bill to show Blymire the source of the *Hex*. Placing the image of George Washington face-up over the palm of Blymire's hand, Knapp recited an incantation, and then told Blymire to remove the dollar bill and gaze into his palm. As if by magic, the dark image of a face appeared in Blymire's palm, which he immediately recognized as the face of Nelson Rehmeyer.[72]

This dollar bill trick is no supernatural display of power, but a common phenomenon known as an afterimage, and it is produced by retinal fatigue. By staring at any image long enough, one will see the image in reverse coloration on a neutral surface. Thus the image of the light-haired George Washington found on the one dollar bill will produce a reverse afterimage as a dark-haired figure with a dark area like a long beard corresponding directly to the white shirt and collar of the first president.[73] Ironically, this image of Washington in reverse coloration appears not unlike the bearded portraits of Nelson Rehmeyer that appeared in local papers after his slaying. Emma Knapp's advice to Blymire was to destroy the curse by means of obtaining a lock of Nelson Rehmeyer's hair and his copy of Hohman's *Long Lost Friend* and to bury them eight feet below the soil.[74]

Also in the summer of 1928, at the same time that Blymire had been visiting with Emma Knapp, he had begun a series of powwowing consultations for the family of Milton Hess at Leader's Heights, near York. Milton believed that the family had been subjected to a curse. Starting in 1926, the family's farm took a turn for the worse with poor yields from crops and livestock, as well as illness among the family. The family initially suspected that their ill-fortune had been caused by their neighbor Ida J. Hess, sister-in-law of Milton Hess, with whom they were actively engaged in a property line dispute. Blymire, going under the pseudonym "John Albright", out of fear from being pursued by the State asylum,[75] convinced the Hess family that they were also victims of Nelson Rehmeyer, who had supposedly been hired by Ida.

Although no one in the family had any direct contact with Rehmeyer, nor had they any reason to suspect a motive for the supposed *Hex*, they believed in Blymire's testimony and engaged his services with a deposit of $10 to assist them in removing the curse.[76] Blymire powwowed for the whole family, and even performed a ritual to find their lost chickens and to restore milk to their cows but to no avail.[77] Blymire would later claim that the $10 was given to him to retrieve a "Queen Elizabeth Root" (Orris root) from the York powwow doctor Samuel Schmuck for the purpose of driving out witches from the house, but he never had the chance to purchase the root.[78]

On Monday evening, November, 26th, 1928, Blymire went with John Curry to gather information at Rehmeyer's Hollow. The hollow was a long dirt farm lane in North Hopewell Township, with a series of properties settled by the Rehmeyer family, descended from early nineteenth-century German-speaking immigrants whose descendants numbered over 400 in the region by the time of the incident.[79] Nelson Rehmeyer was a potato farmer, and due to a recent separation with his wife over his powwowing practice had become somewhat reclusive. On the night of Blymire's visit with Curry, Rehmeyer was not home, so the two men stopped at the home of Alice C. Rehmeyer (1878-1944), who lived with their two children, Beatrice and Florence, just a mile away, and maintained regular contact with him, despite their separation. Alice knew Blymire as a child, and at one time she had been a member of the same church as his mother Agnes.[80] Blymire inquired with Alice about her husband's whereabouts, and she replied that he was likely at the home of a woman named Emma Gladfelter, where Nelson had recently been spending much of his time and called him a "devilish old cock."[81]

Alice Rehmeyer's outburst about her husband was not only due to her suspicions of infidelity, but also a general disapproval of his powwowing activities. She had moved out of the Rehmeyer farm with her two daughters after she was no longer willing to

Above: A comparison of the image of Nelson Rehmeyer and the inverted image of George Washington from a 1928 one dollar bill. *The Evening News*, Harrisburg, Pennsylvania, Saturday, Dec 1 1928.

tolerate the disruptions of clients and strangers coming regularly at strange hours to the home to be powwowed. Rehmeyer was also an ardent socialist, whose ideas were unpopular with his neighbors, and socialist posters and literature were visible throughout the house.[82] Blymire and Curry's inquiry with Alice concerning Rehmeyer's whereabouts was what later allowed authorities to positively identify them as Rehmeyer's killers.

Following the short visit with Alice that evening, Blymire and Curry stopped one last time at Rehmeyer's house, and by this time he was home. Blymire claimed to have been treated by Rehmeyer at least a year prior for his illness, so his stopping by at night was not looked upon unfavorably. Rehmeyer welcomed them into his kitchen and stayed up late talking with Blymire about "the book" – his copy of Hohman's *Long Lost Friend*. Although Blymire never saw Rehmeyer's copy, it was allegedly a paperback pulp edition from the turn of the century, likely printed in Philadelphia or Chicago.[83]

Although the visit was friendly on the surface, Blymire had previously informed Curry and Hess that he would ritually "work on Rehmeyer's mind"[84] in an attempt to overpower Rehmeyer, who was too large to physically subdue under normal circumstances. Although Curry and Blymire had secretly brought rope with them with the intention of tying him to cut a lock of his hair, they made no attempt to do so, as the odds were clearly in Rehmeyer's favor. Instead, they gave no indication of their intentions. Rehmeyer was a generous host, allowing Blymire and Curry to spend the night in the kitchen and feeding them breakfast the next morning.

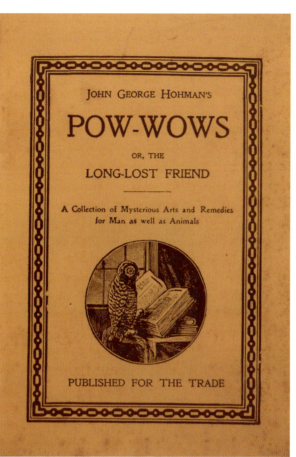

A turn-of-the-century pulp edition of John George Hohman's *Long Lost Friend*, just like the edition allegedly owned by Nelson Rehmeyer. Heilman Collection.

Blymire immediately returned to the Hess Family and called upon them for reinforcements. As Blymire and Curry were no match for Rehmeyer, Milton Hess sent his eighteen-year-old son Wilbert along, believing that their mission would result in the removal of the family's curse. That evening the three men were taken to the Hollow by Wilbert's brother Clayton, who drove them in his car and dropped them off a short distance from Rehmeyer's house.[85] They approached Rehmeyer's home and knocked on the door. Blymire asked to be admitted under the pretense of having forgotten something from the previous evening, and while Rehmeyer fumbled with a flashlight, the emboldened Blymire seized him, initiating his haphazard plan to obtain a lock of hair. What had started off as a quest to secure the means to ritual atonement quickly became a clumsy and frantic fight to the death, with Blymire leading the charge against the physically superior Rehmeyer, and shouting orders to his accomplices. Although none of the defendants had intended to kill Rehmeyer, the robust farmer was not easy prey, and excessive force was employed to subdue him. The accounts of what transpired were later related by the assailants, all of whom told a different variation of the events – and none of them could agree on precisely who had dealt the final blow. By the time that Rehmeyer was dead, he had been bound with ropes around his neck, arms and legs, and beaten with a chair and piece of firewood. In the midst of the pandemonium, no one ever bothered to cut a lock of hair from Rehmeyer's head, but instead took money from him and attempted to conceal the evidence of their crime.

First they poured water around the scene in a mistaken attempt to eliminate fingerprints, then poured kerosene over Rehmeyer's body, and ignited a straw mattress. For any number of reasons, the fire sprung up long enough for the three assailants to run from the scene, but the fire went out and never consumed the evidence, the body, or the house.

Blymire claimed to have seen a ghostly image of Rehmeyer standing in the flames as they fled, suggesting to some that Rehmeyer may have been merely unconscious when the fire was lit.[86] Nevertheless, Blymire, Curry, and Hess walked back to the Hess' home, hoping that the fire would obliterate the whole incident and allow them to escape their deeds.

Within 24 hours, Wilbert had already confessed to his family what had happened, and Rehmeyer's neighbors alerted the authorities two days later after checking on his unfed livestock. Alice Rehmeyer informed investigators of the visit from Blymire, and in the end it was a fellow powwower, Charles W. Dice of Poplar Street, York, who cooperated with authorities to locate Blymire and his accomplice John Curry.[87] Once in custody, Blymire made a series of fragmented statements about his improvement in health since the death of Rehmeyer, suggesting that the curse was lifted.

> Blymire is tranquil. His mind is at rest and he can sleep, he says, because the 'hex' which he says Rehmeyer had put on him was broken with Rehmeyer's death. Blymire failed to obtain the lock of Rehmeyer's hair, which he wanted as a charm to break the 'hex,' because the hair was bloody. But the death of Rehmeyer has had the desired effect.[88]

As the three suspects were prepared for trial and the story went public, newspapers from across the nation focused attention on the ritual motives, unleashing a media frenzy, hungry for any information on powwowing in the region. Scathing headlines attributed the killing to a cult and decried powwowing as a deceptive and predatory practice. These accounts conflated the terms "powwowing," "witchcraft," "voodooism" and "hex" as interchangeable terms with absolutely no regard for their distinctive meanings, and vilified the "ignorance" and "superstition" of the Pennsylvania Dutch of York County.[89] Dubbed "The Hex-Murder," the incident placed the word "*Hex*" into the general American vocabulary as synonymous with "witchcraft" (*Hexerei*) – when in fact the word referred more specifically to the curse that Blymire perceived, or the action of cursing. Thus the use of "*Hex*" in popular parlance of the time (and even among some in the present day) is sometimes marked by the awkward lack of an article, "the" or "a," producing statements like "It is difficult to describe 'hex'..."[90] – a statement which would sound equally ridiculous if the word "curse" were used instead. Such clumsy newspaper accounts focused on exposing powwowing and *Hexerei* to edify an international audience eager to learn of the persistence of "witchcraft" in the twentieth century. Such efforts had begun long before Rehmeyer's murder,[91] but the deluge of media attention emphasized the "York Hex Murder" as the ultimate incident of its kind. Legal historian J. Ross McGinnis described the media attention: "Never before had the York community been swallowed up in a daily avalanche of publicity that was as critical as it was unrelenting."[92]

Handwritten blessings from the personal papers of John H. Blymire, reproduced in the *Philadelphia Inquirer,* Dec 2, 1928.

Such national attention resulted in the reclusive Rehmeyer's funeral hosting over 500 people in the modestly sized sanctuary at St. John's Saddler's Lutheran Church located between Stewartstown and Shrewsbury. The Rev. Bowersox delivered a funeral sermon that was intended both as a comfort to the family, and as a cautionary tale to the community:

It is not our purpose here today to discuss the motives of the crime that brings us here. Nor is it our mission to judge either the living or the dead. We are not called upon to rehearse any of the ugly details of the crime against this man as we gather here. The general light of the community is far above anything we see as the motive given in the confession of the three that have been arrested. Whatever the purpose may have been back of the deed, it is the work of sin and the assailants are prompted by the devil. We are here because of the sinfulness of hard men. We pray on behalf of those because of whose crime and sin we come together, and pray that they may see the light and repent. While much could be found in the world that is of sin and death one of the greatest sorrows of the tragedy was that such a thing is possible in this community...The evil spirit must be wiped out by prompt action on the part of the authorities, that we may not practice evil arts and that we shall follow him who said, 'I am the light of the world.' [93]

While Rev. Bowersox's homily aimed to help his congregation come to terms with the heinous murder through the lens of Christian forgiveness, his sentiments were later echoed by local authorities who were eager to portray the county of York as being above the crime – sometimes through the exclusion of the social context of the crime.

Prosecutor and District Attorney Amos Herrmann admitted that although "powwowing was not necessarily dangerous, the falling of this so-called art into the hands of these men make them a public menace." He went on to officially declare: "I'm going to make a desperate effort to drive these men out of the county, and if we can secure any kind of information against them, they will be prosecuted."[94] At the same time that these threats were made against powwowing practitioners in York County, Herrmann also attempted to obstruct any mention of the words "powwow" or "hex" from the trial of Blymire and his two accomplices, despite the fact that their motives were already clearly established.[95]

The district attorney instead cited the few coins, amounting to a mere three dollars that were taken from Rehmeyer on the night of the incident, as evidence of robbery as the true motive and demanded death or imprisonment for the three men.[96]

As the investigation of the Rehmeyer murder progressed, another York murder case that had previously been unsolved also was brought to the forefront because of a confession from one of Blymire's landlords about his powwowing activities. On November 11, 1927, 16-year-old Gertrude Rudy had been found on the railroad tracks near the border between York County and Maryland, her body described by police as "mutilated" with a wound from a shotgun fired at close range and a crushed skull from the stock of the weapon. The body had been carried there by a car and placed on the tracks in order to destroy the evidence of the murder. She had been pregnant at the time of the murder. Ruby had been a friend of Blymire, who worked in the same factory, and he attended her funeral. According to his landlord, Ruby frequently called the house asking for "John Albright" and she also made visits to his upstairs room alone to be powwowed.[97] Authorities suspected that Blymire was powwowing her in relation to her pregnancy, or that he may have been intimate with her.[98]

Blymire denied any intimacy with Gertrude Rudy, as well as any connection to the murder, citing his inability to operate a car as his alibi. This latter fact was later disputed by the son of Blymire's landlord, who reported that Blymire had rented a car, was not at home the night of the murder, and returned at 3 o'clock the following morning.[99] Despite Blymire's conflicting testimony, police pursued the possibility of Blymire's involvement no further, and although several other suspects were later detained, the murder has never been solved.[100]

The Nelson Rehmeyer homicide trials began on January 7th, 1929, and York County Judge Sherwood and President Judge Niles initially attempted to suppress media coverage of the trial, by declaring that they would limit the number of seats reserved for the press box to only four individuals in the courtroom. This action favored the local newspapers with two of the four seats, sending a message to outsiders that sparked a controversy over the freedom of the press.[101] In the end, all newspaper correspondents were admitted to the courtroom, and while four representatives were given reserved seating, no one was barred from attending the trial.[102]

Because of an appeal from John Blymire's defense Attorney Herbert Cohen, the three defendants were tried separately, in an attempt to acquit Blymire on the grounds of an insanity plea, or at the very least to reduce his sentence. Although at least one physician in the county pronounced Blymire perfectly sane,[103] two other doctors strongly disagreed. Another York physician testified that Blymire was indeed insane for the span of six years or more, and a doctor familiar with Blymire from his brief stay in the State Hospital for the Insane described him as "a feeble-minded, undeveloped individual" unable to distinguish right from wrong."[104]

The prosecution aimed to portray the murder in a different light, that the backdrop of Hexerei was only a veneer to a home invasion and robbery gone wrong. Despite District Attorney Herrmann's repeated objections to any mention of powwowing or witchcraft, eventually the story of Blymire's presumed curse came to the forefront and was central in the defendants' testimony and the testimony of others.[105] By the third day, however, this admission was of no assistance to the defense, and Blymire was found guilty of first-degree murder and sentenced to life in prison on January 9, 1929.

Blymire's response to his attorney, however, was one of relief. Blymire said to Cohen, "I'm happy now, I'm not bewitched anymore, I can sleep and eat, and I am not pining away – the hex is broke and the witch is dead – but I think they went a little strong – yes, that's it – a little too strong."[106] He had narrowly escaped the electric chair, so commonly used in capital punishment of the time, and would later serve only a portion of his life sentence.

John Curry's trial commenced the following day, with former district attorney Walter W. Van Baman as Curry's court appointed defense.[107] Unfortunately for Curry, there was no excuse of insanity, and no distraction from the murder narrative by personal affliction from a perceived curse like that of Blymire. Curry had youth on his side, but he was precocious, with a clear memory of the events of the murder that did not work in his favor to produce the illusion of innocence. Curry had remarked that he had come along "to see some of this witchcraft performed," and that both he and Blymire wore gloves to conceal their finger prints.[108] In the end, he became one of the youngest Pennsylvanians to be convicted of first-degree murder and sentenced to life in prison.[109]

The final trial, of Wilbert Hess began the same day that Curry was sentenced, but would later take a more compassionate tone than the preceding trials of his comrades. His defense lawyer was Harvey Gross, who had represented Wilbert's father Milton Hess as his attorney for over the course of twenty years. He reluctantly accepted the role of Wilbert's defense, and called it "one of the most distasteful cases of [his] life."[110] Gross carefully orchestrated his arguments around a compelling narrative that Wilbert was had not willingly joined the trio that killed Nelson Rehmeyer, but rather was sent by his family to free them from their *Hex*.

Unlike the previous defense attorneys, Gross made a serious impression on the jury and the public. Philadelphia correspondent John McCullough would later describe his closing remarks as "an extraordinary situation, majestic in its immensity and in the tribute which it paid to the humanity, the lucidity, and the pulsing sincerity of the little gray-eyed York County lawyer, Harvey A. Gross."[111]

Instead of relying on Wilbert's age, Gross wisely conjured a narrative that portrayed Wilbert as a "sacrificial lamb" – sent forth into uncertain and dangerous circumstances in the dark of night to deliver the family from their misfortune. After successfully presenting this emotionally charged narrative, Gross concluded the trial by drawing a broader parallel to the whole community and County of York. Appealing to the consciences of the members of the jury, he urged justice for Wilbert, rather further sacrifice.

> York county ought not to feel that it has to be vindicated of a spot – a spot of superstition. It does not have to draw the last drop of blood from this boy's heart, nor wring tears from the throat and break the heart of his mother, merely in order show the world that we do not believe in witchcraft and powwow.[112]

Hess was found guilty of second degree murder and sentenced to 10-20 years imprisonment. He would later be the only one of the three to serve his full sentence of ten years, as both Blymire and Curry had their sentences commuted. Curry was imprisoned for only ten years of his life sentence, and later joined the military, where he became a cartographer in General Eisenhower's staff. He assisted in drafting the maps of the invasion of Normandy.[113] Blymire was released in 1953, and became a night watchman in Philadelphia until 1965. His life escaped further notice by the press until his death in 1972.[114]

Anti-Powwow Crusades

Ironically, throughout the trial, the media continued to proudly proclaim that the incident had generated enough momentum to launch a statewide prosecution of all practitioners of powwow. These stories came to a head in December 1928 in the weeks following the death of Nelson Rehmeyer, when reports were issued from Harrisburg that the State Board of Medical Examination and Licensure would be taking action "to suppress the activities of powwow practitioners in the southeastern counties of the state."[115] State Inspector Charles N. Fry offered the following statement prior to the announcement of the State's initiative:

> There are no doubt many powwowers against whom it will be impossible to find evidence that they had diagnosed, prescribed, or charged fees in connection with healing rites. Many of these are old-time powwowers who do not make a profession of healing and only try their skill occasionally. But there are others who have practiced wholesale frauds and it is these whom we intend to get.

However, no report was ever produced, and the announcement was never followed with any plan of action. It appeared as though this state agency was merely conducting business as usual. It was surely under the agency's purview to identify any practitioners who violated the laws outlined by inspector Fry, and to turn their names over to authorities. In fact, this was not an unusual or irregular occurrence, and had nothing whatsoever to do with the homicide of Nelson Rehmeyer.

As quickly as this bubble of bureaucratic and media attention swelled, it just as rapidly deflated, leaving behind a series of dangling news reports which promised a monumental "Federal Powwow Probe" with absolutely no follow up.

This vacuum was quickly filled, however, with a long-running media fascination with any death or homicide connected with mysterious or ritual elements. Following on the footsteps of the sentencing of the murderers of Nelson Rehmeyer, a new story came to light within two months. The body of 21-year-old Verna Octavia Delp of Farmersville, Northampton County, was discovered in a field near the gun club in Catasauqua, Lehigh County. Delp was pregnant at the time of her death, and was carrying protective inscriptions, created for her by a powwow practitioner named Charles T. Belles of Allentown. Authorities believed that she had been poisoned.[116] Verna lived with foster parents, and had been visiting several powwow doctors on account of both her concealed pregnancy and the belief that she required protection from spirits.

Rumors circulated that Belles, known for treating women seeking to "avoid maternity," had administered medicine to her that resulted in her death.[117] The newspapers prematurely reported that a warrant was obtained for Belles' arrest, alerting him and his family prior to his actual arrest.[118] Thus, Belles was held for over a month, while chemists unsuccessfully tested samples taken from Verna Delp's body for poisons. Being unable to produce any trace evidence to suggest that Delp had been poisoned, or that Belles had any role in her death, the courts of Allentown were petitioned to grant a speedy trial in a habeas corpus writ.[119] Eventually the charges were dropped due to a lack of sufficient evidence.[120] The murder was never solved, perhaps because so much energy was spent in an attempt to prove that the crime was related to powwowing than in searching for additional evidence.

Although numerous cases of "hex murders" and other media sensations occurred throughout the 1930s, one of the most horrific incidents involved the killing of powwow practitioner Mrs. Susan Mummey, of Ferndale, near Ringtown, Schuylkill County, who was shot by an obsessed young man. Described as clean-cut and intelligent, 24-year-old Albert Shinsky of nearby Shenandoah confessed to authorities that he suffered from a seven-year curse laid by Mummey, and admitted to killing her with a 12-gauge shotgun fired through the window of her home. He had worked on an adjacent farm and claimed that Mummey had hexed him with her stare, and later visited him regularly in the form of a demonic cat that would torture him while he slept.

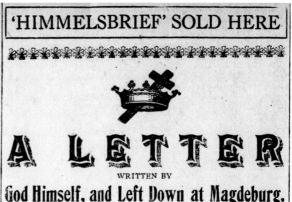

A copy of a *Himmelsbrief* carried by a Reading minister who carried it with him while campaigning against powwowing. *Reading Times*, Dec 25, 1928.

Shinsky suffered from hallucinations, and, like John Blymire, from undiagnosed mental illness.[121]

His story of the cat however, was part of a series of local tales of the supernatural that had begun two decades earlier with the "Hex Cat of Tumbling Run," near Orwigsburg, Schuylkill County. The story ran in local papers across the United States[122] in 1911 and 1912, and outlined the story of the family of Howell Thomas, who claimed to have been plagued by a shape-shifting, "Hex Cat."[123] Howell died as his farm went to wreck and ruin reportedly under the influence of the cat, and his daughter Mary accused her sister living in Orwigsburg of being responsible. This accusation took place at their father's funeral.[124] The sister had allegedly conjured a demon taking the form of the cat, and Mary Thomas and her uncle William were instructed by a hex-doctor to shoot the cat with a bullet made of gold. The cat failed to appear when the bullet was at the ready.

The plot thickened when a man from Schuylkill Haven brought his cat to the Thomas family for aid. A local hex-doctor had deemed his cat to be a "hexahemeron cat,"[125] born on the 6th day of the 6th month in 1906, the sixth of a litter of six, which open its eyes on the 6th day after birth (all other cats, alleged the owner, open their eyes on day nine). Citing the lore of *The Sixth and Seventh Books of Moses*, the owner claimed that the cat was good for warding off all evil and regularly ate serpents and toads.[126]

The Hexahemeron Cat was of no avail, and a neighbor named Charles Lawless eventually captured the feline by throwing a Bible at it. The cat was placed in a steel cage, and exhibited in the storefront window of a business in Pottsville.[127] Thousands of people allegedly came to see the cat before it escaped, and was later found frozen to death on a farm neighboring the Thomas residence.[128]

When murders and demonic cats were in short supply, stories of sick people who died after having been treated by powwowers were the next-best source of media attention. Words like "manslaughter" would appear in such headlines, claiming that powwowers were responsible for death because their

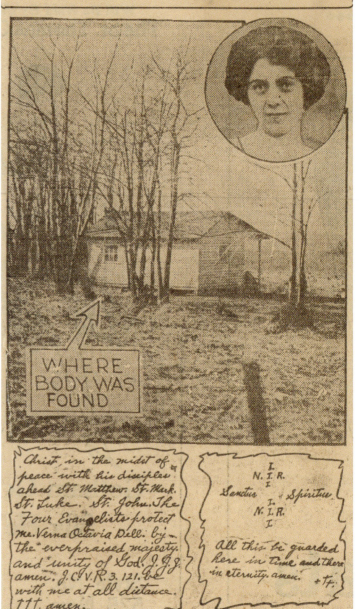

National News coverage of the Verna Delp mystery, dubbed a "Hex Murder" by authorities, showing pictures of her portrait, the location where her body was discovered, and the blessings found on her body. Powwower Charles Belles was accused of poisoning her, but he was acquitted due to a lack of evidence. *Battle Creek Moon Journal.* Battle Creek, Michigan, Friday Mar 29, 1929.

patients had not sought conventional treatments in a timely manner. These types of cases were often easily put to rest, as practitioners could be fined or imprisoned for practicing medicine without a license as a misdemeanor, but healers were not held responsible for the choices made by patients to avoid conventional treatments.[129]

A sideline at the time of the "York Hex Murders" was a widely circulated rumor that "scores" of infants died each year from the negligence of parents who trusted in powwow treatments over conventional doctors.[130] Such reports even found their way into *The New York Times*, and were cited as evidence of the dangers of powwowing in numerous articles over the course of a decade, including the case of Verna Delp.[131]

The York County Medical Society would prove to be the source of the inflation of these statements, and Dr. P. A. Noll, secretary of the Society, gave the following statement to the *Philadelphia Record* on December 4, 1928, shortly after the murder of Nelson Rehmeyer, in "Leaders of civic organizations, women's clubs, and nursing societies open a war of propaganda and education on "Pow wowism"[sic]:

> There is no doubt that the deaths of scores of children can be laid at the door of the 'pow wow' practitioners… in a few cases, convictions have been obtained… it is next to impossible to obtain evidence because of the superstitious dread with which the followers of these men regard them… I do not believe a jury could be obtained which would not include half a dozen jurors who would fear the 'hex' too much to permit them to return a verdict against the defendant.[132]

York County Coroner L. V. Zech, often cited as the source of the information, would later describe this rumor as "ridiculous," stating that "I don't really believe that any children died here from 'pow-wowing.' Those who are listed expired because they had not the proper medical attention, not because [of] their families' belief in 'pow-wowing.' Such cases as I now refer to number three or four."[133]

Nevertheless, such exaggerated stories became the mainstay of the anti-powwowing crusades that continued through the 1930s. Although medical societies claimed a moral prerogative to eradicate superstitious beliefs, this campaign was beyond the scope of law. There never was any organized effort by law enforcement or the judicial system to target powwow practitioners beyond the scope of medical licensing. Civic organizations then turned to allies in the educational sector to provide anti-powwowing and anti-superstition educational programs to regional schools.

Such programs aimed to draw attention to in a wide variety of popular beliefs like fear of black cats and walking under ladders as a means to discredit non-scientific thinking, while powwowing was ridiculed and presented as a dangerous perception.[134] Parody illustrations of powwowing were found in local newspapers, depicting practitioners as classic images of witches, and dubious caricatures of patients mocked the Amish of Lancaster County. While many of these zealous efforts appear petty and laughable by today's standards, there is no telling how effective these efforts were in eradicating or suppressing folk beliefs on a local level.

German Hex Murders

Ironically, this phenomenon was not merely limited to Pennsylvania, but found in North America,[135] and even in Germany and Switzerland from where many of these beliefs proceed.

One of the best, albeit heavily biased sources on these events in Europe, is the Lutheran minister turned Christian-psychotherapist, Rev. Kurt Koch. Koch pioneered a highly experimental and religiously oriented approach to psychotherapy, concluding that insanity was the result of occult influences, and included everything from *Brauchen* to astrology, and even some forms of charismatic healing among Christian fundamentalist denominations.[136] His work was only partially scientific, and even suggested that any occult deeds performed by an ancestor could affect their descendants generations later. Kurt was not only a regional advocate against folk medicine, *Brauche*, and beliefs in Hexerei in Germany and Switzerland, he was instrumental in providing fuel to the American "Satanic Panic" of the 1980s. Koch's work was translated into English, and widely distributed in the United States to eager audiences of evangelical Christians.[137]

From the 1940s-1970s, Rev. Koch collected accounts of *Brauchen* as a means to prove his hypothesis that such behaviors resulted in mental illness. While many of these stories are only marginally reliable because of the biased methods through which they were collected, the detailed stories document the persistence of ritual practices in Germany well into the twentieth century. He describes the use of ritual to remove warts performed by doctors, and even ministers, including the practice of placing an item representative of an illness into a casket at a funeral to remove illness; and even the use of water which has been used to wash a corpse to remove warts by a bishop in Northern Germany – water used for a male corpse to cure warts in women, and vice versa.[138] Rev. Koch also describes the use of *The Sixth and Seventh Books of Moses* and *The Spiritual Shield*, the very presence of which, he claims, would cause spiritual and mental disruptions, including the perception of hauntings. Thus to Rev. Koch, hauntings are in fact real, except that he relegates them to psychotic symptoms of a mind poisoned by the devil. Such mixture of scientific and religious language made his work highly appealing worldwide.[139]

Rev. Koch was also eager to establish connections between Hexerei and murder, death, abuse, and suicide. He cites examples, such as a woman in Glarus, Switzerland who was burned to death in her home by members of her community in 1934 because she was accused of bewitching horses. Two heinous murders in Lower Saxony took place over suspicions of witchcraft 1951, and included a nineteen-year-old man of Lunenburg who killed his father over suspicions of witchcraft and later hung himself. In Brunswick, two men set fire to a woman's house, claiming that she was a witch, and although the woman escaped, two of her relatives died in the fire.[140]

One of Koch's most poignant examples is that of a young woman, identified only as a Ms. L., who married into a farming family in Haltern, Germany. Following the marriage, an illness claimed the lives of the cattle, and the family sought advice from a fortune-teller in Gelsenkirchen. The fortune-teller identified the young woman as a witch and source of the curse. She advised the family in how to remove the curse, which resulted in the young woman's imprisonment in a darkened room on the farmstead, where she was routinely and savagely tortured with beatings and starvation. The family and the fortune-teller were arrested, but the young bride died of her injuries.[141]

For examples such as these, Rev. Koch frequently cited the works of Johann Kruse of Schlesswig-Holstein, who published a book the very same year as the events in Lunenburg and Brunswick, entitled *Hexen Unter Uns?* (Are there Witches Among Us?).[142] The two Germans were on opposite ends of the social and religious spectrum, as Koch was a fundamentalist and Kruse was described as "an anti-clerical Social Democrat" who collected materials to document what he saw as a modern witchcraft craze, beginning in the 1920s. Koch and Kruse could at least agree on one basic premise: folk healing was to blame for such incidents. Kruse however, as an ardent socialist, feared a new incarnation of the witchcraft executions of the Middle Ages, worrying that women, the elderly, and vulnerable people in society would be the victims of violence.[143]

Echoing nearly the voices of members of the Medical Society of York County, Pennsylvania, Kruse claimed, "Still today, in the middle of the twentieth century, every city in Germany has its 'witches' and almost every village has its 'servant of the devil.' Because of their defenselessness, they are ostracized and persecuted, some are mistreated and even killed. Thousands and thousands of women suffer from the effects of this witchcraft delusion."[144] Furthermore, Kruse and his contemporaries were of the belief that 'superstition' – a blanket term for the fears and social anxieties surrounding traditional practices - were to blame for the extremism in Nazi Germany that produced the Holocaust.[145]

In 1954, Kruse urged authorities in the State of Lower Saxony to prosecute Ferdinand Masuch and Heinrich Schnell, proprietors of Planet Verlag, the publishers of *The Sixth and Seventh Books of Moses*, on

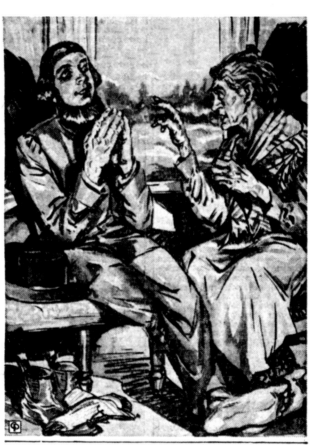

Fictional depiction of a powwow doctor treating an Amish client, from the anti-powwowing campaign in Reading, Pennsylvania. "Conquering Superstition." *Reading Eagle*, Nov 22, 1936.

the grounds of fraud (making of false claims), instigation to criminal offense such as the desecration of cemeteries or the harming or mistreatment of animals in ritual circumstances, and violation of laws regarding sexually-transmitted diseases (on account of old recipes said to cure syphilis).[146] In the end, all criminal charges were dropped in 1960, based on testimony from celebrated German folklorist and ethnologist Dr. Will-Erich Peuckert at the University of Goettingen, who defended the value of such works within the context of early modern, pre-scientific, folk-cultural literature that encompasses agricultural, medical and household knowledge. Peuckert was also likely to have been familiar with the fact that such works were systematically destroyed under the Third Reich,[147] and as well as the legal and moral implications of replicating such censorship in the post-war era.

Nevertheless, even well into the 1950s, statistics were published showing a widely held belief in ritual healing. Kruse's data suggested that there were an estimated 10,000 practitioners in Germany of various forms of ritual healing alleging some form of supernatural power.[148] At the same time, Kruse identifies that while some of these are charlatans, others are sincere. Officials in Lower Saxony were far more conservative in their estimates, claiming knowledge only of their immediate geographic state, said that there were hundreds of individuals holding such beliefs. "You just cannot stamp it out entirely," recalled Dr. Rolf Bunnemann, chief of the State Health Department in 1957 and leader in an official anti-witchcraft campaign. "All the government can do is try to educate the people to the fact that there are no witches."[149]

Much in the same way that the hype of Pennsylvania's twentieth-century conflicts fizzled out, so too did the media coverage of such events in Europe. But why? Part of the answer lies in the fact that such events were marginal, and decidedly few in number. Notions of widespread hysteria existed only on the pages of newspapers. In places where beliefs in powwowing and *Braucherei* were indeed present, such communities were simply unable to sustain the media attention, due to an overall lack of consistently newsworthy behavior. Murder and excess are by no means the inevitable result of beliefs surrounding healing traditions, and are even less likely to motivate criminal violence than religious or political movements.

Throughout the decades that this fascination persisted, media coverage continued to express disbelief at how ideas such as powwow could persist in the twentieth century. Although powwow-related controversies were portrayed as the dregs from a bygone era, the opposite is actually true: conflicting social forces in the early part of the century combined in explosive new ways to produce these isolated events in a manner unlike what had been previously experienced in the culture. As the narratives in this chapter reveal, powwowing merely provided a nuanced cultural veneer to stories that highlighted social issues surrounding poverty and disparities in economic and educational advantage, mental and physical illness, access to healthcare, complicated family conflicts, and neighborly grudges.

At the same time, Pennsylvania Dutch culture was experiencing dramatic transformations as a result of the rapid expansion of industry; the collision of rural and urban landscapes and populations; and the development of institutional authority in areas of education and medicine. These alone were powerful forces of change, but they were coupled with two consecutive world wars in which Germany and the United States were in opposition, which fostered anti-German sentiments and contributed to the decline of the use of Pennsylvania Dutch language in the home.

In communities where powwowing had been interwoven into everyday life, this sense of integration began to unravel. Without the surety of stable, multigenerational farm operations and everyday use of the language, powwowing began to experience the same type of compartmentalization as other customs and traditions that relied on integrative social structure such as community husking bees for shucking corn, rag parties for preparing material for rug making, belsnickeling at the holidays, and collective neighborhood gatherings to help with butchering and the making of scrapple or apple-butter.[150] The breakdown of the social structures that nurtured these traditions also contributed to the illusion that healing was somehow separate from community life – a notion, which has both fundamentally diminished the role of powwowing in Pennsylvania Dutch communities as well as instigated its revival among those seeking a return to community-based and culturally significant alternative healing systems in the present day.

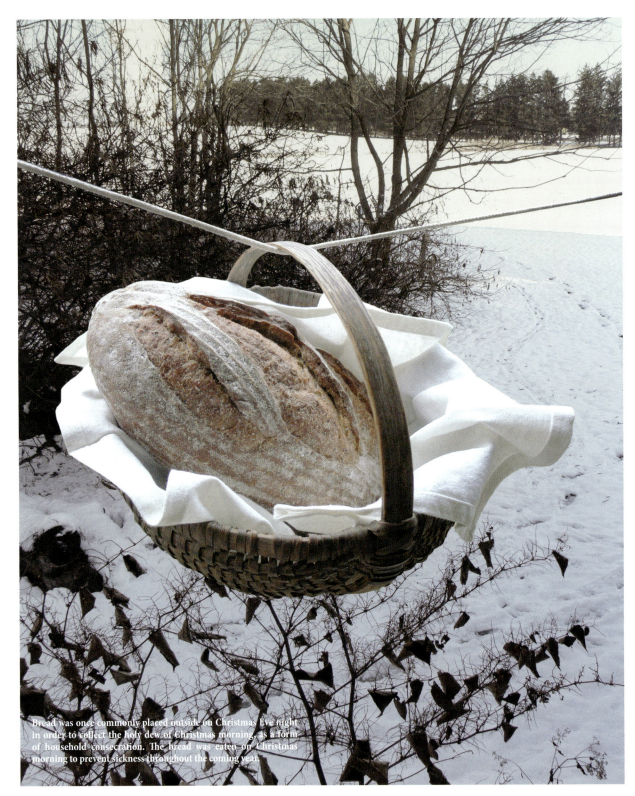

Bread was once commonly placed outside on Christmas Eve night in order to collect the holy dew of Christmas morning, as a form of household consecration. The bread was eaten on Christmas morning to prevent sickness throughout the coming year.

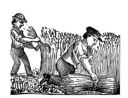 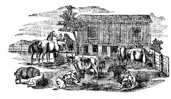 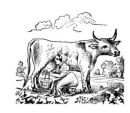

Chapter X

The Ritual of Everyday Life
Domestic, Agricultural, Sacred

One need not be Pennsylvania Dutch or from the core region of southeastern Pennsylvania to appreciate the opportunities that powwowing presents to forge healthy and thoughtful connections between our beliefs and daily life. Although present-day applications of *Braucherei* have become progressively more focused on healing practices, surprisingly few of the traditions integrating ritual with farming, animal husbandry, gardening, and domestic life have survived. In one sense, this is because there has been an overall decline in farming, and our domestic transactions have become increasingly automated.

One element of human experience, however, that is much more stable and less subject to change is the human need to alleviate suffering – which is another reason why the healing traditions have persisted in an ever-changing world. As a result, rituals of daily life have often been downplayed and called "superstitions" – rather than being viewed as functional integrations of belief and life. *Braucherei*, as a collective body of ritual customs and traditions, is necessarily an integrative element of Pennsylvania Dutch life and society, and such traditions present opportunities to bring people together and reinforce cultural identities.

Many ritual traditions of the domestic and agricultural variety are essentially historical, that is, well-documented, but no longer widely practiced throughout the region. Gradual decline in the maintenance of ritual practices has been described for over a century among the Pennsylvania Dutch in the research of early folklorists working in the cultural "twilight" of the early twentieth century, when farm-life began to rapidly change at a faster rate than in previous generations. Even though some of these traditions are perceived to be no longer flourishing or in active use, it is nevertheless highly significant to identify that many diverse practices are actually still alive and well in parts of the Dutch country today. Even when such practices begin to fall into disuse, the preservation of ritual in the form of stories gives these traditions a second-life as family and community narratives of identity.

This study does not mean to suggest that stories about ritual practices and beliefs should be regarded as equivalent to living traditions. Instead, family stories serve as one form of oral tradition that allows for practices to occasionally resurface from disuse and reintegrate into life. Still, any modern reconstructions of historic rituals will be identified as such in this exploration, but it is important to remember that such reinvestigations of ritual practices like *Braucherei* are essential components of any living tradition that is at least partially undergirded by a combination of oral and literary sources.

SUPERSTITIONS OR RITUALS?

In 1915, one of the most comprehensive lists of Pennsylvania Dutch ritual practices was assembled by folklorist Edwin Miller Fogel (1874-1949), in his *Beliefs and Superstitions of the Pennsylvania Germans*.[1] As a byproduct of his time, Fogel's study was based in the accumulation of succinct narrative statements that described a practice, belief, or attitude that appeared culturally distinct, with no accompanying context. All of Fogel's information was collected from oral rather than written sources from among native speakers of Pennsylvania Dutch in fourteen counties and are provided in the original language.

Fogel's use of the word "superstition" is dated, and betrays the bias of his day toward a wholly unscientific way of classifying traditional beliefs. Usually reserved for beliefs in supernatural causation, superstition is a label that lacks any single-agreed upon criteria, and is often arbitrarily assigned to ideas held by someone else – rather than one's own beliefs. Thus, there is no objective way without asserting a bias to determine what is considered a religious belief and what is superstitious.[2] Such designations preclude a deeper understanding of the culture from which such beliefs proceed. While Fogel provides no precise criteria for what beliefs or attitudes were worthy of inclusion in his study, his important research runs the full gamut from beliefs concerning weather to medicine, agriculture to special days and seasons. Perhaps most importantly his work was one of the most comprehensive collections of ritual descriptions described in the Pennsylvania Dutch language.

Ironically, although Fogel's title suggests a somewhat nebulous and far-reaching cross-section of the culture's perceptions and values, his entries can be broadly placed into three distinct categories: rituals, precautions, and omens.[3] Rituals comprise over half of Fogel's collection,[4] and in this case are any prescriptive symbolic actions performed for a distinct purpose such as throwing a dwarf egg over the barn to dispel misfortune,[5] or sowing cabbage seed on Good Friday.[6] Fogel's precautions, comprising less than a quarter of his collection [7] consist of recommendations to ritualize the avoidance of certain behaviors due to the possibility of a negative outcome such as the advice to never thank anyone for plants given as a gift for the garden or they will not grow.[8] In contrast to descriptions of ritual, which is based in action to fulfill a function, this second category describes the rationale behind the deliberate circumvention of certain consequences – essentially, action defined by what is not enacted. Lastly, omens comprise over one quarter of Fogel's entries,[9] and these consist of signs of future events, like "if the stars are remarkably clear and bright, there will be rain the next day."[10] While the first two categories are defined by ritual procedures or abstaining from specific actions, omens provide the context for certain rituals, such as the household practice of breaking a chicken wishbone after dinner – the person who gets the smaller part of the bone that looks like a shovel will outlive (i.e. bury) the person who receives the longer side of the bone.[11]

There are certainly those who would say that domestic ritual practices undergirded by folk belief (such as throwing a dwarf egg over the barn) are not strictly "powwowing" per se – but such a stance needs to be closely examined. In Pennsylvania Dutch, *Braucherei* means "customs, traditions, rituals"[12] – thus, by nature, a wide range of non-healing rituals such as divination with a wishbone fit the description quite well. One could easily contend that omens have little to do with powwowing, but on the contrary, even Hohman and many other authors included omens in their compendiums of ritual procedures, suggesting that such beliefs inform and belong with their ritual counterparts. (see Hohman's *The Friend in Need*, in Chapter V.) While ritual literature may at first glance appear to include many seemingly unrelated recipes, procedures, and statements of belief, the fact is that this perception may also be a byproduct of biases in our present-day society, where daily life does not always go hand-in-hand with ritual traditions. *Braucherei*, by its very nature, tends to resist the constraints of compartmentalization. Thus, beliefs and rituals that may appear distinct and separate to audiences today were once undoubtedly part of the same cultural tapestry that comprised the patterns of daily life. *Braucherei* is not so much an exclusive term to describe only those aspects of ritual behaviors that appear exotic or magical by today's standards: even the mundane rituals are manifestations of the same systems of belief.

When confronted with the vast array of ritual behaviors recorded among the Pennsylvania Dutch, it is safe to say that on a very basic level, ritual suffused all aspects of human life.[13] While certainly not all people practiced each ritual expression in an overarching or comprehensive manner – by no means was this the case – nevertheless, the breadth of ritual applications across the myriad functions of life demonstrates an immense potential for integration of belief into day-to-day affairs, and for such practices to follow throughout the course of one's earthly existence.

Birth & Children

From the very beginnings of life, rituals accompanied each step leading up to and after childbirth. A needle and thread could be used as a pendulum to divine the gender of a child still in the womb, and to predict how many children a mother would have.[14] Special written blessings were carried on pregnant mothers for protection and for safe delivery, and spoken blessings were used throughout pregnancy to reduce the discomfort experienced during the transition.

Ritual blessings were used to treat the symptoms from a wide variety of uterine pains, likely caused by cysts or fibroids, or even early contractions, typically grouped under the polite and ambiguous term *Mudderkrankheit*.[15] Frequently translated with the dated English terms "hysterics" or "mother-fits,"[16] these conditions were perceived to result from a displacement of the womb (*Bärmudder*), which is why many blessings address the uterus, asking it to "take thy rightful place."[17]

A few ritual cures double as both blessings and instructions:

Trink du ein rot Glaß Wein und iß ein schwarz Stick Brot daß ist für Kolig und Bermüter gut. +. +. +

Drink thou a glass of red wine, and eat a piece of black bread, this is good for colic and birthmothers. +. +. +.[18]

While this could be understood literally as a recipe for the benefit of either a pregnant mother experiencing uterine pain or abdominal cramping (colic), it is also written in the original German language with a meter and rhyme, indicating that the words could be used as both a recipe and a poetic blessing invoking the body and blood of Christ through the imagery of the bread and wine. While the three crosses concluding the prayer are further indication that the recipe is to be spoken, certainly, this prayer could also be enacted as a ritual, involving the glass of red wine and piece of black bread as physical elements in a non-sanctioned, folk expression of the Eucharist.[19]

Himmelsbriefe and copies of the Three Kings Prayer were kept close at hand during childbirth,[20] and if topical applications of these blessed documents were insufficient, prayers or the SATOR square could be written upon a plate and washed off with water or wine that could be taken internally.[21] If bleeding after birth was profuse, one would gently tie a red string around the thumb and big toe to help staunch the flow of blood,[22] or a red band of flannel around the leg.[23]

When a child was born, it was once customary for it to be carried up a flight of stairs within the hour, to ensure prosperity,[24] and a child should be nursed first from the right breast to ensure that it becomes right-handed.[25] In Berks Country in the early twentieth century, the umbilical cord was cut with an axe if the child was a boy, in order ensure that he would be good at hewing wood, and a girl's was sewn so that she would become a good seamstress.[26] The placenta should be buried under an elderberry tree to protect the child through life.[27]

Just as written blessings were used in labor, so to were blessings created for babies that were placed in cribs in order to prevent or cure illness,[28] and even an infant's first bath was to be infused with four peony leaves, a little moss and some red wine to prevent infant convulsions (*Gichter*).[29] The first bathwater was to be thrown out the window onto a tree to make the child high-minded.[30] Bathing the child's feet in cold spring water, or allowing children to play barefoot in the first snow was believed to keep one healthy and to prevent frostbite in the extremities.[31]

Herbal bundles used as amulets were assembled for children that were to be weaned, and they consisted of a month's growth of hazelnut leaves, parsley, and the sweepings from the thresholds of three doors placed in an unused piece of gingham fabric and hung around the child's neck over the breast.[32] Children were sometimes weaned in order to avoid certain times of the year such as when fruit trees are in blossom or when the moon was in Leo.[33] If a child were to die before being weaned, the child's shirt should be laid upon the mother's breasts to prevent soreness.[34]

Baptismal rituals in church were often blended with folk practices, such as the gathering of rain water on Good Friday for use in the baptismal ceremony. Good Friday rain water was still brought to church by Berks County families up until very recently, and was considered holy.[35] In other traditions, consecrated baptismal water was thought to be particularly effective for the cure of childhood ailments, and small amounts were brought home to ease the pain of teething.[36] If the baptismal water is poured over a rosebush, it was believed to give the child rosy cheeks.[37]

A child's first diaper should be an old one in order to make it pass its stool more easily, and alternately the first diaper can be burned to ensure luck.[38] The first louse found on the child's head could be crushed on the cover of a hymnbook in order to ensure that the child would become a good singer, or on the Bible, so that the child would be smart.[39]

Childhood ailments, such as thrush, were treated with ritual cures. Thrush was cured by blowing into the mouth of the infant three times, or by drawing three lengths of straw from the household broom through a child's mouth and then depositing the straw into the outhouse, whereupon one would urinate.[40]

In order to prevent childhood ailments, no one was to ever step over a child lying on the floor or rock an empty cradle. Tickling a child too much was believed to cause colic.[41] To cure colic or excessive crying, rituals that mirrored the birthing process were employed, such as passing the child through a horse collar or under an arched branch of a blackberry bush that had grown back into the ground, or around the leg of a table.[42] What is less obvious in these instances are the secondary benefits to the adults,

Passing a child through a horse collar was once a common cure for the infant complaint known as being "livergrown" (*aagewaxe*). Pennsylvania German Cultural Heritage Center, Kutztown University.

who necessarily had to perform these rituals cooperatively. Such processes gave the parents of the child a course of action while dealing with an otherwise inconsolable child.

Youth, Courting & Marriage

Although there is no one single period of a person's life with more potential for ritual activity than birth and infancy, rituals follow in fits and spurts throughout life. For previous generations among many farming families, as children grew up and assumed more responsibility, they would learn to read the almanac, and internalize many of the rituals employed by their parents. Nevertheless, young people had their own reasons to employ rituals, and they were as likely to learn these from their peers as from older members of the family.

Young girls in particular would attempt to remove freckles, birthmarks, or blemishes by waking before sunrise on the first of May, and washing in the dew that had settled on the grass. Some variations of the ritual require one to be absolutely naked. A contact from Lehigh County described that her mother had attempted this form of freckle removal when she was young because of a profuse cluster that spread across her upper back. She went out before dawn, stripped off her clothes, and gathered the dew on her hands. She reached over her shoulder with one hand to wipe at the freckles, only to realize that an older man was standing nearby and saw her nakedness. She quickly ran indoors and throughout her life, she still had her freckles except for the one spot over her shoulder where she managed to wipe before being seen.[43]

A number of rituals surrounded the way in which one was taught to groom, especially regarding the cutting and disposal of one's hair and washing. Hair was to be cut in the increase of the moon, so that it would grow thick, and was not to be casually tossed away, whereby birds could make nests with it or a person wishing one ill could come by

A Bible with a key inserted at the Book of Ruth and tied with a red ribbon for use in divination of a future spouse among young people.

it and use it for *Hexerei*. If a bird's nest was made with one's hair, it causes headaches, but burning of the hair makes one stupid.[44] For boys, trimming of a beard for the first time was likewise timed with the waxing moon, or if one desired a thicker mustache, one would drink milk and let the cat lick the milk off the upper lip, so that the hair would become thick like the cat's.[45] When washing or bathing, using the same water or towel that someone else used would cause a quarrel, unless the second person spits in the water, or turns the towel and uses the opposite side.[46]

When young people entertained the notion of courting and marrying, a wide variety of divination was used to discover who one would marry. There are a number of very simple and whimsical exercises of this sort, such as hanging a four-leafed clover or a wishbone over the door so that the first person to enter would be the future spouse, or paring an apple in one long strip and throwing the paring over the shoulder so that any letter made by the paring would reveal the first initial of the future spouse.[47]

Others are far more complex, involving ritual objects, and divination by dreams. On January 24, St. Agnes' Day, one could invoke the saint before retiring to bed in the hopes to dream of the future spouse:

St. Agnes, sei en Friend zu mir, loss mich die Nacht mei Mann (odder Fraa) sehne.

Saint Agnes, be a friend of mine. Permit me this night to see my future spouse.[48]

A large door key figures in several rituals, such as pouring molten lead through the eyelet into water so that the figures created indicate the occupation of the future husband,[49] or the use of a key or a pair of scissors tied in a Bible to reveal the name of the future spouse. Some sources indicate that the key must be placed at verse 16 of chapter 1 of the Book of Ruth:[50] "And Ruth said, Entreat me not to leave thee, or to return from following after thee: for whither thou goest, I will go; and where thou lodgest, I will lodge: thy people shall be my people, and thy God my God." While others indicate verse 7 of chapter 8 of the Song of Solomon:[51] "Many waters cannot quench love, neither can the floods drown it: if a man would give all the substance of his house for love, it would utterly be contemned." This procedure is to be performed by two friends (girls or boys) who must bind the key to the book with a length of cord, and balance the book with two fingers on other side of the key's loop or the handle of the scissors. The Bible verse must be recited, while a yes or no question is asked, and the book will turn clockwise for a positive answer and counterclockwise for a negative. Other variations suggest that the book will turn when the recited verse reaches a letter that corresponds to the future spouses' name.[52]

For those who might be impatient and wished to ritually rush the prospect of marriage rather than merely wait until the appropriate time, one could swallow the raw heart of a chicken, and whoever one thinks about while doing this will become their future spouse, or one could carry the heart of an owl in their sleeve, or the eye of the European hoopoe bird.[53] If one wished to court a prospective spouse, one might carry the leaves of *Fimfingergraut* (five-finger-grass or cinquefoil) so that their request to court might be granted,[54] or if one's suggestion were spurned, one might crawl underneath a blackberry branch that is rooted on both sides, which is also used for curing infant colic.[55] If one were to count seven stars on seven successive nights, the first person with which one shakes hands will be the other's future spouse.[56]

It was once considered an unlucky thing if a younger daughter married before an older daughter, an attitude reflected in the biblical story of Laban's daughter's Rachel and Leah.[57] If such a thing were to occur among the Pennsylvania Dutch, the older sibling was expected to dance in the pig trough at the wedding, ride the bakeoven, or dance in silk stockings.[58] This practice is rooted in the eighteenth century, and reflected in early Berks County literature as early as 1805 as well as in Hohman's *The Friend in Need* in 1813. Hohman's description of the ritual, however, has the older "sisters" dancing barefoot, "in order to drive out misfortune, and also to help them find husbands."[59] As of 2015, a Berks County resident described that this ritual was performed at a local wedding when a younger sibling was married. The family carried a scalding trough used in butchering into the area designated as the dance floor, and the sibling was forced to dance barefoot in the trough in front of the whole wedding party. While this contemporary example was likely intended for amusement, it was also an expression of identity, as the older members of the family had made the suggestion of performing the ritual. In Hohman's era however, it is clear that the ritual was actually intended to heal a family's misfortune, and to entice prospective spouses for the older sibling. Although such rituals may function purely as a social ritual when adapted in the present day, the ritual clearly addresses healing within the social dimension of the family and community.

In the same manner that such family marital concerns could be cured through ritual, many newlywed couples would proactively bless their union by stepping, hopping, or jumping over a broom as they entered their home for the first time together.[60] The household broom is perhaps one of the best examples of the perception among the Pennsylvania Dutch that the context of everyday life is what empowers an object for use in powwow rituals.

Rituals of the Broom

According to beliefs held even by some in the present day, the household broom, when leaned against the jamb of the front door, or concealed below the threshold, has the capacity to protect the home from anyone wishing spiritual harm upon the occupants. A concealed broom of this sort was recently discovered in a Berks County farm house and was placed there by an occupant within the past few decades. While some have assumed that this custom is related to popular associations of the broom with witchcraft, indeed the opposite is true.

The broom represented the home, and had direct contact with the dust in the home, created by everyday activities. This dust was believed to carry some measure of the essence of the house and family, which fostered a wide range of beliefs surrounding the cleaning of the home. One was not to sweep out the house after dark for fear that the home would be vulnerable to spiritual attack or misfortune.[61] One should not sweep on baking day (Friday), or the bread would not rise. The old broom was customarily the first item placed into a new home, as it brought with it some measure of the essence of the previous dwelling place and established a sense of domestic continuity. During feast days such as the week between Christmas and New Year's Day, one was not to sweep out the house or barn for fear that they would sweep away the blessings that were imparted by the atmosphere during these holy times of year.[62]

Even outside of the sacred calendar, the dust from the home was believed to have important useful properties. It was once common to take dust from the four corners of

Three leaves of "Five-Finger-Grass" (Cinquefoil), picked and carried in one's pocket to curry favor from other people in everyday affairs.

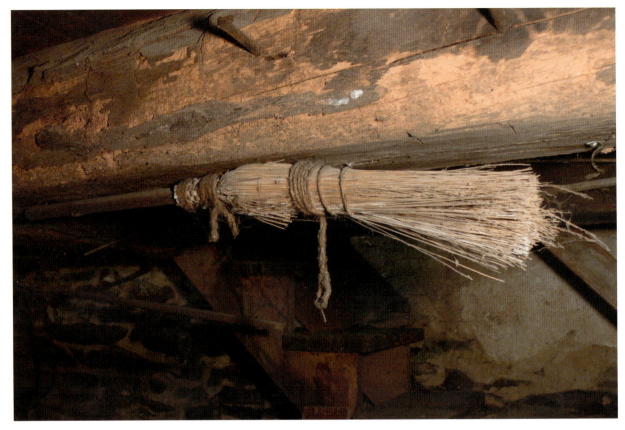

A concealed broom in a Berks County farm house, nailed to a floor joist visible by the basement stairs. Private Collection.

the house and to mix a tiny bit into your coffee or into the flour used to bake bread before one embarked on a long journey in order to avoid homesickness.[63] The person who partook of the coffee or bread was therefore taking the home's essence into their body in order to fortify them against pining for home while away. This type of integrated belief made manifest in domestic ritual lends a whole new level of meaning to the activities of daily life, and links everyday tasks to a broader sense of cosmic order.

Domestic arts

Chores around the house were organized according to the day of the week, and rituals were woven through many aspects of cooking, baking, sewing, ironing, and cleaning. Sewing in particular had strong ritual implications because of the use of thread or cord that had the power not only to mend fabric but to bind things together in a symbolic sense. For instance, clothes should not be mended while a person is wearing them, or the person will become thought-bound or will develop enmity. Ironing was also conducted with care, for ironing the back of someone's shirt could give them backache or make them cross. Sewing was not to be done on Ascension Day and neither should one nail or fasten anything,[64] because it was believed to work against the sacred order of the day, when Christ ascended to heaven. Fishing, however, was appropriate on this day because it agreed with the Great Commission, and was a biblical metaphor for proselytizing.

Clothing itself was once thought to be the carrier or mitigator of illness, as one Berks County powwow practitioner described, "If the ritual doesn't work, take off your clothes and try again."[65] Due to the fact that the clothing was near to the body, it not only carried the essence of a person, but it was also a mirror of their overall health. Just as a scrap of fabric from a person's clothes could be used to curse a person, so too could a person who has been cursed use their clothing to repel a curse. Ritual cures often involved tying or inverting clothing to create a change in the person's state of being. A knot tied in the left side of one's shirt could be used to cure strangury (difficult urination),[66] or if a childhood illness was believed to be the result of witchcraft, the shirt could be pulled off the

Objects deliberately concealed in walls or foundations are part of centuries-old traditions used to protect and bless the establishment of a new building at the time of its construction. These architectural concealments or building offerings (*Bau-Opfer*) are diverse, consisting of both man-made objects as well as animals. Many of these concealments are found at the time that buildings are torn down or renovated, providing evidence today of rituals performed by previous generations of builders and inhabitants from ancient times up until fairly recently. These traditions are well documented throughout Central Europe and the British Isles, as well as in North America, Australia, and many other parts of the world.

A house from the 1930s in Auburn, Schuylkill County underwent a series of renovations beginning in 2012. When the west walls of the house were opened, an extensive concealment of domestic items and animal bones were discovered in the walls, including bottles, broken ceramics, metal cookware, newspapers, fabrics, a scrap of paper with biblical verses, and most striking — the bones of the heads and legs of over a dozen chickens, each carefully wrapped in cement bags from the pouring of the foundation. Many of the chickens' feet were deliberately interlocked, as seen to the right. Below: a needle and thread wound around a scrap of fabric strapping also concealed in the wall. *Courtesy of the Bretzius Family.*

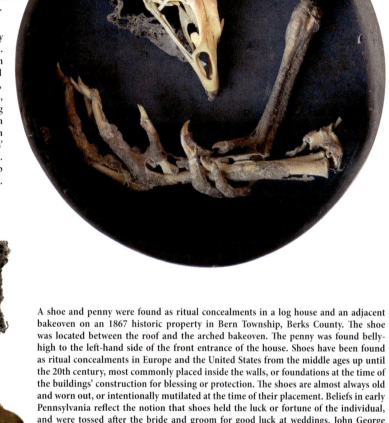

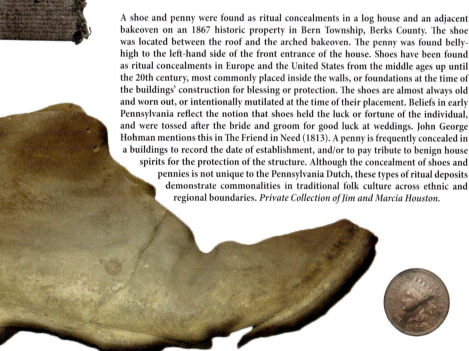

A shoe and penny were found as ritual concealments in a log house and an adjacent bakeoven on an 1867 historic property in Bern Township, Berks County. The shoe was located between the roof and the arched bakeoven. The penny was found belly-high to the left-hand side of the front entrance of the house. Shoes have been found as ritual concealments in Europe and the United States from the middle ages up until the 20th century, most commonly placed inside the walls, or foundations at the time of the buildings' construction for blessing or protection. The shoes are almost always old and worn out, or intentionally mutilated at the time of their placement. Beliefs in early Pennsylvania reflect the notion that shoes held the luck or fortune of the individual, and were tossed after the bride and groom for good luck at weddings. John George Hohman mentions this in The Friend in Need (1813). A penny is frequently concealed in a buildings to record the date of establishment, and/or to pay tribute to benign house spirits for the protection of the structure. Although the concealment of shoes and pennies is not unique to the Pennsylvania Dutch, these types of ritual deposits demonstrate commonalities in traditional folk culture across ethnic and regional boundaries. *Private Collection of Jim and Marcia Houston.*

child inside-out and then slammed in the door to punish the witch.⁶⁷ Hohman describes that one who is cursed or slandered should take off their shirt and turn it inside out while having the verse recited over them:

> If you are slandered to your very skin, to your very flesh, to your very bones, then cast it back upon the false tongues.+++ ⁶⁸

Likewise, the belief was that one could obtain an illness from someone else's clothes, promoting the idea still firmly held today in many Pennsylvania Dutch families that one should not wear a shirt without washing it first out of concern for who else may have tried it on.⁶⁹

Some clothing worn by others, however, could also have favorable effects upon health. A child subject to seizures should be wrapped in the father's shirt, or part of the parent's wedding garments.⁷⁰ Not only were the clothes of a healthy or familial person helpful in providing a cure, one's own clothing could also be used to transfer an illness from the body. Clothes could be burned to remove an illness such as epilepsy.⁷¹ Although there were serious taboos against burying a corpse with the clothes of the living,⁷² there were exceptions for epilepsy⁷³ and some other illnesses, where the sickness was transferred to the dead person, who would carry the illness into the next world.

Likewise, a cloth used in washing a corpse could later be used to remove warts,⁷⁴ a tradition well established in Europe, where a man's warts were treated with a cloth that washed the corpse of a female, and vice versa. Not only were such cloths used, but a wide variety of clothes and personal items that had contact with particular regions of the body would be placed in a casket, such as gloves, undergarments, or socks. ⁷⁵ Such practices are not only informed by attitudes towards death, but also the notion of the church-yard as a sacred space, where the bodies of the community of saints come to rest. These Protestant traditions can be compared to the practice of leaving behind garments or votive offerings at the shrines of the saints for healing in Roman Catholic traditions.

Christmas Dew & the Ritual of Three Things

The use of votive offerings, while largely absent from Protestant traditions in any overt sense, plays an important role in understanding the seasonal customs of the Pennsylvania Dutch, whereby small samples or portions of household goods are blessed on winter feast days, such as Christmas or New Year's Eve (St. Sylvester). On Christmas Eve, it was once customary to place a loaf of bread on the window sill to collect the dew overnight, whereby it was consumed for breakfast the following day with the belief that it would instill good health, protect against fevers, and secure the blessings of this sacred time of year. On the eve of these holy days, the atmosphere itself imparts some measure of the divine upon all things, which is why farmers would leave straw and hay out in the open air in the barnyard overnight, so that the hay would later impart similar blessings to the animals as fodder, and the straw, used as bedding, would fortify the stables against disease.⁷⁶ Between Christmas and New Year's Day, one was not to clean the stables, sweep the house, or even change one's undergarments. The sacred atmosphere was to be allowed to settle, uninterrupted, upon all living things and spaces.

On New Year's Eve, the atmosphere not only imparted blessings, but some indication of the year to come. For this reason, it was common up until fairly recently in Berks County to place *die drei Dinge*, or small samples of "three things" outside on the windowsill on New Year's Eve. The samples represented three substances that would be blessed so that the household would have abundance of these three things, and would not run out of them over the course of the next year. Each family had their own way of interpreting this ritual. One family from Bernville, Berks County, placed a coin, a lump of coal, and a small dish of flour so that the family would have sufficient money, fuel, and food in the

The "Three Things" placed on the window sill overnight on New Year's Eve ensured abundance in the coming year.

coming year.[77] Other local families focused instead upon pantry items so that flour, salt, and lard, or flour, salt, and butter were placed upon the windowsill.

Rituals of the windowsill utilize a liminal domestic space as a convenient location for a specific type of traditional transaction that brings together the inner realm of the house and home and the outside world. The collecting of the atmosphere of a special day remains constant as a passive act of consecration, but the transformations are nuanced. While the Christmas dew would impart health benefits through consumption, the ritual of the "three things" imparts a blessing to samples representing the whole of the family's consumption of household necessities throughout the year. In many rituals of blessing, a portion of something becomes emblematic of the whole, and capable of distributing its blessing throughout. This microcosmic significance imbues the "little picture" with great significance and a sense of agency that is disproportionate with its apparent size. While these domestic rituals are distilled from the notion that all things come proceed from a greater source, nowhere are cosmic beliefs more overt than in agricultural rituals that embrace the celestial and religious calendar.

Agriculture & Foodways

Foodways are necessarily ritual in nature because of the repetition, timing, and precision necessary for growing crops, raising animals, storing and preserving food, and cooking. Each species of plant and animal has its own life rhythm to which humans must adapt in order to effectively secure food. As with many agricultural societies, the Pennsylvania Dutch possess a well-developed system of beliefs concerning the movements of the heavens and their effects on earthly processes as well as on botanical, animal, and human affairs. While the bulk of these beliefs in Pennsylvania proceed from the European traditions of the agricultural almanac, these conceptions have been liberally blended with religious attitudes. Thus, the stars in their courses along with the rising and setting of the sun and the phases of the moon were not only regarded as the clearest indicators of the passage of time, but were emblematic of the belief in a stable, ordered sacred universe.[78]

The progression of the sun, moon, and stars are a central feature in the agricultural almanacs still used in the present day, where celestial activities are charted and interpreted for their influence on the mechanics of earthly life. Each almanac is essentially an annual household reference booklet, and includes the liturgical church calendar of saints' days and festivals, charts of the lunar phases, the day to day progression of the zodiac constellations and planets, as well as calculations for the appearance of comets, eclipses, and other astronomical phenomena.[79] This information was once used to orchestrate the activities of daily life.

Whether in planting or harvesting, felling trees or tilling the soil, baking bread or fermenting vinegar, breeding or slaughtering livestock, bearing children or getting married, there were believed to be appropriate days of the week, times of the month, phases of the moon, saints' days, or alignments of celestial bodies which would either positively or negatively affect the outcome of life events.[80] This system was an attempt to harmonize the progression of human life with the progression of the heavens, and believed to be the manifestation and visible order of the divine will.

In agricultural practices, tilling, planting, and harvesting schedules were planned in accordance with moon-signs (*Muhnzeiche*) or the lunar zodiac. The twelve signs of the zodiac which stretch across the celestial sphere were divided into four basic groups corresponding to the four elements: fire (Aries, Leo, Sagittarius), Air (Gemini, Libra, Aquarius), water (Cancer, Scorpio, Pisces), and Earth (Taurus, Virgo, Capricorn). While practical application of this system varied somewhat, a general rule of thumb was to tend root vegetables in "earth-signs," vines and stems in "water-signs," flowering plants in "air-signs," and fruiting plants in "fire-signs." This rule set into motion a series of correspondences that governed all aspects of tending plants, both domestic and wild.

In addition to the signs of the zodiac, the moon was believed to exert a particular force on the Earth which varied according to its phase: as the moon waxed (*Zunemme*) to full, it was believed to exert a force which pulled away from the Earth, and as it waned (*Abnemme*) to the new moon, it exerted a force towards the Earth. This force was believed to be the strongest at either extreme. A whole series of behaviors and tasks revolved around this belief, especially as it pertained to farm work: the new moon was the time to establish, and the full moon was a time to uproot or harvest.

Thus, common tasks such as planting potatoes, setting fence-posts in the ground, or nailing roof shingles was done in the "dark of the moon" - a time when things are to be fixed in place. Whereas, potatoes were best harvested in the waxing "light of the moon," along with other activities such as pruning trees and trimming one's hair - where the force of the moon was believed to encourage new growth.[81] This system was by no means simple, however, as planting — which at first may seem to be an act of fixing something in place — is usually a task to be done in the "light of the moon" for plants which grow upwards. On the other hand, root vegetables are often planted in the "dark of the moon" as their growth is directed into the Earth.

Not only were gardens and fields planted according to the timing of the moon's phases and the signs of the zodiac, but also to saint's days and religious holidays. One sowed potatoes and cabbage on St. Gertrude's Day (March 17),[82] or cabbages could also be planted along with all manner of flowers on Good Friday.[83] Good Friday is a moveable religious feast day designated as the first Friday after the first full moon following the vernal equinox. The holy significance of Good Friday also carried over into other Friday practices, such as healing,[84] and even planting. One should begin sowing grain on a Friday and end on the following Friday, and if the task is completed beforehand, then the seed-bag should be hung on the fence until Friday arrived.[85]

Likewise, the lard was saved from frying of fasnacht cakes or doughnuts on Shrove Tuesday prior to the commencing of the season of Lent. It was not only used as a salve to heal all manner of sores; it was also saved and employed for agricultural purposes. When hauling in grain, one should grease the hayforks and the axles of the wagon with the lard in which fasnachts have been fried so that the grain will store well without weevils, and greasing the plow in the same manner will rid the fields and soil of pests that spoil the crops.[86] Thus the lard is used in the manner of a holy unction for anointing tools and implements as a form of agricultural consecration. It was not only the lard that imparted a blessing to the grain and the soil, fasnachts themselves were considered beneficial for the crops and the community. It was once commonly believed that if a family did not fry fasnachts, their flax crop would fail. On the contrary, if one were to fry many batches and to give them out generously to their friends, the crop would grow tall and successfully.[87] Thus, the community's sense of abundance was reflected in the quality and success of their crops.

Holy days were even believed to control the price of grain and the weather. The Ember Days were three moveable days of fasting from the liturgical calendar indicated on the farmer's almanac for each season of the year. If the Ember Days fell on days of the month with low numbers, then the price of grain was believed likely to fall, and if the Ember Days were high, so to would the prices rise.[88] The three Ember Days were believed to signify the weather for the next three months, thus the weather on each day would rule each successive month.

Even today, many Berks County farmers still recall the old perception of the influence of the moon upon snow. The number of days observed between the first snow and the next snow following full moon, would indicate how many snows there would be in total for the winter season.[89] The most well-known traditional method of predicting precipitation during the growing season was based on the Virgin Mary "going over the mountain." "*Wann die Mariche iwwer der Barrich geht, un's reggert, kummt sie drucke wider mol z'rick. Awwer wann's net, gebt's sex Woche Regge*" (If it rains when Mary goes over the mountain, she comes back dry. But when it doesn't, six weeks of rain will follow).[90] This statement is used to predict the weather starting on the Visitation of the Virgin in the old liturgical calendar (July 2), or as some say "*Sie geht iwwer der Barrich fer ihre Schweschder bsuche*" (She goes over the mountain to visit her sister).[91] The day of Mary's return is August 15, or the Assumption of the Virgin, according to the Roman Catholic doctrine that Mary ascended to heaven like Christ. The local perception is however, that the mountain in question is no biblical Holy Mountain, but the Blue Mountain, separating Berks, Lehigh and Lebanon, from Carbon, Northampton and Schuylkill counties.

The use of religiously inspired words and phrases could also accompany agricultural processes, especially for certain plants. It was believed that anything planted in God's name would grow,[92] and this can be compared to invocations of the Three Highest Names, the Father, Son, and Holy Spirit, used extensively in healing.

An early American astrological wheel, showing the correspondences of the signs of the zodiac to the parts of the body. The zodiacal signs are not in monthly order, but according to their placement on the human body, with the top of the wheel corresponding to the head (Aries) and the bottom to the feet (Pisces). *Heilman Collection.*

The religious uses of holy names in planting stands in contrast to the ritual use of three names in other domestic contexts – especially those names which are perceived to carry certain qualities. When starting yeast for baking, one should write the names of three capable women on a slip of paper or call their names into the mixture to ensure its activity.[93] The opposite is true of vinegar: one should write the names of the nastiest people one knows on a piece of paper, or take three stems from a grapevine and name them and put them in the vinegar in order that it will become strong. In the same vein of thought, the best vinegar is made when one is angry.[94] The emotional and social implication of these vinegar rituals suggests that all qualities have their function, and even seemingly undesirable experiences and traits can be properly apportioned for human benefit.

Other agricultural procedures involve ritual comparisons, some of which are humorous as opposed to religious. When planting radishes from seed, one should say, "*So long ass mei Aarm, so dick ass mei Aarsch*" (as long as my arm, and as big as my rear).[95] In other similar cases, comparisons are not made through words, but through symbolic actions such as showing one's rear to flax so that it would grow tall.[96] A man should plant cucumbers from seed in order that they should grow large, or plant them on the longest day of the year.[97] Other plants such as thyme, will not grow if a woman does not sit on the seedlings after transplanting.[98] A Lehigh County contact told me that the best way to divine whether the soil was warm enough for planting corn: "*Mer muss net sei Welschkann blantze, bis mer sei Hosse abgeduh kann un uffem grund hocke, unne Kalt waere*" (One should not plant corn until one can take their pants off and sit on the ground without feeling cold).[99] Sitting bare on the soil was also considered a cure for chafing if the soil was newly plowed.[100]

While many rituals pertaining to food, land, and healing may be tailored to specific plants, illnesses, and functions, the blessing of seed and soil was also performed as a comprehensive ritual to ensure the fecundity and usefulness of the land for food. The kitchen garden was not only sown with cabbage, potatoes, and onions on St. Gertrude's Day, March 17, but the day was also designated as a time to bless the garden and rid the land of any moles or vermin that had held out over the winter. As the patron saint of cats, St. Gertrude of Nivelles was often depicted in Late Medieval art accompanied by mice, which she was invoked to eradicate.[101] As late as the 1950s in Pennsylvania, Dutch gardeners would walk around the inside perimeter of the garden fence three times to drive away moles.[102] This is likely to be a survival of a more comprehensive ritual whereby a ceremonial Lenten cake was baked and integrated into the blessing of the garden in honor of St. Gertrude. *Trudisdaag Datsch* or St. Gertrude's Datsch, is a particular type of thick bread (*Datsch*) that is baked slowly "down hearth" in an iron baking pan with a lid, surrounded on top and bottom with hot coals.[103] The bread was eaten and crumbs from the bread were scattered at the four corners of the garden, as indicated in a rhyming blessing recalled by Amanda Baer Stoudt (1857-1942):[104]

Ebbes Griene, ebbes Schwaatze,
Ebbes Weisse fer ihre Katze.
Backt mer Datsch am Trudisdaag
Streu die Grimmle wo sie mag,
Fun Eck zu Eck am Gorderand,
So wachse dei Greider uffem Land.

A little something green, A little something black,
A little something white for her cat.
Bake a Datsch on St. Gertrude's Day
Scatter the crumbs where she directs,
From corner to corner along the garden's edge,
So that your plants will thrive upon the land.[105]

Saints, however, were not the only helpers in the garden. Near Kutztown a local Mennonite farmer recently recalled that his father used to plow the large patch garden in the 1960s with rounded corners, leaving these small areas within the garden fence for perennial wildflowers, as the farmer's father used to say "*wu die Eck-Leitli wuhne*" (Where the little corner people live).[106] These garden spirits were believed to be the equivalents of faeries or the little people, inspiring a wide variety of domestic rituals on both sides of the Atlantic. In Pennsylvania, as well as in Alsace, Austria, Switzerland, and throughout Germany, *'S Bucklich-Mennli* (the Little Hunchbacked Man) was the subject of children's rhymes and folk songs, which described the little spirit of the house and garden as a bringer of mischief.[107] A popular song named after the little scamp, describes his interference with the household chores of the children:

Wann ich in mei Schtibbche kumm,
Fa mei Schtibbche kehre,
Scheht des bucklich Mennli dadd
Un fangt aa zu wehre.

When I enter my little room,
To sweep it out,
The little hunchbacked man is there
and attempts to hinder me.[108]

If freshly planted onion sets were uprooted, impurities found in milk freshly run though the sieve, or dust on a cleanly swept floor, '*S Bucklich-Mennli* was to blame. Celebrated dialect orator John Brendle (1889 -1966) recalled that bakers would blame the imp if a fly were in the pie crust, or it a cake would nicely rise and later fall in the pan. However, if a pie was baked to perfection, "*dann hot sie, uffkors, aa gsaat—'ya well, des muss mer em Bucklich Mennli gewwe, er hot mer mitgholfe fer den Kuche backe,*'" (then, of course, they also said, "Yes, well, I must give a little to the Hunchbacked Man, as he helped me bake this pie").[109]

The Little Hunchbacked Man was often appeased into dutiful service if a member of the household were to place a bowl of milk on the windowsill for him.[110] Brendle also recalled that this particular spirit and his counterparts, "*die gleene Mennlin*" (the Little People), were most active in spring, and that many a housewife would maintain a small section of the hearth unswept, where '*S Bucklich Mennli* was believed to sleep.[111]

Well into the twentieth century, the hearth and its later adaptation, the wood stove, was the proverbial soul of the home. Located in the kitchen, hot coals were always to be kept live as these were used to start each day's cooking fire. This perpetual fire was symbolic of the family's wellbeing and attentiveness, and so rituals surrounded the hearth and the keeping of the fire.

One method for maintaining such a perpetual fire was to perform a ritual at the time that the hearth was constructed by placing three tin boxes in three corners under the stones or bricks of the hearth, each containing the following inscription:

> *Deus Pater, Deus Filius, Deus Spiritus Sanctus in Oel Trinitatis, Sonne und Mond haben ihrem Gang zu Wasser und zu Land, daß kein Feuer und Flammen in diesem Haus ausgang.*
>
> God the Father, God the Son, God the Holy Spirit, in the oil of the Trinity. Sun and Moon have their course over water and land, so that no fire or flames shall go out in this house.[112]

While the hearth was the site of numerous healing rituals, such as the curing of "wound wood" used to lance suppurating wounds,[113] the treatment of jaundice with a carrot,[114] or the "smoking" of the red string used for erysipelas,[115] the hearth was also the source of ashes employed on *Eschemittwoch* (Ash Wednesday) to bless cattle, to protect against lice and topical parasites and to bless the garden to keep away insects. Some even sprinkled the ashes in the shape of a cross, from north to south and east to west in the garden, while others spread a protective circle of ashes around the home to repel snakes.[116] These practices are informed by official liturgical distribution of ashes in Ash Wednesday services in the Roman Catholic, Lutheran, and Reformed traditions, when the sign of the cross is made on the forehead in ashes mixed with oil, as a reminder of mortality: "Remember that you are dust, and to dust you shall return."[117] The domestic and agricultural use of ashes extends this Lenten observation beyond the church and to the whole farm and property. Unlike the distribution of ashes in the church, which utilizes ashes made from palms from the Palm Sunday service, the ashes used around the home, in the garden, and on the farm, were ashes from the family's hearth or cookstove, suggesting that even such a mundane substance could have sacred implications.

The bakeoven is likewise the site of ritual healing. Infants suffering from colic are placed in the mouth of the bakeoven when it is still warm and cooling down, in much the same way that the horse collar is used for a similar cure – both ritually imply a rebirth. Thus the ritual pantomiming of baking the child in the bakeoven was suggestive of the womb and of the child being baked to perfection like a loaf of bread. Bread baked on Ascension Day was believed to be impervious to molding, and bread baked on Good Friday was used in creating healing salves.[118] Bread, symbolic of the body, was not to be turned upside-down, or placed on its round side, or it would foretell a quarrel.

If a person was suspected to have drowned and the body could not be located, it was once common to toss a loaf of bread into the water, with the belief that the loaf (*der Leeb*) would float to the location just above where the body (*der Leib*) of the deceased was submerged.[119] There is doubtlessly a presumed symbolic connection between the bread and the body, which is further compounded by the similarity of the words in both Pennsylvania Dutch and standard German (*der Laib, der Leib*).

If however, it is unknown if a missing person drowned or not, another bread ritual allows for one to remotely determine if the person in question is living or dead:

> Take two little crumbs from a loaf of bread and lay them opposite each other three finger's distance from one another and then also 3 coals also 3 fingers apart, then take a sewing needle and a length of thread half an ell long, thread it, and make a knot in the end. Stick the needle through the bread, and hold it so that it doesn't touch the table and say, "If thou art living, then go to the dear bread, but if thou art dead, then go to the coals. It is certainly true.[120]

A leather amulet, shaped like the silhouette of the dancing figure of '*S Bucklich Mennli*, or the Little Hunchbacked Man, a spirit believed to cause mischief on Pennsylvania Dutch farms, especially relating to dairy activities. This amulet was believed to ward off the influence of the spirit. Found on a milkhouse door in Ruscombmanor Township, Berks County. Private Collection.

The same principles apply to methods of determining if a person is terminally ill, or if they will recover. One particular method again involves bread, which is rubbed on the teeth[121] or the brow[122] of the sick person. If a dog will not eat the bread, then the person is deathly ill. The same ritual is performed with bacon rubbed on the feet of the sick person and then fed to the dog.

Just as the hearth and bakeoven provide ritual space and substance, so too does the table on which the family eats. In a number of domestic rituals, the table is not only a familial space, but a common source of *materia medica*. Scrapings from the four corners of the table were used to treat colic, to keep a servant from becoming homesick, and a dog from straying[123] A more elaborate ritual attributed to St. Albert the Great to protect children from *Hexerei* suggests scraping upwards from three corners of the table, each with a little salt, bread, and goat's beard (salsify), and assembling a bundle with unbleached yarn without talking to anyone. One was to hang the bundle around the child's neck in an uneven hour and say: "N.N. I hang this upon thee as penance in the Name of God the Father, and of the Son, and of the Holy Spirit."[124] Thus the scrapings from the table are representative of the family's gathering place, the identity of the home, and domestic solidarity. This is the same notion that undergirds the ritual of sweeping a piece of bread or bacon from the underside of the table to top so that the dogs under the table do not quarrel.[125] Domestic ritual spaces such as the table are not relegated to human needs and activities, but extend to the animal kingdom as well.

Animals & Livestock

Farm animals and livestock were treated with the same level of interest as humans, and received blessings for their ailments and assistance in difficult transitions. Draft animals were of utmost importance as the primary means of transportation and work for farmers and tradesmen. Families depended upon their horses, mules, and oxen in much the same way that people today depend upon their vehicles. Rituals played an important role in the feeding, working, raising, and even training of draft animals.

A benediction used by the farrier and horse-doctor Conrad Raber in Berks County around 1800 for breaking a foal for use with a halter invokes the Three Kings: "Caspar take thee, Melchior bind thee, and Balthasar lead thee, in the name of the Father, Son and Holy Spirit."[126] In this prayer, the Three Kings are being asked to intercede on behalf of the Foal and calm its immature and inherently wild temperament, allowing the rider or farmer to safely work with the animal and introduce the foal to its future function as a beast of labor. A similar blessing is attributed to St. Francis, patron saint of animals, for when one is yoking oxen for the first time: "Ox, I yoke thee in the name of St. Francis. Ox, I lay the yoke upon thee, bear it with patience, just as Christ bore his cross. + + +"[127]

The health of draft animals was absolutely essential on the farm, and a number of ailments could prevent an animal from being productive. Delays in the use of a draft horse or mule could cause delays in harvesting and processing crops – a potential disaster for the farm family. Another example of one of Conrad Raber's animal blessings incorporates the use of physical gestures to produce a cure for "Sweeny," an archaic term for an atrophy that afflicts overworked limbs of humans and animals. This illness will cause a draft animal to become weak and incapable of working, spelling delays and difficulty for the farmer who depends on the horse for scheduled labor. Raber's healing method requires the practitioner to stroke the underside of the ailing horse with his hand, and speak: "Thou fadest away in in the flesh or in the marrow or in the blood. O, our Lord Jesus, how [much more] mighty thou art in name - x x x." A play on words that is apparent in the original German is found in the verb "to fade away" or "disappear" which is found in the dialect form "*schwinst*," directly related to the name of the disease in German – "*Schwinde*" – meaning both for the body to waste away as well as for the disease to spread. Here the "*Schwinde*" is asked to "*schwinne*" – or for the "Sweeny" to "disappear," or waste away, as it cannot prevail against the power of Christ.[128]

Other common ailments in horses and livestock include foundering, described by Raber as "*zu reh vom Wasser oder Futer*" – "to founder from water or food," and elsewhere as "*aufgessen*" – "to overeat." This disease is caused by an animal's excessive eating of grass or drinking too much water, resulting in severe bloating and in the worst cases immobilization and incapacity to work as draft animals. This archaic use of the word "founder" is not to be confused with another condition, *die Hufrehe*, where foundering in a modern sense can refer to laminitis of the hoof in a horse, causing it to "founder" or fall.[129] Raber's remedy for foundering from water or food was to take a woman's shirt when she is menstruating, and rinse it out with water into the horse feed.[130] Menstruation was not necessarily viewed positively, as women typically avoided a whole range of domestic tasks "*in ihre Zeit*" (in their time) – everything from canning and preserving to making soap; from stirring vinegar to planting the garden.[131] However, each state of being was considered useful in the proper context. Menstruation was considered to be a release from the body, and the body smell of a woman menstruating was believed to help a horse that was congested and bloated from food or water to release its congestion.

Another illness, which Raber refers to as *Gehlwasser*, literally "yellow-water," is edema, or the accumulation of fluid in organ tissue or flesh. This illness was often associated with a deficiency of the liver, as indicated by the archaic humoral designation of "yellow." Accordingly, it was once believed that goading a team of oxen with a willow-switch encouraged the accumulation of water (*gehlwasser*), as willow trees often favor watery growing conditions.[132] Raber's sympathetic cure was to infuse the animal's feed with water in which yellow burdock had been boiled — a yellow cure for a yellow illness.

Animals raised for their meat were no less subject to ritual procedures in their care — everything from the hatching of eggs to the butchering of birds, to the weaning calves. Setting hens for hatching eggs is a delicate process and one that was coordinated with the hour when the blessing was given in church, between 11 o'clock and noon,[133] and was frequently the only work performed on a Sunday aside from feeding the animal and milking the cows. Hens should be set on an odd number of eggs and one should not speak about the eggs while they are being hatched.[134] So that the chicks are all female, eggs should be transferred to the nest for hatching under a brooding hen in a woman's apron by a woman,[135] a symbol of maternity that appears frequently in rituals performed by women.

Just like the News Year's ritual of the "Three Things," three kinds of grain set out on Christmas night and fed to chickens on Christmas and New Year's mornings would protect the chickens from being eaten by hawks, and a rope stretched on Christmas Day from the chicken coop to as far as the chickens tend to roam would define the radius of a safe area where hawks would not cross to prey upon the chickens.[136] Turkeys that would ordinarily foam farther from home were given corn soaked in the lard from frying Fasnachts to keep them nearby when they were laying eggs.[137]

Geese were thought to be particularly useful in predicting winter weather, by means of the breast bone of a goose selected for its certain size, color, and from a certain flock.[138] For some, this was to be a gray goose with a trace of wild blood, that had hatched in spring. The dots on the bone's keel indicated the placement of winter storms and precipitation, while the darker the spots, the colder the weather would be.[139] Willoughby H. Troxell (1870-1945), "The Goosebone Man" of Laurys Station, Lehigh County, predicted the weather by the blade-shaped bones of two white geese, eaten for Thanksgiving dinner.[140] Troxell raised the geese himself at his home at Indian Spring Park and would harvest the bone to use in his prediction, but only from a goose hatched within the year.[141] Troxell would divide the breastbones into sections representing December, January, and February and make his prediction between Thanksgiving and the first week of December for the coming year.[142]

Eggs laid on Good Friday were gathered in the morning without speaking to anyone, and were considered holy. Such *Karfreidaagsoier* (Good Friday eggs) were believed to impart a blessing through eating so that one would not get a fevers or hernia.[143] Some families would collect eggs on Good Friday, Holy Saturday, and Easter and would put some of each into an omelet consumed on Easter morning for breakfast.[144] By placing a Good Friday egg in a crock or other container under the eaves in the attic, the house and its occupants would be protected from fire, storms, lightning, and disaster, as long as the egg remained undisturbed.[145] One Lehigh County contact recently told me that his family had done this every year for as long as he could remember except for last year, when he decided he would no longer keep his own chickens. Thus such traditions are dependent upon maintaining a connection to farming.

Good Friday Eggs were also said to be "*gut fer brauche damit*" (good with which to powwow), and were used in any ritual where an egg was called for in the removal of an illness, especially when the egg was buried outside under the eaves.[146] If one disposes of egg shells, however, they must be crushed, otherwise they served as hiding places for spirits, both bad and good.[147]

Chickens, pigs, or steers, valued for their meat, were typically butchered in the waxing moon, when the animal is most robust, otherwise the meat would shrink and spoil.[148] A method to keep chicken meat from bruising during butchering was to draw a circle intersected by a cross in *Hinkeldreck* (chicken feces) and place the chicken's neck over the cross when cutting off its head, so that the body would lie still and not run without its head.[149] *Hinkeldreck*

Eggs laid on Good Friday were once thought to be blessed, and were concealed in the home for protection, as well as used for the removal of illness. *Pennsylvania German Cultural Heritage Center, Kutztown University of Pennsylvania.*

also featured in one of the most common rituals associated with childhood injury, and spoken over many a skinned knee or bruised elbow:

Heeli, Heeli Hinkeldreck, bis Marriye frieh un all iss weck.

Healing, healing chicken dung, by early tomorrow, it will all be gone.

While it is the general consensus among speakers of the dialect in Berks and Lehigh that these humorous words were merely a parody of powwowing, rather than a serious application of ritual, for a handful of others, this rhyme was used in the removal of all sorts of illnesses and injuries, and occasionally combined with the use of a potato.[150] A number of contacts who could recite the words were completely unaware of their meaning. The language barrier is perhaps responsible for this integration of the rhyme into oral tradition without coterminous meaning. Despite this ambiguity, between satire and blessing, the rhyme and its use for children remains a culturally specific expression of care in Pennsylvania Dutch communities.[151]

Aside from the ubiquitous role of the chicken and the pig for meat, dairy cows were precious for the income that was produced from milk and butter. Processing milk and butter were sensitive activities, and it was not uncommon to perceive that supernatural forces, including a grudge, curse (*Hex*) or envy would cause milk to spoil or cause butter not to form.[152] Aside from all of the ritual forms of retribution such as thrusting a hot poker, scythe, or butcher knife into the milk, or shooting a silver coin out of a gun into the butter churn,[153] these challenges could be overcome in a variety of other ways. If the envy was perceived to be from a neighbor, one could steal or beg a small piece of bread that could be fed to the cow to restore the milk. Just as a dishcloth, stolen from a person that begrudges you, could be used to ensure positive outcomes in baking,[154] likewise water poured through a stolen dishcloth could cure a cow of indigestion. Otherwise, one should get up first thing in the morning without speaking to anyone, milk the cow, pour the milk into the outhouse, and relieve one's self upon it. Or, as Helfenstein suggests:

> If an accident befalls a cow, so that it no longer gives milk or butter, and further becomes gaunt and dry, take the milk, put it in a pot, cook it for one hour, and stab it frequently with a grass-scythe. Then bury it in a hole, and defecate upon it, cover it with earth, and say the following words three times: All evil shall pass away, as dust and dung. From whence the evil cometh, so shall it return. As this milk decays, so shall all sorcery dissipate, in the name of Matthew the Holy Apostle.[155]

Rituals for cattle, however, are not merely concerned with their safety, health and productivity, but also address issues of salability such as one from the manuscript of Peter Hain of Reading, describing a sure way to ensure that a cow is sold at market. To sell a cow at market, one should go to an ant hill, and find the legendary ball of black resin that the ants store in the middle of the hill, and rub the cow with the ball of resin, and it will surely be sold.[156] This ritual ensures that one will not travel the distance to market, only to find that the animal does not sell, and both time, energy, and travel are wasted, an undesirable scenario for a farmer who may be relying on the cash sale. For one who purchases a cow, however, a stone should be taken from the property where the animal formerly dwelled, and placed in the manger to keep the animal from being homesick and curb the desire to stray.[157]

Likewise, a wide range of rituals are employed to locate animals that may have strayed or been stolen, as well as to ensure that animals do not run away. In the case of an animal that has left of its own volition (as opposed to theft), one could call the animal through a knothole in the barn siding three times, on nine mornings in succession, without speaking to anyone and while holding your breath.[158] A widely circulated method to compel a horse or cow that has been stolen to turn from the hands of the thief, using the dung fork:

> *Wan dir ein Vieh gestolen wird so nim die Mistgabel und stich hinein Wo daß Vieh ist gestanden und nene daß Vih mit Namen sprich ich drit dich ich s[t]ich dich bit ich bit dich du solt Wieder kommen und dich wenden auß daß Diebs Händen geschwind gleich wie der Wind als wie den Fisch im Wasser als wie der Vogel in der Luft als wie der Thau über die Blumen sold du hurtig und geschwind wieder in den s[t]all Kommen daß seÿ dir zur Buse gezehlt im N[amen] [Vater, Sohn, Heilig Geist] Amen.*

> When an animal is stolen, then take the dung fork and stick it into the ground where the animal last stood, and call the animal by name. Say: I kick thee, I stick thee, I bid thee, that thou shalt return and turn from the hands of the thief, as quick as the wind, as the fish swims in water, as the bird in the air, as the dew upon the flowers, thou shalt quickly and swiftly return to the

stable, that penance may be reckoned unto thee, in the Name of the Father, Son, and Holy Spirit. Amen.[159]

It is implicit here that one addresses the animal through the pitchfork, which has been in contact with the animal's dung, and therefore carries some measure of its essence. Matching the poetic cadence, the speaker "kick[s]" the pitchfork. The pitchfork "stick[s]" the spot of ground where the horse was last seen, and the "bid[ding]" is meant to reach the animal remotely by means of sympathy. In this case the pitchfork and the ground are meant to serve as intermediaries through which the spirit of the animal is being addressed.[160] This ritual is identical to one found in the eighteenth-century manuscript of Rosina Barbara Werli, of Weisenberg Township, Lehigh County,[161] demonstrating the wide distribution of this particular ritual throughout southeastern Pennsylvania.

This particular ritual was employed in a modern adaptation in 2008 for a man living in Kutztown, who had a particularly friendly cat that he suspected had either wandered off or had been stolen. The cat had already been gone for two weeks by the time he asked me if I knew of any powwowing techniques for retrieving his cat. I recommended the same procedure used for horses that had been included in the Werli manuscript. It was agreed, that since a pitchfork was not applicable to a cat, the scoop used to attend to the cat's litter box would have to suffice. We went to where the cat had last been seen in the yard, between two row homes on Main Street, and we stuck the handle of the scoop into the soil. I recited the words in Pennsylvania Dutch three times, and each time where I came to the words "*Ich dred dich*," we gave the little plastic scoop a soft kick. We were unaware at the time that as we completed the final round the cat had already snuck up behind us and was quietly watching the whole affair unnoticed. When we finished the ritual, the owner asked me, "What's next?" When I responded that we should be patient, I could tell he was disappointed. But when we turned and saw the cat standing there in the moonlight, he was so startled that the cat ran away again. We both walked around the block in vain looking to see where the cat had gone, and after an hour's search, we gave up. The next day, however, the cat came up to the kitchen window when the owner was washing dishes, but when he went outside to retrieve the cat, it was gone. By the third day, the cat came up to him on the porch and never left him again as long as it lived. This incident demonstrates not only the ways in which historical rituals can be adapted to meet the needs of present-day people, but also that there are still many aspects of daily life that are outside of our realm of control for which we may turn to ritual as a means of assistance.

HUNTING, FISHING, WILD ANIMALS

While domesticated animals and livestock receive considerably more attention in *Braucherei* than wild animals, hunters, fishers, and farmers employed ritual as a means to influence positive outcomes with animals that were otherwise wholly unpredictable. For hunters, this took the form of ritually attracting, bating, and binding game:

> To bring many deer together and halt them so that they do not flee: In May, early in the morning on a Monday, in the first hour of the day as soon as the sun rises, gather carline thistle (*Eberwurz*), mountain parsley (*Hirschwurz*), lovage, and camphor. Dry the leaves and roots and make a powder. Take also birch ashes and a newly burned, unused roof shingle, and the placenta of a pregnant doe, and dry them in the same manner. Mix everything together and knead it into a dough with pea-meal and fresh water taken from a stream that flows forth out of a woods. Make the dough into pellets and let them dry, and keep them for use. Its working occurs most powerfully when the sun passes into the twentieth degree of Cancer until the 30th degree, i.e. from about the 10th to the twentieth of July, although otherwise it has proven so powerful that Sylvius was able to assemble twenty-five head of deer by this means. But you must lay the pellets in a place where the game are accustomed to make their path. As soon as one of them eats it, it cannot move from the spot except to go and lead other deer thither – droves of them. If also a man carries the pellets with him, approaches the deer, and the deer already has tried the pellets, they will not run away, but rather stand still so that they can be touched.[162]

This class of ritual is described in the original language as a "*Schtellung*" – an act that binds and holds an animal so that it cannot flee unless released, similar to the use of a *Dieb-Segen*, a binding "Thief-Blessing" used for the same purpose.[163] Ritual bindings are well documented for use with attracting and binding game such as deer, foxes, and birds as well as in protective blessings to be used against snakes, wasps, dogs, and wolves.

A Wolf-Blessing (*Wolfssegen*) attributed to St. Albert the Great was intended for use by shepherds and keepers of livestock, and features Christ, Peter, and Mary:

> **Lord Jesus Christ and St. Peter went out in the morning, and St. Mary went ahead. She said: O dear Lord, whither shall we hie? We shall journey over hill and dale, therefore protect my flock, wherever it may be. St. Peter took his key, and locked the wolves' snouts, that they gnaw no bone. + + +**[164]

Such religious invocations of saints used to stay the predations of wolves are not unlike the function of blessings used for protection from stinging insects such as wasps, where the insect is told that it cannot sting because on account of a sacred truth:

Gehl Wespa, gehl Wespa, gehl Wespa,
dir könnt mich so wennig stecha,
das der Satan der das word Jesus kann sprecha.

Yellow Wasps, Yellow Wasps, Yellow Wasps:
ye can sting me only so much as Satan can speak
the word Jesus.[165]

Not all methods use sacred imagery, however, as one for stopping bumble bees is vulgar:

Hummle brummle ogsafatz
Die angel is drei zoll zu katz.

Bumble-bee buzz an ox's pudendum,
Your rod is three inches too short.[166]

A York County man demonstrated for me a method for keeping brown mud-dauber wasps from stinging, by simply biting his tongue. I watched him handle wasps with his hands, without ever being stung.[167] This is quite similar to an old method to keep a dog from barking, by holding the thumb firmly inside one's fist.[168]

Snake-bite blessings are common, but far less well-recorded are the words (*Schlangensegen*) and means by which one could stop and bind a snake so that it cannot move from the spot or bite. Johannes Spangenberg's method involved the chant "Osii, Osia, Osii,"[169] a variation of a fifteenth century Latin blessing:

Osi + Osi + Osi + Ave admissiva serpens stes in verbis dei sicut stetit ab ea in Jordane cum Johannes Xristum baptizavit. + Tetragramaton + Adonay + Alpha + et O +. Coniuro te serpens per deum meum, per deum verum, per deum sanctum, per deum vivum, qui te et me creavit, per deum qui te dampnavit inter cuncta animalia….

Thou Detested One + Thou Detested One + Thou Detested One + Hail thou welcome Serpent, stand still by the Word of God, just as Christ stood in the River Jordan with St. John the Baptist when he baptized him. Yahweh, Lord, Alpha and Omega. I bind thee, Serpent, through my God, through the True God, through the Holy God, through the Living God, who made thee and me, who cursed thee above all creatures…[170]

This blessing, drawing upon the biblical curse of the snake, is a predecessor to the common blessing used for snake-bite, which addresses the snake, "Cursed art thou, Serpent, and cursed shalt thou remain…" It is possible that the Pennsylvania variation was also intended to bind the particular snake responsible for a bite in order to compel it to remove its venom: "… withdraw thy poison, withdraw thy poison, withdraw thy poison…"[171] This is also suggested by the self-proclaimed "Snake-Charmer" of Reading, Berks County, Michael Heller, who described that he knew words for treating a bite in combination with his herbal remedies, but that, in most cases, he had to actually locate the snake responsible for the bite in order to perform the ritual.[172] The snake however, was not to be killed, but allowed to go free.

It was once commonly believed that a snake that was killed could be used to influence the weather, and by hanging a dead snake over the fence would bring rain.[173] Another method to achieve the same result, without having to take the life of a snake involves taking two stones in one's hand, and clicking them together while chanting a Pennsylvania Dutch blessing:

Raya, raya drupa,
De Boova mus m'r glupa.

Rain, rain drops,
The boys we must paddle.[174]

Snakes were not only believed to affect the weather; they were also feared for their ability to *verhex* a gun, or render it useless when pointed directly at the snake. For this reason, two people intending to kill a snake with a gun would bring along a cane with which to point at the snake first, so that the snake would mistakenly *verhex* the cane, while the one with the gun could take aim and shoot the snake.[175]

The Blessing of Guns and Rifles

For hunters, influence was not only exerted by ritual means over animals and game, but also for assurance that one's firearms would be protected from any outside influence, whether supernatural or ritual in nature. One of the earliest extant Pennsylvania firearm blessings was discovered in an early nineteenth-century rifle, consisting of the first 3 verses of the Gospel of John.[176] The passage was written out longhand and carefully rolled up to occupy a small space between the barrel of the gun and the stock. At the time of the blessing's creation, one's ability to shoot accurately not only depended upon one's skill, but also on correct functioning of the gun and proper combustion of the gunpowder. In a flintlock rifle, if the powder was too moist, if the touch-hole between the flash pan and the barrel was clogged, or if any number of variables were not properly in place, the shot may be to no avail. As each shot was individually muzzle-loaded, the process was time consuming and highly subject to human error. The complex factors affecting a hunter's ability to shoot undoubtedly gave rise to popular aphorisms, like the German phrase, "*Alle Kunst ist umsonst, wann ein Engel in das zündloch brunst*" (All skill is in vain if an angel pisses in the touchhole of your musket).[177]

Such ideas were not merely archaic but carried over long into the twentieth century, when written inscriptions were still used by hunters. An old double-barrel shotgun from Windsor Castle, Berks County, was recently purchased by Donald G. Batz of Topton and taken apart for cleaning. An old inscription was found on a piece of paper tucked inside the stock, featuring long abbreviations attributed to

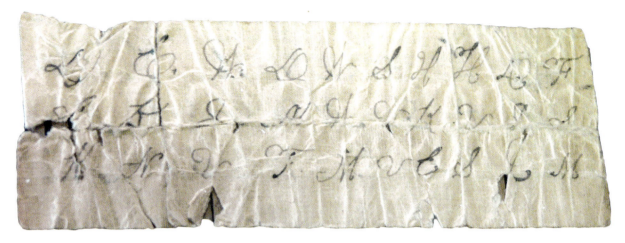

An abbreviated blessing concealed in a Berks County shotgun from Egyptian Secrets of Albertus Magnus. *Courtesy of Donald G. Batz.*

St. Albert the Great. The gun had been last serviced in 1919 by its original owner Robert Hermansader, as evidenced by a fragment of a Reading Eagle newspaper tucked around the blessing, which read as following:[178]

DCWDWSHHDF
SKJMWWKVJS
KNVFMVESLM

Such measures were taken in order to avoid one's gun from being *verhext*, a state whereby shots fired from the gun would always miss the target, no matter how skilled the shooter. Several ways to dispel such misfortune were to immerse the whole gun in running water in a creek to dispel the *Hex*,[179] load the gun with a silver bullet or dime, or stick two pins in the gunstock in the shape of a cross.[180] One could also take asafetida, resin from the storax tree, and water from a flowing source, and mix into a cleaning compound. The rag used for swabbing the barrel should thereafter be smoked in a chimney or dropped into a freshly dug grave.[181]

In order to ensure deadly accuracy with a gun, one could swab the barrel with the heart of a bat,[182] or take a needle used to sew the gown of a corpse, and drive it into the gunstock, or place a wad of communion bread there.[183] Although numerous methods exist for treating the gun, some also focus on the shooter, such as taking the guts of a trout caught between Christmas and New Year's Day and burn them to powder on a copper lid. Instructions were to put a little into the stock of the gun and some in a little bundle to be hung under the right arm.[184]

Likewise, a number of plants were used to construct bundles that were believed to ensure that one could not be shot such as the use of the roots of mouse's ear (Forget-me-not, *Myosotis*) dug at full or new moon and concealed on the person for protection, or by harvesting blue chicory on Peter and Paul Day, the 29th of June, a quarter hour before 12 o'clock and carried in the same manner. The latter ritual also alleges that it will prevent one from being bound or imprisoned.[185]

Rituals to deflect a shot are not only protective, but occasionally competitive. In order to prevent one from hitting a target in a shooting match, one should place a splinter of wood from a tree that was struck by lightning behind the target,[186] perhaps on account of the belief that lightning cannot strike the same spot twice. As shooting matches are social engagements and the outcomes are by no means of dire importance, this latter ritual is an example of how ritual can satisfy one's self interest and be personally-driven.

The same logic applies to other rituals intended to tip the odds in one's favor in gambling, playing cards or dice. One could hold the right thumb in the palm of the right hand in the right trouser pocket when a hanging takes place, in order to bless the hand for card playing.[187] Another method was to carry the heart of an owl, or secure a bat's heart on one's person with a red silk string.[188]

RITUALS OF VIRILITY, INVINCIBILITY & POWER

Although not all of these rituals for self-aggrandizement are harmful or oriented towards *Hexerei*, quite a number are suspiciously oriented toward advantage over others or for demonstrations of feats of strength or invincibility. Most of the rituals of this type were used by men who aimed to increase their status and virility.

A hunter's manuscript describes not only typical rituals applying to attracting and catching animals, but also how to become invincible:

To obtain great strength, take a bottle of red wine, seal it well and bury it in an ant-hill on Green Thursday. Let it remain there a whole year, and on Good Friday of the following year, remove the wine from the hill and drink a little each morning. You will experience wonders…[189]

As ants can lift objects many times their size and weight, this sympathetic ritual involves the person taking on the strength of the ants. Perceivably, some of these types of procedures could be used for helpful purposes especially for soldiers, such as methods to prevent one from tiring while marching by using wormwood leaves and roots gathered on St. Bartholomew's Day and carried in one's shoes and pockets, to hinder perspiration and weariness.[190] Others, however, are distinctly for the purpose of enabling reckless behavior:

To keep one from becoming drunk when you are in company and want to drink a great deal. Swallow a whole freshly laid egg warm from the hen in the morning after fasting and without speaking to anyone, and then eat the marrow from pork.[191]

In the regrettable event that this ritual does not work, a wide variety of hangover cures are documented, such as the use of fungus that grows on the linden tree steeped in equal parts water and old wine, and administered in the morning, noon, and evening,[192] or for those who are not only hung over but still drunk, Ossman and Steel recommend a complex recipe of sulphate of iron, magnesia, peppermint water, and nutmeg extract three times a day, which "prevents that absolute physical and moral prostration that follows a sudden breaking off from the use of stimulating drinks."[193]

And if one's bad behavior were enough to dissuade a sweetheart from marriage, a wide range of rituals were available to remedy the situation. Such rituals could be as simple as borrowing the virility from a rooster by taking three feathers from its tail and pressing them into her hand. If however, virility were not enough to satisfy a sweetheart's affections, a gruesome alternative was to pull out the tongue of a turtledove and put it in one's mouth while wooing. This latter ritual has been documented in Berks County in the middle of the last century.[194]

If the aforementioned rituals intended to inspire love proved ineffective, further recourse could include the concealment of materials in a woman's bedchamber unbeknownst to the woman:

To drive a lover crazy: sneak into her room and mix salt, bread, and soft cheese together and hide it in her bedstead. She will not be able to sleep until she comes to see you.[195]

A Moravian manuscript from the eighteenth century, penned by Johann Christoph Pyrlaeus Jr. (1748-1808) of Bethlehem, offers a number of similar entries, such as carrying the head of a hoopoe bird in order to "Gain One's Love,"[196] or how to get a woman to tell one her secrets in her sleep. For the latter, one was to write the name of the woman in question on a linen rag which is wrapped around the liver of a rabbit, and lay it under her head (presumably while she is in bed), whereby she will answer any question which is asked of her. Pyrlaeus also included instructions for how to use a sympathetic

The heart of a bat (*Schpeckmaus-Hatz*) bound in red flannel and discretely tied with a red silk string around the arm of a gambler ensured a lucky hand at cards or throw of the dice.

mixture of quicksilver and blackbirds' eggs to compel women to leave the bathroom naked. These entries would not have been particularly becoming of a Moravian, or a member of any other denomination for that matter, however, for many personal manuscripts containing these instructions, there is often little evidence to confirm that the writer actually participated in such unethical rituals. Especially considering once again the scarcity of the Old World hoopoe necessary to perform the first of these three entries, it is almost certain that Pyrlaeus was unable to perform some of these procedures for lack of necessary materials.[197] Since disgust and improbability is suggested in the details, perhaps they were a humorous reminder of the limits of these rituals.

Nevertheless, such instructions for ritual predations against women are rare in manuscripts, and only found in one powwow manual, *Egyptian Secrets,* attributed to St. Albert the Great. Even if these processes were not often employed, their presence in ritual writings reflects the kind of insecurities that men may have held concerning their relations with women.

These types of anxieties highlighted in ritual literature were further exhibited in remedies specifically used to restore lost "manhood" such as one remedy for men who fear their wedding nights, who were instructed to urinate through their new wedding ring to alleviate their anxiety.[198] Contrary to this this type of identification of anxiety as a potential cause, some rituals specifically blamed women for male impotence:

> When you are infatuated and bewitched by a woman, so that you may not love another, then take the blood of a billy goat and grease your head therewith, and you will soon be right again.[199]

This remedy, like the use of rooster feathers, aims to transfer some measure of masculinity from an archetypal male animal to compensate for the perceived "missing" or "stolen" qualities in the man. Still others rituals for curing a man of impotence simply aim to ritually overturn the imbalance in the man's condition through acts of phallic inversion, like pulling out an oak stake in a vineyard, urinating in the empty hole, and replacing the stake upside down, in order to symbolically overturn the condition.[200] Ironically, while a number of ritual remedies among men specifically aim to address issues of potency and self-confidence in intimate and social relationships, many rituals designated for women are utilized as damage control for issues arising from unchecked behavior among men, giving women a sense of agency in otherwise difficult situations.

Ritual protection of Women & Families

Just as a wide variety of ritual expressions in *Braucherei* developed around the activities and social roles of men, so too were particular rituals tailored to the needs and empowerment of women. A number of these rituals specifically address concerns over personal safety and the easing of domestic tensions through behavior modification.

One of the primary reasons that men were concerned about their guns becoming *verhext* is because of the power that women were perceived to have over the outcomes of hunting and fishing. For instance, if a man were poaching on someone else's land, all a woman would need to do to prevent a man's gun from firing is to take off her apron and lay it over her shoulder.[201] This ritual posture, suggestive of scolding, was enough to destroy even the best marksman's chances at the hunt and suggests that women had ritual recourse to protect the property even when the odds were not necessarily in her favor physically.

Likewise, if a woman brushes her apron over a hunting dog's nose "*geht er der ganz Daag hinnerscht-vedderscht uff der Schpur*" (all day he goes backwards up the path, i.e. is useless for hunting).[202] The same rule applies for fishermen if a woman is encountered on the way to the water.[203] While one explanation for this gendered advantage is that the woman in question could be a witch, but the simple fact of the matter is that women were perceived to have the power to influence men and therefore sway their luck.

A ritual cure to reform the addiction of a drunkard involved the family discreetely spiking his whiskey with the dirt scraped from under his finger nails. This subtle cocktail, made from the drunkard's own filth, was believed to have the permanent effect of making him ill each time he drinks.

But this influence need not be overstated, as rituals designed to protect women from violence were cultural indicators of the prevalence of inequality. The ritual of the "Three Drops of Blood" in the private manuscript of Rosina Barbara Werli from Weisenberg Township, Lehigh County in 1790 was used to stop molestations at the hands of "*Spisbuwen*" (hooligans).[204] Other variations describe the same ritual as a means to "take the power from a man, so that he cannot harm thee," by taking from the perpetrator "three drops of blood, one from thine heart, one from thine head, and one from thy manhood." These parts of the body are by no means selected randomly, or merely for their poetic effect, but because of their significance in averting violence in the form of sexual assault.

Some rituals were used to protect women and children from husbands with tendencies toward alcoholism and violence. A ritual means of averting domestic abuse of women and children at the hands of a drunkard is to spike his drink with the dirt from under his fingernails when he is in a stupor.[205] The result is that he will become incredibly ill when he drinks, as he will be sympathetically ingesting his own foul nature. The clippings of his fingernails could also be employed so that a man will not beat his wife, when the clippings are placed into a funeral bier.[206]

Another method is to take an apple, place it in the hand of a dying person, and hold it there until the person has passed away. In order to ritually compel a man to cut his drinking back by half, he should be fed half the apple without knowing where it came from. If one wishes for him to completely shun alcohol, the whole apple is given, but he must be unaware that the ritual is taking place.[207]

These rituals involving the dead gave women agency in otherwise dire circumstances. If a woman takes a needle and some dirt from a grave and wraps it in a cloth used at a funeral, "no man can defy her as long as she carries it."[208]

The same type of clandestine operations were employed to break a man of a destructive gambling habit by letting a gambler wash his hands in water with which a corpse has been washed,[209] or by letting him drink the milk of a sow.[210] Both of these are designed that a man would become physically, even deathly ill when he gambles.

These types of rituals used for empowerment and protection by means of behavior modification are by no means the norm for *Braucherei*, but are significant to note, suggesting that earlier generations dealt with the same types of social and domestic challenges affecting our society today.

Women's Rituals

Most of the traditional processes and procedures for women address pregnancy and birth, but a wide range of other procedures and rituals accompany breast-feeding, menstruation, fertility, menopause, and even abortions. The most common of these are related to menstrual cramps. Aside from the use of blessings, like Peter Schlessman's invocation of fire and water utilizing a blue string,[211] a woman could also carry wild ramps to alleviate cramps,[212] or ritually transplant some of the herb southern wormwood,[213] or make tea from the shells of cucumber.[214] A piece of clothing in which a person died could also be tied around the abdomen.[215]

A period was occasionally referred to as "*die monatliche Blume*" (the monthly blossom).[216] This "polite" way to refer to menstruation also undergirded a variety of folk beliefs and rituals, especially the use of flowers in treating women's ailments.[217] It was widely believed that a cloth used by a woman during her period should be rinsed out and the water poured onto the rose bush toward the rising of the sun, so by association, "*blieht's*

A woman's apron (*Schatz*) flung over the shoulder could make a hunter's shot go astray, and biting an apronstring could avert slander.

Weibsmensch wie en Ros" (the woman will bloom like a rose).[218] To encourage a period that is late, one could apply warm compresses of elderberry leaves on the abdomen, or take internally the juice from the bark of elder.[219] Administration of herbal compounds for a late period was to be timed with the waxing moon, as it was believed to be much harder to treat in the waning moon.[220]

Infertility was treated with a fumigation prepared from black caraway and frankincense,[221] and "diseases of the womb" were treated with astringent herbal infusions, including elder flowers, angelica, rue, wormwood, ginger, and cloves that were distilled in wine and tea of St. Benedict's herb (*Geum urbanum*).[222]

One item rarely described in ritual literature but often described in stories told by local people throughout Berks and Lehigh is abortion. These were easily achieved in early pregnancy with recipes for herbal teas, including pennyroyal and tansy, as well as juniper in *Culpeper's Herbal* and a wide range of similar works.[223] Within powwowing manuscripts and printed manuals, these recipes were not frequently recorded, as they were highly discouraged and only used in cases of emergency. Certain powwow doctors were consulted for this purpose,[224] but these services were as extremely confidential as they were controversial. Some early twentieth century recipes for abortives and morning-after contraceptives were dangerous, calling for bichloride of mercury and other lethal chemicals administered in precise doses. Evidence suggests that some recipes and instructions were intentionally destroyed, thus in most cases it is impossible to know what role ritual played in such procedures.[225]

Menopause was also treated by herbal and ritual means, with *Aaron-Wurzel* (Arum, Priest's Hood) soaked in old wine, taken before breakfast and evenings before bed,[226] or as a suspension of powdered amber mixed with fresh well water, mixed with sugar to taste to be taken with meals and during the day to reduce hot flashes.[227] *Braucherei* encompasses ritual expressions throughout all of life, and times of transition were of particular importance with numerous rituals accompanying the aging process.

Rituals of Old Age

By the time one reaches a ripe old age, a wide variety of degenerative illnesses and infirmities are likely to be experienced, and everything from poor eyesight to arthritis, difficulty in walking to the loss of teeth were once addressed by ritual means.

When one's mobility became limited and sure footing was required, a blessing for walking was used with the baptismal name of the person, "*Geht Jesus mit N. N. Er ist mein Haupt; ich bin sein Glied. Drum geht Jesus mit N. N.*" (Jesus walks with N. N. He is my head, I am his limb. Therefore, Jesus walks with N. N.).[228]

For degenerating eyesight or cataracts, greater celandine was once used as an eyewash, also called swallow-wort on account of its growth during the time in March that swallows build their nests.[229] Or a more involved ritual for removing a film on the eye involves digging four or five dandelion roots on St. Bartholomew's Day, and sewing them into a bundle without typing a knot, and suspend the bundle in front of the afflicted eye.[230]

Palsy, epilepsy, neurological disorders, and strokes, were treated in a similar manner through the use of blessings, both spoken and written, as well as the use of ritual agents such as the blood of a dove or the dried roots of beech or wormwood.[231] Blessings used for *Gichter* (convulsions, tremors, or palsy) often addressed both the afflicted person and the illness by name:

> **For convulsions, call the baptismal name of the sick person three times, and each time say the following words:**
>
> **All fits be still, desist, and rest these bones. I appeal for them, and not for the world, but rather for those whom thou hast given to me, for they are thine, that thou guardest them from evil. So truly as Mary was a pure virgin, the fits shall yield, disappear, and harm not, in the name of the Three Wise Men, and the Holy Trinity.**[232]

Chronic arthritic concerns, rheumatism, and gout inspired the carrying of a wide variety of objects as both preventative and curative measures: the eye tooth of a pig, a horse-chestnut, three potatoes, the triangular bone from a ham, a copper cent in one's shoe, a burnt-out carbon from an arc light (*en Schtick Electrisiti*), a horseshoe nail, or a coffin nail.[233] Another method was to let blood from the arm fall into a hole in the ground prepared for a little sprig of willow so that it grows and sprouts.[234] Others tied blue woolen yarn around arthritic joints, in much the same way that red yarn is used to stop inflammation, bleeding, and soreness. Instructions to give gout to the elderberry bush on three successive mornings, included saying:

> **Elder Tree, I have the gout and you do not, take it away… in the name of God the Father, God the Son, and God the Holy Spirit.**[235]

Cancers, tumors, and a wide range of other growths and complaints that afflict the aged are best removed with the hand of a corpse, so that the illnesses were taken to the grave,[236] foreshadowing the final resting place of all and the transition to the next world.

Rituals of Death & Renewal

Death is a unifying experience, claiming young and old, rich and poor, without prejudice for one's achievements or station in life. For centuries among the Pennsylvania Dutch, anticipation of death began at the very beginning of life when infant and childhood mortality was a common fact of life. The average life expectancy from birth even by the turn of the twentieth century was less than 50 years.[237]

Certificates of birth and baptism produced by the thousands throughout Pennsylvania reflected the shortness of life in poetry:

> Our wasting lives grow shorter still,
> As months and days increase,
> And every beating pulse we tell,
> Leaves but the number less.
> The Year rolls round and steals away,
> The breath that first it gave,
> Whate'er we do, whate'er we be
> We are traveling to the grave.
> Infinite joy or endless woe
> Attends on every breath,
> And yet how unconcern'd we go,
> Upon the brink of dead!
> Waken, O Lord! Our drowsy sense,
> To walk this dangerous road;
> And if our souls are hurried hence,
> May they be found with God.[238]

The length of one's life was once commonly believed to be determined, not by human action, but by the hand of the divine[239] as reflected in biblical passages from the Book of Psalms verses from the Book of Psalms: "My time stands in your hands," and "Behold, my days are as a handbreadth to thee."[240] For this reason, the duration of human existence is given special emphasis in sacred material culture. Gravestones recorded the precise length of one's life in years, months, and days.

Unlike the institutional and clinical settings of today's world, death frequently occurred at home or near home. For those dying of illness, especially anyone bedridden for the last part of their life, a number of rituals were performed to determine if indeed the person was dying or if recovery was possible. One method involves a ritual form of questioning:

Das erstenmal wenn du ihn siehest wann er krank ist, dann sag sein Dauf Namen: Willd du sterben so bedenkt dein End und lipf deine Händ, willd du aber länger büssen so lipf deine Füssen.

The first time when thou seest him, when he is sick, then speak thou his baptismal name: Wilt thou to die, then consider thine end, and lift thine Hands. Wilt thou rather suffer longer, then lift thy feet.[241]

These instructions, rhyming in the original German, suggest that either the person is conscious of the inquiry and is responding of their own will, (in a similar manner that one might communicate with a person suffering from a stroke who can no longer speak) or that the sick person is unconscious, and that the raising of the hands or feet are attributed to the power of the words.

Other variations involve the use of specific herbs or other objects that are placed in proximity with the sick person, and their behavior is observed. If a sick person sings when a sprig of *Schellkraut* (greater celandine) is placed under the head, then the person will recover; if however, the sick person cries, it is an omen of death.[242]

If a person was known to be dying, but was seemingly unable to pass away peacefully, the family would unlock all doors, padlocks, drawers, and cabinets to initiate a ritual release throughout the house.[243] Likewise the clock could be stopped, or a New Testament could be placed under the head to aid in a peaceful death.[244]

Not only were objects used in rituals to aid the dying, but the dying were also believed to have a great effect upon other objects and living things. If a person who is struggling to die was a keeper of bees, the hive would need to be moved to release the

---

Funerals were once commonly the venue for a wide variety of healing rituals. Depositis placed in coffins and graves were thought to take the illness to the next world.

person from this world to the next,[245] or if the person dies easily, the hive must be moved before the body leaves the home, so that the bees do not desert the hive or die.[246] If it is the mother or grandmother in the home who is passing away, the vinegar should be stirred to keep the vinegar mother from dying.[247] An old practice, even surviving in the present day, is that a window should be opened when a person dies to allow the passage of the soul outside to the open heavens.[248]

Prior to the widespread practice of embalming, the home was the site of the initial washing and preparation of the body. A parlor or dining room was often partitioned for this purpose, where the body was laid out and would remain there overnight or sometimes for a few days as funeral preparations took place, such as sending notice to relatives and friends at some distance, digging the grave, and securing the services of the minister. Ice for cooling the corpse was brought from a local icehouse, which had been stocked from a frozen pond or creek in winter and insulated with sawdust. In early times, sod was used as a temporary measure to cool the corpse, or cloths soaked in brandy. Family members, sometimes courting couples, would attend to the body and the changing of the cloths in an overnight vigil.[249] A candle was left burning all night until the burial, and mirrors and pictures on the wall were covered with fabric to avoid seeing the image of the dead person in the reflection of the glass.[250]

For Pennsylvania Dutch families, there were three phases of a funeral – a visitation and service in the home, a formal service in the church, and a service of interment at the gravesite.[251] Ritual practices accompanied these three phases of sanctioned funeral services. It was during the period of preparation before the service in the home that many medicinal rituals were enacted such as the passing of a dead person's hand over a goiter, tumor, birthmarks or wart to remove them. A similar procedure involves the borrowing of an undertaker's hammer for the same purpose of removing unwanted growths.[252] These processes could take place in relative confidentiality in these circumstances as opposed to in public services in the church. This was also the time that many family members would create mementos of the dead such as small locks of hair cut from the deceased person, which were braided or tied with a ribbon and stored in family Bibles or carried during the period of mourning.

The corpse had to be dressed in their own clothing, otherwise whoever gives clothing to a corpse is bound to die. The burial shroud was carefully placed on the body in order to avoid the shroud getting into the dead person's mouth. If a person died and several other family members died in rapid succession, it was believed that the grave of the first to die should be opened to see if the veil had been drawn into the mouth of the corpse, and would need to be removed.[253]

Aside from significant personal and family objects, certain items were discretely placed in the coffin with the deceased person. A red piece of string tied around the finger of a corpse during the vigil and then tied around the tumor of a living person could be placed in the coffin to remove the illness,[254] and articles of clothing

Lancaster County gravestone from the Ephrata Cloister cemetery, depicting three flowers, a symbol of resurrection, and a common motif in the poetry of ritual blessings used in powwowing.

could be used in a similar manner.[255] The name of a person afflicted with epilepsy could be written six times on a piece of paper laid under the head of the deceased to take the illness to the grave. The same could be achieved with a hair deposited in the coffin, or a small sample of blood.[256]

Behavior in the funeral processions was thought to portend a subsequent death of one in the community. Everything from a pallbearer stumbling in the procession, to the degree of smoothness of motion was considered suggestive.[257] Certain rituals for removing corns were timed for the tolling of funeral bells during the procession from the church to the graveyard,[258] but in some rituals the funeral had to be for a person of the same or opposite gender, depending on the nature of the illness.[259]

Rituals and practices did not only follow the body of the deceased, but the freshly dug grave was utilized as a space for ritual deposits to cure illness and remove curses before the body was interred. Graves were dug by hand and typically sat empty overnight until the funeral the following day. It was at nightfall before the burial took place that ritual deposits in the grave would be made.[260] If it rained or snowed into the open grave, it portended the person's entrance into heaven.[261] Graveyard plantings often consisted of creeping plants like flocks or thyme, and the plucking and smelling these plantings was believed to destroy or suspend one's sense of smell.[262] Temporary wooden markers were used prior to the placing of a permanent gravestone, which were typically erected after one year had passed. The delay was on account of the belief that someone else in the family would die if the stone were erected soon after death. Traditionally, the stone and the grave would face east, the direction of the rising sun and the very same direction was used to orient the healing rituals of *Braucherei*. Thus the rituals and the grave both reflect an anticipation of transformation – one in an earthly sense of renewal of health and the other through the promise of resurrection of the soul.

As an extension of the church and the sanctity of its space, the churchyard, or God's acre (*Gottes Acker*), play an important role in the poetry of healing blessings. In everything from stopping blood to purging worms, from reducing swelling to easing toothache, from cooling burns to removing warts, the graveyard is one of the quintessential symbolic settings for poetic healing transformations.

A common version fo the Three Worms Blessing describes the plowing of a graveyard: "Our Lord God went to a field, on God's Acre. He plowed three furrows, he found three worms. The one is white, the other is red, the third is death for all ye worms…"[263] In this case, the Lord is plowing the cemetery in order to harvest the three archetypal worms from the remains of the saints interred. The worms are not exclusively worms per se, but representative of the invisible forces of human illness responsible for the decay of the flesh.[264] Each color represents a different state of decay: red, the color of inflammation; white, the color of purulence; and black the color of mortification. Thus, to kill the three worms is to purify the flesh, not only of literal parasites, but of the symptoms of decay, as a victory over death. In other versions it is three men, three apostles, St. Peter, St. Istorius, or the Virgin Mary who strike down the three worms.[265]

In cases of intensifying and progressive illnesses, especially those involving swelling, inflammation, infection, tumors or growths, external or within the body, the imagery of decay and the grave is likened to the withering and destruction of the illness: "…decrease like the dead in the grave," or "…as dead as the dead in his grave."[266]

A blessing for protection from bullets begins, "Here I stand on this grave and beseech the Holy Boys: the first is God the Father, the second is God the Son, the third is God the Holy Spirit…"[267]

The ultimate imagery of the grave is in a classic invocation of three divine virtues embodied by three flowers springing forth from the grave of Christ: "Three flowers grow upon the grave of our Lord Jesus Christ, the first is goodness, the third is humility, the third is God's will…"[268] Typically used for stopping blood, this invocation has been adapted for blessings for protection, toothache, binding thieves, dropsy, and uterine bleeding. The supernal healing virtues of the resurrection are not only reflected in the hereafter, but in the presence of the divine in the earthly process of life.

Paradoxically, while death can be fraught with a wide array of social and emotional struggles, bringing to mind the fragility and mortality of humanity, it is also a time of renewal and healing. Death served as a reminder of the immortality of the soul and also of the temporary nature of human suffering. Healing rituals provide an alternate context for death, rendering the loss of life useful for the preserving of life. From birth to death and back again, ritual has both shaped and been shaped by the whole spectrum of human experiences. Thus, ritual serves as a powerful means of assuring transformative solutions in the most difficult of times.

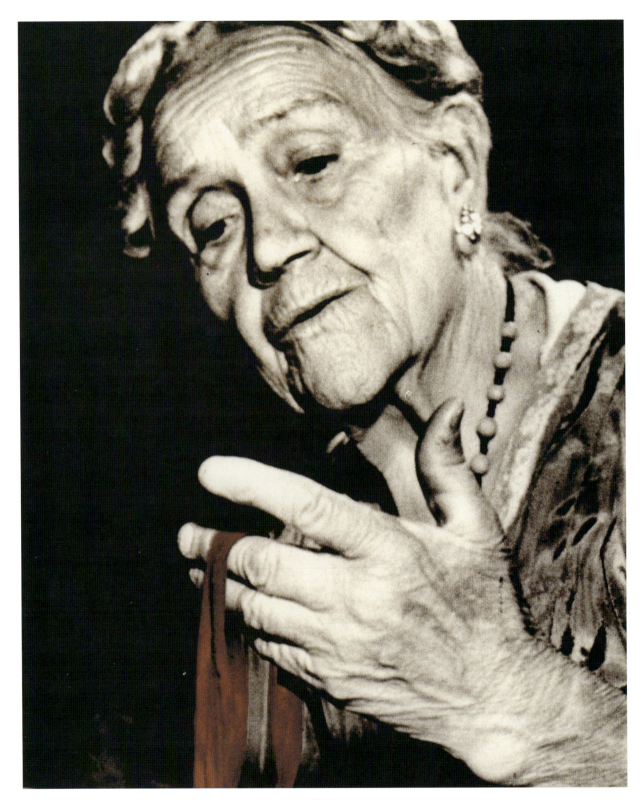

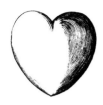 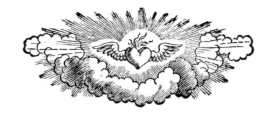 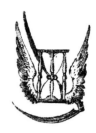

Conclusion

Pennsylvania Dutch folk culture, like many traditional societies across the globe, has demonstrated throughout the centuries a highly integrated system of belief that encompasses domestic and communal life. Powwowing provides an opportunity to witness how ordinary challenges are encountered and constructively engaged within a context of meaningful relationships. Ritual forms the basis for this dialogue, transforming ordinary experience into an expression of cosmic and sacred proportions.

Whether in acts of ritual healing, protection from physical and spiritual harm, or assistance in times of need, powwowing offers a wide spectrum of possibilities to seamlessly blend ritual with all facets of life. Whether in times of emergency or in simple mundane affairs, ritual serves not only as an activity to mitigate and address important personal and communal concerns, but also provides a means to do so in a manner that resonates with the culture's values and needs.

Ultimately, although some of these expressions of ritual culture do not make overt reference to religion, the underlying correspondences and relationships mirror the old sacred hierarchy of heaven and earth. By virtue of this sacred order of the cosmos, the world is positively alive with meaning and capable of communicating. Ritual is the mechanism by which this worldview is both experienced and reinforced, allowing for all people to participate in the unfolding of creation.

The overarching structure of these beliefs, however, is not fixed in one particular temporal or theological moment, but has demonstrated a versatility and flexibility throughout the centuries, providing a meaningful way to adapt to an ever changing world. The historical record indicates that a wide range of ritual practices may exist only in memory, as a relic of the needs and lifestyle of previous generations. While this may indeed be the case for some portions of powwowing, this is by no means an indication that the tradition is dead or dying. In fact the opposite is true - generations in the present day, both young and old, are seeking ways to engage these traditions as part of their cultural identity.

While concerns about the preservation of this important practice of powwowing are justified, it is equally important to remember that these ritual traditions were not observed self-consciously out of a desire for preservation or idealization of the past, but as practical expressions of a community identity. It would obviously be absurd and impractical to advocate for any wholesale, present-day performance of these rituals as some form of veneration of previous stages of a culture's history – that is, without actually sharing the beliefs that shaped and integrated such traditions into a coherent way of life.

At the same time, dismissing such traditions as obsolete would also be missing a unique opportunity to more closely reflect on our dynamic American culture's diversity of spiritual expression, as well as to learn from our difficulties and grow with an awareness of our roots. Powwowing challenges us to become more fully cognizant of the ways in which ritual is still very much an active force in present human endeavor to heal existential concerns and satisfy hunger for meaning.

Although the structure and organization of our lives have changed dramatically in the past three hundred years, powwowing has survived into the present day as evidence of a vibrant spiritual tradition that continues to be a viable expression of the vast potential to discover meaning in everyday experience.

Saint of the Coal Regions, Sophia Leininger Bailer (1870 - 1954) powwowing with a red silk ribbon. *Don Yoder Collection, Pennsylvania German Cultural Heritage Center, Kutztown University of Pennsylvania.*

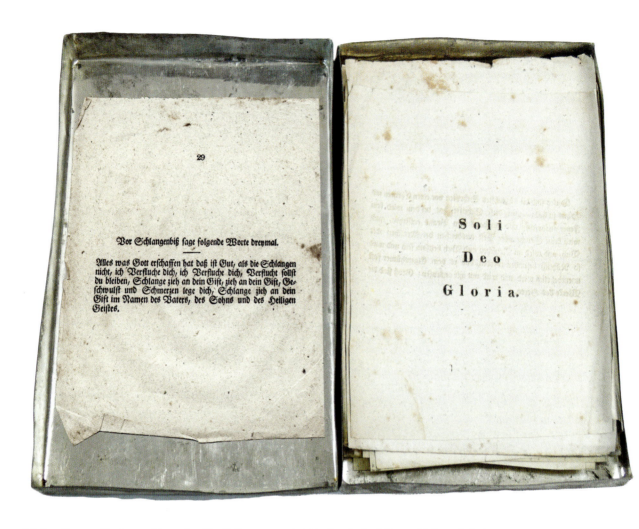

Soli Deo Gloria, or The Secrets of Sympathy of Dr. Helfenstein, ca. 1810, Northumberland County. *Heilman Collection.*

A rare unbound book of cures entitled *Glory to God Alone*, attributed to Dr. Georg Friedrich Helfenstein, a medical doctor educated in the Netherlands, who becomes a practitioner of spiritual healing methods, after a mysterious "gray man" teaches him the "secrets of sympathy" and vanishes before his very eyes. Comprised of three books: the first containing religious blessings to be used in healing the sick; the second, rituals for assistance in times of need, protection from violence, stopping thieves, etc.; the third, blessings for animals and livestock. The introduction is signed "J. H. Helfenstein" and is sealed with two wax seals depicting a fox and a lion. The unbound collection was issued as broadsides, which could be removed from the collection, and used as talismans or applied in healing rituals. Around a dozen copies are known in Pennsylvania, most of which are enclosed in decorative paper or tin boxes for safekeeping.

The signature of J. H. Helfenstein on page 286 is based on a copy in the Pennsylvania Folklife Society Archive in Special Collections and Archives at the Myrin Library, Ursinus College. This signature contrasts strongly with other Helfenstein signatures, such as one in the Heilman Collection, suggesting that the handwriting is artificial, and that Helfenstein was a pen-name. The wax seals on the same page are taken from the lid of the decorative paper box in the Heilman Collection shown on page 142.

Soli Deo Gloria
Dr. Helfenstein's Secrets of Sympathy
Newly Translated by Patrick J. Donmoyer

The following are useful works for a Christian to have in the home: Whoever possesses these writings, unto them no fire will break out, and absolutely no conflagration will occur. Likewise neither plague nor pestilence will erupt among man or beast. It will be found to be both so beneficial and useful for man and beast, that it will become indispensible to the owner, and with me he will proclaim: "Great are the works of the Lord."

Foreword

It is not my intention to begin this valuable book with a great eulogy. The owner will himself be convinced, that neither silver nor gold is as precious as this useful work, which has been revealed for the glory of God alone, and for the wellbeing of man and beast. Every owner of this book be duly warned to make no abuse of it, and to employ everything as called for in each sympathy, so that thou needest not doubt.

A Brief Account of the Life of the Author

I, George Frederick Helfenstein, was born in the year of Our Lord 1730 in Rotterdam in the kingdom of Holland. My parents were poor and could provide little for me, and therefore also little education was I allowed. In my ninth year, my cousin Carl Augustus Helfenstein, took me to live with him. He was quite rich, and my demeanor and thirst for knowledge earned me honor and friendship, as well as veneration and love. In my thirteenth year my parents passed away, and I was now an orphan, left to my heavenly father and my cousin. My cousin sent me to the university, where I studied as a physician. In the twenty-second year of my life, I returned again to Rotterdam as a doctor, where I practiced my vocation with skill, renown, dilligence, and piety. All my patients loved me, and were wholly pleased with me. It was my custom, each time to pray to God, that my medical and healing assistance would bring blessing and prosperity.

One day when I was called to attend a man who had a twisted leg, I was of the mind to visit him, and was already halfway there, when I encountered an old gray man, that I had never seen nor heard anything about before this time. Upon his cryptic and intrusive suggestion, he ordered me to turn back to my house, whereby I told him that I must first visit a sick person. He replied that this was well known to him, but that he would relieve the pain of the sick person with spiritual medicine - that is with sympathy - and afterwords he would teach it to me. I followed this mysterious man, whereupon he said to me: this is thy fortune – I will teach thee to heal with words, as Christ the Lord restored the sick. (Here I wish to mention that as I came to the sick man the next day, he told me that an old gray man had been by him, and had laid his hands upon the bone, and the pain and the sprain ceased.) The gray man led me forth and said: "As he taught in the Gospel of Saint Mark in the eleventh chapter, verses 22 and 23, Jesus answered and spoke to them: 'Have faith in God. For verily I say unto thee, that whosoever shall say unto this mountain, be thou removed, and be thou cast into the sea; and shall not doubt in his heart, but shall believe that those things which he saith shall come to pass; and he shall have whatsoever he saith.' This reference is also found in the Gospel of St. Matthew, ch. 17, v. 20, and we find this throughout the holy scripture." And thus did this mysterious man share with me the secrets of sympathy included herein, through which, with the help of God and firm faith in him, have done much good, and healed many illnesses. And so can thou also, my dear reader and witness - beloved brother or sister, I remind thee once again, to make no abuse of these writings, but instead employ them in the name and in firm faith of the Holy Trinity.

And when this strange and mysterious man made known to me all that is included in this book, he vanished before my very eyes, and I never saw him again. Thus I, the author and a friend of mankind, became aware of this healing art, which is here newly reproduced and dedicated to the alleviation of the sufferings of my fellow men and neighbors, and to the glory of the Holy Trinity.

Soli Deo Gloria.

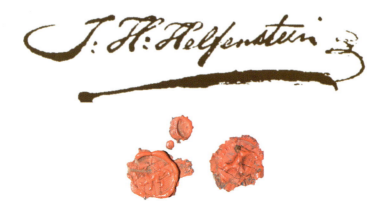

Book I   Erstes Buch

(1)

For a sprain, pass thine hand three times over the affected part of the body, and each time say the following words:

———

Christ upon the cross was hanged, and thy bone is sprained. It harmed him not, thus shall thy sprain harm thee not, in the name of the Father and of the Son, and of the Holy Spirit, Amen, Amen, Amen.

(2)

For a sprain, pass thine hand three times over the affected part of the body, and each time say the following words:

———

Christ hath made the lame to walk, the dead to rise: thus may thy sprain heal. It shall descend into the depths. Jesus alone healeth the sick, and to him alone shall one give praise, in the name of the Father and of the Son, and of the Holy Spirit.

(3)

When a limb twists by accident, as that which is caused by man, so pass thine hand crosswise over the wound and speak the following words:

———

It is banished and it is dispatched. It shall nothing harm, nor nothing lade. It shall heal, and linger not. The wind shall blow it asunder, as dust it shall blow away. It shall descend into the depths of the sea. Pain abate, heal, yield, depart, in the name of the seven guardian angels.

(4)

When one has received a new hernia, then thou must try in the following manner: Take a clean bed sheet, and lay him upon it, and take two doves, bind them, and lay them next to him. Call his baptismal name five times, and each time say the following words, then kill the doves.

———

Jesus heals the hernial-tremors, and in the name of Jesus, thou shalt be healed. As it is written: What ye do in my name, shall come to pass. The death of these doves shall be thy salvation. Thy pains come upon the doves, and they are taken from thee, in the name of the Father, and of the Son, and of the Holy Spirit.

———

(1)

Vor Verrenkung streiche mit der Hand dreymal über den wehen Theil des Körpers und sage jedesmal folgendes Worte.

———

Christus ist ans Kreuz gehenkt und dein Bein ist verrenkt — Schadet ihm sein Henken nichts, so schadet dir dein Verrenken nichts, im Namen des Vaters, des Sohnes und des Heiligen Geistes, Amen, Amen, Amen.

(2)

Für Verrenkung streiche mit der Hand dreymal über den wehen Theil des Körpers und sage jedesmal folgendes Worte.

———

Christus machte Lahme gehen, Todte machte er auferstehn, So heile denn dein Verrenken, In die Tiefe soll es versenken, Jesus allein heilet Kranken, Ihn allein soll man danken - im Namen des Vaters, des Sohnes und des Heiligen Geistes.

(3)

Wenn ein Glied von ohngefehr erkrummt, als wie es durch Menschen gethan, so streiche kreuzweis mit der Hand über den Schaden und sprech folgende Worte Dreimal.

———

Es sei gebant und versandt, Es soll nichts Schaden und nichts Laden, Es soll Heilen und nicht verweilen, der Wind soll es verwehen, Wie Staub soll es verwehen, ins Tiefe Meer soll es versinken, Lege, Heile, Weiche, Vergehe, Schmerz, im Namen der Sieben Schutz-Engeln.

(4)

Wenn eins ein neuer Bruch bekommen hat, denn mußt du auf folgende Art brauchen: Nehme ein sauber Bettuch und lege ihn darauf und nehme zwei Tauben, binde sie und lege sie neben ihn, und nenne seinen Taufnamen 5 mahl und sage jedesmal folgende Worte, und denn tödte die Tauben.

———

Jesus heilte Gichtbrüchige und in Jesus Namen sollst du geheilt sein, wie es heißt, was ihr in meinem Namen thut, soll sein, diese Tauben ihr Tod sey dein Heil, deine Schmerzen sind auf die Tauben kommen, sie sind von dir weggenommen, im Namen des Vaters und des Sohnes und des Heiligen Geistes.

(5)

To stop blood, thou must call the baptismal name for whom thou tryest, and say the following words nine times:

———

Christ hath struggled for us,
He hath wearily contended,
And bled to death upon the cross,
Which is good for all bleeding.
In the name of Christ shall it stand,
And neither run nor further go,
but upon the proper place,
neither surge nor flow.
So healed be the bleeding,
And properly apportioned be,
In the name of the Father, and of the Son,
and of the Holy Spirit.

(6)

To stop blood, thou must call the name for whom thou thou tryest, and three times say the following words:

———

The name of Jesus was annunciated at Nazareth. Christ our God, Jesus was killed at Jerusalem. As true as this is, so stand thou blood, or this I steal, as it is called, and bring him the Holy Spirit, the blood, in the name of the Father, and of the Son, and of the Holy Spirit.

(7)

A blessing, if something ails a person and thou knowest not what it is, so call his baptismal name and say the following words three times:

———

Hast thou recovered health and God? So I lead thee back to God the Father, Son and Holy Spirit. I know not what has befallen thee, or what ails thee, therefore so help thee Father, Son and Holy Spirit. Our Lord Jesus gladly blessed, and shalt thou blessed be, as the chalice and the wine, and the holy bread, that our Lord Jesus Christ offered to his beloved disciples at night on Maundy Thursday. Therefore, help thee in the name of him who suffered for thee death upon the cross.

(5)

Für Blut zu stillen muß du den Taufnamen nennen von dem du Brauchen willst, und spreche folgende Worte neunmahl.

———

Christus hat für uns gelitten,
Er hat sich müde gestritten.
Am Kreuze Todt geblut,
Das ist vor alles Bluten gut,
In Christus Namen soll es stehn,
Nicht rinnen oder weiter gehn,
Am rechten Orte bleiben,
Nicht fließen oder Treiben,
Daß Bluten sei geheilt,
Im rechten sich vertheilt,
im Namen des Vaters und des Sohnes
und des Heiligen Geistes.

(6)

Für Blut zu stillen, nenne den Taufnamen von dem du Brauchen willst, und sage folgende Worte dreymahl.

———

Der Name Jesus ward zu Nazareth verkündet, Christus unser Gott, Jesus ward zu Jerusalem getödtet, so wahr das ist, so steh du Blut, oder stehl ich diesen wie es heißt, und bring ihn den Heiligen Geist, daß Blut im Namen des Vaters und des Sohnes und des Heiligen Geistes.

(7)

Ein Seegen, wann en Mensch etwas fehlt und du weiß nicht was es ist, so nenne seinen Taufnamen und sage folgende Worte dreimal.

———

Bist du gesund worden und Gott so führe ich wieder zu Gott dem Vater, Sohn und heiligen Geist, ich weiß nicht wie dir geschehen oder was dir gebricht, darum so helf dir Vater, Sohn und heiliger Geist, unser Herr Jesus Christus gern, und sollst du sowohl gesegnet sein, als der Kelch und der Wein, und das heilige Brod, daß unser Herr Jesus Christ am hohen Donnerstag zu Nacht, seinen Lieben Jüngern anbat, dazu helfe dir der Name, der dir den Tod am Stamme des Kreuzes gelitten hat.

(8)

When a child is Livergrown or has Cardialogy, so anoint the child with thy saliva from the sternum to the lower body and from the shoulders to the lower back, six times in one half-hour - and speak each time the following words:

―――

Livergrown and Cardialogy withdraw from my child's rib, just as Christ the Lord departed from his crib: God the Father, Son, and Holy Spirit.

(9)

To alleviate pains, so call the baptismal name for whom thou triest five times, and each time say the following words:

―――

Ye pains, I banish you, I rebuke you, I expell you. Let these limbs have rest and peace. Be ye expelled to the highest mountain and sunk into the deepest sea.

Through Mary's pains was Jesus born,
Therefore all pains will be forlorn,
In the names of the Guardian Angels.

(10)

For burns received by a man, say the following words, and each time blow three times and pass thine hand over the wound, and wait ten minutes between each of the three times.

―――

There goes a man over land,
and he found a hand,
and the hand extinguished the brand.

(11)

For burns received by a woman, say the following words, and each time blow three times and pass thine hand over the wound, and wait ten minutes between each of the three times.

―――

There goes a woman over land,
and she found a hand,
and the hand extinguished the brand.

(8)

Wenn ein Kind angewachsen oder das Herzgesperr hat, so schmiere es mit deinem Speichel in der Herzgrube bis am Underleib und denn von die Schultern bis am hintern, in einer halben stunde sechsmal - und sage jedesmal folgende Worte.

―――

Anwachs und Herzgesperr geh weg von meinem Kind sein Rip, wie Christus der Herr ist gegangen aus seine Krip, Gott Vater, Sohn und heiliger Geist.

(9)

Für Schmerzen zu nehmen, so nenne den Taufnamen von dem du Brauchen willst, 5 mahl und sage jedesmal folgende Worte.

―――

Ihr Schmerzen ich banne euch, Verweise euch, treibe euch zurück, laß diese Glieder Ruh und Frieden, sei auf den höchsten Berg verweisen und in das tiefe Meer versenkt.

Maria hat Jesus in Schmerzen geboren,
Hirdurch gehn alle Schmerzen verloren.
Im Namen der Schutz Engeln.

(10)

Für Brennen bei ein Mans Person, sage folgende Worte neunmahl, bei jede dreimal blase und streiche mit der Hand über den Schaden und zwischen jede dreimal warte zehn Minuten.

―――

Es geht ein Mann über Land,
und fand eine Hand,
und die hand thät den Brand.

(11)

Für Brennen bei ein Weibsperson sage folgende Worte neunmahl, bei jede dreimal blase und streiche mit der Hand über den Schaden, und zwischen jede dreimal warte zehn Minuten.

―――

Es geht eine Frau über Land,
und fand eine Hand, und die
Hand thät den Brand

(12)

For a wen in the eye, blow nine times into the eye, and say the following words each time, and place the person for whom thou tryest on the threshold of the home:

———

Jesus said, What wilt thou that I should do unto thee? Lord, that I might receive my sight. It be so, see, in Jesus' name thine eyes shall become bright, pure, clean, clear, as the moon and stars in the firmament of heaven.

(13)

If the rest is taken from a child, make an inscription and therein write the following words, and hang it on the child:

———

Mara :)⊂(**Martha**)⊂(
]⊂[**Inri**]⊂[

all that was done to him, be banished, dispatched, chased, driven out, done away, turned about. Come thou sweet rest, in peace, that this portion be alloted to him.

Johannes * **Estferis**

_ S ; V ; R ; G ; X ; W ; _

(14)

If a person is troubled or plagued in his his sleep, make an inscription as follows, and put it in a linen cloth and hang it by the sternum:

———

S S X O V A Q C J L

Sola Maxima Gratia

Depart ye wicked spirits far away, never return. Be ye banished in the name of the Father, be dispelled in the name of the Son, and never return in the name of the Holy Spirit.

X F : ⚖ F X :

---

(12)

Für eine Schußblätter im Auge blase neunmahl ins Auge, und bei jedesmal sage folgende Worte, und setze dich mit dem du Brauchst in die Hausthüre.

———

Jesus sprach was willst du, das ich dir thun soll, Herr das ich sehen kann, es sei so sehe, in Jesu Namen werde deine Augen helle, rein, sauber, klahr, wie der Mond und Sterne am Firmament das Himmels.

(13)

Wenn ein Kind die Ruhe genommen ist, so mache einen Brief und schreibe folgende Worte darin, und Hänge es dem Kinde an.

———

Mara :)⊂(**Martha**)⊂(
]⊂[**Inri**]⊂[

alles was ihm angethan ist sei verbannt, verfant, verjagt, vertrieben, abgethan umgewandt, komme Liebe Ruh in Frieden, dieses Theil sei ihm Beschieden.

Johannes * **Estferis**

_ S ; V ; R ; G ; X ; W ; _

(14)

der Geplagt
ein Leinen

(15)

For pains in the limbs, pass thine hand over the afflicted member, and say the following words seven times:

The wounds of Christ
Have bound all things.
The blood of Christ
Is good for all pains.
The limbs of Christ
Shall heal again.
The bone of Christ
Shall make us clean.
The life of Christ
Must give strength.

(15)

Für Gliederschmerzen, streiche mit der Hand über den Leidenden Theil un sage siebenmahl folgende Worte.

Christi Wunden,
Hat alles verbunden,
Christi Blut,
Ist vor alle Schmerzen gut,
Christi Glieder,
Heilen wieder,
Christi Bein,
Macht uns rein,
Christi Leben,
Muß Kraft geben

(16)

If a child is livergrown, or has cardialogy, then undress him, and lay him on on his belly, and pass thine hand from the head to the feet, and say the following words three times and anoint the child with candle soot three times.

And Jesus said, suffer the children to come unto me, and he blessed them the very same hour. Therefore, shalt thou also recover thine health. May the livergrowing from this child heal, redirect, turn away, and remember thy name. Blessed be this child of heart, Therefore shall these pains depart.

(16)

Wenn ein Kind angewachsen oder das Herzgesperr hatt, so Kleide ihn nakend aus, und lege ihn auf den Leib, und streiche ihn mit der Hand, vom Kopf bis an die Füsse und sage folgende Worte dreimahl und Schmiere dem Kinde mit die Schwärze vom Lichte dreimal.

Und Jesus sprach, laß die Kindlein zu mir kommen, und er Seegenete Sie zu der Selbigen stunde. " " --darum sollst du auch gesund werden, der Anwachs von diesen Kind, Heile, Lenke, Schwenke und dein Namen gedenke, Gesegnet ist das Kind von Herzen,Darum vergehen diese Schmerzen.

(17)

For the gripes or the belly-ache of a small child, pass thine hand from the neck to the knees five times, and say the following words each time:

Golgotha! Golgotha! Thou wicked place, where Jesus Christ was Crucified, there His blood was shed, which is good for all pains, in the name of the Twelve Holy Disciples of Jesus.

(17)

Vor Bauchgrimmen oder Leibschmerzen, vor ein Kleines Kind, streiche mit der Hand, vom halse bis an die Knie fünfmal, und sage jedesmal folgende Worte.

Golgotha ! Golgotha ! du Böser Ort, wo Jesus Christus gekreuziget ward, da ist vergossen sein Blut, das ist vor alle Schmerzen Gut, im Namen der Heiligen zwölf Jünger Jesus.

(18)

For a headache, pass the hand before the head, and say the following words seven times:

Jesus bowed his head and died upon the beam of the cross. He was patient as a lamb. He shed for us His blood, which is good for the head and nerves, in the name of the Holy Guardian Angels.

(18)

Vor Kopfweh, Lege die Hand vor den Kopf, und sage folgende Worte siebenmahl.

Jesus neigte sein Haupt, und Starb am Kreuzes Stamm, Er war geduldig wie ein Lamm, Er vergoß vor uns sein Blut,das ist für Kopf und Nerfen Gut, im Namen der Heiligen Schutz Engeln. --

(19)

For weak and blurry eyes, go to flowing water before sunrise, and wash the eyes five times with the left hand, and each time say the following words, and then throw a handfull of salt into the water. Then take seven steps backwards and then go home forwards, for three days in succession.

———

As this salt shall disappear,
So shall my eyes be clear.
Christ is he who can help me,
Herewith begins the blessing.

(20)

For sweeny in the limbs, rub with thine hand nine times over the afflicted member, and each time say the following words:

———

In Jesus' name, I try for thee, in the name of the Holy Trinity, this shall depart to the high mountains, into deep chasms, to high trees, into the deep sea. The angel came, the man went forth, and so he taketh away the sweeny forever.

(21)

So that no raging animal, or snake, or wild beast can harm thee, write the following inscription and carry it always with thee.

———

Montusa: Slamiel

W N V B Z W X W

Rebbe Sorech cum

Yield, Animals and Snakes in the Name of the Father, Yield, Wicked Beasts in the Name of the Holy Spirit, Yield, all wickedness, in the name of Jesus Christ the Son, **Inri.**

E N N J L L D M Æ Y

(22)

For wildfire (for a man) blow nine times over the afflicted part of the body, and each time say the following words:

———

Three men from the east went out for the Wildfire-Stone to seek: They search, they find, they come, they go, they run, they jump. Wildfire, withdraw, and nevermore return. Fly out into the deep sea, be as a stone. In the name of Jesus, it shall be.

(23)

For wildfire (by a female) blow nine times over the afflicted part of the body, and each time say the following words:

———

Three women from the east went out for the Wildfire Stone to seek: They search, they find, they come, they go, they run, they jump. Wildfire, withdraw, and nevermore return. Fly out into the deep sea, be as a stone. In the name of Jesus, it shall be.

(24)

For the bite of a snake, say the following words:

———

Everything that God made is good, except for the snake. I curse thee, I curse thee, I curse thee, cursed thou shalt remain. Snake withdraw thy poison, withdraw thy poison, swelling and pain abate, Snake withdraw thy poison in the name of the Father, of the Son, and of the Holy Spirit.

(25)

For fever, call the baptismal name of the sick person three times and each time say the following words:

———

Heaven and Earth were created, and everything was good. Everything made by God is good, only the fever is a plague. Therefore, yield from me, depart from me, remove thyself, and vanish from me. Fly to the highest mountains and thou shalt withdraw into the depths. Withdraw from me in the name of John the Holy Apostle, and Jesus Christ the Son of God.

(26)

For convulsions, call the baptismal name of the sick person three times, and each time say the following words:

―――

All fits be still, desist, and rest these bones. I appeal for them, and not for the world, but rather for those whom thou hast given to me, for they are thine, that thou guardest them from evil. So truly as Mary was a pure virgin, the fits shall yield, disappear, and harm not, in the name of the Three Wise Men, and the Holy Trinity.

(27)

For headaches, place thine hand in front of the head, and speak the following words five times:

―――

Jesus bowed his head and died, whereby he granted salvation to many. He also shed his precious blood, which is good for all pains. At the time, far and wide, great and small, only he can alleviate pains in every heart, in the name of St. Anthony.

(28)

For a whitlow, hold thy finger out the window, and the person who is trying for thee must stand under the open sky and say the following words seven times:

―――

Thus shall this felon be slain, and this finger mend, through the finger of God, and the Lord worked great wonders through the finger of Paul. So truly as Christ was born in a manger, so shall this felon be doomed. Jesus said: Take this wine - with it thou must be attended, in the name of the Trinity.

(29)

For swelling, make the sign of the cross three times with the hand over the afflicted part, and each time say the following words:

―――

Swelling, thou shalt vanish, and ye pains, depart. Just as we are one body in Christ, but each members of one another, swelling, thou shalt vanish, and ye pains, depart in the name of Jesus Christ of Nazareth. So truly shalt thou be attended, as truly as the Three Wise Men of the East worshipped Jesus first.

(26)

Vor die Gichtern, Nenne den Taufnamen des Kranken dreymal und sage jedesmal folgende Worte.

―――

Alle Gichtern, werden Schüchtern, lasset ab, und Ruhen diese Glieder, ich Bitte für Sie und Bitte nicht für die Welt, sondern die du mir gegeben hast, den Sie sind dein, daß du Sie bewahrest vor dem Uebel, so wahr Maria eine Reine Jungfrau war sollen die Gichtern weichen, Fortgehen, Verschwinden, un nicht Schaden, im Namen der drei Weisen, un der Heiligen Dreyeinigkeit.

(27)

Vor Kopfweh, Lege die Hand vor den Kopf und spreche folgende Worte fünfmahl.

―――

Jesus Beute sein Haupt und starb, Womit er viel Heil erwarb, Auch hat er vergossen sein Theures Blut, daß ist vor alle Schmerzen Gut, Weit und Breit, zu der Zeit, Groß und Klein, nur allein, Lindre alle Schmerzen, und jeden Herzen, im Namen des heiligen Antonius

(28)

Vor Fingerwurm, halte deinen Finger, aus dem Fenster, und der dir braucht muß unterm freien Himmel stehen und sprechen folgende Worte siebenmahl

―――

Also soll dieser Wurm getödtet sein, und dieser Finger bessern, durch den Finger Gottes, und der Herr wirkte Große wunder durch die Finger Pauli So wahr wie Jesus ist in eine Krippe geboren, so gehe dieser Wurm verloren, Jesus sprach nimmt hin den Wein, Damit muß dir geholfen sein im Namen der Dreieinigkeit.

(29)

Vor Geschwulst, Fahre dreimahl mit der Hand Kreuzweis über den Leidenden Theil und sage jedesmahl folgende Worte.

―――

Geschwulst du solst verschwinden, Ihr Schmerzen fahret fort, --Also sind wir ein Leib in Christo, aber unter einander ist einer des andern Glied. Geschwulst du solst verschwinden, Ihr Schmerzen fahret aus, im Namen Jesus Christ von Nazaret, so wahr sollst du geholfen sein, so wahr es ist das die drei Weisen von Morgenland Jesus zuerst angebeten haben.

(30)

For a sore throat, take a woolen band, wind it around the neck five times, and each time say the following words:

———

For I long to see thee, that I may impart unto thee some spiritual gift, that thou may be strengthened. In the name of Jesus the Crucified, shall these pains depart from thee. Throat and neck, ye are consecrated unto God, from now on until eternity.

(31)

For colic and mother-pains, take salt, bread, and camphor, as much of each as a hazelnut, and sew it into a linen rag, and hang it over the pit of the stomach, and write the following inscription and hang it thereupon:

———

Minchen Seibal al Ponecho,

So that also from his body were brought unto the sick handkerchiefs or aprons, and the diseases departed from them

Neficho Lefoney

Colic and mother-pains abate, in the name of Jesus Christ, Amen.

(32)

If a child cries too much, place thine hand upon the mouth, and say the following words three times:

———

O dear Lord Jesus Christ,
Thou didst die upon the cross,
In thy name help this child,
Swiftly in this very hour.
Jesus helps all the children,
And so shalt thou be atended in his name,
Jesus Christ of Nazareth.

(33)

For earache, rub the ear seven times with thy two forefingers, and each time say the following words:

———

And he touched his ear and it was healed that very hour. The ear hears the wonders of heaven. Pains, yield in the name of Jesus Christ, and be sunk into the deep sea, in the name of the Holy Angels. Be healed in the name of the Twelve Apostles.

(34)

When one cannot sleep, then say the following words three times:

———

Unrest depart, Rest settle in. So shall it be, sweet rest return and depart not. The members come from the Great Spirit, as it is written. Unrest, thou canst not remain, Rest will drive thee away. Rest come, Rest settle in, Rest remain, in the name of the Father, of the Son, and of the Holy Spirit.

(35)

To treat wildfire, thou must call the name of the sick person seven times, and each time say the following words:

———

I command thee Wildfire, thou shalt abate, by the precious blood of Jesus Christ. Thou shalt stand still, and go no further. So truly as Mary maintained her maidenhead, thou shalt depart and not return. So truly as Jesus Christ was taken from the cross, withdraw in the name of the Father, abate in the name of the Son, and never return in the name of the Holy Spirit.

(36)

For mortification, take dead wood-coals, seven in number and tap with each one on the wound, and speak to each the following words, and afterwards, thou must grind them to powder, and strew them over flowing water:

———

As this coal was once ablaze, and now burns no more, so shall this mortification be extinguished. Body and soul stand in the hand of God, therefore all evil be banished. The Blood of Christ atones for all. All flesh will perish, and the mortification cannot endure the stars so far, blue as heaven, as clear as the sun, in the name of John the Baptist.

(37)

For wounds, bruises, punctures, and lacerations, take four pieces of pine-wood of equal length, and tap with each upon the wound and say to each one, the following words five times and then burn the wood:

———

Upon Golgatha, upon Golgatha, upon Cyprus, upon Cyprus, upon Arrorat, upon Arrorat thy pains shall flee, into the deep sea thy pain shall descend, and by the wounds of Christ I lay thine. As this wood doth burn, so thy pains be drowned.

(34)

Wen einer nicht Schlafen kan, so sage folgende Worte dreimal.

———

Unruh weiche, Ruh kehr ein, so soll es sein, Süsser Schlaf kom zurück und weiche nicht, die Glieder kommen vom Großen Geist, oder wie es heißt, Unruh kannst nicht bleiben, Ruh wird dich vertreiben, Ruhe komme Ruhe kehr ein, Ruhe bleibe, im Namen des Vaters, des Sohnes, und des Heiligen Geistes.

(35)

Wildfeuer zu Brauchen, mußt du den Namen des Kranken siebenmal nennen, und jedesmal folgende Worte sagen.

———

Ich gebiete, dir Wildfeuer, du solst dir legen bei Jesus Christus Theures Blut, du sollst stille stehen und nicht weiter gehn, so wahr Maria hatte ihre Jungfrauschaft, du solst, weichen und nicht wieder kommen, so wahr Jeus Christus ist vom Kreuz genommen, ziehe aus im Namen des Vaters, laß ab im Namen des Sohns und kehre nie zurück im Namen des Heiligen Geistes.

(36)

Für kalter Brand, nehme Todte Holzkohlen, sieben an der Zahl und duppe mit eine jede einzeln auf den Schaden, und spreche zu eine jede folgende Worte, und nachher mußt du sie sein zu Pulver machen und vor Sonnenaufgang aufs Fließende Wasser streuen.

———

Wie diese Kohle Feuer war, und jetzt nicht mehr Brent, so soll dieser Brand getödtet sein, Leib und Seele stehen in Gottes Hand, drum alles Böse sei verbannt, Christus Blut macht alles Gut, alles Fleisch muß vergehen, und der Brand kan nicht bestehen, Sterne, Ferne, Himmelsblau, Sonnenklar, im Namen Johannes des Täufers.

(37)

Für Wunden, Quetschen, Stoßen, Schneiden, nehme fier Peint Hölzer von gleicher länger duppe mit ein jedes auf den Schaden und sage bei ein jedes folgende Worte fünfmal und den Verbrenne diese Hölzer.

———

Auf Golgatha, auf Golgatha, auf Ciprus, auf Ciprus, auf Arrorot, auf Arrorot, sollen deine Schmerzen Fliehen, ins Tiefe Meer soll dein Schmerz versinken, und bei Jesus wunden lege ich deine. Wie dieses Holz Brennt, Sei dein Schmerz versenkt.

(38)

When a woman hath not her monthly course or cycle, or is congested, then call her baptismal name three times, and each time say the following words three days in succession:

———

And she touched his garment, and was healed. Thus I command thee blood, by the precious blood of Christ, to take thy regular course. I command thee congested blood, by the flowing wounds of Christ, to take thy regular course. So truly as Paul was bound, this sickness shall be overcome, in the name of the Father, of the Son, and of the Holy Spirit.

(39)

When a woman hath too much of her monthly course or cycle, so that the flow will not cease, then call her baptismal name three times and each time say the following words three days in succession:

———

And the bleeding ceased and he healed her at that very hour. Now, cease to flow in the name of Jesus Christ. So truly as Jesus hath turned water into wine, shall this flow take its proper course. The Lord hath made everything well, and considered humankind good, in the name of the Father, and of the Son, and of the Holy Spirit.

(40)

For swelling, blisters, and erruptions, call the baptismal name of the afflicted person seven times, and each time speak the following words:

———

So truly as Jesus healed the lepers, so also shalt thou be pure. In the name of the Holy Trinity, shall this flesh become clean. So truly as the wise men came, shall this plague be taken from thee, in the name of the Twelve Apostles of Jesus Christ.

The End of the First Part.

(38)

Wen ein Weibsbild ihre Zeit oder monatliche Reinigung nicht hat, oder verstopft ist, so nenne ihren Taufnamen dreymal und sage jedesmal folgende Worte drey Tage nacheinander.

———

Und sie Rührte sein Kleid an, und ward gesund, also gebiete ich dier Geblüht bey Jesus Christus Theures Blut, nehme deinen rechten Lauf ich gebiete dier verstopftes Blut, bei Christus Fließende Wunden, nehme deinen rechten Lauf, So wahr Paulus war gebunden, Sei diese Krankheit überwunden, im namen des Vaters, des Sohnes und des Heiligen Geistes.

(39)

Wen ein Weibsbild ihre Zeit oder Monatlich Geblüt zu viel hat, so daß ein Fluß daraus entstanden ist, so nenne den Taufname des Kranken dreymal und sage jedesmal folgende Worte, drey Tage nacheinander.

———

Und der Blutgang hörete auf und er Heilete sie zu der Selbigen Stunde, Nun so höre den auf zu Fließen, in Jesus Christus Namen, So wahr wie Jesus aus Wasser hat gemacht Wein, Soll der Fluß sich stellen zu rechter Zeit Ein, Der Herr hat alles Wohl gemacht, und hat den Mensch gut bedacht, im Namen des Vaters, des Sohnes, und des Heiligen Geistes.

(40)

Für Geschwüre, Blattern und Ausschlag nenne den Taufnamen des Kranken siebenmal, und spreche jedesmal folgende Worte.

———

So wahr wie Jesus die Aussätzigen Heilete, solst auch du Rein sein, im Namen der dreifaltigkeit, soll dieses Fleisch Sauber werden, so wahr wie die drei Weisen sind kommen, Sei diese Plage von ihm genommen im Namen der zwölf Aposteln von Jesus Christus.

Ende des Ersten Theils.

Book II

As I begin the second part, it is absolutely necessary in advance to offer a small foreword. If the dear reader regards everything as here prescribed, so willt thou with the help of Christ enjoy the benefit which Jesus Christ has promised to all pious Christians and true followers. But since the second part addresses different matters, so I caution thee dear reader to make no use of thereof, when it is not absolutely necessary.

By the Grace of God.

(1)

When thou wishest to take the power from the gunpowder of another, so that he can hit nothing, say the following:

———

Christ's fire was dear,
Thy fire is severe,
Vexation marks thy shot,
So shall it miss, and reach thy target not.
I invoke you by the wind, lead, iron, and powder, that ye shall go astray without power, and reach not your aim, dispersed and commanded by the wind.

(2)

To take the power from a man, so that he cannot harm thee, say the following words:

———

In the name of Jesus of Nazareth! I take from thee three drops of blood: one from thine heart, one from thine head, and one from thy virility. In the name of the Seven Angels that guard Christ, shalt thou be powerless, stand still, and harm me not. This I command thee by the power of God, who orchestrates and creates all.

(3)

If something is stolen from thee, then take a horseshoe with three nails in it, make it red hot, and sprinkle salt and pepper on it, and let it cool at the spot where the stolen item was located. Lay three black chicken feathers on it, cover it with a black rag, and make three white crosses on it, and say the following words three times:

Five evil angels shall pursue thee. Thy conscience shall despair. I conjure thee in the name of the Holy Trinity: Bring back what thou hast stolen at this very time. Thou shalt burn as fire, wander as a monstrosity. The Seventh Commandment condemns thee to hell and flames of fire. I command thee by the power of Heaven, bring back what thou hast taken away. The Earth shall devour thee, if thou dost not bring it back. Restlessness shall afflict thee, Lucifer shall chase after thee, and thou shalt become lame and immobile, until thou bringest what thou hast stolen. In the name of the Twelve Holy Apostles of Jesus Christ.

———

And after this, take a red onion, and stick the three nails which have been made red-hot by fire into the onion, and say the following three times:

———

As red as this onion is, so is thy corrupted heart. In the Name of the father, I drive a glowing nail into thine heart. In the name of the Son, I drive a glowing nail into thy lungs and liver. In the name of the Holy Spirit, I drive a glowing nail into thy virility, until thou returnest what thou hast stolen, by the will of Jesus Christ and in the names of the Twelve Apostles.

———

When a thief returns the stolen goods, then thou canst release him by the following means and retrieve all related things, by saying the following words three times:

———

I release thee from thine anguish and vexation in the name of the Father, Son, and Holy Spirit, and take all heavy bonds placed upon thee, and commend them to be sunken into the deep sea in the Name of the Power of Jesus Christ of Nazareth.

(4)

To stop bleeding for man or beast, take a fresh egg, and let the white run out of it, and thereafter allow it to be filled to the yolk with blood from the wound, and place it in hot embers. One will see a wonder, for as the egg sets, so shall the bleeding stop by saying the following words three times:

———

Jesus' wounds have bound all things, Jesus blood makes all things good.

(5)

When the milk is spoiled, so that it will give neither cream nor butter, go to the ground-ivy and speak before thou breakest the herb, and pass thine hand in a circle. Take the herb and say the following words:

———

Ground-ivy, Christ hath given thee grace. He hath created the clouds, and brings back the milk to me - to me mine, and each his own in the name of the Father, Son, and Holy Spirit. Then break the herb, and give it to the cow with salt to eat " " --- thus will it again give cream and butter.

(6)

So that no witch nor spirit may harm thy property: take rue, bread, salt, and oaken coals. Bore a hole in the door sill, where the cattle go in and out, and put the powder into a rag and stuff it into the hole with the tine of a harrow, thus the cattle will be safe.

(7)

When an accident befalls thee, whether by means of sorcery or otherwise a wicked person, then take thine own urine, and put it into a bottle sealed tightly, and lock it up. Thou must keep it locked up for nine days. Give or lend nothing from thine house, and speak the following words each day three times:

———

Just as Paul was bound, so be thou defeated. In Jesus' name, thou shalt burn, in the name of Peter thou shalt burst. Make good what thou hast harmed, or else the bonds of hell will rest upon thee. Thine heart shall burn in thy body, thy blood shall run away like water. Thou shalt grow lame and crooked, deaf, and dumb. Thy bladder shall burst. In the air thou shalt be scorched, in the name of the Holy Spirit, and the Holy Guardian Angels.

(5)

Wan die Milch Veruntreut ist das es weder Rahm noch Butter geben will, so geh zu Gunt Beerenkraut und sprich ehe du das Kraut abbrichst, und fahre Scheibenweis mit der Hand, so nim das Kraut und sprich folgende Worte.

———

Gunt Reben, Christus hat dir Gnade geben, Der hat erschaffen die Wolken, und Bring mir die Milch wieder, mier das meine, und jeder das seine im Namen des Vaters, Sohn und Heiliger Geist, dan brich das Kraut, und gieb es der Kuh mit Salz zu fressen " " --- so geibt es wiede Rahm und Butter.

(6)

Das keine Hexe noch Gespenst dein Gut mag Schaden so nim Rauten und Brod und Salz, und Eichene Kohlen, bohr ein Loch in der Thür Schwelle, wo daß Vieh aus und eingehet, und das Pulver in einen Lumpen Thu, in das Loch, und Verschlage es mit einem Eggen Zahn, so ist dein Vieh sicher.

(7)

Wenn dier etwas von ohngefähr angethan ist es sei von Zauberei oder sonst Böse Menschen, so nehme dein eigen Wasser, thue es in eine Botelji fest zugestoft, und verschließe es, du mußt es neun tage Verschlossen halten, nichts aus dein Haus geben oder ausleihen, und den spreche folgende Worte jeden Tag dreymal.

———

So wie der Paulus war gebunden, So sey du uberwunden, In Jesus Namen solst du Brennen, In Petrus Namen solst du verspringen Mache gut was du geschadet hast, Sonst liegt auf dier die Höllen Last, dein Herz im Leib soll brennen, wie Wasser soll dein Blut verrennen, du solst verlahmen und verkrummen, Vertauben und Verstummen, die Blase im Leib soll dir verspringen, In der Luft solst du versengen, im Namen des Heilligen Geistes, und der Heiligen Schutz Engeln.

A veritable tale, or proven art, to use in danger of fire and also in times of pestilence. It was devised by a Christian Choirmaster named King from Egypt. It came to pass in the year 1714 on the 10th day of June, in the Kingdom of Prussia, that 6 gypsies, or so called heathens, were sentenced to hanging, but a seventh man of 80 years of age, was sentenced to be executed by the sword right thereafter on the sixteenth day. Meanwhile, by his luck, a terrible conflagration broke out, so that the old man was quickly unfettered and taken to the conflagration to practice his art, which he also did to great amazement, so that in one quarter-hour the fire was done, and well and completely ceased and extinguished, whereupon after this test, his life was pardoned and he was set free.

———

One must walk around the fire three times, that the sun riseth behind him, and speak the following:

———

Thou art welcome, thou fiery guest, seize no further than what thou hast; this I reckon to thee as penance, in the name of God the Father, the Son and the Holy Spirit. I command thee Fire, by the power of God, that doth all and createth all, thou wouldst stand still and go no further, so truly as Christ stood in the Jordan, where the Holy Man John baptized him. This I reckon to thee Fire as a penance in the name of the Holy Trinity. I command thee by the power of God, thou wouldst lay down thy flames, so true as Mary maintained her maidenhead before all all seed, this she maintained so chaste and pure, stop here thy flames, Fire. This I reckon to thee as a penance, in the name of the Holy Trinity. I command thee, Fire, thou wouldst lay down thine heat, by the precious blood of Jesus Christ, that he shed for us, for our sin and misdoing. This I reckon to thee, Fire, as penance in the name of God the Father, the Son and the Holy Spirit. Jesus of Nazareth, a King of the Jews, help us out of this fiery-strife and guard this land and border, from all plague and pestilence.

———

Whoever hath this inscription in his house, by him no conflagration will break out nor arise. Also in the same way, if a pregnant woman carrieth this inscription with her, neither sorcery or evil spirits can harm her or her baby. Also, the house will be safe against the infestation of plague.

End of the Second Part

Book III

It is necessary at the beginning of the third part to set forth a brief admonition, thus I will say only so much as that the third and last part contains the correct remedies for animals. Indeed, thou must make use of everything in firm faith in God and the Trinity, but under no circumstances shouldst thou use the Holiest Names when treating an animal.

Remedy Proved By Grace.

(1)

When a horse has botflies, lead him to a stone, and say the following words nine times, and between each three times thou must strike the horse on the belly with the stone. Each of the three times thou must wait one quarter-hour, and then lay the stone back at the same spot where it once laid.

―――

Peter plowed an acre with his golden plow, and under the plow lie three stones. The first is white, the second black, and the third red - thus I seize them, and strike the worms dead.

(2)

When a horse has colic, rub him with thine hand from the head to the tail, and say the following words three times:

―――

Jerusalem, Jerusalem, city of the Jews,
Where Jesus was crucified,
There he shed his precious blood,
Which for all pain in animals is good.

(3)

If a horse has ring-bone, then first burn the sore with a hot iron, and wait a half-hour, then rub the wound from the top downwards, and say the following words seven times.

―――

Upon Golgotha Jesus suffered,
There he sufferend unto death.
From all pains and suffering,
Shall this animal be relieved.
The Blood of Christ
Is good for all wounds.

(4)

If a horse has sweeny, then rub the wound with thine hand from the top downwards three times. Thou must do this three times each day for nine days in succession in the light of the waxing moon, and each time say the following words:

———

Marrow and bone,
Flesh and blood,
For the sweeny is all good.
Just as Paul did escape,
So the pain from this animal take.
Strengthen flesh and bone,
Restore it unto thee.

(5)

If a horse cannot urinate, then rub over the ribs with the hand seven times, and say the following words three times:

———

Great is the help from above, the heavens bestow mercy. He who hath created the animals, must also restore their health. Water flow, water flow, water stream, water take thy proper course, and remove this illness. Just as the sun doth rise and set, so let thy pains abate.

(6)

If a horse has worms, then rub from the breast to the belly with the hand five times, and each time say the following words:

———

Worm withdraw from this beast,
Here is not thy dwelling place.
Now withdraw away and stay away,
Worm thou shalt wither,
And not endure.
I do conjure and demand
That thou shalt wither and waste.
Relieved be thy pains,
And never come again.

(4)

Wen ein Gaul die Schwinne hat, so streiche mit der Hand, 3 mal, von oben, bis unten, über den Schaden, dieses mußt du dreymal, jeden tag, neun Tage hinter einander, im zunehmende Licht thun, und sage jedesmal folgende Worte.

———

Mark und Bein,
Fleisch und Blut,
Ist vor alles Schwinden Gut.
So wie Paulus ist entkommen,
Sey dem Thier der Schmerz genommen.
Sterke Fleisch und Bein,
Stelle dich wieder ein.

(5)

Wen ein Pferd nicht Wassern kann, so streiche mit der Hand, siebenmal über die Rippen und sage folgende Worte dreimal.

———

Gros ist die Hülfe von oben, der Himmel Thut Barmherzigkeit, der die Thiere Erschaffen hat, der muß sie auch gesund erhalten, Wasser Fließe, Wasser Fließe, Wasser Ströhme, Wasser nehme deinen Rechten Lauf, und hebe diesen Schaden auf, So wie die Sonne geht auf und ab, so lasse deine Schmerzen ab.

(6)

Wen ein Pferd Würme hat, so streiche mit der Hand von der Brust bis am Leib fünfmal und sage jedesmal folgende Worte.

———

Wurm ziehe aus von diesem Their,
Dein Verbleibsplatz ist nicht hier,
Nun ziehe fort und bleibe fort,
Wurm du solst vergehen,
Und nicht bestehen,
Ich Thu beschwören, und begehren,
Du solst vergehen und verzehren,
Deine Schmerzen sind genommen,
Und sollen nicht wieder kommen.

(7)

If a horse has collar boils, then take a bone from a dead horse that was found by accident, and rub the boil with the underside of the bone seven times, and each time say the following words:

———

In six days the heavens and the earth were created, and it was good. Therefore all that has been created good shall be kept good. Jesus hath banished all evil, and the good shall remain. So shalt thou be healed in Jesus' Name.

(8)

If a horse is constipated, then rub him with the hand seven times over the ribs, and say each time the following words:

———

The disciples of Christ have healed all diseases by man and beast. In the name of John thou shalt be opened, in the name of Peter all things shall take their proper course. I bespeek thee in faith: thou shalt recover thine health. In the name of Paul shall thy pains abate.

(9)

If a horse has colic, treat him with the following words three times, and each time strike him on the ribs:

———

All colic, all pains shall wither away in the name of Caspar, Melchior and Balthasar. I adjure thee colic - thou shalt wither away and never return. With the Holy Word, I bespeak thee, with the Holy Creed, I banish thee, with the Holy Power, I expell thee.

(10)

If an accident befalls a cow, so that it no longer gives milk or butter, and further becomes gaunt and dry, take the milk, put it in a pot, cook it for one hour, and stab it frequently with a grass-scythe. Then inter the milk in a hole, and defecate upon it, cover it with earth, and say the following words three times:

———

All evil shall pass away, as dust and dung. From whence the evil cometh, so shall it return. As this milk decays, so shall all sorcery dissipate, in the name of Matthew the Holy Apostle.

———

(7)

Wenn ein Gaul Kummetblatter hat, so nehme einen Knochen von en Todes Pferd, von ohngefähr gefunden und reibe es mit der Bodenseite, des Knochens siebenmahl untersich, und sage jedesmahl folgende Worte.

———

In sechs Tage ist Himmel und Erde gemacht und es ward Gut, also wiel alles Gut Geschaffen ist, soll alles Gut erhalten warden, Jesus hat alles Böse Vertrieben, und das Gute muß bleiben, so solst du geheilet sein in Jesus Namen.

(8)

Wen ein Pferd verstopft ist, so streichen ihm mit der Hand siebenmal an die Rippen und sage jedesmal folgende Worte.

———

Christus seine Jünger haben alle Krankheiten geheilet an Menschen und vieh, im Namen Johannes solst du öfnung haben, im Namen Petrus soll alles sein Rechten gang gehn, ich bespreche dier im Glauben, du solst gesund warden, im Namen Paulus sollen dier deine Schmerzen verlassen.

(9)

Wen ein Pferd die Colik hat, so brauche es mit folgende Worte dreimal, und schlage jedesmal an die Rippe.

———

Alle Colik, alle Schmerzen sollen vergehen im namen Caspar, Melchior, und Baster, ich beschwöre dier Colik du solst vergehen und nicht wieder kommen, mit das Heilige Wort, bespreche ich dier, mit den Heiligen Glauben Banne ich dier, mit der Heiligen Kraft vertreibe ich dier.

(10)

Wen eine Kuh von ohngefähr etwas angethan ist, so daß es kein Milch oder Butter mehr giebt und sonst Mager und Derr wird, nehme die Milch und thu es in ein Topf und koche es eine Stunde und stoße mit eine Gras-Sens Fleißig darin herum, und den Grabe die Milch in ein Loch und thu deine Nothdurft dazu, und decke es mit Erde zu, und sage folgende Worte dreimal.

———

Alles Uebel soll vergehen wie Staub und Mist, wo das Uebel herkommt, soll es wieder hinziehen. Wie diese Milch vergeht soll alle Zauberkraft vergehen, im Namen Matheus des Heiligen Apostels.

If a cow or a horse has dysentery, then speak the following words softly in the morning to the animal, three days in succession:

———

He who hath created and made all things, hath considered all things good. But take this illness from this animal, or as it is said: Paul's crown will persist, but this disease shall vanish. Dysentery I adjure thee by the power of faith, withdraw from this animal, the sufferings of Christ are enough.

End of the Third Part

A Farewell to the Reader

My dear reader and friend, male or female, this work was not revealed out of the desire for profit, but instead out of compassion alone, because it was intended only for the wellbeing of man and beast. It was compiled for the use of everyone and will be considered a treasury of the most useful writings ever to see the light of day. Also wilt thou, my dear reader, consider this collection a precious treasure, a gem, better than silver or gold, however one that is not expensive to obtain. It happened that a benefactor underwrote the first edition for one thousand dollars, so that it has been made available to the dear reader at half the cost it would have been otherwise. I am completely confident that thou wilt not regret the purchse of it, but instead, that it will bring thee great joy. Thou wilt consider it a friend to thine house, a deliverer in times of danger, a relief in pain and suffering, and a comforter of body and soul. Thus, I bid thee, dear reader, farewell, and commend thee to the protection and assistance of Holy Trinity.

The Compiler.

Wen eine Kuh oder ein Gaul den Durchlauf hat, so spreche dreimal des Morgens unbeschrien bey den Viehe folgende Worte drei Tage nacheinander.

———

Der alles Schaft und alles macht, hat alles Wohlbedacht, aber diese Plage nimm weg diesem Vieh, oder wie es heißt, Paulus Krone wird bestehen, nur diese Seuche soll vergehen, Durchlauf ich beschwöre dir mit der Kraft des Glaubens, laß ab von diesen Vieh, Christo Leiden sind genug.

Ende des zweiten Theils.

Abschied vom Leser

Mein geliebter Leser oder Leserin, Freund oer Freundin, dieses Werk ist nicht aus Geldgewinn ans Tageslight gekommen, sondern allein aus Menschenfreundschaft, dieweil es nur allein bestimmt ist zum wohl der Menschen und Vieh, und ein jeder der Gebrauch davon gemacht hat, hat es als ein Schatz, eins der nützlichen Schriften befunden, die jemals ans Tageslicht gekommen sind, und so wirst auch du, mein' geliebter Leser oder Leserin, dieses als ein köstlicher Schatz, als ein Kleinod, der besser ist als Silber und Gold, diese Schrift würde nicht so theuer kommen, es hat aber ein Menschenfreund vor die Erste Abschrift müssen Tausend Thaler bezahlen, sonst würde es dem geliebten Leser um die Hälfte billiger können geliefert wer den, ich bin völlig überzeugt, daß es dir nicht gereuen, sondern große Freude machen wird, und du wirst es als ein Hausfreund, ein Retter un Gefahren, eine Zuflucht in Schmerz und Pein, ein Tröster von Leib und Seele betrachten, indem ich dir Lebewohl wünsche geliebter Leser, empfehle ich dir den Schutz und Beistand der Heiligen Dreieinigkeit.

Der Verfasser.

To eliminate mouth decay, one shall take three glasses completely filled with flowing water. This must take place in the light of the waning moon, in the morning without speaking for three days in succession. One must take the first glass and cleanse the mouth with it, and say the following words five times after cleansing:

———

Just as Christ was clean!	Blessed be this hour,
So will the mouth be clean and clear:	God's salvation in the mouth!
John baptised the Lamb of God!	The mouth that praiseth all
That took affliction from the world.	Father, Son, and Holy Spirit.

When thou hast emptied the first glass, thereupon take the second glass, cleanse the mouth with it, and say the following words three times:

———

Just as Mary was a virgin pure	Clean, hale, and pure
So will the mouth be clean and clear:	This mouth of God shall be,
Born in purity was Christ:	No decay shall endure,
So the mouth rot shall be lost.	In the name of the guardian angels three.

When thou hast emptied the first two glasses, thereupon take the third, cleanse the mouth with it, and say the following words three times:

———

Just as the moon doth decrease,	Blessed be this hour,
So shall the mouth rot decease,	God's salvation in the mouth!
What God created pure and clean,	The mouth that praiseth all
So must the mouth also be.	Father, Son, and Holy Spirit.

ENDNOTES

Chapter I. Ritual Traditions of the Pennsylvania Dutch

1. Although the study of powwowing was pioneered by early twentieth-century folklorists such as Edwin Miller Fogel (*Beliefs & Superstitions of the Pennsylvania Germans*, 1915), Dr. Ezra Grumbine ("Folklore and Superstitious Beliefs of Lebanon County," 1905), Rev. Thomas R. Brendle and Claude W. Unger (*Folk Medicine of the Pennsylvania Germans*, 1935), it was fundamentally transformed by the founders of the American Folklife Studies movement Alfred L. Shoemaker and Don Yoder (see: *Discovering American Folklife*, 2015, 11; *Hohman and Romanus: The Origins and Distribution of the Pennsylvania German Powwow Manual*, 1976, & *Official Religion Versus Folk Religion*, 1965) who studied powwow as a living expression of a folk tradition. In more recent years, powwowing has also been integrated into the ethnographic study of alternative and complementary medicine, in works by Barbara Reimensnyder (*Powwowing in Union County*, 1982), David J. Hufford (*Folk Medicine in Contemporary America*, 1992), Bonnie Blair O'Connor (*Healing Traditions: Alternative Medicine and the Health Profession*, 1995), and David Kriebel (*Powwowing Among the Pennsylvania Dutch: A Traditional Medical Practice in the Modern World*, 2007). Powwowing has also taken an important role in esoteric studies and charm literature, in works by Daniel Harms (*The Long Lost Friend: A 19th-Century American Grimoire*, 2012), Joseph Peterson (*The Sixth and Seventh Books of Moses*, 2008), and Natacha Klein Käfer ("German healing prayers in a transcontinental perspective: the case of the '*Dreyerley Würm Segen*,'" 2014).

2. Fogel, Edwin M, and C. Richard Beam. 1995. *Beliefs and Superstitions of the Pennsylvania Germans.* Millersville, PA: Center for Pennsylvania German Studies, Millersville University; Shoemaker, Alfred L. 2000. *Eastertide in Pennsylvania: A Folk Cultural Study.* Mechanicsburg, PA: Stackpole Books; Donmoyer, Patrick J. 2012. *The Friend in Need: An Annotated Translation of an Early Pennsylvania Folk Healing Manual.* Kutztown, PA: Pennsylvania German Cultural Heritage Center, Kutztown University.

3. Yoder, Don 1965, 234-36.

4. For more about each of these regions, see: Montgomery, Jack G. 2008. *American Shamans: Journeys with Traditional Healers.* Ithaca, N.Y: Busca, Inc, ; Gandee, Lee R. 1971. *Strange Experience: The Autobiography of a Hexenmeister.* Englewood Cliffs, NJ: Prentice-Hall, ; Cavender, Anthony P. 2003. *Folk Medicine in Southern Appalachia.* Chapel Hill: University of North Carolina Press; Randolph, Vance. *Ozark Magic and Folklore.* New York, NY: Dover Publications, 1964; Dorson, Richard M. 1952. *Bloodstoppers & Bearwalkers: Folk Traditions of the Upper Peninsula.* Cambridge: Harvard University Press; Arends, Shirley F. 1989. *The Central Dakota Germans: Their History, Language, and Culture.* Washington, D.C: Georgetown University Press; McKegney, Pat. 1989. *"Charm for Me, Mr. Eby": Folk Medicine in Southern Ontario 1890-1920.* Bamberg, Ont: Bamberg Press; Yoder, Don. 2015 "Brazilian Journals." *Discovering American Folklife* (2015):297-329; Kloberdanz, Timothy J., and Rosalinda Kloberdanz. 1993. *Thunder on the Steppe: Volga German Folklife in a Changing Russia.* Lincoln, Neb: American Historical Society of Germans from Russia.

5. For information on "Passing," also called *Benedicaria*, see: Weaver, Karol K. 2011. *Medical Caregiving and Identity in Pennsylvania's Anthracite Coal Region 1880-2000.* University Park, PA: Pennsylvania State University Press; For Rootwork, see: Montgomery, Jack 2008; For Santeria, see: González-Wippler, Migene. 1989. *Santería, the Religion: A Legacy of Faith, Rites, and Magic.* New York: Harmony; For Curanderismo, see: Kiev, Ari. 1968. *Curanderismo: Mexican-American Folk Psychiatry*, New York: The Free Press; For granny doctors, see: Montgomery, Jack. ibid; Milnes, Gerald. 2007. *Signs, Cures, & Witchery: German Appalachian Folklore.* Knoxville, TN. University of Tennessee Press; For Cajun healing, see: Veillon, Berk. 1998. *Cajun Healing: Les Traiteur et Les Traiteuse.* Antonio, TX: Acclaim Publishing.

6. For a thorough examination of modern American vernacular healing systems, see Hufford 1992.

7. Kriebel 2007, 18.

8. Brendle and Unger 1935, 68; KJV John 3:30-31; Luther Bibel 1912: *Er muß wachsen, ich aber muß abnehmen. Der von obenher kommt, ist über alle. Wer von der Erde ist, der ist von der Erde und redet von der Erde. Der vom Himmel kommt, der ist über alle.*

9. Hohman, Johann Georg. 1820. *Der lange Verborgene Freund, oder Getreuer und Christlicher Unterricht für jedermann...* Reading, PA: C. A. Bruckmann, 23.

10. Fogel 1995, 203.

11. Fogel 1995, 179; Randolph 1964, 133; Donmoyer 2012, 81.

12. Fogel 1995, 225.

13. Wintemberg 1950, 15; Fogel 1995, 205.

14. Yoder 2015, 322.

15. KJV Psalm 147:4.

16 KJV Genesis 15:5.

17. Yoder 1976, 248.

18. Beam 2004-2006, II(145-146), IV(17-18).

19. Beam 2004-2006, V(87-89).

20. Donmoyer 2016.

21. Beam 2004, 1(12, 35).

22. Cavender 2003, 138.

23. My grandmother's process can be likened to a hybridization of Grumbine's description (1905, 277) of anointing and powwowing with words for infant colic documented in Lebanon where my grandmother lived.

24. Brendle 1995, 53.

25. Helfenstein broadsides, 21.

26. For a range of authors who wrote about their first-hand experiences working with powwowers for ethnographic field work and discussed ethical considerations about confidentiality and the oral tradition, see: Graves 1985; Kriebel 2000; Donmoyer 2012.

27. *Powwow* literally implies a healing ritual, having been derived from the Algonquin title for a shaman or medicine man, meaning "he

dreams." Harper, Douglas. 2015 *Online Etymological Dictionary*. <www.etymonline.com>

28. Eliot & Mayhew 2008; Lyman 1928, 364; Liebman & Mayhew, 2008, 21.

29 Webster, Noah. 1861. "Powwow." *The American Dictionary of the English Language.* Springfield, MA: George and Charles Meriam.

30. Klepp, Whitehead, & Büttner 2006, 86-87.

31. Confusion of Pennsylvania Dutch practices with the widespread American phenomenon of the popular commercial image of the "Indian Healer" is offered as an explanation for the origin of the word "powwow" among the Pennsylvania Dutch, in Weaver 2011.

32. This theme of exoticism is echoed in many North American titles: *The Egyptian Secrets of Albertus Magnus (Albertus Magnus'... Egyptische Geheimnisse).* 1869. Allentown, PA: Harlacher and Weiser; *The Magnificent Book of the Gypsies (Das Vortreffliche Zigeuner Büchlein.* c.1810, Reading, PA: Heinrich Sage); *The Sixth and Seventh Books of Moses (Das sechste und siebente Buch Mosis.* 1871. New York: Wilhelm Radde.

33. *Various Sympathetic and Secret Formulae (Verschiedene sympathetische und geheime Kunststücke).* c.1800. [Egypt]: Stofel Ehrlig, for the Gypsy King.

34. Fogel 1995, 225.

35. Peterson 2008.

36. See Chapter II: Powwowing and the Clergy.

Chapter II. Who Powwows? Practitioners & Facilitators

1. Interview in Lower Macungie, Lehigh County, 2015.

2. Lebanon City Directory 1945, 1948, www.ancestry.com; "William Reppert" in Lebanon Borough, U.S. Federal Census 1940.

3. Oral History with Anabell Karnes, Lebanon, PA 2017.

4. KJV Job 5:18, Matthew 10:7-8.

5. Oral History with Anabell Karnes, Lebanon, PA. April, 2017.

6. Interiew in Cornwall, Lebanon County, November, 2013.

7. "William Reppert" in Lebanon Borough, US. Federal Census 1920.

8. See, Donmoyer 2016, 29-37; "Bewitched Children. A Strange Case of Superstition and Witchcraft in Windsor, Pa." April 1, 1885. *St. Louis Post Dispatch*; see also Chapter IX: Dr. Joseph H. Hageman.

9. Ledgers of Isaac W. Zwalley, Landis Valley Museum, Pennsylvania Historic and Museum Commission. See also: *Consolidated Lists of Civil War Draft Registration Records, Provost Marshal General's Bureau; Consolidated Enrollment Lists, 1863-1865,* III(110): 4213514; National Archives and Records Administration, Washington, D.C.;

10. Isaac Zwalley obituary, *Ephrata Review* (Ephrata, Pa.), Friday, February 3, 1899, p. 1, col. 6

11. Oral History with John Messner, Shartlesville, Berks County, 2012.

12. For more on Doc Brunner, see the recent volume *Good Land, Good People.* 2014. Kempton, PA: Albany Township Historical Society.

13. Yoder, Don. 1952. *Sophia Bailer Speaks II. Transcript of interview at 3nd Annual Kutztown Folk Festival.* Unpublished papers.

14. Ibid.

15. Waldenberger, Johan Daniel. 1796. Manuscript, Don Yoder Collection, Pennsylvania German Cultural Heritage Center, Kutztown University of Pennsylvania. See also Brendle 1935, where Waldenberger is listed throughout the text as source MS11.

16. For examples of edible blessings printed on starch paper with images of the saints and blessing inscriptions, see Wunderlin 2005, 24-25; See also Chapter III: Brauchen &Transatlantic Emigration for edible written blessings by Johannes Ernst Spangenberg.

17. Chapter on "Sympathie" in Oley Valley Doctor's Ledger, ca. 1830. Manuscript, Heilman Collection.

18. Oley Township, US Federal Census 1850, located with the assistance of Michael Emery of Landis Valley Museum, Lancaster, Pa.

19. For a less than flattering biography of Rev. Georg P. Mennig, see Early 1902, 11, and for discussion of his broadsides, see Yoder 2005, 123-124.

20. Patterson, James. 1835. *Lutheran Observer and Weekly Religious Literary Visitor.* Baltimore. Feb 20, 1835. New Series, II(26).

21. Yoder 2005, 125.

22. Munro 1981, 79.

23. Yoder, Don. Unpublished research conducted at the Evangelical & Reformed Historical Society, Lancaster, PA, date unknown. I was able to examine Herrmann's ledgers in 2017, but was unable to find any evidence of what Don Yoder documented, however at least half a dozen pages appear to have been excised from Herrmann's ledger, and the contents are missing from the original document as well as the microfilm.

24. Helffrich 1906. 345.

25. Originally published in *The Guardian* in 1868, reprinted in the *Pennsylvania Dutchman*, 5:14, March 15 1954, Lancaster, PA: Pennsylvania Dutch Folklore Center, Franklin & Marshall College.

26. *Diary of J. Spangler Kiefer,* Friday Aug 27, 1886, Manuscript, Historical Society of the Evangelical and Reformed Church, Lancaster PA. Volume for 1884-1887.

27. Morris & Sprague 1861, 98.

28. "Pow-Wow Doctor." *Reading Times*, Reading, PA. Fri, Oct 8, 1880, 1.

29. From "Medico-Religious Quackery" a scathing editorial by "Medicus," in *The Lebanon Advertiser,* Dec 28, 1870.

30. Raber, W. B. 1855. *The Devil and Some Of His Doings.* Canton, OH: United Brethren in Christ.

31. Several broadside Ezekiel 16:6 cures exist: one from the Roughwood Collection at the Library Company of Philadelphia, and several more in the collection of Russel D. Earnest Associates. A manuscript of the verse was also found in a Fegley family Bible from Berks County, PA (Heilman Collection). The family Bible of Dr. Joseph H. Hageman of Reading, PA (Private Collection) has a mark in the margin by the verse in Ezekiel. At least one Bible known to the author has the verse cut out of the book.

32. Yoder 1965, 234-36

33. Interview with Berks County practitioner, Wernersville, PA, 2010.

34. Interview with Chester County practitioner, Elverson, PA, 2009.

35. Hufford, David. "Folk Medicine" in Dorson, Richard Mercer. 1995. *Handbook of American Folklore.* Bloomington, In: Indiana University Press. Handbook of American Folklore.

36. Fogel, 1995, 42.

37. For a wide range of cultural responses to children born with the caul, see Hovorka & Kronfeld 1909, II: 593-594; Forbes, T. R. 1953. "The Social History of the Caul." *The Yale Journal of Biology and Medicine.* 25(6), 495–508; Rich, C. (1976). "Born with the Veil: Black Folklore in Louisiana." *The Journal of American Folklore,* 89(353): 328-331; Wilson 2004, 334; Ginzburg 2011.

38. Fogel 1995, 40.

39. Oral History Interview with Great-Granddaughter of H. Edward Swope, 2017.

40. Fogel 1995, 187.

41. My primary contact for stories of Marty Springer is Anna Mae Peterson of Brecknock Township, who helped me to understand the community's outlook on his healing. She supplied information as well for Goodling, Evans C., Jr. 2015. *Brecknock: Early History and*

Biographical Annals of Brecknock Township, Berks County, Pa. Reading: Reading Eagle Press, 526-531, 682-684; Robert Springer obituary clipping, *New Holland Clarion*, Dec 3 1887.

42. Clipping, *Reading Eagle*, April 14, 1885.
43. Goodling 2015, 526-531, 682-684.
44. Fogel 1995, 210.
45. Ibid, 201.
46. Ibid, 201; see also Hand. Wayland. 1968. "Folk Medical Inhalants in Respiratory Disorders." *Medical History,* XII(2) April.
47. Fogel 1995, 42.
48. ibid, 212.
49. ibid, 212-213.
50. ibid, 212.
51. Montgomery 2008.
51. Listed in 1883 and 1884 City Directories as a physician: Philadelphia, Pennsylvania, City Directory, 1884: 1565. <www.ancestry.com>
52. Proof of Death Registers 1875-1893, Chester County Archives and Record Services, West Chester, PA; Local Daily News Editorial, "Education Needed" Geo. G. Groff. 10-8-1900; *Evening Public Ledger* (Philadelphia, Pennsylvania) Mon 23 Nov 1914, 8.
53. Montgomery 2008.
54. Interview with Anna Mae Peterson in Brecknock in 2015.
55. Louden 2016, 54-56.
56. York, Pennsylvania, US Federal Census 1930.
57. Lewis 1970, 34.
58. Phillips, Lockwood. 1928. "York Murder Stirs Officials to War on Powwowism" *Reading Times*, Thu, Dec 13, 1928, 8.
59. Lewis 1970, 34-35.
60. Phillips 1928, 8.
61. "Conjuration: How it is Practiced in Lancaster." *Lancaster intelligencer,* Feb 13 1869.
62. Laydom, Levi. 1859. Manuscript in the private collection of Gregory Wonder & Family.
63. Strassburger & Hinke 1992, 471.
64. Rutherford, Hiram. 1894. "French Jacob… Wizard of Lykens Valley." *Notes and Queries: Historical, Biographical and Genealogical, Chiefly Relating to Interior Pennsylvania.* Ed. William Henry Egle, Harrisburg, PA: Harrisburg Publishing Co. VI: 171.
65. Ibid.
66. Ibid.
67. Carr, James C. 2005-2015. *French Jacob*. Pendleton County Genealogy Project. <www.kykinfolk.com/pendleton\>
68. *Kurzgefasstes Arznei Büchlein für Menschen und Vieh.* Ephrata, PA: Solomon Meyer, 1791.
69. Boyer, Dennis. "Jake, Der Holzman," *Hollerbier Haven.* Kutztown: Three Sisters Center for the Healing Arts. 1:2, August 2007, 9.
70. Also spelled Wash Frau, Wascht Fraa, Wurst Frau, Woorst, etc. See also: Gibbons 2001, 402.
71. Iskra-Chubb, Joanne Flores. 2003. "Reading's Wash Fraus: Powwowing for Three Generations." *Historical Review of Berks County,* LXVIII(3): 130-134.
72. Discussion of learning from her father is included in "Something about the Wash Frau." *Reading Eagle* Nov 23 1874; information on her father's occupation and status in *Württemberg, Germany, Lutheran Baptisms, Marriages, and Burials, 1500-1985* [database on-line]. Provo, UT, USA: Ancestry.com Operations, Inc., 2016. *Heimerdingen: Taufen, Tote und Heiraten* 1566-1968, Wuertt. Evang. Landeskirche, Evang. Dekanatampt Leonberg, Film Nr. KB 532, pg 307, 882.
73. "Sketch of a Well-Known Female Celebrity – Brauche Method of Curing." *Reading Times,* May 15, 1899.
74. Reading Eagle July 26, 1903.
75. "Something about the 'Wash Frau'-The History and Achievements of this Famous Person-A visit to Her Home-The Origin of the Peculiar Name" *Reading Times.* 23 Nov 1874.
76. Catherine Hess Obituary, *Reading Eagle* July 26, 1903.
77. Iskra-Chubb 2003, 132
78. "... Brauche Method of Curing." *Reading Times,* May 15, 1899
79. "Something about the 'Wash Frau'..." *Reading Times.* 23 Nov 1874.
80. "A Victim of Powwow Folly." *Lancaster Daily Intelligencer.* Apr 10, 1890, 4.
81. "The Wurst Frau Arrested." *Reading Eagle* April 9, 1890, p 1; "Mrs. Eberth's Defense." *Reading Eagle* April 10, 1890, 1.
82. "Large Turnout at Mrs. Eberth's Funeral-Rev. Huntsinger's Tribute to the Deceased, Who Was Popularly Known as the 'Wash-Frau.'" *Reading Eagle,* July 23, 1903.
83. "New Trial Refused." *Reading Times,* Mar 13 1906
84. Iskra-Chubb 2003, 134.
85. "Something about the 'Wash Frau'..." *Reading Times.* 23 Nov 1874.
86. Listed as "Sophyia" in the 1880 US Federal Census in Tremont, Schuylkill County, PA.
87. Bailer, Sophia. 1947. *The Leininger Family: One of the Oldest in the State and Nation.* Tremont, PA: Mrs. Charles Bailer.
88. Yoder, Don. ca. 1960 "Occult Folk Medicine Among the Pennsylvania Germans." Keynote Address given for the Department of Folklore & Folklife, University of Pennsylvania. No date, 3.
89. *Publications of the Historical Society of Schuylkill County*, 1910. Pottsville, PA: Daily Republican Print, II:132.
90. Bailer, 1947, np; This information is confirmed on her PA Death Certificate 1954, no. 54163.
91. Bailer 1947, np.
92. Later listed as Mrs. Mark West on Sophia's PA Death Certificate 1954.
93. Tremont, Schuylkill County, PA, U.S. Federal Census 1920.
94. "Braucha Healing." *Phillidelphia Inquirer,* June 22, 1952.
95. Sophia Bailer Manuscripts, Heilman Collection.
96. Yoder, Don. 1952. "Sophia Bailer Speaks Transcripts" Unpublished, part II, 1952,4.
97. Ibid.
98. Yoder address, ca. 1960, 11.
99. Yoder 1952, II: 3.
100. Harms 2012, 153.
101. Harms 2012, 153, 47.
102. Harms 2012, 93.
103. Sophia Bailer Manuscripts, Heilman Collection. The word "whare" is likely to be a variation of *wahre* (true) or possibly *Harr* (Lord).
104. Yoder, Don. 2015. "The Saint's Legend in the Pennsylvania German Folk Culture." *Discovering American Folklife.* Kutztown, PA: Pennsylvania German Cultural Heritage Center, 199-229.
105. Brown, Frank. 1966. "New Light on Mountain Mary." *Pennsylvania Folklife.* 15:3 Spring 1966, 10-15.
106. Hollinshead in Stoudt 1974, 11-12.
107. Hollinshead, Benjamin M. 1965. "Mountain Mary (*Die Berg Maria*)." In Preston Barba's "*Es Pennsylvaanisch Deitsch Eck,*" Allentown *Morning Call.* Nov. 20 and 27 1965.
108. See Boyer 2004.
109. Lewis 1972, 10. (see Chapter X)
110. A full reprint of this work is available in Stoudt 1974.
111. Yoder 2015, 213.

Chapter III. European Origins

1. Yoder 1976, 248.
2. For more on the development of the cult of the saints in early Christianity, see: Brown 1981.
3. Yoder, Don. 2015, 199.
4. Bainton 1972, 26-27.
5. Clebsch & Jaekle 1964, 174.
6. Beitl 1978.
7. For a the most comprehensive treatment of the use of blessings in both sanctioned and folk-cultural settings in the Middle Ages, see: Franz 1960
8. *Ein Sehr Kräftiges Gebet* (*A Very Powerful Prayer*) ca. 1880, Kutztown, PA: Urich & Gehring. Pennsylvania German Cultural Heritage Center, Kutztown University, Don Yoder Collection.
9. Yoder 2005, 221-222.
10. *Abschrift aus einen Geistlichen Schilt.* Manuscript from Manheim, PA. ca. 1850. Private collection of Michael Emery.
11. Yoder 2016, 111.
12. For St. Lawrence and Cyprian in published and manuscript prayers, see Yoder 2015, 202; St. Blaise in prayers for menstrual disorders, see Donmoyer 2012, 99; St. George & St. Martin in Georg Henninger, 1775, Albany Township, Berks County. Manuscript, Heilman Collection.
13. "Three Holy Women" or "Three Virgins" are frequently mentioned in North American and European ritual literature and rarely identified. Hohman names them as Saints "Elisabeth, Brigitta und Mechtildis (Matilda)" in his 1819 apocryphal work *Das Evangelium Nicodemus*, printed by C. A. Bruckman in Reading. See Yoder 2016, 141.
14. Yoder 2015, 203; Donmoyer 2012, 88-91.
15. Hoffman 1976.
16. McCain, Dau & Bente 2009. *Luther's Large Catechism*, I:11.
17. Yoder 2015, 200.
18. Kolb, Wengert & Arand. 2000. *Augsburg Confession,* Article 21.
19. Marty 2004.
20. Klein 2011, 55.
21. Hoffman 1976.
22. Luther & Hazlitt 1990.
23. Luther & Hazlitt 1990, DXCIII.
24. For a modern translation of the ritual , see Weller 1964.
25. Luther, Bachmann & Lehmann 1965, XXV: 96-101, and Spinks 1976, XIII(1).
26. Seyfarth 1913, 17.
27. Lea 1957, III: 1051.
28. Luther & Hazlit 1990, DLXXVII.
29. Luther, Lehmann & Hillerbrand 1965, LII: 159-286; Also in the Weimar edition, X: 555-728.
30. Luther 1910, 319-320. As a continuation of the previous entry on "*Zauberei*" (Sorcery), the original language suggests, rather than merely a literal reading of "*die Todten, die wandelnden Geister*" (the dead, the wandering ghosts), that the eighth and last category concerns those who consult the dead, i.e. Necromancers.
31. For more on Luther's Sermon in relation to charmers within the Pennsylvania German community, and particularly those in Ontario, see the upcoming article by Reginald Good in the Waterloo Historical Society publication, *Romanus-Büchlein (Little Romani or Gypsy Book): An eighteenth Century Collection of Mystical or Sympathetic Folk charms*, Donated to the Waterloo Historical Society in 1930-31.
32. Bayer 1733, 101; see also Muhlenberg & Schipper 1812. "*beschweeren*," np.
33. Portions of this sermon were published in two separate editions of a tract entitled: *The Difference Between True and False Worship*, Dr. Martin Luther, 1522, and 1646. Other portions were published in a separate tract: *An Exposition and Explanation of the Papacy in Its Own Colors*, by Dr. Martin Luther, 1522.
34. Hutton 2012, 247. These estimates are conservative. Levack (2016, 19) says "no more than 90,000."
35. Lea 1957, III: 1075. The present work owes a debt of gratitude to H. C. Lea's exhaustive treatment of primary and secondary sources in witchcraft prosecution in central Europe.
36. *Polizeiordnung* (Police Order) of Saxony in 1556, and in Wittgenstein in 1573, see Dickel, Horst. 1979. "Wortzauber in Wittgenstein."*Blätter für Wittgensteiner Heimatvereins*, XLIII: 50-52.
37. Käfer, Natacha Klein. 2014. "German healing prayers in a transcontinental perspective: the Case of the 'Dreyerley Würm Segen'" TEEME, third annual conference: Contemplating Early Modernities: Concept, Content & Context. Freie Universität Berlin, For documentation of the *Vergichtsegen, Diebsegen, Krongebet, Poppensegen, and Chrismbündlein* see Lea 1957, 1109, 1099, 1103, 1100.
38. Levack 2016, np.
39. Hutton 2012, 241.
40. Burr 1907, III(4).
41. Levack 2014, 78.
42. Mackay & Kramer 2009, 170.
43. Levack 2014, 79.
44. Lea 1957, III: 1078.
45. ibid, 1063.
46. Mackay & Kramer 2009, 446.
47. Ibid, 446-447.
48. Ibid, 448.
49. Donmoyer, Patrick 2016, 29-37; See Chapter IX.
50. Mackay & Kramer 2009, 267-268.
51. Lea 1957, III: 1052.
52. Laycock 2015, 99.
53. Lea 1957, III: 1079-1080; see also Thurston 2013.
54. Fischer 1791, 113-134.
55. Lea 1957, III: 1051.
56. See: Shulman & Stroumsa 2001, 160-161.
57. Menghi, Girolamo. 1576. *Flagellum Daemonum*. Bologna: Johannes Ross; Menghi, Girolamo. 1584. *Fustis Daemonum*. Bologna: Johannes Ross.
58. Lea 1957, III: 1056
59. Ibid, 1060.
60. "Painted Prints: Renaissance and Baroque Hand-Colored Engravings, Etchings, and Woodcuts." Baltimore Museum of Art, 2002-2003, no. 17.
61. *Die gewisse und wahrhafte Länge unsers Herrn Jesu Christi*. ca. 1780. Broadside, Heilman Collection. See also Kreissl 2014, 6, 28.
62. HDA IV: 902.
63. Brugsch 1888, 447.
64. HDA 5:902.
65. HDA 5:902.

66. Wilson 2004, 330.

67. Sexton 1992, 237-248. Two Jewish friends living in Berks County described to me in 2017 their experiences with the use of red string in rituals of blessing.

68. Fogel 1908, 286-314.

69. Yoder 2005, 209.

70. Ibid 210.

71. See the upcoming article from the Waterloo Historical Society on the Himmelsbrief of St. Michaelsburg by Reginald Good in Ontario, Canada, entitled "Peddling Protection: A Talismanic Form of Homeowners Insurance Sold by Peddlers in nineteenth Century Waterloo County."

72. Troxell, William. 1941. "Es Pennsylfawnisch Deitsch Eck: Der Himmelsbrief." *Morning Call.* 4 Oct 1941. Allentown, PA. This copy of the Himmelsbrief was issued just prior to the entry of the United States into World War II, and, it has been suggested by local author Richard Shaner that newspaper clippings of William (Pumpernickel Bill) Troxell's *Himmelsbrief* was carried overseas in the war.

73. Yoder 2016, 135-143.

74. Suter 1989, 1-2.

75. *Die Sieben Heiligen Himmelsriegel und Unserer Lieben Frauen Traum.* No imprint, likely Ignatius Kohler of Philadelphia ca. 1880, based on typographical evidence. Broadsheet, Heilman Collection. Author's translation.

76. Donmoyer 2011.

77. Ibid.

78. Mitterauer 2000, 83.

79. "Die Sieben Schloss darin sich die Seel sicher verschlissen kan." Closing prayer in 1771 Roman Catholic Manuscript prayer-book of Andonia Gerth, Heilman Collection.

80. *Die Sieben Heiligen Schluss,* Jerusalem. Ca.1800. Chapbook, Heilman Collection.

81. Regine Grube-Verhoeven. 1966. "Die Verwendung von Büchern Christlich-Religiösen Inhalts zu Magischen Zwecken." *Zauberei und Frömmigkeit.* Tübingen: Tübinger Vereinigung für Volkskunde, 23-28.

82. *Andachtiges Seelen Regal, Bestehend ein Morgens-, Abends-, Mess, Beicht-, und Communion-, den Divers anmüthige-Gebether!* 1797. Manuscript belonging to Sexaphin Antoni Oberdorfer, Heilman Collection.

83. *Geistlicher Schild, gegen geist- und leibliche Gefaerlichkeiten allzeit bei sich zu tragen…* 1747. Prag: Wenzeslaus Nowodni. Heilman Collection.

84. *Der Wahre Geistliche Schild, so vor 300 Jahren von dem heil. Pabst Leo X. bestätigt worden, wider alle gefährliche böse Menschen sowohl, als aller Hexerei und Teufelswerk entgegengesetzt.* Reading [Reutlingen]: Louis Ensslin, 1840. Heilman Collection.

85. KJV John 1:1-14.

86. G. S. Ensslin 1840, 2-4.

87. G. S. Nowodni 1747, np.

88. ibid, np.

89. Kreissel 2014, 29.

90. KJV, Matt 24:42; Mark 13:33.

91. G. S. Nowodni 1747, np.

92. Author's translation of inscription from, Spamer & Nickel 1958, 24.

93. Herbermann 1973, "Sts. Romanus."

94. Ibid; *Baer's Agricultural Almanac for the Year of our Lord* 2017, Lancaster, PA: John Baer's Sons.

95. Brewer 1894, 240.

96. Spamer & Nickel 1958, in Harms 2012, 18-19.

97. Kreissl 2014, 48.

98. Private collection of Reginald Good, Ontario, Canada.

99. Hohman, 1820, 12.

100. Harper 2001-2017. "Rominy."

101. *Romanus-Büchlein vor GOtt der HErr bewahre meine Seele, meinen Aus- und Eingang; von nun an bis in alle Ewigkeit, Amen. Halleluja. Gedruckt zu Venedig.* ca. 1800. Heilman Collection.

102. Free translation of Nowodni 1747, np.

103. KJV Job 2:7-8: "So went Satan forth from the presence of the LORD, and smote Job with sore boils from the sole of his foot unto his crown. And he took him a potsherd to scrape himself withal; and he sat down among the ashes."

104. Author's translation of Ensslin 1840: 147.

105. Roper 2005, 111-12.

106. *Ein Morgen Segen* (*A Morning Prayer*), ca. 1860, carried by Nathan Fernsler Krall, Rexmont, Lebanon County, Pennsylvania. Manuscript, Heilman Collection.

107. Heeger 1936, 20, and Lommer 1878, 5.

108. Grimm 1883, III: 1151.

109. Bayer 1733, "*Brauch,*" "*Brauchen.*" 126-127.

110. Adelung 1970, I:1161 and DWB II: 315.

111. *Diccionari de la Llengua catalana Segona edició*. Barcelona: Institut d'Estudis Catalans. http://dlc.iec.cat

112. "Bruja." *Diccionario Etymológico español en línea.* < http://etimologias.dechile.net/>

113. "List of Spanish words of Celtic origin." *World Heritage Encyclopedia.* World Public Library Association. 2017. http://worldbooklibrary.net/articles/list_of_spanish_words_of_celtic_origin

114. Breul 1906, 121.

115. PfWB I: 1167; RWB I: 926.

116. PfWB I: 940-942

117. Dickel 1979, 50-52.

118. ibid 50.

119. Heeger 1936, 19.

120. Shivley 1953, 9; Brendle & Troxell 1944, 50.

121. Heeger, op cit.

122. Dickel 1979, 50-52.

123. Heeger, op cit.

124. Lommer 1878, 35.

125. Dickel 1979, 50-52.

126. ibid.

127. Fischer 1791, 185-193; Stadler 2005; See Bernheimer 1952 for the Wild Man.

128. Fischer 1791, 186.

129. [Dr. Medicus]. 1830. *Der Hausarzt und die Hausapotheke, welche in allen Fällen Hulfe schaffen, oder die Kunst in 24 Stunden sein eigener Arzt zu werden. Ein lehrreiches Noth und Hülfsbuch für Jedermann.* (The Domestic Doctor and House Apothecary, Providing Assistance in All Circumstances, or the Method to Become Your Own Doctor in 24 Hours). Reutlingen: J. N. Enßlin.

130. Ibid. 5

131. HDA I: 1162

132. HDA Nachtrage (Supplement Volume): 257

133. Klepp, Whitehead, Frederick, & Büttner 2006, 86-87.

134. HDA III: 264-265

135. HDA I: 1162

136. HDA I: 1163

137. [Dr. Medicus] 1830, 6.

138. Ibid. 22, author's translation.

139. Ibid. 23, author's translation.

140. Ibid. 23, author's translation. Herb Robert refers to *Geranium Robertiana,* Cranesbill.

141. Ibid. 24, author's translation.
142. Breier, Eduard. 1873. *Der Freimüthige. Volkskalender für das Jahr 1873*, Von Eduard Breier, Neubau: Wiener Vereins-Buchdruckerei, 80-83.
143. Author's translation of Breier, 80.
144. Author's translation of Breier, 81.
145. Author's translation of Breier, 83.
146. Fischer 1791, i.
147. Author's translation of Breier, 13.
148. Agapkina, Karpov & Toporkov 2013, 43-59.
149. Free translation of "*Pro Nessia*" German text from the 9th Century Munich MS, featured in Kerr & Stewart 1983, 32.
150. Seyfarth 1917, 17; Hovorka & Kronfeld II: 891-892.
151. Seyfarth 1917, 82.
152. Ms. Dresden, Heilman Collection.
153. KJV Mark 5:1-16.
154. Other variations read: "*Alle Psalmen sind gesungen, Alle Glocken sind verklungen, Alle Evangelien sind gelesen, Alle Heiligen sind gewesen, Das Feuer in meinen Zähnen soll verwesen.*" in Grube-Verhoeven 1966, 32.
155. Hovorka & Kronfeld II: 406.
156. ibid. II: 406
157. Donmoyer 2012, 64.
158. Author's translation of Nürnberg Manuscript, Heilman Collection. This manuscript has similar contents to two manuscript collections from Saxony featured in Tetzner 1902, 346.
159. Author's translation of Seyfarth 1917, 77.
160. Author's translation of Nürnberg MS. Heilman Collection.
161. Author's translation of Seyfarth 1917, 77.
162. Author's translation of Seyfarth 1917, 79.
163. Author's translation of Seyfarth 1917, 80.
164. Yoder 1976, 240.
165. HDA I: 1160-1161
166. Yoder 2005, 221-222; Donmoyer 2012, 134-136.
167. Donmoyer 2012, 112.
168. Peterson 2008.
169. Author's translation of "A Veritable Tale" in Donmoyer 2012a, 136-138.
170. Fogel 1908 304-306.
171. Author's translation of undated Nürnberg MS. Heilman Collection.
172. Lea 1957, III: 1536-1537
173. Tetzner 1902, 346.
174. HDA I: 1163.
175. For a thorough assessment of the relation of the Christophell Thommass manuscript to the Northampton County line of practitioners Saylor and Wilhelm, see Heindel 2005.
176. Author's transcription and translation of Christophell Thommass & Jacob Wilhelm Manuscript, Williams Township Historical Society, 135.
177. For a detailed account of sources surrounding the life of Serenus Sammonicus, see: Champlin 1981, 189-212. For speculation about the linguistic origins of the phrase, see Ohrt 1922, 86-88; Budge 1961, 220-221; Bischoff 1903, 94-95, Buchholz 1956, 257-259.
178. Thommass & Wilhelm MS, author's transcription and translation, 131.
179. ibid, Author's transcription and translation 132.
180. ibid, Author's transcription and translation 136.
181. Seyfarth 1917, 21.
182. "Feibel" DWB, III: 1432.
183. Entry for "*Feifel*" in Leib 1842, 8-9.
184. "Strangles in Horses." 2002. Equinews. Lexington: Kentucky Equine Research.
185. Thommass & Wilhelm MS, author's transcription and translation, 137.
186. "Christoph David Thomas." *Germany, Select Births and Baptisms, 1558-1898* [Database online]. Provo, UT: Ancestry.com Operations, Inc. 2014; "Christoph David Thomas." *Wuerttemberg, Germany, Lutheran Baptisms, Marriages, and Burials, 1500-1985* [Database online]. Provo, UT: Ancestry.com Operations, Inc. 2016.
187. Heindel 2005, 101-104.
188. Fabian 1972, 2-14; Yoder 2016, 118-121.
189. Thommass & Wilhelm MS, author's transcription and translation, 170-171. See also: Heindel 2005, 103-104.
190. *Merkwürdige Dinger zugehörig an Johannes Stecher (Extraordinary Things, belonging to Johannes Stecher)* Transcribed by Edward Quinter, 2010. Translated by Patrick J. Donmoyer 2017. Pennsylvania German Cultural Heritage Center, Kutztown University.
191. Photograph of Johannes Stecher's tombstone from the Mary Abel Eyer Schuler Collection of Abel Family Papers and Artifacts, Pennsylvania German Cultural Heritage Center, Kutztown University.
192. Earnest, Earnest & Rosenberry 2005, 101-102.
193. Merrifield 1988, 142-144.
194. This spelling of the SATOR formula is atypical, although not uncommon in early Pennsylvania printed sources, such as *Kurzgefaßtes Weiber-Büchlein*, printed in 1799 by Meyer of York, and *Nützliches und sehr bewährt befundenes Weiber-Büchlein* printed at Ephrata in 1822. Spangenberg merely supplants the "T" in the first line with an "H."
195. KJV Rev 1:8
196. Fishwic 1964, 39-53.
197. Fennell 2010.
198. Donmoyer 2012, 88-91
199. Fishwick 1964, 50.
200. Robert Zoller, Scholar of Latin and Medieval astrology of Rosedale, New York, has kindly provided this insight into the dynamics of AREPO as two words within a larger poetic arrangement: A REPO (A REPA) – literally, "by the bank." Latin poetry, with heavy emphasis on rhyme and structure, is notorious for altering word endings or the gender of a word to conform to poetic arrangements, thus a feminine word is inflected with a masculine ending to complete the palindrome; see: Donmoyer 2012, 88-91. For a description of the complications of the structures of Latin poetry, see the detailed footnote on 182 in: Ellicott, Charles John. 1897. *An Old Testament Commentary for English Readers*. London: Cassell.
201. Pewter plate with SATOR Square Inscription. Plate by Thomas Compton, London, ca. 1800, inscription date unknown. Nancy & Abe Roan Collection, Schwenkfelder Library and Heritage Center, Pennsburg, PA.

Chapter IV. Healing, Cosmology & Ritual

1. For more discussion of the diverse ways to define ritual and its functions within broader systems of beliefs, see: Asad, Talal. 1997. *Genealogies of Religion: Discipline and Reasons of Power in Christianity and Islam*. Baltimore, MD: Johns Hopkins Univ. Press; Bell, Catherine M. 2010. *Ritual Theory, Ritual Practice*. New York: Oxford University Press; Geertz, Clifford. 2009. *The Interpretation of Cultures: selected essays*. New York: Basic Books.
2. HDA VIII:619-628; Erich, Oswald A. & Beitl, Richard. *Wörterbuch der deutschen Volkskunde*. Leipzig: Alfred Kroner Verlag, 1936, 699; Most, George Friedrich. *Die Sympathetischen Mittel und Curmethoden*. Rostock: Eberstein and Otto, 1842, 51.
3. To compare two different views of the ethnographer's role in systematizing diverse ritual practices within a specific culture, see: Kemp, P. *Healing Ritual; Studies in the Technique and Tradition of the Southern Slavs*. London: Faber and Faber limited, 1935, 12. Compare this with the introduction of Wilson 2004.
4. To see one author's categorization of powwow according to levels of complexity and the distribution of ritual features, see: Kriebel, David. 2007. *Powwowing Among the Pennsylvania Dutch: Traditional Medical Practice in the Modern World*. University Park, PA: Pennsylvania State University Press.
5. Reimensnyder 1982, 90.
6. Fogel 1995, 179; Donmoyer 2012, 81.
7. For a closer look at the subtle differentiations between conjuration, blessing, and prayer within the realm of European folk cultural expressions of healing, see: Hampp, Irmgard. 1961. *Beschwörung, Segen, und Gebet: Untersuchungen zum Zauberspruch aus dem Bereich der Volksheilkunde*. Stuttgart: Silberburg Verlag.
8. For one common written variation, see: Hohman 1820, 63.
9. Harms 2012, 86.
10. See Appendix II for the full text and translation of: Soli Deo Gloria, or The Secrets of Sympathy of Dr. Helfenstein, ca. 1820 [Sunbury, Northumberland Co.], 12. Heilman Collection.
11. KJV Romans 1:11.
12. Helfenstein, 35.
13. Helfenstein, 14.
14. Conrad Raber his Docter [sic] Book. Ca. 1800, Tulpehocken, Berks County, PA. Pennsylvania German Cultural Heritage Center. Two versions of this prayer can be found in Egyptian Secrets of Albertus Magnus.
15. Brendle & Unger 82;
16. Author's translation of MS. Raber, 11; compare with Grumbine 1905, 277. Raber says "*Back dich so wennig als du willst...*" (Bake thou as much as desired...), but compare with Grumbine's "*Buck dich...*" (depart thou...), asking the illness to abate.
17. *Kalendar-Bilder: Illustrationen aus schweizerischen Volkskalendern des 19. Jahrhunderts*. Basel, CH Schweizerisches: Museum für Volkskunde. 1978(79).
18. A fragment from an eighteenth century edition of Albertus Magnus' *Book of Aggregations*, 97. PA German Cultural Heritage Center, Kutztown University.
19. Massage plays a minor, but not infrequent role in the repertoire of some practitioners. For a Northampton example: "The Powwow Doctor. Hundreds visit Wilhelm when the Moon is Right." *Allentown Leader*, Mon, July 1, 1901, 2. For an account among the Volga Deitsch of the Dakotas, see: Kusler, Ruth Weil and Peggy Sailer O'Neil. 1998. *Tender Hands: Ruth's Story of Healing*. Fargo, ND: Germans from Russia Heritage Collection, North Dakota State University Libraries.
20. This term "blowing for burns" appears in Don Yoder's typed transcription of a late 18th-century English healing manuscript penned by Farrier George Brinton of Chester County ca. 1790, suggesting that this English idiom was already well established in early Pennsylvania, and the possibility that such rituals were likely to have been common to both English and German-speaking Pennsylvanians.
21. For Appalachian cures involving inhalation see: Wigginton, Eliot. 1972. *The Foxfire Book*. Garden City, NY: An Anchor Book: Bantam Doubleday Dell Pub, 357-358. For Pennsylvania cures involving blowing, see Chapter II: Laydom, Levi. 1859. Manuscript in the private collection of Gregory Wonder. A similar variation is found in Brendle & Unger 114.
22. KJV Acts 2:2.
23. Recollection of John Messer, Shartlesville, Berks County, 2012.
24. Recollection of Keith Brintzenhoff, near Topton, Berks County in the 1950s; compare with Brendle & Unger, 127.
25. Manuscript of Georg Henninger, 1775. Albany Township, Berks County. Heilman Collection.
26. Brendle & Unger 149.
27. From the papers of Nathan Fernsler Krall, Rexmont, Lebanon County, Ca. 1900.
28. Fogel 1995, 101.
29. Brendle & Unger 111: suggests that objects from the home carry the protective spirit of the home or "*Schutzgeist*."
30. Fogel 1995, 97; for other similar methods, see Donmoyer 2012, 81 & 85.
31. Brendle & Unger 65.
32. This story was related to me by a contact in Schaefferstown, Pennsylvania in 2012.
33. The "Three Things" ritual occurs in many forms, and I've recorded several variants in Berks County. See Chapter X.
34. Lutz, Gladys. 2014. *Folk Art Memories: The Folklife Illustrations of Gladys Lutz*. Kutztown, PA: Pennsylvania German Cultural Heritage Center, 114.
35. Fogel 1995, 14.
36. AM 1869 I: 25.
37. Fogel 1995, 29.
38. This important piece of folklore was documented by E. Reginald Good of Kitchener, Ontario among the Old Order Amish and some Mennonites in Canadian and Pennsylvanian populations. Personal correspondence, 2016.
39. For more on found and begged objects, see Chapter VIII; for begged nails, see Donmoyer 2012, 59; begged wood, AM 1869 II: 72.
40. "Powwower J. H. Wilhelm: The News in General" *The Shippensburg Chronicle*, Shippensburg, PA: Fri 18 Jun 1886, 2.
41. *Allentown Leader*, Mon July 1 1901.
42. See Chapter II.
43. See Chapter VII.
44. Fogel 1995, 164.
45. See recipe for plaster made under a lunar influence, recorded by Conrad Raber in Chapter VII.
46. Brendle & Unger 95.
47. Helfenstein Broadsides, 67.
48. Ensminger 2003, 13.
49. Story collected from former resident of Lenhartsville, Berks County,

2009.

50. Heindel, Ned D. 2009. *Hexenkopf: History, Healing, and Hexerei*. Easton, PA: Northampton County Historical & Genealogical Society.

51. Zentler, Conrad. 1793. *Amerikanische Stadt- und Land-Calendar*. Philadelphia, Pa. Conrad Zentler.

52. According to former Windsor Township Supervisor Ernest Heckman, the township was asked to officially name the road in the 1970s, which had formerly been a significant artery between Virginville and Hamburg yet had no other name than the local name of "*Hexebarrich*" in the dialect. The township decided upon the name "Witchcraft Road" after careful consideration of the Pennsylvania Dutch name.

53. Helfenstein Broadsides, 24.

54. See Chapter I.

55. KJV Mark 5:13

56. Yoder 2015, 327.

57. Frederick A. Weicksel Death Certificate 1948. *Pennsylvania State Death certificates, 1906–1963*. Series 11.90, Records of the Pennsylvania Department of Health, Record Group 11. Pennsylvania Historical and Museum Commission, Harrisburg, Pennsylvania.

58. Schreiber 1976, 12.

59. Donmoyer 2012, 93.

60. Yoder 1976, 244.

61. A present-day practitioner living near the border of Schuylkill and Carbon Counties subscribes to the notion that belief is necessary, but that the power of the divine knows no boundaries concerning the precise religion to which one adheres.

62. Yoder 1976, 244; Leib1841.

63. KJV Matthew 18:18

64. KJV Gen 3:14.

65. Arndt 1835.

66. Tillich 1951.

67. KJV Num 21:8

68. Yoder, Don. 1952. *Sophia Bailer Speaks*, Unpublished Transcripts II, 1952, 4.

69. KJV Mark 5:41

70. KJV Mark 7:34

71. Ingram 2007.

72. Deigendesch1837.

73. Helfenstein Broadsides, 4.

74. Yoder, Don. 1951. *Sophia Bailer Speaks*, Unpublished Transcripts I, 1951.

75. KJV Mark 1:21.

76. KJV John 11:43.

77. KJV Mark 1: 41.

78. KJV Mark 6:5.

79. KJV Mark 5:30.

80. KJV Matt 14:36.

81. KJV Acts 19:12.

82. KJV II Kings 5:11.

83. KJV Mark 7:31.

84. KJV John 9:6-7.

85. See Chapter III for more on the origins of this practice.

86. KJV John 8:1-11.

87. Christ is depicted writing words on the ground in two classic Bibles: The 1704 Merian folio Bible, printed at Frankfurt am Main, and in engravings by Julius Schnorr von Carolsfeld, featured in the popular Victorian German *Familien-Bibel* of A. J. Holman in Philadelphia, and in another Philadelphia publication of *Die Bibel in Bilder* by Ignatius Kohler, a copiously illustrated, bilingual picture Bible, with verses in English and German below each plate.

88. KJV Mark 10:51.

89. Helfenstein Broadsides, 17.

90. Helfenstein Broadsides, 7.

91. Helfenstein Broadsides, 6.

92. Donmoyer 2012, 64-65.

93. A rhyming cure for burns found tucked between the pages of a dual edition of Hohman and Helfenstein from Scheffer and Beck, 1853. Heilman Collection. This cure was also included in a broadside in English and German by William Woomer, entitled "*Für den Brand zu tödten*," and "To Cure Mortification and Burns."

94. Hohman 1820, 28.

95. MS. Peter Schlessmann 1816, Heilman Collection.

96. Helfenstein broadsides, 42-43.

97. Küffner 1866, 5-6.

98. Yoder 2005, 123-124.

99. Mennig, Georg. ca. 1840. *Pfarrer Mennigs Chur fürs wilde Feuer. Geschrieben von George Mennig*. Library Company of Philadelphia, Roughwood Collection.

100. ibid.

101. Harms 2012, 61.

102. Manuscript inside of Kutztown High School Note Book, ca. 1920, Kutztown Historical Society.

103. Harlacher & Weiser, Albertus Magnus II: 7.

104. NIV Lev 14:1-7

105. KJV Gen 38:28

106. KJV Jos 2:18-21

107. Jowett, J.H. 1920. *Christian Century*. Mar 25, XXXVII (13): 20-21: "There is nothing needed to perfect the work of Christ said the preacher There is no deficit no adverse balance in his account It is impossible to bring anything to Calvary and enrich it but a man can take up his own cross and surrender his own life and strength to the glorifying of the Cross Wherever we touch the life of Christ we touch the spirit of sacrifice .There is a red thread running through from end to end. Break it where you will you could find a crimson streak. In Christ's life there is an unfailing continuance of sacrificial passion. The apostles also had a crimson line running through their lives. Everywhere they went carrying the Evangel they carried their own sufferings. Can we find the crimson streak in the Church's life today?"

108. M'Clintock 1889, 739.

109. KJV Matt 14:36.

110. See Chapter III for the True Length of Chris, and see Wilson 2004,

112. This phrase is used by powwow & hoodoo practitioner Jack Montgomery, author of American Shamans; Journeys with Traditional Healers. 2009. Ithaca, NY: Busca Inc.

113. KJV I Kings 17:20-23)

114. KJV Matt 24:27.

115. KJV Ezek 43:2.

116. KJV Ezek 43:17.

117. A comment made by a practitioner from the border of Schuylkill and Carbon counties in 2006.

118. This perception described in the oral tradition is echoed by directions accompanying a snake bite prayer, contained in a Lehigh County manuscript, which describes in German that the motions of the hands must move always away from the heart, so as not to drive the poison inward.

119. Sophia Bailer was known to schedule appointments via the telephone, as well as to receive calls from those seeking assistance. In times of emergency no such easterly orientation was required. See Chapter II: Sophia Bailer.

220. While the word "trance" is not commonly associated with powwow

except in an academic sense, this is a term used by Lee R. Gandee, powwow doctor from the Dutch Fork, documented in the work of Montgomery 2005, 72-122; as well as in Gandee's 1971 autobiography, *Strange Experience: Autobiography of a Hexenmeister.*

221. Story from a Lebanon County contact who was powwowed between 2012 and 2013.

222. Kriebel 2009, 35.

223. Apprentice is by no means a formal term, but one that accurately describes any person who studies with a master, whether it be a carpenter, a painter, or a powwower.

224. Menstruation is a complicated factor for female practitioners, and perspectives are by no means unanimous. One female powwow practitioner I personally know confided to me that she had only once attempted to powwow while menstruating. Originally thinking that any taboo on the subject must have been a relic from a bygone era, and certainly not a rule made by women, she had powwowed for a client anyway. Afterwards, she described feeling ill and claimed that the temporary, residual feeling of her client's imbalance clung to her much longer than usual, producing an overall unpleasant encounter.

225. The word "secret" is used frequently, although historically it was most often used as a way to enhance salability in popular published works such as *Verschiedene Sympathetische und Geheime Kunst-Stücke* (*Various Sympathetic and Secret Ritual Arts*) or Helfenstein's *Secrets of Sympathy*. I do not know of any living practitioners who describe their work as a "secret." Although one could say that an element of "secrecy" surrounds aspects of the prayers used for healing, it is equally apropos to use the word "discretion." David Kriebel described a "widespread reticence to discuss powwowing" among people he asked while conducting ethnographic research. He attributed it to social factors (Kriebel 2009, 33). My experience has been that knowledgeable people are willing to speak about such matters, but only to those who are trusted or from within the same community, congregation, or family.

226. KJV Matt 6:5-6.

227. Grumbine 1905, 279. See Chapter II for a solo ritual for removing warts with the morning dew. Such rituals are also used for removing freckles or growths; see Chapter X.

228. Reimensnyder 49-50.

229. Oral History with Anabell Karnes, Lebanon, PA 2017.

230. Schreiber 1976, 12.

231. *Allentown Leader.* Allentown, PA. (Jul 1, 1901).

232. See the case of Dennis Rex in Chapter IX.

233. Fogel 1995, 239.

234. Ibid, 212; See also Chapter VIII.

235. Ibid, 131.

235. Ibid, 57.

236. Reimensnyder, 49.

237. Boyer 2007, 9.

238. See the chapter on folk medicine in Arends 2016.

239. KJV II Kings 5:16.

240. KJV II Kings 5:27.

241. KJV Matthew 10: 1, 7-9.

242. KJV Acts 8:18-20.

Chapter V: Ritual Literature

1. These three names refer to *Egyptian Secrets* of St. Albert the Great; *The Ladies Book of Midwifery* printed in York and Ephrata attributed to St. Albert the Great and Aristotle; *The True Spiritual Shield* attributed to Pope Leo X; and *The Sixth and Seventh Books of Moses.*

2. See discussion in Chapter III on the Merseberg Incantations of the 10th century.

3. Burgert 1992, Also Henninger's gravestone at Old Zion Lutheran Church in Grimsville, Berks County reads that he was "Born in 1737, in Germany, in Hatten, in Alsace."

4. A 1681 book under the same name was printed by a Samuel Mueller in Dresden, according to Holzmann, *Deutsches Anonymen-Lexicon*, in: Arndt & Eck 1989, 323.

5. Henninger, Johann Georg. 1775. *Arzneÿ Büchlein für Menschen und Vieh, gehört mir Georg Henninger, ANNO 1775*. Albany Township, Berks County. Manuscript, Heilman Collection.

6. See Chapter VIII for ritual objects, and Henninger's ritual knife.

7. Donmoyer 2012, 72-75.

8. KJV Ephesians 4:9

9. Shively, John. 1837. The property of John Shively his paper a cure for sick cows when they have the blood. Northampton County. Manuscript, Heilman Collection.

10. Shoemaker 1951, 1.

11. For the most recent and comprehensive assessment of the history and present state of the language, see: Louden 2015.

12. Donmoyer 2012, 78.

13. Kauffman, Johann. 1789. *Dieses Buch gehört mir Johann Kauffman.* Lancaster County. Manuscript, Private collection of Clarke Hess.

14. KJV Genesis 3:15

15. Author's deciphering & translation of Kauffman 1789.

16. Although this word has been translated in many ways, and even I used the phrase "Magical Formulae" in my translation of *The Friend in Need* (2012), This simple phrase does not translate easily into English while maintaining its original connotation in early German. While literally implying "formulae of the ritual arts," the modern German term has changed over time to mean "secrets," "stunts," "tricks," even "deceptions." See Donmoyer 2012a, 57.

17. From the introduction included in all variants of the *Kunst-Stücke*.

18. Printed by Carl Andreas Bruckman, 1805; Johann Ritter, 1812 & 1813; Heinrich B. Sage 1815.

19. Hohman, Johann George, *Der Freund in der Noth, oder Sympathetische Wissenschaft.* [Pennsylvania]: *Gedruckt für die Käufer*, (Printed for the buyer) 1826; American Antiquarian Society. Likely from the press of Friedrich Goeb at Schellsburg, based upon the typographical cover which is comparable to Daniel Ballmer's *Neue Recepte* 1826.

20. Zittle, Michael, Jr. 1845. *The Friend in Need.* Boonsboro, Md.: Josiah Knodle. Sole surviving copy in Boonsborough Museum of History, collection of Doug Bast. A self-published edition was released recently: Empedocles, Drogo. 2015. *Friend In Need: Sympathetic Knowledge.* CreateSpace Independent Publishing Platform(Amazon Books).

21. Donmoyer 2012, 79.

22. Ibid. 88-89

23. Yoder 2016, 135-136.

24. 1798. *Kurzgefasstes Weiber-Büchlein. Enthaelt Aristoteli und A. Magni Hebammen-Kunst.* Ephrata, PA: Benjamin Meyer.

25. KJV. Exodus 1:21

26. One copy in the collection of the Pennsylvania German Cultural Heritage Center features these recycled papers on the interior of the book's paper wraps, and another 1799 edition in the collection of the Library

27. Copy of the Remeli midwifery book is in the Harvard College Library. George Remeli (1751–1827) died in Heidelburg Twp., Northampton Co., Pa. (present day Lehigh); married Maria Magdalena Kocher, son Heinrich Remeli. Henry Remeli is buried at the Salem Union Church, Moorestown, Northampton Co., PA., 10 Jul 1777 and died 24 Apr 1836.

28. A will in the Lehigh County Courthouse, for Georg Remelÿ of Heidelberg Township, Lehigh County on July 23, 1827, co-signed by Adam Gilbert and Henry Leh, bears the signature of Georg Remeli [sic] and the writing is identical to that in the midwifery manual.

29. Inscription found inside the fly leaves of an 1827 copy of Daniel Ballmer's New Receipts, printed by Friedrick Goeb at Schellsburg.

30. Albertus Magnus' bewährte und approbirte sympathetische und natürliche Egyptische Geheimnisse. Allentown: Harlacher and Weiser, 1869, 1:5.

31. Harms 2012, 18, and HDA 242-243. Peuckert also suggests the text is from the nineteenth-century, see: Peuckert 1954, 40-96.

32. Peuckert 1954, 40-44.

33. AM Radde 1:18.

34. AM Radde 2:12, Author's translation

35. AM Radde 2:68.

36. AM Radde 2:16, Author's translation

37. AM Radde 2:5, Author's translation

38. English edition of *Egyptian Secrets*, Egyptian Publishing co., circa 1910, iv-vi.

39. For more discussion of the confusion surrounding the term "Gypsy," see: Peterson 2008.

40. Based on a copy in the Heilman Collection; also available in numerous online formats.

41. Author's translation, from Helfenstein Broadsides, 4-5.

42. Only two copies are known to exist, both of which were located by Dr. Don Yoder. One presently resides at Winterthur, and another in the Heilman Collection.

43. Good, 1899; Good, James I. & William John Hinke, and John Philip Boehm. 1903.

44. Miller 1906.

45. Beissel, William I. 1938. *Secrets of Sympathy*. Klingerstown, PA: William Beissel; Bohr, Nicholas. 1901. *Secrets of Sympathy*. Shamokin, Pa.; Press of E[lmer]. E. Scott. Elmer E. Scott (1862-1909) appears in the 1880 US Census as a printer's apprentice in Shamokin, and is buried at the Shamokin Cemetery. His death certificate locates him at 701 N. Liberty Street, Shamokin, according to the Common Wealth of PA Vital Statistics Certificate # 77444, 1909).

46. "Ebenezer, masc. proper name, from Hebrew '*ebhen ezar*' - 'stone of help,' from *ebhen* 'stone' + *ezer* 'help.' Sometimes also the name of a Protestant chapel or meeting house, from name of a stone raised by Samuel to commemorate a divinely aided victory over the Philistines at Mizpeh (I Samuel vii.12)." Harper 2017.

47. Helfenstein broadsides, 69.

48. Ibid, 44.

49. KJV Mark 5:25-34

50. Helfenstein broadsides, 43.

51. Ibid, 15-16.

52. Ibid, 27-28.

53. Ibid, 58.

54. Ibid, 41.

55. Ibid, 42

56. Ibid, 30.

57. Heindel 2005.

58. KJV: Mark 11:22-23.

59. KJV: Mark 11:14, 20.

60. See Chapter VIII: The Iron Horseshoe

61. See Chapter VI: Borrowing, Lending, and the Witch Bottle

62. See Chapter III, pg 90.

63. Helfenstein broadsides, 48.

64. Donmoyer 2012, 54.

65. AM 1869 1:57.

66. Donmoyer 2012, 54.

67. Yoder, 1976, 97.

68. Helfenstein broadsides, 64.

69. Ibid, 65.

70. Yoder, 2015, 161, 164

71. KJV Matt 16:19

72. See Peter Paul Rubens' *Descent from the Cross*, 1612-1614, Cathedral of Our Lady, Antwerp, Belgium.

73. KJV Galatians 4

74. Helfenstein broadsides, 68

75. KJV Phil 4:1

76. I Thes 2:19

77. Helfenstein broadsides, 69.

78. For the most recent, complete edition of Hohman's Long Lost Friend, see: Hohman, Johann Georg, and Daniel Harms. 2012. *The Long-Lost Friend: A nineteenth Century American Grimoire.* Woodbury, MN: Llewellyn Publications. In all cases where the standard 1850 edition in German from Harrisburg is used, I have cited Harms 2012. In other cases, where English is provided that appears different from the Harrisburg edition (1850) provided by Harms, I have provided a new translation, noted accordingly from the 1820 edition.

79. Yoder, 1976, 244.

80. A story related to me by Dr. Don Yoder in 2012 confirmed that Alfred Shoemaker had been aware of a copy of Hohman that had been discovered in the Philippines, likely having been brought there by a Mennonite missionary.

81. Strassburger & Hinke 1992, 120-121.

82. Ibid,

83. Dell, Eugene. Date unknown. "John George Hohman." Unpublished paper, 7-8. This portion of Hohman's story was discovered by Eugene Dell, citing the work of Marion Dexter Learned, who found reference to a Hohman and Krick who left Halberstadt for America. The document bore the date of 1802, but this date was not related to the date of departure. Johann Friedrich Hohmann and Friedrich Krich arrived on the same boat in 1800, corroborating the Halberstadt document. Don Yoder had a copy of Dell's unpublished paper on Hohman, but the title page was lost. Yoder's copy of this paper was in the form of photographs from the Pennsylvania Folklife Society Archives, which were greatly purged in 1961-1962, due to the Society's bankruptcy. The whereabouts of Eugene Dell's paper is unknown.

84. Harms 2012, 5-6.

85. Wellenreuther 2013, 72, 286.

86. Hohman regularly began passages with "I Hohman…" See: Harms 2012, 41.

87. Bötte, Tannhof, Arndt, & Eck 1989.

88. Oda, Wilbur H. 1948. "John George Hohman." *The Historical Review of Berks County.* Reading, Historical Society of Berks County, XIII (3): 67.

89. Donmoyer 2012, 18

90. Ibid, 16.

91. Hagan, Chet. 1994. *Berks Authors Collection*, Friends of the Reading-Berks Public Libraries. I: 12.

92. Donmoyer 2012, 14.

93. Hohman, Johann Georg. 1818. *Die Land- und Haus-Apotheke, oder, Getreuer und gründlicher Unterricht für den Bauer und Stadtmann.* Reading, PA: Carl Andreas Bruckman, Introduction, i.

94. Ibid, 7. While not all carrots are yellow, in Pennsylvania Dutch, the word is *Gehl-Riewe*, literally meaning "yellow turnip." Historically, many heirloom varieties of carrots were yellow, and not orange like today.

95. Ibid, 41.

96. Ibid, 22; Also in Eugene Dell, op cit., 10.

97. This book can be found in the Pennsylvania Folklife Society Archive at Ursinus College Myrin Library. The first part of this book is missing, but portions of it have been reproduced and translated in The Friend in Need (2012), edited by Patrick Donmoyer.

98. Hohman, Johann Georg. 1819. Der kleine Catholische Catechismus : oder kurzgefasste nothwendige Glaubens-Fragen, welches absonderlich ein Catholischer Christ wissen und glauben soll. Nebst einem kleinen Anhang Einiger nothwendiger Gebeter. Zum erstenmal in dieser Form herausgegeben / von Johann George Homan, nahe bey Reading, in Berks Caunty. Mit erlaubnis Geistlicher Obrigkeit. Reading, PA: Carl A. Bruckman.

99. The biblical story of Nicodemus can be found in John 3:1.

100. Yoder 2016, 134-143.

101. Hohman 1819, 85-86.

102. *Der Wahre Geistliche Schild*, Maynz, 1647, 64-68.

103. Yoder, 1976, 244.

104. Ibid, 238.

105. The only known copy of this rare edition of *Das vortreffliche Zigeuner-Büchlein* is at the Library Company of Philadelphia, attributed to the press of Heinrich B. Sage of Reading, Pennsylvania, ca. 1810. The subtitle matches European imprints of the Romanus-Büchlein, bearing the false imprint of "*Venedig: Gott der Herr bewahre meine Seele, meinen Aus- uud [sic] Eingang; vor nun an bis in alle Ewigkeit, Amen. Halleluja.*" See also, Spamer & Nickel 1958, 26.

106. See Chapter III for more on the identity of *Romanus*.

107. Harms 2012, 19.

108. English translated text from the Harrisburg edition of 1850, in: Harms 2012, 44.

109. Hohman 1820, 9.

110. Harms 2012, 43

111. Ibid, 44.

112. Ibid, 40.

113. Ibid, 39; Donmoyer 2012, 34.

114. Ibid, 41.

115. Hohman 1820, Introduction 6; author's translation.

116. Oda 1948, 67.

117. Located on page 90 of the original edition.

118. Hohman 1820, 89.

119. Harms 2012, 277-278, cites: *Juvenal and Persius*. With an English Translation by G.G. Ramsay (Cambridge: Harvard University Press, 1965), 361.

120. Hohman 1820, 23, 38, echoed in Helfenstein broadsides, 64.

121. Hohman, Johann Georg. 1840. *Der Lang Verborgene Freund, oder Getreuer Unterricht für Jedermann…* Harrisburg, PA. [no publisher], 27, and the English in quotes from the 1850 Harrisburg edition.

122. Author's translation (A.t.) of Hohman 1820, 35.

123. Ibid, 50. A.t.

124. Ibid, 50. A.t.

125. Ibid, 15. A.t.

126. Ibid, 72. A.t.

127. Ibid, 14, 93. A.t.

128. Ibid, 20-21. A.t.

129. Ibid, 50-51. A.t.

130. Ibid, 54. A.t.

131. Ibid, 36-37. A.t.

132. Quitman 1810, 8.

133. Patterson 1835. II(26 New Series).

134. Literally, flow-herb, *Plumbago L.* See: "*Flöhkraut,*" Adelung II: 216.

135. Don Yoder hand-typed transcription of Manuscript Account Book, 1831 ff., of *Frederick Sheeder, Jr., Stage Driver from Kimberton to Morgantown along the Philadelphia & Lancaster Mail Stage*, 1831.

136. "Magic Healing," *Reading Eagle*. Reading, PA. (July 24, 1895).

137. Other sources suggest that Maria Margaretha Croll, wife of Pvt. Michael Croll (1762-1822) may be buried with her husband in New Bethel Zion Church in Grimsville, Berks County, however her stone is located at St. John's Hamburg.

138. Chelule, Mokgatle, Zungu, & Chaponda 2014, 54–60.

139. Croll, M. Margaretha. 1826. *Eine Sammlung Auserlesener Rezepte heilsamer Mittel bey krankheiten der Menschen und des Vieh zu gebrauchen.* Reading, PA: Heinrich B. Sage, 3, 16, 17.

140. Ibid, 18.

141. See: Grimm's DWB: "*katzenspur*" XI: 301- 302: "*Fuszspur einer katze; in der Wetterau sagt man von einem der an der fuszsohle einen schwären hat, er habe in eine katzenspur getreten.*"

142. Croll 1826, 4.

143. Ibid, 17; Author's translation.

144. Ibid, 18.

145. See Chapter IV: Sympathy.

146. Croll 1826, 14.

147. PfWB: I: 953 -955.

148. See Chapter 3, and Hovorka & Kronfeld II: 406.

149. Croll 1826, 19; Author's translation.

150. See: Philadelphia Free Library: Birth and Baptismal Certificate (*Geburts und Taufschein*) for [blank] Heulein (No: frk01254); Birth and Baptismal Certificate (*Geburts und Taufschein*) for Aaron Will (No. frk01144); and Birth and Baptismal Certificate (*Geburts und Taufschein*) for Maria Anna Neukommer (No: frk01164).

151. See Chapter II: Levi Laydom, Adams County.

152. Ballmer, Daniel 1827. *Eine Sammlung von Neuen Recepten und Bewährten Curen für Menschen und Vieh.* Schellsburg, PA: Friedrich Goeb, 17-18.

153. Diary of James L. Morris, Episcopalian storekeeper of Morgantown, Berks County (1837-1844) Yoder original transcription, later republished in *Pennsylvania Dutchman*, March 1, 1953, IV(13): 14.

154. Ballmer, Daniel. 1827. *A Collection of New Receipts and Approved Cures for Man and Beast.* Shellsburg, PA: Frederick Goeb.

155. PfWB: "Neu-licht" V: 130 - 131; Lambert 1977, 12, in PfWB: "Alt-licht," I: 190.

156. Ballmer 1827, 31, 24.

157. Fogel 1995, 155.

158. Ballmer [English]1827, 24.

159. Both of Paul Bolmer's later editions can be found in the Pennsylvania Folklife Society Archive, Myrin Library, Ursinus College.

160. Ballmer [English] 1827, 13, 21-22.

161. Hohman, Johann Georg. 1837. *Der lange Verborgene Schatz und Haus-Freund.* Skippacksville, PA: A. Puwelle.

162. Hohman 1820, 28. Elsewhere, Hohman does cite a cure for rabies by the name of a man named Valentine Kettring of Dauphin County. See Harms 19.

163. Hohman 1837, 4.

164. George Allen Collection, Library Company of Philadelphia: Hohman, Johann Georg. 1840. *Der lange verborgene Freund: oder getreuer und christlicher Unterricht für Jedermann, enthaltend: wunderbare und probmässige Mittel und Künste sowohl für Menschen als Vieh. … Herausgegeben von Johann George Homan … Dritte durchaus verbesserte Auflage.* [Reading]: *Gedruckt in diesem Jahre.*

165. Hohman, John. G. 1846. *The Long Secreted Friend, or a True and Christian Information for Every Body; Containing Wonderful and Approved Remedies and Arts for Men and Beast*. Harrisburg, PA: n.p.

166. Ibid. A copy with this fine cloth binding and stamped leather plate is at the Library Company of Philadelphia.

167. Ibid, 47.

168. This Harrisburg edition was used by Daniel Harms to prepare his newly edited and complete edition in 2012.

169. The social movements towards English-only education and other institutions are discussed in: Donner, William. 2017. "Education." *Pennsylvania Germans: An Interpretive Encyclopedia*. Edited by Simon J. Bronner, and Joshua R. Brown. Baltimore, MD.: Johns Hopkins Press, 397; and Louden 2015.

170. Earnest & Earnest 2005, 228.

171. Kelker 1907, 351-352.

172. KJV Mark 11: 22 & 24

173. Hohman, Johann Georg. 1853. *Der lang verborgene Freund : enthaltend wunderbare und probmässige Mittel und Künste, für die Menschen und Vieh, Herausgegeben von Johann Georg Hohman. Demselben is beigefügt Dr. G. F. Helfenstein's vielfältig erprobter Hauschatz der Sympathie*. Harrisburg, PA: Scheffer und Beck.

174. See Chapter III.

175. Quinter & Donmoyer 2012.

176. For Hohman's Nockamixon advertisement, see: Donmoyer 2012, 14; Hohman's 1811 Easton broadsides, see: Yoder 2005, 212.

177. I had the opportunity to examine this manuscript when it was offered for sale through M & S Rare Books, Inc. Providence, RI, confirming that it was indeed a pre-Hohman copy of Romanus, penned in the United States. Church records of Christ Lutheran, Upper Mouth Bethel supply information about a Tobias Schick born 17 April 1782 in Springfield, Bucks County, baptized 24 Apr 1802; and Tobias Schick, corporal in War of 1812, 71 Regiment (Hutter's) Pennsylvania Militia.

178. Beers, J. H. 1914. *Armstrong County, Pennsylvania; Her People, Past and Present: Embracing a History of the County and a Genealogical and Biographical of Representative Families*. Chicago, Illinois, J.H. Beers & Co, 287.

179. Prützmann, Daniel. 1855. *Die Wunder der Sympathie, zum zwecke für Heilungen an menschen, thieren, und pflanzen von Hein. Hassendang*. Canton, Oh.: John Saxton un Sohn. Heilman Collection. Prützmann is listed in the 1881 city directory for Canton Ohio (Canton News Co. 1881), and is buried at Loudonville, Ashland County, Ohio. John Saxon is the grandfather of President William McKinley's wife, Ida Saxton McKinley; see: Lehman 1916, 395.

180. Cazden 1975, 57-77: "Father Henni lashed out at Boffinger in no uncertain terms for publishing this "abomination" in the first place, let alone for being so cowardly as to publish it anonymously. "We leave it to the public," he wrote, "to judge what to think of such a man who, even if short of cash, degrades his press-which should be devoted only to education, and for which the truth should be sacred-by disseminating lies and superstition among simple creatures."

181. Yoder, 2016, 28-29. The Erie imprint appears to be modeled closely after the work of Ensslin in Reutlingen, distributed by Radde in New York.

182. The imprint is unlikely to be genuine, because of its over-corrective statement "in Austria" – no European imprint would need to specify where Vienna is located. The work is signed with the name Georg Henninger, and was connected with his father's 1775 manuscript.

183. Reading imprint bearing the name Louis Ensslin, from Reutlingen, Germany, Heilman Collection.

184. National Park Service. U.S. Civil War Soldiers, 1861-1865 [database on-line]. Provo, UT, USA: Ancestry.com Operations Inc, 2007, M554 roll 117; Isaac D. Steel is buried at Calvary United Methodist Cemetery, Wiconisco, Dauphin County.

185. Ossman & Steel. 1894. Ossman & Steel's *Guide to Health or Household Instructor*. Wiconisco, PA: Ossman & Steel. Page 83 attributes a remedy to Mr. Steel for closing an ulcer with condensed carpenter's glue, following his return from military service; And again, 87: another remedy attributed to "one of the authors" consists of a method for drying wounds with ash from burned shoe-leather.

186. Romberger, Gene and Capitol Area Genealogical Society. 2002. *Selected Dauphin County Pennsylvania Death Records*. Apollo, PA: Closson Press, 293.

187. A current resident of Lykens, known to the author, collects imprints from local estate and farm sales, and has found multiple copies of Hohman's *Der Freund in der Noth* (1813) in the Lykens Valley and the surrounding region.

188. Introduction to Ossman & Steel, 17-19.

189. Ibid, 28; and 51, 79, 99.

190. Ibid, 77-78.

191. Ibid, 88; Lambert 1977, "horse-kimmel" a hybrid English and Pennsylvania Dutch word for – Jimsonweed, *stramonium datura*, 22. This entry, like several others, has corrections in pencil, inserting the word "horse" before "kimmel." Elsewhere in the text are several other corrections, such as "urine" written over "wine." It is possible, that since Ossman & Steel's Guide was locally distributed by mail order, that these corrections were at the suggestions of the author. Two editions owned by the author have the same corrections in identical handwriting.

192. Ibid, 82.

193. Ibid, 70, 69, 92, 74.

194. Ibid, 94.

195. Yoder, Don. ca. 1960. "Gallows Lore," Signs of Folklife Themes at the Kutztown Folk Festival, signs hand-painted by Emmaus commercial painter William Schuster: "In eighteenth century Pennsylvania, public hangings were festive occasions. As they did throughout the country, these events attracted hugh[sic] crowds. Every county seat had it's 'Gallows Hill.' The PA Dutch expression *Ar hut dar Shitvvel[sic] Dons-ga-doo*, [*Er hot der Schtiwwel-Danz geduh*] means "He danced the boot dance." After the hanging, everyone wanted a piece of the rope, which was believed to have great powers. One inch lengths were sold for a high price. The PA. Dutch believed that if this rope were worn around the neck, it would prevent epileptic seizures. Another belief was that if a piece of rope were inserted into whipstocks, the horses would be easier to break."

196. Ibid, 83.

197. Ibid, 68-69.

198. Ibid, 50.

199. Ibid, 45.

200. Ibid, 40-41; compare with Chapter I: Of Warts and Waning.

201. Ibid, 53.

202. See: Chapter I: Learning to Powwow; compare with Esther Heilman's cure.

203. Ibid, 54.

204. Ibid, 48.

205. Ibid, 26.

206. Ibid, 65.

207. Ibid, 32.

208. Bohr's contents include entries present in the Helfenstein broadsides that are not present in Scheffer & Beck's Harrisburg edition, suggesting that Bohr owned the original edition and did not base it on Scheffer & Beck's. Nicholas R. Bohr 18 S. Market St, Shamokin in 1901, in: Boyd, William H. 1901. *Boyd's Directory of Shamokin: Containing the Names of the Citizens, Compendium of the Government, and of Public and Private Institutions... Together with a Classified Business Directory, and Alphabetical Business Directories of Locust Gap, Mt. Carmel, Northumberland, Sunbury and Trevorton...* Shamokin, PA: William H. Boyd, 60; Listed as Bar tender in 1900 US Federal Census at the same address; Died Oct 17, 1901 in

Shamokin, from Asthma, aged 48 years, 3 months, 18 days, in: Eveland, Tracy & David Donmoyer. 2011. *Shamokin Cemetery Company Burial Records, Northumberland, PA*; Baptismal records list a Nichlaus Bohr, baptized on 29 Jun 1852, in Detzem, Germany, son of Nicolai Borh & Barbara Kollmann, in: *Germany, Births and Baptisms, 1558-1898*. Salt Lake City, Utah: FamilySearch, 2013; Another Nicholas Bohr (1879-1950), second-generation immigrant born in Schuylkill County, farmed in Shamokin, and appears on the census beginning in 1920, but is an unlikely fit for the publication.

209. Listed in Shoemaker, Alfred. Pennsylvania Folklife Society Card Catalog entry "Powwow": "*Secrets of Sympathy*, Newly Published and Improved by Wm. C. Kline. Shamokin, Pa. Press of Shamokin Daily News. 1928."

210. Beissel, William in Commonwealth of Pennsylvania Death Certificates: No. 34741; US Federal Census 1940 shows William Beissel living in Coal Township, just outside of Shamokin, and lists his native language as [Pennsylvania] "Dutch."

211. Beissel, William. 1938. *Secrets of Sympathy*. Klingerstown, PA: William Beissel, 2-4.

212. Advertisement for the Louis de Claremont edition of Hohman's *Long Lost Friend*, featured in the Pittsburgh Courier, April 29, 1939.

213. A copy of this edition is in the collection of the Pennsylvania German Cultural Heritage Center, Kutztown University, and is possibly the earliest edition to use the term "Powwows" in the title. See also: Harms 2012, 22.

214. Rix, Alice. "The Reading Witch Doctor's Sway Over the Trusting and the Ignorant." *North American*. Philadelphia, PA: (May, 22, 1900):16; Brubaker, Henry C. "Witch Murderer Under Suspicion in Girl's Slaying." *Philadelphia Inquirer*. Philadelphia, PA.(Dec 2, 1928).

215. Interest in the murder case was largely due to the classic journalistic account by Philadelphia author Arthur Lewis in *Hex* (New York: Trident Press, 1969), and later revisited, see: McGinnis, J. Ross. 2000. *Trials of Hex*. Davis/Trinity Co. McGinnis' work recently served as the basis for a feature-length independent motion picture called Hex Hollow (2016). See Chapter IX for an overview of the Rehmeyer murder.

216. My paternal grandmother warned me of this book's ill effects when I informed her of my research in 2009 and she asked me "aren't you afraid of being read fast?"

217. Bachter, Stephan. 2005. "Anleitung zum Aberglauben: Zauberbücher und die Verbreitung magischen „Wissens" seit dem 18. Jahrhundert" Dissertation in fulfillment of doctorate in philosophy, University of Hamburg.

218. Scheible, Johann. 1849. *Das 6te und 7te Buch Moses. Bibliothek der Zauber-Geheimniss- und Offenbarungs-Bücher, und der Wunder-Hausschatz-Literatur aller Nationen in allen ihren Raritäten und Kuriositäten*. Vol. VI. Stuttgart: Johann Scheibel. Unbound edition in Heilman Collection. See also: Peterson 2009.

219. Receipt from Christoph Pierson 1872 for two copies of "Books of Moses" from Wm. Radde, New York. A list of publications can be found on the back of the receipt.

220. *Das 6te und 7te Buch Moses*. Weissensee nahe Berlin: E. Bartels, .ca. 1900. Edition with red and black paper seals of the skull and crossed bones, Heilman Collection.

221. *Das Achte und Neunte Buch Moses*. Weissensee nahe Berlin: E. Bartels. ca. 1900. Edition with black wax seals of the skull and crossed bones, along with the rod of Asclepos, Heilman Collection.

222. *Verbrannte und Verbannte; Die Liste der in Nationalsozialismus verbotenen Publikationen und Autoren*. <http://verbrannte-und-verbannte.de/list/4069>

223. Berks County account in Oley, PA, of a friend whose grandfather's powwow books were all burned, including a copy of *The Sixth and Seventh Books of Moses*, following his death in the 1970s.

Chapter VI: Hexerei and Ritual Harm

1. Brendle & Unger 136-137: defines Hex as: "A person who works evil through an alliance with the devil, or who casts spells by means of a book or otherwise." See also, Beam, C. Richard, Josh Brown & Jennifer L. Trout. 2004-2006. "*Hexerei*," "*Hex*," "*Hexedoktor*." *Pennsylvania German Dictionary*. Millersville, PA: Center for Pennsylvania German Studies, IV: 87-90.Beam's dictionary citations run the gamut from folklorists to popular humorists – with no context for readers to determine the tone of the writer's use of the word. While some of his entries equate Hexerei with satanic practices (a view held by religiously conservative portions of the population), others discuss belief or disbelief in witchcraft, while still others are from humorous editorials from the late nineteenth and early twentieth century dialect writers, such as Boonestiel (T.H. Harter), who ridicule belief in witches. There are several entries that directly discuss the notion of Hexerei as relating to malice ("*Hex*"), abuse ("*Hexe*"), and violence ("*Hexegluppe*," "*Hexeschuss*"), but this connotation is not communicated throughout. Beam's use of the negative word "bewitch" is perhaps not strong enough to evoke the same emotions to new generations. In X: 61, in the entry "*verhext*" Beam equates "bewitched" with "cursed." It is unusual that the word "curse" would be avoided throughout the entries pertaining to the concept of a "*Hex*" – as it is the most precise meaning in common parlance. Scholars of witchcraft, have likewise pointed to the historical use of the word *Hexerei* as implying malice, as opposed to ceremonial uses of magic. See Levack 2014, 4.

2. Yoder 2015, 98.

3. Beam IV: 87-90; X: 61.

4. *Minutes of the Provincial Council of Pennsylvania*. 93, 94-96.

5. Shivley 1953, 9. The US census 1880 corroborates the proximity of people featured in Shively's story in Millmont, where Elizabeth Heilman appears on the census.

6. Hartman 1949, 2.

7. "Where Witches Flourish in this Twentieth Century: New York Woman Haled to Court as a Magician in Allentown." New York Times (1857-1922); Sep 10, 1911; ProQuest Historical Newspapers: The New York Times, pg. SM3.

8. Adams, Charles J., III. 2017. "Pennsylvania Dutch farmers feared the 'Thaustreicher.'" *Reading Eagle*. Wed May 3; Wakeman, Edgar L. 1887. "Pennsylvania Dutch: The Folk-Lore and Superstitions Prevalent In Our State." *Philadelphia Times*. Sun June 12, 1887, 11.

9. For the Altmark tradition, see: Grimm, *Teutonic Mythology* II: 786-787.

10. See Chapter VII: *Allermansharnisch-Wurzel* and Ramps

11. Donmoyer 2013:87

12. Ibid. 87.

13. Shoemaker 1955, IV(18):1-3.

14. A coffin-shaped blessing features the same progression of stars, crosses, and abbreviations, including "J.N.R.J." Heilman Collection.

15. Donmoyer 2013, 87-89.

16. Hohman 1850, 37.

17. Mahr 1935, 215–225.

18. Hufford 1976, 73–85.

19. Hohman 1850, 37.

20. Grimm & Grimm DWB: "*Trude*" XXII: 1233

21. AM Radde, 5.
22. DWB "*Trudenfusz*" XXII: 1240.
23. "*Groddefuss*" and "*Gensefuss*" in Fogel, 92; discussion of "*Hexefuss*" in Henry Chapman Mercer Collection, Archaeological Research Notes. Folder 17. Madrid, Delaware Valley, Yucatan Field notes. Including notes for Tamanend article, draft of Lehigh Hills papers for magazine, sunbonnets, Powwow formulae, Macungie notes -FH 150]. 1863-1930.
24. Fogel 1995, 92.
25. Weaver 1993, 106. Photo of Hubbard Squash found by Ivan Glick and William Woys Weaver at a Lancaster County farmstand. The Amish grower of the squash, according to Weaver was eager to be rid of the squash, because he believed it portended an evil omen. While this story is by no means representative of the Old Order Amish as a whole, it confirms that the idea of a "*Hexefuuss*" was still alive and well at the end of the twentieth century.
26. DWB indicates that *Trudenfusz, Alpfusz* and other variations of the same idea are not only a ritual marking, but also the footprint of a demon or spirit.
27. See Chapter III.
28. Nutting 1924, 4. Nutting warns that his book is pictorial, and not intended to be a scholarly survey of Pennsylvania culture and architecture: "… nor is this volume at all a work of history or a story of Eastern Pennsylvania. It is a book of pictures primarily and principally. Any observations regarding these pictures are made as there may seem to be a necessity for them, or as the incidents of travel urge them…")
29. For information on the origin of Nutting's story, see discussion of W. Ellison Farrell's notes about the informant from Bethlehem. According to Graves, the notes have subsequently disappeared. See: Graves 1985.
30. Nutting 1924, 28.
31. Donmoyer 2013.
32. Graves 1985, 49-52.
33. See "Milton Hill" in Donmoyer 2013.
34. In the summer of 2008, I surveyed over 500 decorated barns in Berks with the intent to document evidence of ritual traditions associated with the protection of the barn by means of powwowing, and to determine what relation these traditions had with artistic traditions in the past and present. Although there were many differing and sometimes contradictory opinions about the relation of powwowing and hex signs, all of these stories were second-hand, and demonstrated a fundamental lack of understanding of both the art and the nature of powwowing. Only one particular story was first-hand: Eric Claypoole and his Father Johnny Claypoole (1921-2004) were both asked at different times to paint a barn star over a prayer written on the surface of the barn siding in pencil. The Claypooles however, were not powwowers, but artists cooperating with the wishes of barn owners. The author has also painted two stars in a similar manner over hand-written prayers on a barn in Lower Macungie in 2016.
35. Cowen, Dick. 1962. "Johnny Ott: A showman of deep religious faith." The Morning Call. Allentown, Pa. July 31 1964.
36. Donmoyer, Barn Star Archive (2008-2017): Examples in Alsace (1), Brecknock (2), Center (1), Hereford (2), Oley (1), Robeson (3). Instances of this pattern are exceedingly rare, while starts of eight, twelve, and six points are found in the hundreds throughout the region.
37. Donmoyer 2013.
38. Discussion of house blessing stones with John Baer Stoudt in "Odd Phase of Pennsylvania History of 131 Years Ago." Reading Eagle, Sept 14, 1930, 4. Cites the stone's location in "Worcester Township, deciphered in 1904" - likely by Stoudt himself.
39. AM Radde I:20, 60; II:29-30; Fogel 1995, 117; AM Radde II:79
40. Author's translation of Börstler, Georg. ca. 1795. Folio manuscript, Heilman Collection.
41. Everhart 1868, 12-14.
42. Gravestone in Buffalo Valley Church of the Brethren: "Elizabeth Wife of Frederick W. Heilman Died June 23. 1897 Aged 77 years."

43. 1950. "Witchcraft in York County: Strange Doings." *The Pennsylvania Dutchman*. II(9): 3; Chrastina, Paul. County Notebook: York Believe it or not, Part 20. Mon Oct 31, 1994, *York Dispatch*.
44. Possibly Henry G. Gusler (1808-1881) a horse farrier from Monaghan, York County, buried at Fileys Christ Lutheran Church Cemetery, Dillsburg, and listed in 1880 US Federal Census as the husband of Mary Gusler in Siddonsburg.
45. The Couple is likely to be Amanda Nestor Nesbit (1851-1884), buried in Fileys Christ Lutheran Church Cemetery, Dillsburg, York County, and Civil War veteran Joseph B. Nesbit (1843-1916) buried in Paxtang Cemetery, Dauphin County, who are listed in the 1870 US Federal Census as tenants living next door to William Speck. Speck is listed as living in very close proximity to two properties of a W. Ross, (where the couple is likely to have rented, according to the original account in the *Lebanon Courier*) on the Map of York County, Pennsylvania, 1860, by W. O. Shearer & D. J. Lake, Publishers, 517, 519, & 521 Minor Street, Philadelphia, 1860. In 1880, following the incident, the couple relocated to Upper Allen, Cumberland County, where they are listed as having three children: Ellsworth (age 10), Annie (8), and Sara (6). Sara was likely the infant in the crib featured in the 1875 incident.
46. Cresswell 1957.
47. 2016 Discussion with contact in the Gehris Family, Bowers, Pa., who described the family fallout because of the article on Aunt Sybilla.
48. Lea 1957, III: 1056
49. Mackay & Kramer 2014.
50. See Chapter III.
51. Discussion with Anonymous Berks County Powwow Practitioner 2008.
52. Discussion with Anonymous Berks County contact from the greater Reading area, 2012.
53. Discussion with Anonymous contact, Macadoo, 2016.
54. See "*ligaturae*" in: Lea 1957, III: 1066.
55. Humenick, Martha Jane Edward. *Descendants of Henry Fronk*: unpublished papers from the Cambria County Historical Society.
56. Nelson, Barry. 1984. "Pow-Wows and Faith Healers in the Mifflin Area." Governer Mifflin Area History. 4:1 April 1984. Mohnton, PA: Governer Mifflin Historical Society, 12.
57. Yoder 1951, 8-9.; Yoder 1952, 2; Don Yoder 1964.
58. Bailer, Sophia. 1952, 8.
59. Yoder 1951, 2
60. Merrifield 163-175.
61. Ibid.
62. Mather, Cotton. 1689. *Late Memorable Providences Relating to Witchcrafts and Possessions.* Boston: R. P. & Sold by Joseph Brunning; see also similar the works of his father, Increase Mather from 1684: *Remarkable Providences Illustrative of the Earlier Days of American Colonisation.* Reprinted by Reeves and Turner of London, 1890.
63. Harms 2012, 48.
64. Ossman & Steel 1894, 61.
65. Helfenstein broadsides, 54.
66. *Ruhkbrief*, received by Don Yoder from Sophia Eberly, ca. 1961; Heilman Collection.
67. Bailer 1952; . Yoder, Don. 1951, 8-9.; Yoder 1952, 2; Yoder 1964.
68. Interviews with Bill Unger of Lebanon, beginning 2012, 2013, and 2015.
69. Shivley 1953.
70. Brendle & Unger 1935.
71. Helfenstein broadsides, 47.
72. Fogel 1995, 163.
73. Ibid, no. 1283.
74. Shaner, Richard. 1973. *American Folklife*. I (6)Apr.

Chapter VII. Herbal Rituals

1. Larson, Duane H. "Martin Luther's Influence on the Rise of the Natural Sciences." *Oxford Research Encyclopedia of Religion*. 29 Jul. 2017.
2. KJV Gen 1:29
3. Weaver, William Woys. 2001. *Sauer's Herbal Cures: America's First Book of Botanic Healing,* 1762-1778. New York: Routledge, xxi.
4. ibid, xx.
5. Hoffman, W. J. "Folk-Medicine of the Pennsylvania Germans." Proceedings of the American Philosophical Society 26, no. 129 (1889),340.
6. Fogel 1995, 175.
7. *Egyptische Geheimnisse, oder das Zigeuner-Buch genannt.* 1844. Harrisburg, PA: Gustav S. Peters, 4.
8. ibid; see also Grumbine 1905, 281.
9. Manuscript recipe, Schuylkill County, PA; for other inflammatory diseases, see: Hoffman 1889, 338-339.
10. Interview with former resident of Hamburg, Berks County, 2016.
11. AM 1869, III: 11.
12. Clipping on Superstition from Lebanon Advertiser, 12-28-1870
13. Eliza Leslie. 1833. *Atlantic Tales: Or, Pictures of Youth.* Boston: Munroe & Francis, 233.
14. HDA, IV: 262.
15. Holböck 2002, np. See St. Leopold.
16. Seymour 1898, 94-95.
17. Grien, Hans Baldung 1516. *Das Blumenwunder der heiligen Dorothea,* tempera on Linden Wood, National Gallery of Prague.
18. HDA, IV: 262.
19. ibid.
20. Harper 2001-2017. "Holland."
21. Yoder 2015, 96.
22. HDA, IV: 262.
23. ibid, 955.
24. ibid, 262.
25. Names of herbs used in this chapter can be found in: Beam and Trout 2012; For European associations with the calendar of the saints, see: Höfler 1899.
26. Shoemaker 2000, 13; Fogel 1995, 163-164.
27. Shoemaker 2000, 15; Fogel 1995, 163.
28. Shoemaker 2000, 15.
29. Fogel 1995, 162.
30. Donmoyer 2012c.
31. Neff & Weiser 1979.
32. Gourley, Norma Mae. 1936. "Some Phases of Witchcraft Among the Pennsylvania Germans." M.A. Dissertation, University of Illinois.
33. Hain, Peter. ca. 1800. Berks County. Manuscript, Heilman Collection.
34. Woyts 1761, 2408.
35. HDA I: xx
36. Kreissl 2005, 5.
37. Copy in the Heilman Collection.
38. Roan, Donald (Abe). 1964. "Deivel-Dreck (Asafoetida): Yesterday and Today." *Pennsylvania Folklife*. Lancaster, PA: Pennsylvania Folklife Society, XIV(2): 32.
39. Author's translation of Romanus-Büchlein. Ca. 1880, Leipzig: Phillip Hulseman, 7; Also included in the manuscript of Jacob Finsi, for Tobias Schick, 1819, Northampton County, Pennsylvania (whereabouts unknown).
40. Helfenstein, 52. See Appendix II.
41. Yoder 2016, 136-143.
42. AM 1869 II: 68, and AM Radde II:74-75. There is much confusion surrounding the use of this particular word throughout the ritual literature in Pennsylvania and Europe. Some souces say "*mit Elfenbeinen Holz*" (ivory wood) (Harms 447), while others say "*mit Elzenbäumen-Holz*" (Romanus, MS Finsi). Still other sources suggest using an "*Egenzahn*" (Helfenstein) or "*Erdbohrer*" (Harms 264) for pushing the bundle into the hole and forcing the peg in place. The compounding of these ideas is found in the synonym for *Elze(r)nbaum, Egel-baum,* listed by Woyts, 927: *Frangula =Zapholz* (plug-wood); see also *Elsenbaum* (*Frangula alnus*). The use of the term "lignum vitae" is exclusive to the English translation of Hohman. Albertus Magnus (Radde II: 74) uses the term "*Oelfenboettenholz*" (literally, elf-bed-wood), and the Allentown edition (1869) uses "*Eisenbötten-Holz*" (iron-bed-wood).
43. Folkard 1884, 261.
44. Donmoyer 2012, 91.
45. Weaver 2001, 246.
46. ibid, 295.
47. "Akron has a Powwow Doctor." *Pittsburg Dispatch*, Sat Sept 28, 1889.
48. Helfenstein, 52; see Appendix II.
49. Heeger 1936, 10.
50. Marzell 2002, 196.
51. Author's translation of Heeger 1936, 55.
52. Author's translation of Marzell 2002, 197.
53. Dickel 1975, 54.
54. "*Maul-fäule.*" PfWB IV:1234.
55. Marzell 2002, 195.
56. Chacon & Mendoza 2012, 452.
57. Harms 2012, 96.
58. AM 1869, III: 57.
59. Undated manuscript fragment, Heilman Collection., formerly from the Roughwood Collection of Dr. Don Yoder. Matches the handwriting of Dr. Johan Peter Saylor of Williams Township, Northampton County. For examples of Saylor's writing, see Heindel 2009, 40. Matches verbatim the toothache cure found in Ballmer 1827, 24.
60. See: Shoemaker 1951, 3; also in the Ozarks, in Randolph 1964, 143,170.
61. Fogel 1995, 155-156.
62. Powwower J. H. Wilhelm in "The News In General" *The Shippensburg Chronicle,* Shippensburg, PA: Fri 18 Jun 1886, 2.
63. Hartland 1895, 178 -183.
64. Yoder, Jacob H. 1952. "Proverbial Lore From Heggins Valley." *The Pennsylvania Dutchman.* II(16):3.
65. Ash, Charles W. 1885. "Communicated: Superstition, Sweeny." *Daily Local News.* West Chester, PA: Nov 13.
66. "A Queer Tradition." *The Medical and Surgical Reporter.* Oct 5, 1885. LIII: 486-487.
67. *Wer Gott Vertraut,* ca. 1800. Broadside, Heilman Collection.
68. Author's translation of Albertus Magnus, I: 7. Wilhelm Radde's New York edition, says "*Zasam*" instead of *Zapfen* (Plug).
69. Author's translation of AM 1869, I: 36.
70. AM 1869 I: 7.
71. HDA V: 955.

72. Author's translation of Marzell 2002, 249.
73. Leslie, Eliza. 1833. *Atlantic Tales: Or, Pictures of Youth*. Boston: Munroe & Francis, 233. Although this book is a work of fiction, it features examples of plausible ritual procedures for the time period, and as with many of Leslie's local-color stories, they are likely based at least partly in reality.
74. Josephus, Flavius. 1820. *Bellum Judaicum.* Philadelphia, PA: Kimber & Sharpless, vii. 6. 3 ; R.K. Harrison. 1956. "The Mandrake And The Ancient World," *The Evangelical Quarterly* 28.2 (1956): 87-92.
75. "Berks Hills and Dale Boast over 200 Plants of Medicinal Value" Reading Eagle, Jan 3 1926, 15.
76. Harrison 1956, 88-89.
77. ibid.
78. *The Goschenhoppen Region*, II(2): 2.

Chapter VIII. Ritual Objects of Power

1. For more info on Mountain Bummy, see: Weaver 1993, 104-105.
2. Walch, Robert S. 1973. "Oley Valley Can Maker." *American Folklife*. April, 1:6..
3. These canes are described in detail in the catalog of the Mercer Museum and the Historical Society of Bucks County, Doylestown, Pennsylvania, RoloPac: Object IDs 13405, 17897, 25051.
4. Sigerist 1961, 54, 65.
5. KJV Num 20:8-9.
6. Jung & Franz 1968, 152-153.
7. Troxell, William S. 1931. "Strange Serpent Canes Used By Paul Heym, First Penna. Witch Doctor in 1755, Unearthed by *Morning Call* Staff Writer." Allentown *Morning Call*, 1 Feb, 1931, 4, 16.
8. Lecture by Honorable Judge D. C. Henning of Schuylkill County, 1911, in Troxell 1931.
9. Troxell 1931, 16.
10. Troxell 1931, 4.
11. KJV Exod 7:9-12.
12. KJV Num 17:8.
13. Mercer Museum Catalog, RoloPac 13405
14. AM Radde, II: 37.
15. AM Radde 1872, II: 12.
16. AM Radde 1872, I: 20, 60; II: 29-30.
17. There is some confusion about the term "*Scherhaufen*" in *Egyptian Secrets,* and English editions suggest the curious "witches-ladder or scissors," when in fact the term is synonymous with a mole-hill. See: Grimm's *Deutsche Wörterbuch*, "*Scherhaufen*."
18. Radde 1872, I:20, 60.
19. Mercer Museum Catalog, RoloPac 17897.
20. Radde 1872, I:20, 60
21. HDA VI:195; Brinckmeier, Eduard. 1850. "*Kreuzmesser - ein mit einem oder drei Kreuzen gezeichnetes Messer.*" *Glossarium Diplomaticum zur Erläuterung Schwieriger einer Diplomatischen Historischen Sachlichen oder Worterklarung Bedürftiger Lateinischer Hoch und Besonders Niederdeutscher Wörter und Formeln.* Wolfenbüttel: Brinckmeier, 1106.
22. Beitl, Klaus. *Volksglaube: Zeugnisse Religiöser Volkskunst.* Salzburg: Residenz Verl, 1978. pp. 42-43
23. See "*Trudenmesser*" DWB XXII: 1241; Kreissl 2014, 61.
24. Author's translation: MS. Henninger 1775 – *Arzneÿ Büchlein für Menschen und Vieh*, Albany Twp., Berks County, 26.
25. Landis 1969, 6-7.
26. Robert Wood reprinted Landis's article almost in entirety with only a few original additions from an oral history conducted with Landis. See; Wood, Robert. 2014. "Three Cross Knife." *Berksmont News*. 03/23/2014. http://www.berksmontnews.com/article/BM/20140323/NEWS/140329978
27. Fischer 1908, II: 360. "*Drei kreuz messer, n. ein Taschenmesser mit 3 Kreuzen ist zur Stillung von Blutungen usw gut.*"
28. Seeligman 1909, 16.
29. Ibid.
30. Fogel 117; Radde 1872, II:79.
31. Seligman 16.
31. Ibid; LEA III: 1371.
32. Author's translation: John Rohrer, Abraham and Jacob Rohrer Mss, ca 1810, Heilman Collection.
33. AM Radde 3:22. Some popular English translations erroneously suggest "alderwood" as opposed to the correct term "elderberry" from the original German "*Holderstock.*"
34. Norman, 2016. Author's Note: Stories of the mythic black dog are not uncommon even today. My grandfather claimed to have seen a black dog cross the street prior to a cataclysmic automobile accident that he was involved in shortly before his death in 2009.
35. Author's translation: AM Radde I: 8.
36. KJV 1 Cor 6:19.
37. KJV Matt 3:11.
38. HDA, VII: 838.
39. KJV Matt 26:26
40. Compare the German, Albertus Magnus Radde 1:8 to trade paperback edition, Chicago Publishing Co. ca. 1900, 1:7.
41. Wakley, Thomas. 1833. *The Lancet*, London: Mills & Jowley. XI: 578-579.
42. AM Radde I: 12.
43. AM Radde III: 26.
44. AM Radde I:28; see also "*Scharlachkraut*" in *Kruenitz Oeconomische Encyclopädie online*, http://www.kruenitz1.uni-trier.de/
45. AM Radde I:12.
46. No author. 1791. *Erdmann Hülfreichs bewährtes Handbüchlein für Bauersleute*. Wien: Aloys Dollischen Buchhandlung, 176.
47. Weaver, 2016.
48. *Drei-Keenich Kreitzer,* in Pennsylvania Dutch, from an interview with a native speaker from Lehigh County in 2009.
49. Mathers 2012, 100.
50. Merrifield 1987, 161-162. Also cited in Davies & Easton 2016, 228.
51. Harms 2012, 86.
52. Harms 2012, 273.
53. This inscription is omitted in the late nineteenth century editions by Wilhelm Radde of New York, but the inscription is featured in Harlacher & Weiser's Allentown imprint, II: 72.
54. Freudenthal 1931; Erich & Beitl, 154.
55. HDA IV: 438.
56. Author's family's discussion, ca. 1990, Lebanon County.
57. Author's 2014 fieldwork with Historic Gettysburg, Adams County.
58. HDA IV: 438-439.
59. Erich & Beitl, 339.
60. HDA IV, 438.

61. ibid.
62. Fogel 1995, 175.
63. Fogel 1995, 209.
64. ibid.
65. Erich & Beitl 207.
66. Fogel 1995, 206; Also in Grumbine 1905.
67. See Chapter X: Rituals of Death and Renewal.
68. HDA IV: 439
69. Helfenstein broadsides, II:3.
70. HDA IV: 440.
71. HDA IV: 442.
72. Beitl 1978, 78-81.
73. Merrified 11-13.
74. Author's amendment of Pennsylvania Dutch entry in Fogel 1995, 169.
75. Fogel 1995, 169.
76. Ibid, 11.
77. Grumbine 1905, 287.
78. Johanson 2009, XLII: 129-174.
79. Stevens 1973, 254- 274.
80. Woyts, 309.
81. Goodrum 2008, 482-508.
82. Marvin, Ursula B. 1992. "The Meteorite of Ensisheim - 1492 to 1992." *Meteoritics*. Cambridge, MA: Harvard University, Harvard-Smithsonian Center for Astrophysics, XXVII: 28-72.
83. Goodrum 482-508.
84. Skeat 1912, 45-80.
85. Translation in Merrifield, 11; Original Latin text from Evans 1887, 64.
86. HDA: VIII: 1174, II: 327
87. Woyts, 309.
88. Skeat 65-69; Rupp 1842, 355.
89. Hufford 2010.
90. Merrifield, 161-162; Johanson 129; Duffin 2011, 84-101.
91. Appearing in English as "the bed-goblin" in twentieth century translations of Albertus Magnus. For a broad study of these entities, see Mahr 1935, 215-225.
92. Goodrum 17

93. Interview with family member in December 2013 at St. Paul's Evangelical Lutheran Church, Fleetwood, Pa.
94. Robacker, Earl F. 1976. "Ancient of Days – Plus Tax!" *Pennsylvania Folklife*. XVI (4).
95. The powwow paddle and wafer iron in Earl F. Robacker's collection appear in *Pennsylvania Folklife* Summer 1966, XV (4). Dr. Don Yoder told me in a personal conversation that he was not convinced of the alleged ritual use of the object, believing instead that it was a paddle used for pressing cheese or butter.
96. Shaner, Richard H. 2006. "Pennsylvania German Powwow Carvings and the Occult," *Historical Review of Berks County*. Reading: Historical Society of Berks County, LXX (1); For additional pictures of Machmer's carvings, see also: Yoder, Don & David J. Hufford. 1998. "The Healing Traditions of the Pennsylvania Dutch" in *North American Healing Traditions*. Westmount, QB: Reader's Digest Association of Canada.
97 Shaner 2006, 13-14.
98. Shaner 2006, 14; also in Shaner, Richard H. 1972. "Recollections of Witchcraft in the Oley Hills." *Pennsylvania Folklife* XXI: Folk Festival Supplement.
99. Thomas Brendle Museum object label, Powwow Chair. Historic Schaefferstown Inc.
100. Ibid.
101. The traditional notion of the two pillars of the church is associated with the Apostles Peter and Paul, but since the three vertical rungs also invoke Paul, Peter, and Jesus, it is also possible that the "two pillars" refers to the two greatest commandments from Matthew 22:36-40: "Jesus said unto him, Thou shalt love the Lord thy God with all thy heart, and with all thy soul, and with all thy mind. 38. This is the first and great commandment. And the second is like unto it, Thou shalt love thy neighbor as thyself. 40. On these two commandments hang all the law and the prophets." (KJV)
102. When the first exhibition of *Powwowing in Pennsylvania* was held at the Schwenkfelder Heritage Center and Library, one of the most frequent concerns voiced to me by colleagues from visiting institutions about the chair was that it appeared to be an ordinary chair. These comments suggest that a humble, everyday object does not always exude the appearance of otherworldliness that is often expected from ritual objects.

Chapter IX. Powwowing & The Authorities

1. "Dr. Joseph H. Hagenman" in Biographical Publishing Company. 1898. *Book of Biographies: This Volume Contains Biographical Sketches of Leading Citizens of Berks County, Pa.* Buffalo, NY: Biographical Pub. Co.
2. For more examples of Joseph Hageman's blessings, see: Donmoyer 2014, 179-195; Donmoyer 2013a. Donmoyer 2012b. Mahr 1935, 215-225.
3. Examination of witness Maggie Hohl, in *Hageman vs. The North American*, it is discovered that Hageman does not speak Pennsylvania Dialect. "Witnesses Heard in Hageman Case." *The North American.* Philadelphia, Pa. (Mar 13 1903):13.
4. "Henrich Herman Hageman" *Germany, Select Births and Baptisms, 1558-1898* [database on-line]. Provo, UT, USA: Ancestry.com Operations, Inc., 2014.
5. *Passenger Lists of Vessels Arriving at Philadelphia, Pennsylvania - Records of the United States Customs Service, 1745-1997*; Record Group Number: 36; Series: M425; Roll: 041 The National Archives at Washington, D.C; *Passenger Lists of Vessels Arriving at Philadelphia, Pennsylvania, 1800-1882*. Washington, D.C.: National Archives and Records Administration. Micropublication M425, rolls 1-71.
6. *Baptismal Records of Salem German Reformed Church Philadelphia in Historic Pennsylvania Church and Town Records*, Reel 166. Philadelphia, Pennsylvania: Historical Society of Pennsylvania.
7. Obituary "Dr. Joseph H. Hagenman" *Reading Eagle.* Reading, PA. (Jun 19 1905).
8 Grave of Elisabeth Hageman (1800-1857) Saint John's U.C.C. Cemetery Pricetown, Berks County.
9. Historic Pennsylvania Church and Town Records. Reel 974. Philadelphia, PA. Historical Society of Pennsylvania.
10. Heinrich Hageman, Reading North West Ward Reading, U.S. Federal Census 1860.
11. "Death of a Widely-Known Herb Doctor" Reading Eagle, Reading, PA. (Jun 21 1882)
12. Charles Kistler, "Powwow Doctor" Allentown City, U.S. Federal Census 1910.
13. "Dr. Joseph H. Hagenman." Book of Biographies: This Volume Contains Biographical Sketches of Leading Citizens of Berks County, Pa. Buffalo, NY: Biographical Pub. Co, 1898.
14. Boyd's U.S. City Directories – Reading, PA 1877-1891 "Joseph H. Hageman, Corner of N. 10th and Pike Sts.; Henry Hageman, 836 Elm St., Physician" (1877) & "Joseph H. Hagenman, Physician 836 Elm" (1891).
15. 1858 cited in Hageman's own words in "Witch Doctor's Case Against North American Withdrawn By Counsel" *The North American.* Philadelphia, PA. (Mar 13 1903): 5. Obituary "Dr. Joseph H. Hagenman." *Reading Eagle.* Reading, PA. (Jun 19 1905).
16. "Reading's 'Woorst-Frau' – Sketch of a Well-Known Female Local Celebrity – 'Braucha' Method of Curing." *Reading Times*, Reading, PA. (May 15 1899):4.
17. "Witch Doctor's Case Against North American Withdrawn By Counsel" *The North American.* Philadelphia, PA. (Mar 13 1903):5.
18. Ermentrout 1876.
19. Obit. J. H. Hagenman, Reading Eagle; John Winters, Farmer. Donegal Township, Lancaster County. U.S. Federal Census. 1880.
20. "Witch Doctor's Case Against North American Withdrawn By Counsel" *The North American.* Philadelphia, PA. (Mar 13 1903): 5.
21. "Witnesses Heard in Hageman Case." *The North American*, Philadelphia, PA. (Mar 13 1903):12-13.
22. "*Der Readinger Hexendoktor*" (*Readinger Adler*, Ca. 1885) Transcribed German-Language Newspaper clipping in the Powwow files of Dr. Don Yoder (1921-2015).
23. Rix, Alice. "The Reading Witch Doctor's Sway Over the Trusting and the Ignorant." *The North American*, (May 22 1900):16.
24. "Where Witches Flourish in this Twentieth Century." *The New York Times.* New York, NY: (Sep 10 1911):39. For more background on this article, see also: Adams, Charles J., III. "Pow-wow Practice in Berks County Gains the National Spotlight." *Reading Eagle*, Reading PA.(Jan 5, 2011).
25. "Witchcraft in Berks" *The Adams Sentinel.* Gettysburg, PA. (Jul 15 1862):1.
26. Rix, Alice. "The Reading Witch Doctor's Sway Over the Trusting and the Ignorant." *The North American*, (May 22 1900):16.
27. Bertolet, John M. 1899. "Witch-Doctors and Their Deceptions." *Philadelphia Monthly Medical Journal.* Philadelphia, PA. Dec 1899. "After Witch Doctors. Berks Physicians May Prosecute Them." *The Allentown Leader.* Allentown, PA. (Mar 14 1900):2.
29. "Witnesses Heard in Hageman Case." *The North American*, Philadelphia, PA. (Mar 13 1903): 13.
"Dr. Hageman's Patients That They Have Faith in Witchery and Spells." *The North American*. Philadelphia, PA. (Mar 11 1903):1.
30. "Where Witches Flourish in this Twentieth Century." *The New York Times.* New York, NY: (Sep 10 1911): 39. For a fascinating look at the twentieth century popular press and its effect on folk medicine, as well as a synopsis of the Hageman case see: Davies 2013.
31. Lewis 1972.
32. "Twenty-Five Years Ago: June 20, 1905." *Reading Times*. Reading, PA. (Jun 20 1930):10
33. Author's translation of Emma Jane Weidner's blessing, made by Dr. Hageman in 1887. *Heilman Collection.*
34. *Slatington Times.* Slatington, PA. (Oct 23, 1914):1.
35. *The Morning Call.* Allentown, PA. (Oct 29, 1914): 5.
36. *Evening Ledger*, Philadelphia, PA. (Nov 23, 1914).
37. *Slatington Times.* Slatington, PA. (Oct 23, 1914).
38. *The Morning Call.* Allentown, PA. (Aug 29, 1930): 5.
39. *Slatington Times.* Slatington, PA. (Oct 23, 1914).
40. Interviews with descendants of Dennis Rex 2013-2017
41. *Slatington Times.* Slatington, PA. (Oct 23, 1914).
42. Unpublished report provided by the family of Denis Rex: "More on Dennis Rex…from various family sources conveyed to Rev. Brian Haas."
43. *Slatington Times.* Slatington, PA. (Oct 23, 1914).; *The Allentown Leader.* Allentown, PA. (Oct 19, 1914): 5.
44. *Slatington Times.* Slatington, PA. (Oct 23, 1914).
45. *Evening Ledger*, Philadelphia, PA. (Nov 23, 1914).
46. *The Morning Call.* Allentown, Pennsylvania (Apr 27, 1929): 5.
47. Smith 2016, 153.
48. *Slatington Times.* Slatington, PA. (Oct 30, 1914). *Evening Ledger*, Philadelphia, PA. (Nov 23, 1914).
49. *The Morning Call.* Allentown, PA. (Feb 28, 1918): 12.
50. *The Morning Call.* Allentown, PA. (Apr 27, 1929): 5.
51. *The Morning Call.* Allentown, PA. (Jun 12, 1929): 5.
52. "Dennis Rex accused by woman 'patient.'" *The Morning Call.* Allentown, PA. (Aug 29, 1930): 5.
53. "Hex Case Dismissed." *Reading Eagle*, Reading, PA. (Sept 5, 1930).
54. ("Wife's Testimony Helps Rex." *The Morning Call.* Allentown, PA.

(Sep 5, 1930): 5, 18.
55. Interview with Mark Kuntz, conducted by Rev. Brian Haas 2016.
56. Farm sale notice, *The Morning Call*. Allentown, PA. (Apr 27, 1944): 18.
34. *Slatington Times*. Slatington, PA. (Oct 23, 1914): 1.
35. *The Morning Call*. Allentown, PA. (Oct 29, 1914): 5.
36. *Evening Ledger*, Philadelphia, PA. (Nov 23, 1914).
37. *Slatington Times*. Slatington, PA. (Oct 23, 1914): 1.
38. *The Morning Call*. Allentown, PA. (Aug 29, 1930): 5.
39. *Slatington Times*. Slatington, PA. (Oct 23, 1914): 1.
40. Interviews with descendants of Dennis Rex 2013-2017.
41. *Slatington Times*. Slatington, PA. (Oct 23, 1914): 1.
42. Unpublished report provided by the family of Denis Rex: "More on Dennis Rex…from various family sources conveyed to Rev. Brian Haas."
43. *Slatington Times*. Slatington, PA. (Oct 23, 1914): 1; *The Allentown Leader*. Allentown, PA. (Oct 19, 1914): 5.
44. *Slatington Times*. Slatington, PA. (Oct 23, 1914): 1.
45. *Evening Ledger*, Philadelphia, PA. (Nov 23, 1914).
46. *The Morning Call*. Allentown, PA. (Apr 27, 1929): 5.
47. Smith 2016, 153.
48. *Slatington Times*. Slatington, PA. (Oct 30, 1914); *Evening Ledger*, Philadelphia, PA. (Nov 23, 1914).
49. *The Morning Call*. Allentown, PA. (Feb 28, 1918): 12.
50. *The Morning Call*. Allentown, PA. (Apr 27, 1929): 5.
51. *The Morning Call*. Allentown, PA. (Jun 12, 1929): 5.
52. "Dennis Rex accused by woman 'patient.'" *The Morning Call*. Allentown, PA. (Aug 29, 1930): 5.
53. "Hex Case Dismissed." *Reading Eagle*, Reading, PA. (Sept 5, 1930).
54. ("Wife's Testimony Helps Rex." *The Morning Call*. Allentown, PA. (Sept 5, 1930): 5, 18.
55. Interview with Mark Kuntz, Rev. Brian Haas 2016.
56. Ibid.
57. Farm sale notice, *The Morning Call*. Allentown, PA. (Apr 27, 1944): 18.
58. *Philadelphia Inquirer*. Philadelphia, PA. (Dec 2, 1928.)
59. McGinnis 5; Lewis 31. The following treatment of the Rehmeyer Murder will follow closely the work of retired York County lawyer and historian of the York Hex Trials, J. Ross McGinnis, and the work of Philadelphia journalist, Arthur Lewis. While Lewis's narrative style has often come under criticism and sources are not cited, many of his facts are indeed supported by local reporting in York and Philadelphia in 1928-1929.
60. Lewis 54
61. Lewis 23
62. McGinnis, 209.
63. Soukhanoff, Sergius. 1906. "On Hypochondriacal Melancholia in Russian Soldiers." *Journal of Abnormal Psychology*. Boston: Gorham Press, I(Aug):135-138.
64. *Philadelphia Inquirer*. Philadelphia, PA. (Jan 9, 1929).
65. Gravestone in Red Lion Cemetery bearing the names of John Blymire and his two children, Richard H. (1918-1918) and Josephine L. (1920-1923); The one surviving child was Thomas Irvin Blymire (1923-2003), obituary in *York Daily Record*, York, PA. (Oct 27, 2003).
66. "Man Accused of Voodoo Murder Escaped Insane Hospital Here in 1923" *The Evening News*, Harrisburg, PA. (Dec 3 1928).
67. *Philadelphia Inquirer*. Philadelphia, PA. (Jan 9, 1929).
68. *Philadelphia Inquirer*. Philadelphia, PA. (Dec 01, 1928): 6; McGinnis 6; "York Murder Stirs Officials to War on Powwowism" *Reading Times*. Reading, PA. (Dec 13, 1928): 1; Lewis 38.
69. "Gertrude Rudy, Since Murdered, Visited the Room of 'Pow-Wow' Doctor." *The Evening News*. Harrisburg, PA. (Dec 4, 1928): 1.
70. McGinnis, 18.
71. PA Commonwealth Death Certificate No. 27455.
72. *Reading Times*. Reading, PA. (Jan 9, 1929).
73. Try this at home: Take a one dollar bill, and place it face-up on your palm. Relax your eyes and stare at it without blinking as much as possible for about 3-5 minutes. Then take the dollar bill away, and stare at a neutral surface (like the palm of your hand or a white wall). The optical afterimage effect is unmistakably the picture of George Washington with inverted colors, i.e white becomes black, black becomes white, and green becomes red, etc. The white of Washington's collar appears dark, like a beard, much like Rehmeyer's.
74. McGinnis 7-8.
75. McGinnis 223.
76. *The Philadelphia Inquirer*. Philadelphia, PA. (Dec 1, 1928): 6.
77. *The Philadelphia Inquirer*. Philadelphia, PA. (Dec 1, 1928): 6, and again on (Jan 13, 1929): 7.
78. McGinnis 222-223.
79. *The Gazette and Daily* York, PA. (Oct, 2 1935): 7.
80. Lewis, 54.
81. McGinnis 217.
82. McGinnis 25.
83. According to some sources, local historian J. Ross McGinnis owns Rehmeyer's copy of the book. See: "York County's Hex murder: 5 quick facts about the forever fascinating witchcraft case" Posted on October 8, 2012 by Jim McClure: <http://www.yorkblog.com/yorktownsquare/2012/10/08/york-countys-hex-murder-5-quick-facts-about-the-forever-fascinating-witchcraft-case/>
84. *The Evening News*. Harrisburg, PA. (Jan 10, 1929): 1.
85. *The Philadelphia Inquirer*. Philadelphia, PA. (Dec 1, 1928): 6.
86. McGinnis 35.
87. *The Evening News*. Harrisburg, PA. (Nov 30 1928): 21.
88. "Theft Believed Murder Motive." *The Evening News*. Harrisburg, PA. (Dec 3 1928): 13.
89. McGinnis, 56.
90. McGinnis xv. This statement by a Philadelphia journalist highlights the clumsy linguistic adaptation of the PA Dutch word *Hex* into English.
91. *Evening Public Ledger*. Philadelphia, PA. (Nov 23, 1914): 8.
92. McGinnis xvii.
93. McGinnis 45-46, copied from *The York Dispatch*, York, PA. (Dec 4, 1928); *Philadelphia Inquirer*. Philadelphia, PA. (Dec 4, 1928).
94. "Scores of Deaths Are Laid at Door of Pow-Wow Cult." *Philadelphia Inquirer*. Philadelphia, PA. (Dec 4 1928): 1.
95. *Pittsburgh-Post Gazette*. Pittsburgh, PA. (January 8, 1928), in McGinnis 95-96.
96. *Philadelphia Inquirer* Philadelphia, PA. (Jan 13, 1929): 7.
97. *The Evening News*. Harrisburg, PA. (Dec 4, 1928): 24.
98. *Mount Carmel Item*. Mount Carmel, PA. (Dec 5, 1928): 2.
99. *Pittsburgh-Post Gazette*. Pittsburgh, PA. (Dec 5, 1928): 2; *The Los Angeles Times*. Los Angeles, CA. (Dec 5, 1928): 8.
100. A recent documentary called *Hex Hollow* (2015 Freestyle Flicks) based largely on J. Ross McGinnis's research of the Rehmeyer murder, includes further speculation on the role of Blymire in the murder of Gertrude Rudy. While some have perpetuated the notion that Blymire may have been the murderer, presumably, police would have had no reason to go lightly on Blymire in the investigation, given the fact that he was already in custody for the murder of Nelson Rehmeyer when he was questioned.

101. *Philadelphia Record*. Philadelphia, PA. (Jan 8, 1928).
102. McGinnis 77-78.
103. Ibid, 69.
104. Ibid, 173, 179.
105. Ibid, 93.
106. Ibid, 246.
107. Ibid, 247.
108. *Philadelphia Inquirer*. Philadelphia, PA. (Jan 12, 1929)
109. ibid.
110. McGinnis 67
111. *Philadelphia Inquirer*. Philadelphia, PA. (Jan 13 1929): 1.
112. Ibid, 7.
113. McGinnis, 440.
114. "John Blymire dies at 76; principal in 'hex' Slaying." *York Daily Record*. York, PA. (May 12, 1972).
115. *The Evening News*. Harrisburg, PA. (Dec 11, 1928): 17.
116. *The Morning Call*. Allentown, PA. (Mar 24, 1929): 5; *Pittsburgh-Post Gazette*. Pittsburgh, PA. (Mar 18, 1929).
117. *Reading Times*. Reading, PA. (Mar 23, 1929): 1.
118. *The Morning Call*. Allentown, PA. (Mar 23, 1929): 22.
119. *The Morning Call*. Allentown, PA: (Apr 4, 1929): 9.
120. *Mauch Chunk Times-News*. Mauch Chunk, PA. (Jun 3, 1929): 1.
121. "Witch Lore Motive for Killing." *Pottsville Republican*. Pottsville, PA. (Mar 22, 1934).
122. *Staunton Daily Leader*, Staunton VA; *Star Ledger*, Kosciusko, Mississippi; *Evening Kansan-Republican*, Newton, Kansas, etc.
123. *Mount Carmel Item*. Mount Carmel, PA. (Sep 28, 1911): 3.
124. *The Allentown Democrat*. Allentown, PA. (Oct 10, 1911): 5.
125. The newspapers claimed: "the word 'hexahemeron' is taken from two Greek words, 'hex' and 'hemera' and means a completion of six parts. It is usually used in referring to the six days' labor of creation, as described in the first chapter of Genesis."
126. *The Indiana Weekly Messenger*. Indiana, PA. (May 22, 1912): 7.
127. *The Allentown Democrat*. Allentown, PA. (Oct 3, 1911): 3.
128. *The Allentown Democrat*. Allentown, PA. (Oct 10, 1911): 5.
129. ."District Attorney Reviews Evidence on Pow-Wowing: No Basis for Manslaughter Charge, He Says; Will Continue Probe." *Reading Times* Reading, PA. (Oct 13, 1926): 12..
130. *The Philadelphia Inquirer*. Philadelphia, PA. (Dec 4, 1928).
131. "Death of 5 Babies Laid To Witch Cult: Pennsylvania Coroner..." *New York Times*. New York, NY. (Dec 4, 1928): 14.
132. *Philadelphia Record*. Philadelphia, PA. (Dec 4, 1928).
133. *The York Gazette and Daily*. York, PA. (Jan 14, 1929), cited in McGinnis 60.
134."Conquering Superstition." *Reading Eagle*. Reading, PA. (Nov 22, 1936).
135. "Canada to stamp out witchcraft in North, Vancouver." *La Grande Observer*. LaGrande, OR. (Oct 21, 1924): 1; "Negro Obsessed by Hex Killed in Gunfight, Nashville, Tennessee." *The Morning Call*. Allentown, PA. (Jul 5, 1947): 7.
136. Koch 1969.
137. Ellis 1995, 77-94.
138. Koch, 122, 28-33, 37.
139. Ellis 1995.
140. Koch, 123
141. Ibid, 105.
142. Kruse 1951, 7.
143. Black 2016, 165.
144. Ibid, 165.
145. Ibid, 160, citing Baumhauer 1984, 168-171.
146. *Daily Independent Journal*. San Rafael, CA. (Jul 28, 1960): 40; and Black 166.
147. See Chapter V: The Sixth and Seventh Books of Moses
148. Interestingly enough, these German statistics were picked up in American Newspapers, such as: "German Finds Key to Old Witchcraft." *Daily Independent Journal*. San Rafael, CA. (Jul 28, 1960): 40.
149. *The Corpus Christi Caller-Times*. Corpus Christi, TX. (July 5, 1957): 19.
150. Both corn husking bees and rag parties (*die Lumpe Parties*) are relics of a bygone era, especially the latter, which was a special type of social gathering centered around cutting and sewing household rags into long strips used for weaving (and later braiding) rag rugs.

Chapter X. The Ritual of Everyday Life

1. For the most useful edition, see: Fogel, Edwin. 1995. *Beliefs and Superstitions of the Pennsylvania Germans.* Ed. C. Richard Beam. Millersville, PA: Center for Pennsylvania German Studies, Millersville University. The original 1915 edition utilizes phonetic spelling of the Pennsylvania Dutch language that is difficult even to some advanced readers and speakers of the language today. Furthermore, Fogel's original edition omits a large section from his original 1915 edition concerning "Sex," and instead produced a rare supplement that is extremely difficult to find, marked "For Private Distribution. Not for Public Perusal." This section is not merely about sex, but covers a wide range of topics, everything from pregnancy to menstruation: "A pregnant woman cannot churn butter"; fertility to postpartum, "If a man visits a woman in confinement he must buy a dress for the child"; with only a few entries actually addressing the topic of intercourse. Beam's updated edition includes the full contents of this valuable chapter.
2. Yoder 2016, 74.
3. Only a handful of the remaining entries are narratives that do not fit the three main categories I've used for this analysis, and all of these are in Fogel's "Miscellaneous" chapter.
4. My statistical analysis of Fogel's work found evidence of descriptions of ritual in 51% or 1070 of 2084 entries. 2085 are listed, but entry 1733 is missing from both 1915 and 1995 editions.
5. Fogel 1995, 119.
6. Ibid 127.
7. 17% or 359 entries.
8. Ibid 131.
9. Over 31% or 660 entries.
10. Ibid 150.
11. Ibid 60.
12. see Chapter I for a definition of "*Braucherei*," and "*brauche*." See Chapter III for a discussion of European origins of the words.
13. In addition to Fogel (1995) the following sections owe a great deal to the works of Thomas Brendle and Claude Unger (1935), Thomas Brendle (edited by C. Richard Beam, 1995) and Ezra Grumbine (1905). While many of these authors were collecting what they called "beliefs" or "superstitions" a large majority of their entries were precise descriptions of the specific procedures and timing of ritual process. Collectively these three works form the largest repository of domestic

and agricultural accounts of ritual for the Pennsylvania Dutch.
14. Interview 5 Sept 2016 with female contact from northern Lehigh County.
15. Harms 2012, 153.
16. Ibid 47.
17. Ibid 47.
18. Conrad Raber his Docter Book. ca. 1800. Pennsylvania German Cultural Heritage Center.
19. Donmoyer 2012c.
20. The Magdeburg *Himmelsbrief*, Philadelphia printings of *Sieben Heiligen Himmelsriegel*, and the Kutztown edition of the *Three Kings Prayer* by Urich & Gehring all explicitly indicate that they are to be used in this manner. See also Chapter III.
21. An entry not included in the original German, but adapted in later editions of *Albertus Magnus' Egyptian Secrets*, ca. 1900. Chicago, IL: Egyptian Publishing Company, 91.
22. 1798. *Kürzgefasstes Weiber Büchlein…* Ephrata, PA: Benjamin Mayer, 32.
23. Fogel 1995, 12.
24. Ibid 31.
25. Ibid 28.
26. Fogel 221.
27. See Chapter VII.
28. Donmoyer 2016, 33-34.
29. *Gichttrophenblätter* in AM 1869, III: 18.
30. Fogel 1995, 37.
31. Interview with contact in Berks County, also echoed by a friend from Vorarlberg, Austria; See also Fogel 1995, 216.
32. AM 1869, III: 20.
33. Fogel 1995, 38.
34. Ibid 43.
35. Carl Arner of Berks County donated to the Pennsylvania German Cultural Heritage Center, 5 ½ gallon mason jars of Good Friday rainwater that had been collected for baptism, along with several dozen Good Friday eggs saved by an aunt for powwowing.
36. Fogel 1995, 29.
37. Ibid 37.
38. Ibid 33.
39. Ibid 34.
40. Interview 4 July 2012, with Michael Yarnall from Yellow House, Amity Township, Berks County, concerning great grandfather Michael Hertzog of Boyertown, Pa.
41. Fogel 1995, 30.
42. Ibid, 175 12, 179; Grumbine 1905, 277.
43. Story from the 1940s shared in 2017 by a woman in Old Zionsville, Upper Milford, Lehigh County. Compare with Grumbine 1905, 279.
44. Fogel 1995, 213-215.
45. My grandfather from Lebanon County suggested this to me when I was sporting a particularly pathetic moustache in high school, and I originally thought he was making fun of me, as opposed to offering a helpful ritual suggestion. See also: Fogel 1995, 232.
46. Ibid 62.
47. Ibid 47-49.
48. Ibid 44.
49. Gibbons 2001, 398; Fogel 48.
50. Hoffbower, Henry F. (Lee Raus Gandee) 1968. "You Too Can Be A Hex." *Fate*, XX (2):215. This valuable article is one of many written under a pen-name by Lee Gandee of the Dutch Fork.
51. Fogel 1995, 48.
52. Gibbons 2001, 398.
53. Quinter & Donmoyer, 2012.
54. Harms 2012, 51; Fogel 1995, 47.
55. Ibid 222.
56. A tradition carried to Ontario with the Pennsylvania Dutch documented by Wintemberg 1950, 19.
57. KJV Genesis 29:26.
58. Fogel 1995, 52; Grumbine 1905, 285.
59. *Verschiedene Sympathetische un Geheime Kunst-Stücke.* 1805. Reading, PA: Jungman & Bruckman; Donmoyer 2012, 93.
60. Fogel 1995, 53.
61. Ibid 75.
62. Ibid 165.
63. Donmoyer 2012, 91; Meyer, Elard Hugo. 1900. *Badisches Folksleben im Neunzehnten Jahrhundert*. Strassburg, Germany: Karl J. Trübner, 374; Fogel 100-101.
64. Brendle & Beam 1995, 80, 89, 92-3.
65. Conrad Raber his Doctor Book, ca. 1800, in cure for "Rotlauf." Pennsylvania German Cultural Heritage Center, Kutztown University.
66. Brendle & Unger 189.
67. Fogel 1995, 93.
68. Harms 2012, 48.
69. Fogel 1995, 83-84; Belief still widely held throughout Pennsylvania.
70. Ibid 210.
71. Ibid 129.
72. Ibid 90.
73. Ibid 192.
74. Ibid 202.
75. Koch 122, 28-33, 37.
76. Lutz 114.
77. Collected in 2017 from two native speakers of the dialect in Berks County.
78. See Donmoyer, 2013, 53-64.
79. The Agricultural Almanac series started by printer and publisher Johann Baer (1795-1858) of Lancaster, Pennsylvania has been in print for over two centuries, and issued in both English and German under the titles *Agricultural Almanac for the Year of Our Lord…* and *Neuer Gemeinnütziger Pennsylvanischer Calender Auf das Jahr…* The firm was later called Johann Baer & Sons, and eventually Johann Baer's Sons. *Baer's Almanac* is still widely distributed today in English Only as one of the classic almanacs in the German almanac tradition.
80. Grumbine 1905, 282; see also Fogel 1995, section on Special Days.
81. Grumbine 1905, 282-284.
82. St. Gertrude's day was later replaced by another patron saint of potatoes, St. Patrick, also observed on March 17.
83. Fogel 1995, 127
84. For discussion of the significance of Friday, see Chapter IV: Features of Ritual Performance and Chapter V: Margaretha Croll.
85. Fogel 1995, 131.
86. Ibid 122.
87. Bean, Theodore. W. 1884. *History of Montgomery County, Pennsylvania*. Philadelphia: Everts & Peck, 336-337.
88. Owens 1891, 123; Grumbine 1905, 285.
89. Fogel 1995, 142.
90. Interview in 2014 with two Berks County dialect speakers, regarding "*wann die Mariche* (Maria) *iwwer der Barrich geht.*" See also Fogel 1995, 143.
91. Recorded in Berks County 2014. Found also in Fogel 1995, 143.
92. Ibid 133.
93. Ibid 122.
94. Ibid 123-125.
95. Ibid 126.
96. Ibid 127.
97. Ibid 130, 134.
98. Ibid 131.
99. Interview in 2016 with Layla Loch of New Smithville, Lehigh County.
100. Fogel 1995, 179.
101. St. Gertrude is depicted with rats on her shoulders in the *Liber*

Chronicarum (The Nuremburg Chronicle) of 1493, by Hartmann Schedel.
102. Werner, William I. 1951. "Folk Beliefs." *Pennsylvania Dutchman.* II (16): 8.
103. Weaver, William Woys. 2016. *Dutch Treats: Heirloom Recipes from Farmhouse Kitchens.* Pittsburgh, PA: St. Lynn's Press, p103-105.
104. Mother of Rev. John Baer Stoudt (1878-1944) and grandmother of folklorist Rev. John Joseph Stoudt, appears in the 1880 census as the wife (23) of John Stoudt (32), in Maxatawny, with son John (Baer) Stoudt (1). The obituary of her son, John Baer Stoudt, suggests that they were residents of Topton, in *The Morning Call,* Allentown, PA (Apr 10, 1944) 5.
105. Weaver 2016, 105.
106. Don Yoder noted the unusual use of the singular diminutive ending "-li" at the end of "Leit" which is normally regarded as a plural noun.
107. Wood 1986, 3-12.
108. Brinton 1955, 2.
109. Brendle, John. 2012. "'*S Katz Deitsch Schtick: 'S Bucklich Mennli*." *Hiwwe wie Driwwe* Online. Editor Michael Werner. Ober Olm: Private Archive of Pennsylvania German Literature. < https://hiwwewiedriwwe.wordpress.com/tag/bucklich-mennli/>
110. Stoudt 1973, 164.
111. Brendle 2012.
112. AM 1869, I: 42.
113. See Chapter V: *The Long Lost Friend*.
114. See chapter V: Ossman & Steel; Fogel 1995, 183.
115. See Chapter IV: Ritual Performance.
116. Shoemaker 1960, 14.
117. KJV Gen 3:19.
118. Fogel 1995, 176.
119. Don Yoder's notes contain a hand-typed story regarding the use of this particular method of locating a deceased person among police in Perry County at the turn of the twentieth century.
120. "A Collection of Hunters' Charms." Yoder Translation of document marked Am 88 95 "German Papers," No 7.
121. Donmoyer 2012, 85.
122. AM 1869, 2:28.
123. Grumbine 1905, 280; Fogel 171, 101-102, 98.
124. AM 1869, II: 30.
125. Donmoyer 2012a, 84-85.
126. Donmoyer, Patrickb. 2012.
127. Author's translation, Am 1869, II: 36.
128. Donmoyer, op cit.
129. Ibid.
130. "*Wann ein Pferd zu reh ist.*" Ms. Conrad Raber his Docter Book. ca. 1800. Pennsylvania German Cultural Heritage Center; Fogel 111.
131. Fogel 1995, 220.
132. Ibid 763.
133. Ibid 120.
134. Ibid 120.
135. Ibid 121.
136. Ibid 119.
137. Ibid 119.
138. *The Philadelphia Inquirer*, Philadelphia, Pa., 7 Jan 1914. This is the most common description of good selection, but there was scarcely any agreement on the particulars.
139. Fogel 1995, 120-121.
140. *The Evening Sun*, Hanover, Pennsylvania, 13 July 1945.
141. *The Plain Speaker*, Hazleton, Pennsylvania, 19 Oct 1937, Tue, pg 2.
142. *The Morning Call,* Allentown, Pennsylvania, 07 Dec 1933, Thu, 10.
143. Fogel 1995, 176, 184.
144. Interview in 2017 with male contact from Lehigh County, Weisenberg Township.
145. Described by contacts in Berks and Lehigh 2015-2017; See also: *The Dutchman* Sept 15, 1951, 3.
146. Fogel 1995, 195.
147. Ibid 121.
148. Ibid 126.
149. Grumbine 1905.
150. Interviews with two Berks County contacts in 2015, one male and one female, who could recite the rhyme, and recalled it being used by relatives in powwowing.
151. Bronner 2006. Note that there are several renderings of the word *Heeli* (pronounced HAY-li, meaning "healing") that have led to some ambiguity about the definition of the word. A similar word *Heilich* means holy, but this is not the common pronunciation in Berks and Lehigh among native speakers of the dialect. I have also interviewed several Germans from the central and south Rhine who have recited identical rhymes, with the sole variation that they invoked *Heeli, Heeli Meisli-Dreck* (healing, healing mouse-dung), and even *Katze-Dreck* (cat-dung).
152. Grumbine 1905, 267. This echoes statements in Luther's Table Talks. See Chapter III: Martin Luther & Ritual of the Reformation Era. Also Fogel 116-117.
153. Helfenstein Broadsides, 67; Fogel 1995, 116-117.
154. See Chapter IV, compare with Fogel 1995, 102.
155. Helfenstein Broadsides, 67.
156. Hain, Peter. ca. 1800. Berks County. Manuscript, Heilman Collection.
157. Fogel 1995, 114.
158. Ibid 97; Owens 1891, 123.
159. Transcription from the oldest known American variant of the dungfork blessing, from 1789 cypher manuscript of Johann Kauffmann, courtesy of Clarke Hess. See also, Donmoyer 2012,
160. Donmoyer 2012, 51.
161. Manuscript in private collection; unpublished translation by Edward E. Quinter, 9.
162. Yoder, Don. Ca. 1960. "A Collection of Hunter's Charms." Unpublished translation.
163. See the thief blessing in Chapter VII: Horseshoe.
164. Am 1869 II: 33.
165. Donmoyer 2012, 103.
166. Author's translation of Alfred Shoemaker's hand-typed card, collected on March 5, 1955 from Mrs. George Schroeder, Albany Eck, Berks County.
167. I observed this in 2002 in Felton, York County, Pennsylvania. Compare with holding one's breath in Brendle & Unger 207.
168. Owens 1891, 123.
169. See the Jacob Wilhelm and Johannes Stecher manuscripts by Johannes Spangenberg in Chapter 3: Brauchen & Immigration Ritual.
170. Galllee 1887.
171. See Chapter IV: Cosmology of the Ritual Blessing.
172. *The Cincinnati Enquirer.* Sat, Jul 10, 1880, 10.
173. Hertzog, Phares H. 1967. "Snake Lore" *Pennsylvania Folklife.* XVII(4), Summer.
174. Mumaw, John R. 1960. Pennsylvania Folklife XI(1), Spring.
175. Hertzog 1967.
176. A beautifully written example reposes in the archive of the Lehigh County Historical Society at the Lehigh Valley Heritage Museum.
177. A photocopied example of this aphorism was found in the papers of Dr. Don Yoder.
178. I had the opportunity to photograph the gun-blessing, courtesy of Donald G. Batz of Topton, Berks County.
179. Fogel 1995, 95.
180. Ibid 94.
181. Am 1869, II: 40
182 Fogel 1995, 231.
183. Needle AM 1869 II: 28; communion bread in Grumbine 1905, 267.

184. Ibid II: 28.
185. Ibid II: 11-12.
186. Ibid II: 8.
187. Ibid II: 12.
188. Donmoyer 2012, 21; Harms 2012, 83.
189. "A Collection of Hunters' Charms." Yoder Translation of Am 88 95 "German Papers," No 1.
190. Ibid 2.
191. Ibid 6.
192. Am 1869 II: 39
193. Ossman & Steel 109.
194. Dick Shaner of Kutztown found an envelope containing turtle-doves tongues, marked "Turtle dove tongue Aug 22, 1912, used" in the attic of the home of his aunt Annie J. (Buchert) Bieber and uncle Freddie Bieber in the 1960s. See Shaner 1972, 39.
195. AM 1869, II: 11-12
196. Pyrlaeus, Johann Christoph, Jr. *Book of Instructions: Memoranda Book*. Ms., Moravian Archive, Bethlehem, PA. 107-108.
197. Quinter, Edward E. & Patrick J. Donmoyer. "The Book of Instructions by Johann Christoph Pyrlaeus Jr.: A Folklife Study of Early Process and Belief. " Unpublished paper, presented at the Bethlehem Conference on Moravian History & Music, 2012.
198. Thomas Brendle Papers, citing *Das Buch d. Geheimnisse*. 1852, Boston, 7. Special Collections and Archives, Franklin and Marshall College.
199. Albertus Magnus' Egyptian Secrets. ca. 1900. Chicago, Il.: DeLawrence Publishing Company, 75. (AM 1900)
200. Brendle Papers, *Buch d. Geheimnisse*, 2.
201. Fogel 1995, 230.
202. Ibid 265. Fogel also describes that biting one's apron string would avert slander, i.e. make the slanderer bite their tongue, ibid,
203. Donmoyer 2012, 95; Fogel 1995, 265.
204. This word literally translates to "pricks" or "cocky boys." For another version of the same ritual, see Chapter V: Helfenstein, and Appendix I.
205. Fogel 1995, 171-172.
206. Eighteenth-century, European book of *Kunst-Stücke*, no title page. Containing CCCCLXXXIX entries No. XCVI. Heilman Collection.
207. Grumbine 1905, 280; AM 1869, II: 32.
208. AM 1900, 149
209. *Das Nützliche Haus und Kunst-Buch, Für allgemainen Gebrauch*. Allentown, 1819, 12.
210. AM 1869, II: 31.
211. See Chapter IV: Cosmology of the Ritual Blessing.
212. Ms Hain, 9.
213. Fogel 1995, 137.
214. Ibid 181.
215. Ibid 183.
216. AM 1869 II: 11.
217. *Kurzgefaßtes Weiber-Büchlein*. Ephrata, PA: Benjamin Meyer 1798, 11.
218. Fogel 1995, 218.
219. AM 1869 II: 11.
220. 1798 *Weiber Buchlein*, 40-41.
221. AM 1869 II: 19.
222. Am 1869 II: 22.
223. Potts, Diggory & Peel 1977, 169-171; Culpeper 2011.
224. According to locals, a Kutztown practitioner in the 1970s used to keep a yard full of tansy for this purpose; See also Chapter IX: Dennis Rex.
225. MS recipes in the fly leaves of an 1894 copy of Ossman & Steel's Guide to Health from Dauphin County. At least one page contiguous with similar contents appears to have been intentionally torn out; for a European book of ritual medicine which has recipes entitled "*Abortieren*" cut out from the pages, see Gerstenberg 1850, Heilman Collection.
226. AM 1869 II: 40.
227. Ibid III: 4.
228. Harms 2012, 55.
229. Ibid, 252.
230. Ibid, 66.
231. Brendle & Unger 104 – 105.
232. Helfenstein Broadsides, 31.
233. Fogel 1995, 206-207.
234. Brendle & Unger 161.
235. Ibid.
236. Fogel 1995, 187.
237. CDC/NCHS, National Vital Statistics System; Grove RD, Hetzel AM. Vital statistics rates in the United States, 1940–1960. Washington, DC: U.S. Government Printing Office, 1968.
238. Certificate of Birth and Baptismal Certificate, Printed and For Sale at the "Eagle" Book Store, No. 542 Penn Street, Reading, PA. ca. 1880.
239. Brendle & Unger, 25.
240. KJV Psalms 31 & 39.
241. Donmoyer 2012, 102.
242. AM 1869 II:29.
243. Fogel 1995, 89.
244. Ibid 89.
245. Ibid.
246. Ibid 90.
247. Ibid 125.
248. Ibid 90.
249. Yoder 2016, 126; Brendle & Unger, 25.
250. Fogel 1995, 91-92.
251. Yoder 2016, 126.
252. For the dead person's hand for warts and tumors, see. Brendle & Unger 63, 79-80 and Fogel 1995, 187; For undertaker's hammer, see Grumbine 1905, 278.
253. Fogel 1995, 87.
254. Brendle & Unger 79-80; Fogel 1995, 177.
255. Brendle & Unger, 106.
256. AM 1869 I: 52.
257. Fogel 1995, 85-87.
258. AM 1869 III: 15.
259. For a member of the same sex, see Am 1869 I: 13. The same ritual appears in reverse in some European sources for members of the opposite sex, Koch 1972; Brendle & Unger, 189, cite that one cures incontinence by urinating into a fresh grave dug for a member of the opposite sex.
260. Fogel 1995, 199; Brendle & Unger 189; see Chapter II: Powwowers in Public Office.
261. Fogel 1995, 90.
262. Ibid 88.
263. Donmoyer 2012, 67. Compare with an alternate version, Ibid 101.
264. For more discussion of *Krankheitsdaemonen*, see Chapter III: The Poetry of the Blessing.
265. For the most recent study of the three-fold worm blessing, see the work of Natacha Klein Käfer. 2014. "German healing prayers in a transcontinental perspective: the case of the 'Dreyerley Würm Segen'" TEEME, third annual conference, "Contemplating Early Modernities: Concept, Content & Context", Freie Universität Berlin.
266. AM 1869, I:13; AM 1869, III: 15; Brendle & Unger 153, 114.
267. Donmoyer 2012, 70-71.
268. AM 1869 II: 40.

BIBLIOGRAPHY

--- ---. 1791. *Erdmann Hülfreichs bewährtes Handbüchlein für Bauersleute*. Wien: Aloys Dollischen Buchhandlung.

--- ---. 1810. *Das vortreffliche Zigeuner-Büchlein, vor Gott der Herr bewahre meine Seele…* Gedruckt zu Venedig. [Reading, Pa] Heinrich B. Sage.

--- ---. 1842. *Das Herz des Menschen*. Harrisburg: Theo. F. Scheffer.

--- ---. 1869. *Albertus Magnus' Bewährte und Approbirte Sympathetische und Natürliche Egyptische Geheimnisse*. Allentown: Harlacher and Weiser.

--- ---. ca. 1900. *Albertus Magnus, Being the Approved, Verified, Sympathetic and Natural Egyptian Secrets*. Chicago: Egyptian Publishing Co.

--- ---. 1902. *Church Book for the Use of the Evangelical Lutheran Congregations*. Philadelphia: General Council Publication Board.

--- ---. ca. 1880. *Ein sehr kräftiges, heiliges Gebet, welches zu Cöln am Rhein in goldnen Buchstaben geschrieben und aufbehalten wird*. Kutztown: Urich & Gehring.

--- ---. 1799. *Kurzgefaßtes Weiber-Büchlein, Enthält Aristoteli und A[lberti]. Magni Hebammen-Kunst mit den darzu gehörigen Recepten*. York: Salomon Mayer.

--- ---. 1803. *Kurzgefasstes Weiber-Büchlein : welches sehr nützlichen Unterricht für Schwangere Weiber und Haushälterinnen…* Reading: Gottlob Jungman und Carl Andreas Bruckman.

--- ---. 1822. *Nützliches und sehr bewährt befundenes Weiber-Büchlein*. Ephrata, PA: Samuel Bauman.

--- ---. 1822. *The Heart of Man*. Reading: Henry B. Sage.

--- ---. *Romanus-Büchlein*. Leipzig: Ph. Hülsemann, date unknown. Niedersächsische Staats- und Universitätsbibliothek Göttingen, GDZ, 2010.

--- ---. *Verschiedene sympathetische und geheime Kunst-stücke*. Egypt [Reading]: Stofel Ehrlig, undated. PGCHC Collection.

--- ---. *Verschiedene sympathetische und geheime Kunst-stücke*. Offenbach am Mayn [Reading]: Kalender-Fabrike, 1790. The Library Company of Philadelphia. Evan's Early American Imprints, Series 1, no.46082, American Antiquarian Society and Newsbank, 2002.

--- ---. *Verschiedene sympathetische und geheime Kunststücke*. Offenbach am Mayn [Reading]: Kalender-Fabrike, 1790. (MS.) Heilman Collection.

Adelung, Johann Christoph. 1970. *Grammatisch-kritisches Worterbuch der hochdeutschen Mundart: mit bestandiger Vergleichung der ubrigen Mundarten, besonders aber der oberdeutschen*. Hildesheim: G. Olms. Online 2011-2017. Trier Center for Digital Humanities <www.woerterbuchnetz.de>

Agapkina, Tatiana, Vladimir Karpov and Andrey Toporkov. 2013. "The Slavic and German Versions of the Second Merseburg Charm." *Incantatio: An International Journal on Charms, Charmers and Charming*. (3):43-59.

Albany Township Historical Society. 2014. *Good Land, Good People*. Kempton, PA: Albany Township Historical Society.

Arends, Shirley Fischer. 2016. *The Central Dakota Germans: Their History, Language, and Culture*. [United States]: SFA Publishing.

Arndt, Johann. 1835. *Sechs Bücher vom wahren Christenthum*. Allentown, PA: Augustus Gräter.

Biographical Publishing Company. 1898. *Book of Biographies: This Volume Contains Biographical Sketches of Leading Citizens of Berks County, Pa.* Buffalo, NY: Biographical Pub. Co.

Bötte, Gerd-J., Tannhof, Werner, Karl John Richard Arndt, and Reimer C. Eck. 1989. *The First century of German language printing in the United States of America*. Gottingen: Niedersächsische Staats-und Universitatsbibliothek.

Bailer, Sophia. 1952. "Witches I have known…" *The Pennsylvania Dutchman*. Lancaster, PA: Pennsylvania Dutch Folklore Center, Franklin and Marshall College, IV(1): 8.

Bailer, Sophia. 1947. *The Leininger Family: One of the Oldest in the State and Nation*. Tremont, PA: Mrs. Charles Bailer.

Bainton, Roland. H. 1972. *The Reformation of the Sixteenth Century*. Boston: Beacon Press.

Ballmer, Daniel. 1827. *A Collection of New Receipts and Approved Cures for Man and Beast*. Shellsburg, PA: Frederick Goeb.

Ballmer, Daniel 1827. *Eine Sammlung von Neuen Recepten und Bewährten Curen für Menschen und Vieh*. Schellsburg, PA: Friedrich Goeb.

Baumhauer, Joachim Friedrich. 1984. *Johann Kruse und der "neuzeitliche Hexenwahn": zur Situation eines norddeutschen Aufklärers und einer Glaubensvorstellung im 20. Jahrhundert : untersucht anhand von Vorgängen in Dithmarschen*. Neumünster: Wachholtz.

Bayer, Jacob. 1733. *Paedagogus Latinus Germanae Juventutis sive Lexicon Germanico-Latinum et Latino-Germanicum*. Mainz: Ex Officina Typographica Mayeriana.

Beam, C. Richard, Jennifer L. Trout and Joshua Brown. 2004-2006. *The Comprehensive Pennsylvania German Dictionary*. Vol I-XII. Millersville, PA: Center for Pennsylvania German Studies.

Beam, C. Richard, and Jennifer L. Trout. 2012. *Pennsylvania German Treasures*. Millersville, PA: Center for Pennsylvania German Studies.

Beissel, William. 1938. *Secrets of Sympathy*. Klingerstown: William Beissel.

Beitl, Klaus. 1978. *Volksglaube: Zeugnisse Religiöser Volkskunst*. Salzburg & Wien, AT: Residenz Verlag.

Bentley, James. *A Calendar of Saints*. New York: Facts on File Publications, 1986.

Bernheiser, Richard. 1952. *Wild Men in the Middle Ages*. Cambridge, MA: Harvard University Press.

Bilardi, C. R. 2009. *The Red Church or the Art of Pennsylvania German Braucherei*. Sunland, CA: Pendraig Publishing.

Bischoff, Erich. 1903. *Die Kabbalah: Einführung in die jüdische Mystik und Geheimwissenschaft*. Leipzig: Grieben.

Black, Monia. 2016 "Witchdoctors Drive Sportscars, Science Takes the Bus: An Anti-Superstition Alliance Across a Divided Germany." *Science, Religion, and Communism in Cold War Europe*. Eds. Paul Betts & Stephen A. Smith. London: Palgrave Macmillan.

Boyer, Dennis. 2004. *Once Upon a Hex: A Spiritual Ecology of the Pennsylvania Germans*. Oregon, Wis: Badger Books.

Brendle, Thomas. 1995. *The Thomas R. Brendle Collection of Pennsylvania German Folklore*. Ed. C. Richard Beam. Schaefferstown, PA: Historic Schaefferstown, Inc.

Brendle, Thomas R. and William Troxell. 1944. *Pennsylvania German Folk-Tales, Legends, Once-Upon-a-Time Stories, Maxims, and Sayings: Spoken in the Dialect Popularly Known as Pennsylvania Dutch*. Norristown, PA: Pennsylvania German Society.

Breul, Karl. 1906. *Heath's German and English Dictionary*. Boston; New York; Chicago: D. C. Heath & Co.

Brewer, Ebenezer Cobham. 1894. *A Dictionary of Miracles: Imitative, Realistic, and Dogmatic*. Philadelphia, J. B. Lippincott Co.

Brinton, George. 1955. "Des Bucklich Mennli." *Pennsylvania Dutch Folk Songs*. LP record, Album No. FA 2215. New York: Folkways Records and Service Corp, 2.

Bronner, Simon. 2006. "'Heile, Heile, Hinkel Dreck': On the Earthiness of Pennsylvania German Folk Narratives." *Preserving Heritage: A Festschrift for C. Richard Beam*, ed. Joshua R. Brown and Leroy T.

Hopkins, Jr. Lawrence, Kansas: Society for German-American Studies, 77-100.

Brown, Carleton F. 1904. "The Long Hidden Friend," *The Journal of American Folklore*. American Folklore Society & University of Illinois. XVII (65). <http://www.jstor.org/stable/533169>

Brown, Peter. 1981. *The Cult of the Saints: Its Rise and Function in Latin Christianity*. Chicago, IL: University of Chicago Press.

Brubaker, Henry C. 1928. "Witch Murderer Under Suspicion in Girl's Slaying." Philadelphia, PA: *Philadelphia Inquirer*, 2 Dec.

Brugsch, Heinrich. 1888. *Religion und Mythologie der alten Aegypter*. Leipzig: J. C. Hinrichs'sche Buchhandlung.

Buchholz, W. 1956. "ABRACADABRA." *Zeitschrift Für Religions- Und Geistesgeschichte*, VIII(3), 257-259.

Budge, E. A. Wallace. 1961. *Amulets and Talismans*. New York: University Books.

Burgert, Annette K. 1992. *Eighteenth Century Emigrants from the Northern Alsace to America*. Camden, ME: Picton Press.

Burr, George Lincoln. 1907. "The Witch-Persecutions." *Translations and Reprints from the Original Sources of European History*. Philadelphia, PA: Dept. of History, University of Pennsylvania. III(4).

Cazden, Robert E. 1975. "The German Book Trade in Ohio Before 1848" *Ohio History Journal*, LXXX4:(1 & 2) 57-77.

Chacon, Richard J. and Rubén G. Mendoza. 2012. *The Ethics of Anthropology and Amerindian Research: Reporting on Environmental Degradation and Warfare*. New York: Springer.

Champlin, E. 1981. "Serenus Sammonicus." *Harvard Studies in Classical Philology*, 85, 189-212.

Chelule, P. K., Mokgatle, M. M., Zungu, L. I., & Chaponda, A. 2014. *Caregivers' Knowledge and Use of Fermented Foods for Infant and Young Children Feeding in a Rural Community of Odi, Gauteng Province, South Africa*. Health Promotion Perspectives, 4(1), 54–60.

Clebsch, William A., and Charles R. Jaekle. 1964. *Pastoral Care in Historical Perspective: An Essay with Exhibits*. Englewood Cliffs, NJ: Prentice-Hall.

Cavender, Anthony P. 2003. *Folk medicine in southern Appalachia*. Chapel Hill: University of North Carolina Press.

Christmann, Ernst, Julius Krämer, Rudolf Post, and Josef Schwing. 1965. *Pfälzisches Wörterbuch*. (PfWB) Wiesbaden: Franz Steiner.

Cresswell, Elsie Gehris. 1957. "Aunt Sybilla." *The Pennsylvania Dutchman*. VIII(2). Lancaster, PA: Pennsylvania Dutch Folklore Center, Franklin and Marshall College.

Croll, M. Margaretha. 1826. *Eine Sammlung Auserlesener Rezepte heilsamer Mittel bey krankheiten der Menschen und des Vieh zu gebrauchen*. Reading, PA: Heinrich B. Sage.

Culpeper, Nicholas. 2011. *Culpeper's Complete Herbal & English Physician*. Bedford, MA: Applewood Books.

Davies, Owen and Timothy Easton. 2016. "Cunning Folk and the Production of Magical Artefacts." *Physical Evidence for Ritual Acts, Sorcery and Witchcraft in Christian Britain: A Feeling for Magic*. Ed. Hutton, Ronald. Houndmills, Basingstoke, Hampshire: Palgrave Macmillan.

Davies, Owen. 2013. *America Bewitched: the Story of Witchcraft After Salem*. Oxford: Oxford University Press.

Deigendesch, Johannes. 1837. N*achrichter's Nützliches und Aufrichtiges Pferd- oder Roßarzneybuch*. Lancaster, Pa.: Johann Baer.

Dickel, Horst. 1979. "Wortzauber in Wittgenstein."*Blätter für Wittgensteiner Heimatvereins*, XLIII.

Donmoyer, Patrick J. 2017. *Powwowing in Pennsylvania: Healing Rituals of the Dutch Country*. Kutztown, PA: Pennsylvania German Cultural Heritage Center, Kutztown University of Pennsylvania & Glencairn Museum.

Donmoyer, Patrick. 2016 "Joseph H. Hageman: Doctor, *Braucher*, Legend in *Hexe-Schteddel*." *Historical Review of Berks County*. 81(1) Winter 2015-2016. Reading, PA: Berks History Center.

Donmoyer, Patrick J. 2015. *Powwowing in Pennsylvania: Healing, Cosmology and Tradition in the Dutch Country*. Kutztown, PA: Pennsylvania German Cultural Heritage Center, Kutztown University of Pennsylvania & Schwenkfelder Library and Heritage Center.

Donmoyer, Patrick J. 2014 "The Concealment of Blessings in Pennsylvania Barns," *Historical Archaeology: Manifestations of Magic: The Archaeology and Material Culture of Folk Religion*. Montclair, NJ: Society for Historical Archaeology, XL(6):179-195.

Donmoyer, Patrick J. 2013. *Hex Signs: Myth and Meaning in Pennsylvania Dutch Barn Stars*. Kutztown, PA: Pennsylvania German Cultural Heritage Center, Kutztown University of Pennsylvania.

Donmoyer, Patrick J. 2012a. *Der Freund in der Noth, or The Friend in Need: An Annotated Translation of an Early Pennsylvania Folk-Healing Manual*. Kutztown: Pennsylvania German Cultural Heritage Center, Kutztown University of Pennsylvania.

Donmoyer, Patrick J. 2012b. "A Translation of Dr. Hageman's Estella May Boyer Blessing Manuscript." *Heritage Center News*. No 54, Winter/Spring. Kutztown, PA: Pennsylvania German Cultural Heritage Center, Kutztown University of Pennsylvania.

Donmoyer, Patrick J. 2012c. "Conrad Raber His Docter Book" A Translation of an Early Berks County Veterinary Healing Manual. *Heritage Center News*, No 55, Spring/Summer. Kutztown, PA: Pennsylvania German Cultural Heritage Center, Kutztown University of Pennsylvania.

Donmoyer, Patrick. 2011. "The Pennsylvania German Broadsheet *Frauen Traum & Himmelsriegel*." *Heritage Center News*, No 52. Pennsylvania German Cultural Heritage Center, Kutztown University of Pennsylvania.

Donmoyer, Patrick J. 2010. "An English Translation of a Kutztown Broadside." *Heritage Center News*, No 50. Kutztown: Pennsylvania German Cultural Heritage Center, Kutztown University of Pennsylvania.

Dorson, Richard M. 1983. *Handbook of American folklore*. Bloomington: Indiana University Press.

Duffin, Christopher J. 2011. "Herbert Toms (1874-1940), Witch Stones, and "Porosphaera" Beads." *Folklore* CXXII(1): 84-101.

Dyer, T. F. Thiselton. 1881. *Domestic Folklore*. London: Cassel, Petter & Galpin.

Early, J. W. 1902. *Lutheran Ministers of Berks County: Sketches of the Lives of Those Who Have Lived and Labored in this County*. Reading, Pa. Central Lutheran League.

Earnest, Russell D., Corinne P. Earnest, and Edward L. Rosenberry. 2005. *Flying Leaves and One-Sheets: Pennsylvania German Broadsides, Fraktur, and Their Printers*. New Castle, DE: Oak Knoll Press.

Eliot, John and Matthew Mayhew. 2008. *Tears of Repentance: or, A Further Narrative of the Progress of the Gospel Amongst the Indians in New-England...* Ann Arbor, MI & Oxford, UK: Early English Books Online <http://name.umdl.umich.edu/A84357.0001.001>

Ellis, Bill. 1995. "Kurt E. Koch and the '*Civitas Diaboli*': Germanic Folk Healing as Satanic Ritual Abuse of Children." *Western Folklore* LIV(2): 77-94.

Ensminger, Robert F. 2003. *The Pennsylvania Barn Its Origin, Evolution, and Distribution in North America*. Baltimore: The Johns Hopkins University Press.

Erich, Oswald A. & Beitl, Richard. 1936. *Wörterbuch der deutschen Volkskunde*. Leipzig: Alfred Kroner Verlag.

Ermentrout, John S. 1876. 1776-1876 A Centennial Memorial Historical Sketch of Kutztown & Maxatawny, Berks County, Penn'a. Kutztown, PA: Urick & Gehring's Steam Job Print.

Earnest, Russell D. and Corrine P. Earnest. 2005. *Flying Leaves and One-Sheets*. New Castle, De.: Oak Knoll Press.

Evans, John. 1887. *The Ancient Stone Implements, Weapons, and Ornaments of Great Britain*. London & Bombay: Longmans, Green & Co.

Everhart, James B. 1868. Poems. Philadelphia: J. B. Lippincott & Co,

Fabian, Monroe H. 1972. "The Easton Bible Artist Identified." *Pennsylvania Folklife*. Lancaster, PA: Pennsylvania Folklife Society, XXII(2): 2-14.

Fennell, Christopher C. 2010. *Crossroads and Cosmologies: Diasporas and Ethnogenesis in the New World*. Gainesville, FL: Univ. Press of Florida.

Fischer, Heinrich Ludwig. 1791. *Das Buch vom Aberglauben*. Leipzig: Schwickertschen Verlag.

Fishwick, Duncan. 1964. "On the Origin of the Rotas-Sator Square." *The Harvard Theological Review*. Cambridge: Cambridge University Press, LVII(1) 39-53.

Fogel, Edwin Miller. 1995. *Beliefs and Superstitions of the Pennsylvania Germans*. Editor C. Richard Beam. Millersville, PA: Center for Pennsylvania German Studies, Millersville University.

Fogel, Edwin Miller. 1995. *Proverbs of the Pennsylvania Germans*. Editor C. Richard Beam. Millersville, PA: Center for Pennsylvania German Studies, Millersville University.

Fogel, Edwin M. 1908. "The Himmelsbrief." *German American Annals*, X: 286-314.

Folkard, Richard. 1884. *Plant Lore, Legends, and Lyrics: Embracing the Myths, Traditions, Superstitions, and Folk-lore of the Plant Kingdom*. London: Sampson Low, Marston, Searle, and Rivington.

Franz, Adolph. 1960. *Die Kirchlichen Benediktionen im Mittelalter*. Band I & II. Graz, AT: Akademische Druck- und. Verlagsanstalt.

Freudenthal, Herbert. 1931. *Das Feuer im deutschen Glauben und Brauch*. Berlin & Leipzig: Walter de Gruyter & Co.

Galllee, J. H. 1887. "Segensprüche" *Germania: Vierteljahrsschrift für deutsche alterthumskunde*, XXXII. Wien: Verlag von Carl Gerold's Sohn.

Gandee, Lee R. 1971. *Strange experience; the Autobiography of a Hexenmeister*. Englewood Cliffs, N.J.: Prentice-Hall.

Gerstenbergk, Heinrich von. 1850. *Buch der Wunder und der Geheimnisse der Natur*. Leipzig: Otto Spamer.

Gibbons, Phoebe Earl. 2001. *Pennsylvania Dutch and Other Essays*. Edited and with a foreword by Don Yoder. Stackpole Books, Mechanicsburg.

Ginzburg, Carlo. 1992. *The Night Battles: Witchcraft and Agrarian Cults*. Baltimore: Johns Hopkins University Press.

Good, James I. 1899. H*istory of the Reformed Church in the U.S., 1725-92*. Reading, Pa.

Good, James I. & William John Hinke, and John Philip Boehm. 1903. *Minutes and letters of the Coetus of the German Reformed congregations in Pennsylvania, 1747-1792 Together with Three Preliminary reports of Rev. John Philip Boehm, 1734-1744*. Philadelphia: Reformed Church Publication Board.

Goodling, Evans C., Jr. 2015. *Brecknock: Early History and Biographical Annals of Brecknock Township, Berks County, Pa*. Reading: Reading Eagle Press.

Goodrum, Matthew R. 2008. "Questioning Thunderstones and Arrowheads: The Problem of Recognizing and Interpreting Stone Artifacts in the Seventeenth Century." *Early Science and Medicine*. XIII(5): 482-508.

Graves, Thomas E. 1985. *The Pennsylvania German Hex Sign: A Study in Folk Process*. Dissertation, University of Pennsylvania.

Grimm, Jacob, and Wilhelm Grimm. 1854. *Deutsches Wörterbuch von Jacob Grimm und Wilhelm Grimm*. (DWB) Leipzig: S. Hirzel. Online 2011-2017. Trier Center for Digital Humanities <www.woerterbuchnetz.de>

Grimm, Jacob. 1883. *Teutonic Mythology*. Translated by James Steven Stallybrass. I-III. London: George Bell & Son.

Hampp, Irmgard. 1961. *Beschwörung, Segen, Gebet; Untersuchungen zum Zauberspruch aus dem Bereich der Volksheilkunde*. Stuttgart: Silberburg-Verlag.

Harms, Daniel and John George Hohman. 2012. *The Long-Lost friend: A Nineteenth Century American Grimoire*. Woodbury, Mn: Llewellyn Publications.

Harper, Douglas. 2001-2017. "Powwow," *Online Etymological Dictionary*. <http://www.etymonline.com/index.php?term=powwow>

Hartland, Edwin S. 1895. *The Legend of Perseus: A Study of Tradition in Story Custom and Belief*. London: Nutt, 178 -183.

Hartman, George. 1949. "A Hex, the Devil, and a Farmer." *The Pennsylvania Dutchman*. Lancaster, PA: Pennsylvania Dutch Folklore Center, Franklin and Marshall College. I(1): 2.

Heeger, Fritz. 1936. *Pfälzer Volksheilkunde: Ein Beitrag zur Volkskunde der Westmark*. Verlag Daniel Meiniger, Neustadt an der Weinstraße.

Heindel, Ned. 2005. *Hexenkopf: History, Healing, and Hexerei*. Easton, PA: Williams Township Historical Society.

Helfenstein, Georg Friedrich. [1810]. *Soli Deo Gloria*. [No publishing place], PA: G. F. Helfenstein.

Helfenstein, Georg Friedrich. [1830]. *Georg F. Helfenstein's Sympathie; Eine Sammlung verzüglicher Heilmittel und Rezepte Für verschiedene Krankheiten der Menschen und des Viehes und andere Fälle, Gedruckt für den Herausgeber*. [No publishing place], PA: G. F. Helfenstein.

Helfenstein, Georg Friedrich. 1853. *Vielfältig Erprobter Hausschatz der Sympathie, Oder Enhüllte Zauberkräfte und Geheimnisse der Natur*. Harrisburg: Scheffer & Beck.

Helffrich, William A. 1906. *Lebensbild aus dem Pennsylvanisch-Deutschen Predigerstand: Oder Wahrheit in Licht und Schatten*. Allentown, PA: N. W. A. & W. A. Helffrich.

Herbermann, C. G. 1973. *The Catholic Encyclopedia: An International Work of Reference on the Constitution, Doctrine, Discipline, and History of the Catholic Church*. New York: Encyclopedia Press. <http://www.newadvent.org/cathen/13163a.htm>

Herr, Karl. 2002. *Hex and Spellwork: the Magical Practices of the Pennsylvania Dutch*. York Beach, ME: Red Wheel/Weiser.

Heywood, John. *The Proverbs, Epigrams, and Miscellanies of John Heywood*. Farmer, John S., editor. London: Early English Drama Society, 1906.

Hirte, Tobias. *Der Freund in der Noth, Oder Zweyter Theil, des Neuen Auserlesenen Gemeinnützigen Hand-Büchleins*. Philadelphia: Peter Leibert, 1793, The Library Company of Philadelphia.

Heatwole, Lewis. J. 1908. *Key to the Almanac, and the Sidereal Heavens*. Scottdale, PA: Mennonite Pub. House.

Höfler, Max. 1899. *Das Jahr im oberbayerischen Volksleben, mit besonderer Berücksichtigung der Volksmedicin*. München: F. Bassermahn.

Hoffman, Bengt R. 1976. *Luther and the Mystics: a Re-Examination of Luther's Spiritual Experience and his relationship to the mystics*. Minneapolis: Augsburg Pub. House.

Hoffmann-Krayer, E., and Hanns Baechtold-Staeubli. 1975. *Handwoerterbuch des deutschen Aberglaubens*. (HDA) Berlin: De Gruyter.

Hohman, Johan Georg. 1813. *Der Freund in der Noth, oder: Geheime Sympathetische Wissenschaft*. Reading, PA: Johann Ritter.

Ho[h]man, Johann George. 1818. *Die Land- und Haus-Apotheke*. Reading, PA: Carl A. Bruckman.

Hohman, Johan Georg. 1819. *Das Evangelium Nicodemus: oder: Gewisser bericht von dem leben, leiden und sterben, unsers heilands Jesu Christi…* Reading, PA: Carl.A. Bruckman.

Hohman, Johann Georg. 1819-1820. *Der lange Verborgene Freund, oder: Getreuer und Christlicher Unterricht für jedermann…* Reading, PA: Carl A. Bruckmann.

Hohman, Johann Georg. 1837. *Der lange Verborgene Schatz und Haus Freund*. Skippacksville, PA: A. Puwelle.

Hohman, John George. 1846. *The Long Secreted Friend*. Harrisburg, PA: John George Hohman.

Hohman, Johann Georg. 1853. *Der Lang Verborgene Freund.* Harrisburg, PA: Scheffer & Beck.

Hohman, John George. 1856. *The Long Lost Friend.* Harrisburg: Theo. F. Scheffer.

Holböck, Ferdinand. 2002. Married Saints and Blesseds Through the Centuries. San Francisco: Ignatius Press.

Hovorka, Oskar von, and A. Kronfeld. 1908. *Vergleichende Volksmedizin; eine Darstellung volksmedizinischer Sitten und Gebräuche, Anschauungen und Heilfaktoren, des Aberglaubens und der Zaubermedizin.* Stuttgart: Strecker & Schröder.

Hufford, David J. 1992. "Folk Medicine in Contemporary America." In *Herbal and Magical Medicine: Traditional Healing Today.* Ed. James Kirkland, Holly F. Matthews, C. W. Sullivan III, and Karen Baldwin. Durham & London: Duke University Press.

Hufford, David J. 1982. *The Terror that Comes in the Night: an Experience-Centered Study of Supernatural Assault Traditions.* Philadelphia: University of Pennsylvania Press.

Hufford, David J. 1976." A New Approach to the 'Old Hag': The Nightmare Tradition Reexamined." *American Folk Medicine.* Ed. Wayland D. Hand. Berkeley, Ca.: University of California Press, 73–85.

Hutton, Ronald. 2012. "Writing the History of Witchcraft: A Personal View." *The Pomegranate.* Sheffield: Equinox Publishing LTD, XII(2): 247.

Ingram, Helen. 2007. *Dragging Down Heaven: Jesus as Magician and Manipulator of Spirits in the Gospels.* Dissertation, University of Birmingham.

Iskra-Chubb, Joanne Flores. 2003. "Reading's Wash Fraus: Powwowing for Three Generations." *Historical Review of Berks County,* LXVIII:3 Summer.

Johanson, Kristina. 2009. "The Changing Meaning of 'Thunderbolts.'" *Folklore,* XLII:129-174.

Julian, John. 1892. *A Dictionary of Hymnology: Setting Forth the Origin and History of Christian Hymns of All Ages and Nations.* New York: Charles Scribner's Sons.

Jung, C. G., and Marie-Luise von Franz. 1968. *Man and His Symbols.* Garden City, N.Y.: Doubleday.

Käfer, Natacha Klein. 2014. "German healing prayers in a transcontinental perspective: the Case of the 'Dreyerley Würm Segen'" TEEME, third annual conference: Contemplating Early Modernities: Concept, Content & Context. Freie Universität Berlin.

Kelker, Luther Reily. 1907. *History of Dauphin County Pennsylvania.* New York & Chicago, IL: Lewis Publishing Co., 351-352.

Kemp, P. 1935. *Healing Ritual; Studies in the Technique and Tradition of the Southern Slavs.* London: Faber and Faber Limited.

Kerr, Kurt and John Stewart. 1983. "*Deutsche Zaubersprüche in Virginia und West Virginia (U. S. A.): Schriftliche Tradition und Mündliche Tradierung.*" *Hessische Blätter für Volks- und Kulturforschung.* Giessen: Wilhelm Schmitz Verlag.

Klein, Holger A. 2011. "Sacred Things and Holy Bodies: Collecting Relics from Late Antiquity to the Early Renaissance." *Treasures of Heaven: Saints, Relics, and Devotion in Medieval Europe.* Ed. Martina Bagnoli, Holger A Klein, C. Griffith Mann, and James Robinson. New Haven & London: Yale University Press.

Klepp, Susan, Whitehead, John Frederick, and Johann Carl Büttner. 2006. *Souls for Sale: Two German Redemptioners Come to Revolutionary America: The Life Stories of John Frederick Whitehead & Johann Carl Büttner.* University Park, PA: Pennsylvania State University Press.

Kloberdanz, Timothy J., and Rosalinda Kloberdanz. 1993. *Thunder on the Steppe: Volga German Folklife in a Changing Russia.* Lincoln, Neb: American Historical Society of Germans from Russia.

Koch, Kurt E. 1969. *The Devil's Alphabet.* Grand Rapids, MI: Kregel Publications.

Kolb, R., T. Wengert, and C. Arand. 2000. "Of the Worship of the Saints." Article 21, *Augsburg Confession.* Minneapolis, MN: Augsburg Fortress.

Kriebel, David W. 2000. *Belief, Power and Identity in Pennsylvania Dutch Brauche, or Powwowing.* Dissertation, University of Pennsylvania. Ann Arbor, MI, UMI Dissertation Services.

Kreissl, Eva. 2014. *Aberglauben Aberwissen: Welt ohne Zufall.* Graz: Universalmuseum Joanneum.

Kruse, Johann. 1951. *Hexen Unter Uns. Magie und Zauberglauben in unserer Zeit.* Hamburg: Verlag Hamburgische Bücherei.

Küffner, Carl. 1866. *Inaugural Dissertation Der Medicinischen Facultät zu Würzburg Nachträglich vom Jahre 1858.* Würzburg: CJ Becker'schen Buchdruckerei.

Kusler, Ruth Weil and Peggy Sailer O'Neil. 1998. *Tender Hands: Ruth's Story of Healing.* Fargo, ND: Germans from Russia Heritage Collection, North Dakota State University Libraries.

Laycock, Joseph P. 2015. *Spirit Possession Around the World: Possession, Communion, and Demon Expulsion Across Cultures.* Santa Barbara, California: ABC-CLIO.

Lambert, M. B. 1977. *Pennsylvania-German Dictionary.* Exton, PA: Schiffer Ltd.

Landis, Gerald. 1969 "Drei Kreizer Messer," *Der Rumlaefer*, Lenhartsville, PA: Pennsylvania Dutch Folk Culture Society, 6-7.

Lea, Henry Charles, Arthur C. Howland, and George Lincoln Burr. 1957. *Materials Toward a History of Witchcraft.* New York: Yoseloff.

Lehman, John H. 1916. *A Standard History of Stark County, Ohio.* Chicago, Il.: Lewis Pub. Co.

Leib, Isaac. 1841. *Wohlerfahrner Pferde-Arzt: enthaltend Mittel für die Heilung aller bekannten und verschiedenartigen Krankheiten und Seuchen der Pferde; welche nach einer fünf und zwanzigjährigen Ausübung der Ross-Heilkunst bewährt und untrüglich befunden wurden.* Lebanon, PA: Joseph Hartman.

Levack, Brian P. 2016, *The Witch-Hunt in Early Modern Europe,* 4th Edition. Abingdon, UK: Routledge, Taylor & Francis Group.

Levack, Brian P. 2014. *The Oxford Handbook of Witchcraft in Early Modern Europe and Colonial America.* New York: Oxford University Press.

Lewis, A. H. 1969. *Hex.* New York, Trident Press.

Liebman, Laura Arnold and Matthew Mayhew. 2008. *Mayhew's Indian Converts: A Cultural Edition.* Amherst, MA: University of Massachusetts Press.

Lindnern, Benjamin. 1745. *Des Hocherleuchteten Mannes Gottes D. Martin Luthers Geist- und Sinn-reiche auserlesene Tisch-Reden un andere erbauliche Gesprache.* Salfeld: Weidemann.

Lommer, Victor. 1878. *Volksthuemliches aus dem Saalthal.* Orlamuende: Verlag von J. F. Heyl.

Long, Amos, Jr. *The Pennsylvania German Family Farm.* Breinigsville: Pennsylvania German Society, 1972.

Louden, Mark. 2016. *Pennsylvania Dutch: The Story of an American Language.* Baltimore: Johns Hopkins University Press.

Luther, Martin. 1910. *Dr. Martin Luthers Sämmtliche Schriften.* St. Louis: Concordia Publishing House.

Luther, Martin. 1828. *Die Bibel, oder die ganze Heilige Schrift des alten und neuen Testaments.* London: W. Clowes.

Luther, Martin. 1828. *Der Psalter des Königs und Propheten David, verdeutscht von Dr. Martin Luther, mit kurzen Summarien oder Inhalt jedes Psalmen.* Philadelphia: Georg. W. Mentz.

Luther, Martin, E T. Bachmann, and Helmut T. Lehmann. 1965. *Luther's Works.* Philadelphia: Fortress Press, XXV.

Luther, Martin, Helmut T. Lehmann, and Hans J. Hillerbrand. 1965. *Luther's Works: Sermons II*, Philadelphia: Fortress Press, LII.

Luther, Martin, and William Hazlitt. 1990. *The Table-Talks of Martin Luther.* Grand Rapids, MI: Christian Classics Ethereal Library.

Lyman, George. 1928. *Witchcraft in old and New England.* Cambridge, Mass: Harvard University Press.

Mackay, Christopher S., and Heinrich Kramer. 2014. *The Hammer of Witches: A Complete Translation of the Malleus Maleficarum.* Cambridge, UK: Cambridge University Press.

Marzell, Heinrich. 2002. *Geschichte und Volkskunde der deutschen Heilpflanzen.* St. Goar: Reichl Verlag.

Mathers, S. Liddell MacGregor. 2012. *The Key of Solomon the King (Clavicula Salomonis).* Cambridge: Cambridge University Press.

M'Clintock, John. 1889. *Cyclopedia of Biblical, Theological and Ecclesiastical Literature,* New York: Harper & Brothers, X: 739.

McCain, Paul Timothy, W. H. T. Dau, and F. Bente. 2009. "Luther's Large Catechism, 1:11." *Concordia: the Lutheran Confessions: A Reader's Edition of the Book of Concord.* St. Louis: Concordia Publishing House.

McGinnis, J. Ross. 2000. *Trials of Hex.* Fawn Grove, PA: Davis/Trinity Pub. Co.

Merrifield, Ralph. 1988. *The Archaeology of Ritual and Magic.* New York: New Amsterdam.

Meyer, Elard Hugo. 1900. *Badisches Volksleben im neunzehnten Jahrhundert.* Straßburg: Karl J. Trübner.

Miller, Daniel. 1906. *Early History of the Reformed Church in Pennsylvania.* Reading, PA: D. Miller.

Mitterauer, Michael. 2000. *Dimensionen des Heiligen: Annäherungen eines Historikers.* Wien: Böhlau Verlag, 83.

Montgomery, Jack G. 2008. *American shamans: journeys with traditional healers.* Ithaca, N.Y.: Busca, Inc.

Morris, John G. 1861. In William B. Sprague. *Annals of the American Lutheran Pulpit.* New York: Robert Carter & Bros.

Moss, Kay. 1998. *Much That May Be Called Domestic: Southern Folk Medicine, 1750-1820.* Columbia, SC: University of South Carolina Press.

Mueller, Joseph. 1928. *Rheinisches Wörterbuch.* (RWB) Bonn: Fritz Klopp.

Muhlenberg, Henry, and B. J. Schipper. 1812. *English-German & German-English Dictionary.* Lancaster, PA: Printed by William Hamilton.

Munro, Joyce Clemmer. 1981. *Willing Inhabitants: A Short Account of Life in Franconia Township, Montgomery County, Pennsylvania.* Franconia, PA: Horace W. Longacre, Inc.

Neff, Larry M. and Frederick S. Weiser. 1979. "Manuscript Powwow Formulas." *Der Reggeboge: Quarterly of the Pennsylvania German Society.* Breinigsville, PA: Pennsylvania German Society. XII (1):3.

Nemec, Helmut. 1976. *Zauberzeichen: Magie im volkstümlichen Bereich.* Wien: Scholl.

Norman, Mark. 2016. *Black Dog Folklore.* London: Troy Books.

Nutting, Wallace. 1924. *Pennsylvania Beautiful.* Framingham, MA: Old America Company Publishers.

Oda, Wilbur H. 1948. "John George Hohman." *The Historical Review of Berks County.* Reading, Historical Society of Berks County, XIII(3).

Ohrt, F. 1922. "Abracadabra." *Journal of the Royal Asiatic Society of Great Britain and Ireland,* (1): 86-88.

Ossman, [Ann] and [Isaac D.]Steel. 1894. *Ossman & Steel's Guide to Health or Household Instructor.* Wiconisco, PA: Ossman & Steel.

Patterson, James. 1835. *Lutheran Observer and Weekly Religious and Literary Visitor.* Baltimore, MD: II(26 New Series).

Pennsylvania, and Samuel Hazard. 1852. *Minutes of the Provincial Council of Pennsylvania: From the Organization to the Termination of the Proprietary Government.* Philadelphia: J. Severns.

Peterson, Joseph H. 2008. *The Sixth and Seventh Books of Moses, or, Moses' Magical Spirit-Arts.* Lake Worth, FL: Ibis Press.

Pfaff, Fridrich. 1892. "Alte Segen Wider Feinde, Wehr, und Waffen." *Allemania: Zeitschrift für Sprache, Kunst und Altertum.* Vol. XIX. Bonn: P. Hansteins Verlag.

Potts, Malcolm, Peter Diggory, and John Peel. 1977. *Abortion.* Cambridge: Cambridge University Press.

Quinter, Edward. E. 2006. *Rosina Barbara Werli Büchlein.* Unpublished translation of the eighteenth Century MS. Lehigh County, Pennsylvania, 2006.

Quinter, Edward E. and Patrick J. Donmoyer. 2012. "The Book of Instructions by Johann Christoph Pyrlaeus Jr.: A Folklife Study of Early Process and Belief. " Unpublished paper, presented at the 2012 Bethlehem Conference on Moravian History and Music.

Quitman, Frederick Henry. 1810. *A Treatise on Magic, or the Intercourse between Spirits and Men.* Albany, NY: Balance Press.

Peuckert, Will-Erich. 1954. "Die egyptischen Geheimnisse." *Journal of Scandinavian Folklore (Tidskrift för Nordisk Folkminnesforskning).* X(10): 40-96.

Raber, W. B. 1855. *The Devil and Some Of His Doings.* Canton, OH: United Brethren in Christ.

Radde, Wilhelm. 1872. *Albertus Magnus bewährte und approbirte sympathetische und natürliche Egyptische Geheimnisse für Menschen und Vieh.* New York: Wilhelm Radde. (AM Radde)

Randolph, Vance. 1964. *Ozark magic and folklore.* New York, N.Y.: Dover Publications.

Rix, Alice. 1900. "The Reading Witch Doctor's Sway Over the Trusting and the Ignorant." Philadelphia, PA: *North American,* 22 May, 129:16.

Roan, Donald. 1964. "Deivel-Dreck (Asafoetida) Yesterday and Today." *Pennsylvania Folklife.* Lancaster, PA: Pennsylvania Folklife Society, XIV(2): 32.

Roper, Jonathan. 2005. *English Verbal Charms.* Ff Communications, No. 288. Helsinki: Suomalainen Tiedeakatemia.

Rupp, Israel Daniel. 1842. *The Farmer's Complete Farrier.* Lancaster, PA: Gilbert Hills.

Sachse, Julius Friedrich. 1970. *The German Pietists of provincial Pennsylvania, 1694-1708.* New York: AMS Press.

Schaff, Philip. 1878. *The Creeds of Christendom: with a History and Critical Notes,* Vol. I. New York: Harper and Brothers Publishers.

Shaner, Richard. 1972. "Recollections of Witchcraft in the Oley Hills." *Pennsylvania Folklife,* XII: Folk Festival Supplement, 39.

Scheible, Johann. 1849. *Das 6te und 7te Buch Moses. Bibliothek der Zauber-Geheimniss- und Offenbarungs-Bücher, und der Wunder-Hausschatz-Literatur aller Nationen in allen ihren Raritäten und Kuriositäten.* Vol. VI. Stuttgart: Johann Scheibel.

Schmid, Johann Christoph. *Schwabisches Wörterbuch.* Stuttgart: E. Schweizerbart's Verlagshandlung, 1831.

Schwan, Christian Friedrich. 1784. *Nouveau Dictionnaire de la Langue Allemande et Françoise,* Vol. II. Mannheim: Schwan et Fontaine.

Scofield, C. I., and Doris Rikkers. 2009. *The Scofield Study Bible: King James Version.* New York: Oxford University Press. (KJV)

Seeligman, Siegfried. 1909. *Der Böse Blick und Verwantes: Ein Beitrag zur Geschichte des Aberglaubens aller Zeiten und Völker.* Berlin: Hermann Barsdorf Verlag.

Sexton, Rocky. 1992. "Cajun and Creole Treaters: Magico-Religious Folk Healing in French Louisiana." *Western Folklore,* Western States Folklore Society, LI(3/4): 237-248.

Seyfarth, Carly. 1913. *Aberglaube und Zauberei in der Volksmedizin Sachsens.* Leipzig: Wilhelm Heims Verlag.

Seymour, William Wood. 1898 *The Cross in Tradition, History, and Art.* New York & London: G. P. Putnam's Sons, The Knickerbocker Press, 94-95.

Shivley, Jacob. 1953. "Betz Heilman, 'Witch'" *The Pennsylvania Dutchman.* Lancaster, PA: Pennsylvania Dutch Folklore Center, Franklin and Marshall College, V(7): 9.

Shoemaker, Alfred Lewis. 2000. *Eastertide in Pennsylvania: A Folk-Cultural Study.* Mechanicsburg, PA: Stackpole Books.

Shoemaker, Alfred. 1960. *Eastertide in Pennsylvania.* Lancaster, PA: Pennsylvania Folklife Society, Franklin & Marshall College.

Shoemaker, Alfred L. 1955. "The Status of Witchcraft in the Pennsylvania Dutch Country Today." *The Pennsylvania Dutchman.* Lancaster, PA: Pennsylvania Dutch Folklore Center, Franklin and Marshall College. IV(18):1-3.

Shoemaker, Alfred Lewis. 1953. *Hex, No!* Lancaster, PA: Pennsylvania Dutch Folklore Center, Inc.

Shoemaker, Alfred L. 1951. "Some Powwow Formulas from Juniata County." *The Pennsylvania Dutchman.* XIII(10): 1.

Shulman, David Dean and Guy G. Stroumsa. 2001. *Self and Self-Transformation in the History of Religions.* NY: Oxford University Press.

Sigerist, Henry E. 1961. A History of Medicine. New York: Oxford University Press.

Skeat, Walter W. 1912. "'Snakestones' and Stone Thunderbolts as Subjects for Systematic Investigation." *Folklore* XXIII(1): 45-80.

Smith, Frank Joseph. 2016. *Religion and Politics in America: An Encyclopedia of Church and State in American Life.* Santa Barbara: ABC-CLIO.

Spinks, Brian D. 1976. "Luther's *Taufbüchlein*." *Liturgical Review.* May XIII(1) Church Service Society. Edinburgh: Scottish Academic Press.

Stadler, Andrea. 2005. *Neuigkeiten aus dem Marktund Schaustellermuseum.* Nr. 4. Essen: Arbeitskreis Kultur und Brauchtum Essen e.V.

Strassburger, Ralph Beaver, and William John Hinke. 1992. *Pennsylvania German pioneers: A Publication of the Original Lists of Arrivals in the Port of Philadelphia from 1727 to 1808.* Camden, Me: Picton Press.

Stine, E. S. 1996. *Pennsylvania German Dictionary.* Birdsboro, PA: The Pennsylvania German Society.

Strassburger, Ralph Beaver, and William John Hinke. 1992. *Pennsylvania German Pioneers: A Publication of the Original Lists of Arrivals in the Port of Philadelphia from 1727 to 1808.* Baltimore: Genealogical Pub. Co.

Spamer, Adolf, and Johanna Nickel. 1958. *Romanusbüchlein: historisch-philologischer Kommentar zu einem deutschen Zauberbuch.* Berlin: Akad.-Verlag.

Stevens, G. R. 1973. "Jurassic belemnites." *Atlas of Palaeobiogeography.* Amsterdam: Elsevier.

Stoudt, John Joseph. 1973. *Sunbonnets and Shoofly Pies: A Pennsylvania Dutch Cultural History*. New York: Castle Books.

Stoudt, John Joseph. 1973. *Sunbonnets and Shoofly Pies: A Pennsylvania Dutch Cultural History*. New York: Castle Books.

Summers, Montague. 1956. *The history of witchcraft and demonology.* New Hyde Park, NY: University Books.

Suter, Paul. 1989. "Himmels- und Schutzbriefe im Baselbiet." *Zeitschrift Schweizerisches Archiv für Volkskunde: Fest und Brauch: Festschrift für Eduard Strübin zum 75. Geburtstag.* Archives suisses des traditions populaires, LXXXV: 1-2.

Tetzner, Friedrich. 1902. "Werdauer Altertümer." *Mittheilungen des Vereins für Sächsische Volkskunde.* II(11).

Thurston, Robert. 2013 *The Witch Hunts: A History of the Witch Persecutions in Europe and North America.* NY: Routledge.

Tillich, Paul. 1951. *Systematic Theology.* Chicago, IL: University of Chicago Press.

Tillich, Paul. 1968. *A History of Christian Thought.* New York: Harper & Row.

Trachtenberg, Joshua. 1939. *Jewish Folk Magic and Superstition.* New York: Behrman's Jewish Book House.

Weaver, William Woys. 2013. *As American as Shoofly Pie: the Foodlore and Fakelore of Pennsylvania Dutch Cuisine.* Philadelphia: University of Pennsylvania Press.

Weaver, William Woys. 2001. *Sauer's Herbal Cures: America's First Book of Botanic Healing, 1762-1778.* New York: Routledge. English translation of Sauer, Christopher. 1762-1778. *Kurtzgefasstes Kräuterbuch.* Germantown, PA: Christopher Saur.

Weaver, William Woys. 1993. *Pennsylvania Dutch Country Cooking.* New York: Abbeville Press.

Webster, Noah. 1861. "Powwow." *The American Dictionary of the English Language.* Springfield, MA: George and Charles Meriam.

Weller, Philip T. 1964. *Rituale Romanum: Complete Edition.* Milwaukee, WI: The Bruce Publishing Company.

Wellenreuther, Hermann. 2013. *Citizens in a Strange Land: A Study of German-American Broadsides and Their Meaning for Germans in North America, 1730-1830.* University Park: Penn State Press.

Wilson, Stephen. 2004. *The Magical Universe: Everyday Ritual and Magic in Pre-Modern Europe.* London: Hambledon and London.

Wintemberg, W. J. 1950. "Folklore of Waterloo County, Ontario." *National Museum of Canada Bulletin No. 116,* Anthropological Series No. 14. Ottowa, CA: Department of Resources and Development.

Wood, Robert. 2014. "Three Cross Knife." *Berksmont News.* 03/23/2014. http://www.berksmontnews.com/article/BM/20140323/NEWS/140329978

Wood, Ralph Charles. 1986. "*Das bucklige Maennlein.*" Historic Schaefferstown Record. Schaefferstown, PA: Historic Schaefferstown, Inc., XX(1): 3-12.

Woyts, Johan Jacob. 1761. *Gazophylacium Medico-Physicum oder Schatz-Kammer medicinisch- und natürlicher Dinge.* Leipzig: Lankischens Buchhandlung.

Wunderlin, Dominik. 2005. *Mittel zum Heil: Religiöse Segens- und Schutzzeichen in der Sammlung Dr. Edmund Müller. Haus zum Dolder, Sammlung Dr. Edmund Müller.* Beromünster: Wallimann Druck & Verlag AG

Yoder, Don. 2016. *The German Bible in America: An Exploration of the Religious and Cultural Legacy of the First European-Language Bible in America.* Ed. Patrick J. Donmoyer. Kutztown, PA: Pennsylvania German Cultural Heritage Center, Kutztown University of Pennsylvania.

Yoder, Don. 2015. *Discovering American Folklife: Essays on Folk Culture and the Pennsylvania Dutch.* Kutztown, PA: Pennsylvania German Cultural Heritage Center, Kutztown University of Pennsylvania

Yoder, Don. 2005. The Pennsylvania German Broadside: A History and Guide. University Park: Penn State University Press.

Yoder, Don, and Thomas. E. Graves. 2000. *Hex signs: Pennsylvania Dutch Barn Symbols and Their Meaning.* Mechanicsburg, PA: Stackpole Books.

Yoder, Don. 1976. "Hohman and Romanus: Origins and Diffusion of the Pennsylvania German Powwow Manual," American Folk Medicine: A Symposium. Ed. Wayland D. Hand. London: University of California Press.

Yoder, Don. 1965. "Official Religion Versus Folk Religion." *Pennsylvania Folklife* 15(2) (Winter 1965-1966): 234-236.

Don Yoder. ca. 1964. *Occult Folk Medicine Among the Pennsylvania Germans.* Transcript of an address at the University of Pennsylvania, unpublished paper.

Yoder, Don. 1952. "Sophia Bailer Speaks II." Recorded at the Third Annual Pennsylvania Dutch Folk Festival, Kutztown, 1952: A Transcript.

Yoder, Don. 1951. "Sophia Bailer Speaks …" Recorded at the Second Annual Pennsylvania Dutch Folk Festival, Kutztown, 1951: A Transcript.

INDEX

abracadabra   92, 152

Adams County   47, 48, 157, 223, 317, 322

Albert the Great, St.   102, 103, 116, 127, 135, **137-141**, 150, 155, 159, 161, 162, 167, 172, 179, 200, 211, 218, 220-222, 237, 251, 269, 272, 274, 276, 308, 313-316, 321-323, 327-329, 331, 335,

Albertus Magnus (see Albert the Great, St.)

alder buckthorn   139, 141, 204, 205

Algonquian language   29

Allentown   84, 111, 162, 177, 181, 217, 222, 241, 243. 244. 251, 308, 309, 311, 313, 315,316, 319, 321, 322, 324-326, 328, 329, 331, 333,

Allermansharnisch-Wurzel (see Victorialis)

almanac   24, 83, 86, 102, 127, 131, 135, 136, 157, 174, 197, 260, 265, 266, 311, 327, 333

Amish   18, 29, 199, 253, 254, 313, 320

Alsace   29, 148, 226, 267, 315, 320, 332.

Anabaptist   29, 83

angel   23, 63, 73-77, 100, 101, 106, 115, 127, 129, 132, 135, 141, 145, 149, 192, 241, 273, 278, 287, 289, 291, 292, 295, 298, 299, 300, 306

animals, healing of & use in ritual   33, 38, 49, 65-67, 69, 85, 86, 92, 102, 106, 108-109, 138-141, 144-146, 151, 154-157, 163, 166, 175, 177, 178, 203-204, 210-211, 219, 227, 255, 263-264, 269-274, 284, 292, 302-303

Anne, St.   63

ant   271, 275

apple   198-199, 211, 255, 260, 277

archangel   77, 100, 106, 139, 277

asafetida   94, 177, 204, 274

asaphoetida (see asafetida)

Ascension Day   105, 199, 262, 268

asperfidity (see asafetida)

attic   23, 106, 270, 329

baby   50, 52, 90, 135, 177, 185, 188-190, 198, 213, 238, 258-260, 301

bacon   26, 33, 104, 199, 215, 269

Baer, Johann   267, 311, 327, 332

Bailer, Sophia (nee Leininger)   20, 38, 51-54, 98, 111, 112, 117-119, 130, 156, 159, 191-193, 283, 308-309, 314, 320, 331

bakeoven   56, 102, 106, 108, 207, 261, 263, 268, 269

baking   16, 104, 261, 262, 265-268, 271

Ballmer, Daniel   136, 157-159, 163, 315, 317, 321

baptism   40, 41, 64, 66, 102, 105, 113, 118, 120, 137, 139, 144, 146, 157, 169, 259, 278, 287, 288, 312, 324, 327, 329

bark   49, 86, 154, 197, 198, 210, 211, 278

barn   18, 19, 20, 23, 26, 59, 83, 99, 103-106, 119, 144, 158, 177-179, 180-182, 205, 207, 221, 223-225, 232, 258, 261, 264, 271, 320

barn blessing   177-183

barn star   19, 20, 180-183, 320

bat   274, 275

bean   24, 204, 208

Beissel, William   20-21, 168-169, 316, 319

bell, church   88, 105, 281

bepispeln   81

Berks County   13, 16, 18, 19, 26, 30, 35-39, 42, 45, 46, 49, 51, 54, 56, 57, 103, 107-109, 115, 116 120 122, 125, 128, 129, 133, 134, 137, 148, 149, 154, 155, 157, 158, 163, 174, 177, 179-187, 190, 195, 198, 199, 202-205, 208, 212, 214, 216, 217, 219-229, 231-232, 234-236, 259, 261, 262-264, 266, 269, 271, 273-275, 278, 308, 309, 310, 311, 313, 315-317, 319-324, 327, 328, 331-336

beschwatze   82

Bible   29, 34, 41, 45, 54, 60, 63, 65, 91, 93, 94, 105, 108, 112, 113, 118, 120, 124, 127, 130, 135, 136, 163, 166, 167, 192, 215, 217, 218, 227, 228, 235, 252, 259, 260, 261, 280, 308, 314

bier, funeral   277

blood   36, 37, 39, 40, 41, 48, 54, 59, 66, 77, 79, 85, 86, 87, 88, 90, 91, 95, 100, 104, 109, 110, 116, 129, 130, 136, 137-140, 143-145, 149, 153, 154, 156, 158, 177, 178, 182, 186, 191, 192, 199-222, 229, 239, 240, 244, 248, 258, 259, 269, 270, 276, 277, 278, 281, 288, 291, 294, 296-303, 307, 315

blowing burns   48, 49, 157,

Blymire, John H.   47, 56, 230, 244-250, 252, 325, 326

Blymyre (see Blymire, John H.)

337

Bohr, Nicholas   167, 168, 316, 318, 319

Bolmer, Paul   159, 317

brauche   26, 29, 81, 82, 83, 257, 258

Brazil   9, 16, 21, 24, 108, 307,

bread   19, 37, 38, 60, 82, 94, 101, 104, 105, 109, 138, 204, 205, 220, 221, 256, 258, 259, 261, 262, 264, 265, 267, 268, 269, 271, 274, 275, 279, 288, 295, 300, 329

Brethren   29, 39, 40, 146, 185, 197, 234, 308, 320, 335

Breverl (*Brevia, Brief*)   62, 70, 76, 224

Brigid, name   82

Brigid, St.   60, 144, 149, 150

broadside   39, 41, 61, 65, 72, 73, 77, 79, 83, 90, 114, 116, 127, 141, 142, 144, 146, 147, 149, 162, 168, 210, 211, 284, 307, 308, 310, 313, 314, 316, 317, 318, 320, 321, 328, 329

broom   15, 23, 65, 99, 103, 215, 259, 261, 262

Bruckman, Carl A.   134, 136, 147-149, 150, 307, 310, 315, 316, 317, 327

Brunner, Dr. Stanley A.   36, 38, 88, 94, 114, 130, 308, 252, 274, 281

bullet   160, 184, 185, 195, 208

Bumbaugh, Lamar (Mountain Bummy)   214, 216, 229

burns   23, 37, 48, 49, 50, 60, 63, 64, 67, 70, 82, 85, 86, 103, 104, 107, 108, 114, 115, 117, 129, 135, 143, 144, 152, 153, 154, 156, 157, 160, 172, 173, 183, 185, 186, 187, 189, 192, 224, 281

butchering   26, 49, 50, 109, 255, 261, 270, 271

butter   37, 38, 65, 105, 138, 176, 177, 183, 202, 206, 217, 219, 220, 228, 255, 265, 271, 300, 304, 323, 326

cancer   35, 45, 85, 243, 278

cane   105, 214-219, 227, 273, 322

Carbon County   40, 241, 243

carving   215-219, 227, 228, 323

Caspar, Melchior, Balthasar (see Three Kings)

cat   14, 170, 184, 221, 251, 252, 260, 267, 272, 311, 328, 338

cemetery (see graveyard)

chair   14, 29, 120, 122, 123, 185, 229, 247, 250, 323

chicken   26, 94, 153, 213, 224, 258, 261, 270, 271, 298

childhood   13, 15, 28, 34, 42, 46, 64, 85, 109, 187, 193, 198, 199, 223, 228, 244, 259, 262, 271, 279

chimney   108, 115, 116, 207, 274

Christ, Jesus   28, 40, 50, 52, 54, 59, 61, 63, 64, 65, 69, 72, 73, 75, 76, 79, 81, 86-91, 94, 95, 101, 102, 106, 108, 110, 111-114, 118, 119, 124, 125, 129, 136, 143-146, 149, 150, 152, 156, 160, 182, 192, 198, 207, 210, 211, 219, 221, 224, 229, 240, 241, 258, 262, 266, 269, 272, 273, 281, 286-306, 308, 314, 317, 318, 320, 335

Christmas   105, 138, 152, 195, 221, 256, 261, 264, 265, 270, 274

church   9, 13, 18, 29, 38, 39, 40, 42, 44, 49, 50, 57, 64, 67-71, 73, 75, 77, 79, 80, 88, 91, 93, 94, 96, 105, 120, 125, 129, 131, 138, 149, 150, 155, 160, 181, 185, 192, 193, 199, 216, 220, 223, 229, 232, 240, 246, 248, 259, 264, 265, 268, 270, 280, 281, 308, 315-318, 320, 323, 324,

coals   102, 103, 144, 204, 205, 267, 268, 296, 300, 338

colic   15, 28, 39, 64, 82, 89, 100, 167, 188, 204, 258, 259, 261, 268, 269, 295, 302, 304, 307

communion   39, 77, 105, 120, 120, 274, 311, 329

corn   25, 103, 108, 155, 255, 267, 270, 326

cow   103, 105, 145, 146, 177, 178, 183, 186, 192, 207, 221, 222, 271, 300, 304, 305

Croll, M. Margaretha   155, 156, 317, 327, 332

cross   13, 18, 24, 28, 29, 60, 64, 69, 71, 75, 76, 77, 79, 80, 83, 87, 89, 95, 96, 100-103, 110, 114, 121, 122, 146, 149, 161, 171, 181, 198, 209, 219-223, 228, 238-240, 258, 262, 268, 269, 270, 274, 287, 288, 291, 294-296, 314, 316

crossroads   26, 38, 106, 195, 208, 219, 220

crown of thorns   149, 205

Cumberland County   177, 320

currant   199

Curry, John   230, 244-248, 250

curse   18, 27, 47, 60, 64, 65, 71, 73, 107, 108, 11, 125, 132, 139, 144, 169, 175, 176, 183, 184, 185, 186, 187, 188, 189, 190, 191, 194, 218, 219, 220, 229, 238, 244-251, 254, 262, 264, 271, 273, 281, 293, 319

cypher   131, 132, 135, 210, 328

dandelion   148, 199, 278

Datsch   267

days of the week   77, 265

death   28, 43-45, 47, 59, 60, 61, 69, 75, 77, 81, 88, 90, 101, 109, 125, 147, 149, 176, 184, 189, 190, 191, 203, 226, 249, 251, 253, 254, 264, 279-281, 287, 288, 302, 325, 326

de Claremont Publishing Co.   169, 170, 319

DeLawrence Publishing Co.   169, 329

Delp, Verna   251-253

demon   71, 179, 252, 320

devil   40, 42, 59, 62, 64-66, 69, 70, 85, 87, 132, 138, 139, 141, 171, 175, 177, 191, 192, 193, 195, 203, 210, 211, 219, 220, 240, 249, 254, 308, 319

dew   33, 105, 124, 177, 256, 260, 264, 271, 315

dialect (see Pennsylvania Dutch language)

dish cloth   15, 26, 104, 177, 215, 271

dog   30, 38, 60, 81, 92, 94, 104, 108, 109, 138, 147, 202, 212, 220, 224, 269, 273, 276, 322

dogwood   197, 198

doll   124, 146, 147, 165, 212, 213, 236, 245, 246, 249, 305, 322

DRAGON   87, 88, 135, 164

Dream, Our Dear Lady's (Frauentraum)   76, 77, 79, 150, 179

drunkard, cures for   276, 277

east   14, 90, 120, 122, 123, 136, 143, 167, 194, 209, 212, 245, 268, 281, 293, 294, 314

Easton   9, 94, 162, 314, 318, 322, 332, 333

eaves   13, 25, 89, 105, 106, 107, 156, 229, 270

Eberly, Sophia Leininger (Niece of Sophia Bailer)   51-54, 191

Eberth, Catherine   49, 50, 51, 234

egg   85, 99, 103, 213, 258, 270, 275, 299

Egyptian Secrets   127, 137-139, 141, 145, 150, 151, 154, 162, 167, 171, 173, 179, 205, 219, 220, 222, 276, 308, 313, 315, 316, 322, 327, 329, 331

elderberry   197, 198, 199, 211, 220, 259, 278, 322

Ember Days   43, 266

erysipelas (Wildfeier)   35, 39, 85, 86, 88, 98, 102, 115, 116, 117, 135, 136, 137,143, 156, 166, 198, 199, 220, 221, 268, 293, 296

exorcism   64, 66, 68-72, 101, 116, 138, 186

Ezekiel   36, 39-41, 54, 102, 120, 308

farrier   49, 102, 116, 202, 269, 313, 320, 335

fasnacht   23, 158, 266, 270

feet   26, 65, 72, 85, 86, 88, 102, 106, 119, 120, 129, 153, 155, 156, 166, 167, 179, 193, 194, 204, 209, 229, 259, 261, 263, 266, 269, 279, 291, 311, 320

fingernails   24, 158, 277

fire   49, 59, 60, 62, 64, 66-68, 74, 75, 80, 85, 88, 90, 97, 98, 102, 105, 108, 114-117, 130, 135, 144, 147, 152, 155, 156, 167, 169, 185, 186, 194, 195, 195, 199, 221, 223, 224, 225, 229, 248, 254, 265, 268, 270, 277, 285, 296, 298, 299, 301

fish   16, 70, 108, 109, 194, 262, 271, 272, 276

food & foodways   20, 65, 105, 190, 197, 218, 264, 265, 267, 269, 332

foundering   156, 269

four elements   114, 115, 229, 265

Frantz, Rev. Orville R.   40

Frauentraum (see Dream, Our Dear Lady's)

Frederick III the Wise   63, 65

Friend in Need (*Freund in der Noth*)   20, 134, 148, 152, 162, 258, 263, 307, 315, 317, 332

Furst, Anna Maria   101

gambling   274, 275, 277

Garden of Eden   112, 149, 197

Gertrude, St.   267, 327

Goeb, Friedrich   157, 315, 316, 317, 331

Good Friday   9, 23, 105, 106, 139, 156, 210, 218, 223, 258, 259, 266, 268, 270, 275, 327

Good Friday egg   9, 23, 105, 106, 270, 327

Gospel of Nicodemus   144, 148, 149, 160, 205, 310, 317, 333

grain   158, 202, 266, 270

grave (see graveyard)

gravestone (see tombstone)

graveyard (cemetery, *Gottes Acker*)   42, 57, 95, 105, 106, 149, 166, 185, 280, 281, 316, 318, 319, 320, 324, 325

Green Thursday   23, 101, 105, 199, 275, 288

ground-ivy   91, 103, 206, 207, 208

Grumbine, Ezra   226, 227, 307, 313, 315, 321, 323, 326, 327, 328, 329

guns (see shooter's blessings)

Gypsy King   90, 134, 308

Hageman, Heinrich H.   231-234

Hageman, Joseph H.   9, 35, 50, 69, 179, 180, 227, 231-242, 308, 324, 332

Hain, Peter and Samuel   203, 204, 223, 271, 321, 328, 329

hair   24, 38, 73, 93, 99, 106, 109, 149, 156, 186, 188, 189, 190, 209, 211, 228, 230, 244, 246-248, 260, 265, 280, 281

hands   14, 33, 34, 41, 45, 60, 68, 69, 81, 101-103, 106, 112, 120, 121, 122, 125, 139, 143, 146, 156, 161, 165-167, 186, 209, 218, 224, 235, 241, 243, 249, 260, 261, 271, 273, 277, 279, 286, 313, 314, 334

harrow   204, 205, 300

hazel   86, 103, 177, 183, 218, 219, 259, 295

339

heaven   25, 26, 34, 59, 60, 63, 73,-77, 81, 85, 89-91, 95, 103, 110, 114, 125, 129, 130, 135, 136, 139, 141, 144, 145, 147, 148, 150, 152, 160, 164, 173, 178, 182, 224, 227, 240, 241, 262, 265, 266, 280, 281, 283, 285, 290, 293, 295, 296, 299, 303, 304, 333, 334

Heilman, Betz   176, 177, 185, 194, 335

Helfenstein, Georg Friedrich   127, 141-146, 153, 161-164, 167-169, 192, 194, 204-207, 224, 271, 284, 285, 307, 313-318, 320, 321, 323, 328, 329, 333

hell   75, 130, 152, 164, 183, 192, 205, 220, 223-225, 240, 299, 300

Henninger, Johann Georg   128, 129, 163, 219, 220, 310, 313, 315, 318, 322

herbs   86, 154, 197, 198, 200, 203, 204, 206, 207, 212, 213, 214, 2116, 231-234, 277, 278, 300, 311, 317

hernia   141, 211, 270, 287

Hess, Catherine Schmidt   49, 51, 309

Hess, Wilbert   230, 244-250

Heym, Paul   217, 218, 322

hex sign (see barn star)

Hexenhammer (see Malleus Maleficarum)

Hexenkopf Hill   106-108, 144, 174, 314, 333

Hexerei   19, 27, 70, 127, 152, 171, 173, 175-195, 208, 248, 249, 253, 254, 2690, 269, 274, 311, 314, 319

Himmelsbrief   Himmelsriegel (see Bolts of Heaven)   75, 76, 311, 327, 332

Hohman, Catharina   146, 151

Hohman, Johann Georg (John George)   45, 54, 81, 97, 134, 135, 141, 146-155, 158-164, 166-170, 178, 191, 192, 208, 221, 222, 230, 244, 246, 247, 258, 261, 263, 264, 307, 310, 311, 313-319, 321, 333, 334, 335, 336

hooligans   277

hoopoe   140, 261, 275, 276

Horati, Pleni   139, 141, 148, 150

horse   14, 23, 28, 38, 45, 46, 49, 87, 89, 91, 92, 93, 103, 104, 105, 110, 112, 116, 129, 144, 145, 146, 148, 154, 155, 156, 166, 177, 178, 185, 193, 203, 204, 209, 223, 224, 225, 241, 254, 259, 268, 269, 271, 272, 278, 298, 302-305, 312, 318, 320

horse collar   259, 268

horseshoe   105, 177, 185, 223-225, 278, 298, 316

house blessing   76, 97, 182, 183

hunting   16, 104, 152, 153, 160, 194, 195, 272-274, 276, 277

hymn   28, 60, 127, 129, 131, 259

inflammaton   38, 60, 85, 88, 92, 102, 104, 108, 115, 116, 119, 121, 137, 156, 198, 199, 203, 205, 206, 220, 278, 281

inquisition   16, 66, 68, 71

INRI (Jesus Nazarenus Rex Judeorum)   23, 69, 79, 100, 152, 178, 204, 241

iron   60, 65, 177, 182, 195, 215, 219, 223, 225, 228, 267, 298, 316

Job, Book of   34, 81, 308, 311

John, the Evangelist   69, 71, 79, 90, 106, 188, 125, 144, 145, 146, 240, 293, 301, 304, 306, 307, 314

Jung, Maria   54, 57, 294, 296, 306

Jungman, Gottlob   134, 136, 147, 327

Kauffman, Johann   131, 132, 135, 315, 328

knife   13, 129, 198, 219, 220-223, 271, 315, 322

knothole   271

Koch, Rev. Kurt   253, 254

Krall, Nathan Fernsler   104, 311, 313

Lancaster County   35, 45-47, 69, 110, 112, 113, 131, 132, 154, 160, 179, 192, 203, 204, 206, 213, 225, 229, 234, 240, 253, 280, 308, 309, 311, 315, 317, 320, 321, 324, 327

Landis, Gerald   219-222

Laydom, Levi   47, 48, 157, 158, 309, 313, 317

laying on of hands   33, 41, 103, 125, 241, 243

Lebanon County   13, 18, 20, 28, 34, 35, 40, 104, 109-111, 114, 120, 122, 124, 179, 182, 185, 193, 199, 204, 209, 210, 217, 220, 223, 225, 226, 266, 307, 308, 311, 313, 315, 320-322, 327

Lehigh County   14, 40, 54, 136, 153, 179, 181, 183, 199, 202, 224, 227, 228, 231, 241, 251, 260, 266, 267, 270-272, 277, 278, 308, 314, 316, 320, 322, 327, 328

Leib, Isaac   110, 312, 334

Leininger, Sophia Fessler   51, 52, 193

Length of Christ (*Laenge Christi*)   72, 118, 119

Length of Mary (*Laenge Maria*)   72, 73

Livergrown (colic, *Aagewaxe*)   28, 34, 89, 119, 237, 259, 289, 291, 303, 304

Long Lost Friend (*Lange Verborgene Freund*)   45, 81, 97, 127, 141, 146-148, 151, 152, 154, 155, 159-164, 166, 167, 169, 170, 221, 222, 230, 244, 246, 247, 307, 316, 319, 328, 333, 334

Long, Henry Schuler   39

Lord's Prayer   60, 69, 81, 87, 129, 219

Luke, the Evangelist   28, 106, 240

Luther, Dr. Martin   60-65, 70, 73, 93, 179, 307, 310, 321, 328, 333, 334, 335, 336

Lutheran   13, 18, 29, 39, 40, 41, 49, 60-65, 70, 73, 93, 105, 109, 120, 124, 129, 141, 146, 154, 155, 157, 179, 188, 240, 248, 253, 268, 307, 308, 309, 310, 312, 315, 318, 320, 321, 323, 328, 331-336

magic   18, 19, 30, 31, 62, 65, 66, 82, 84, 116, 127, 138, 162, 168, 169, 171, 179, 181, 203, 218, 221, 234, 246, 258, 307, 315, 317, 319, 332-336

Malleus Maleficarum (*Hexenhammer*)   68, 69, 186, 335

Man of Signs   102

mandrake   212, 213, 322

manure   107, 205, 206

manuscript   14, 15, 17, 20, 21, 29, 37, 47, 48, 54, 77, 79-90, 92-96, 102, 110, 114, 127, 129-131, 133-136, 140, 145, 154, 155, 157, 158, 162, 171, 184, 203, 204, 207, 210, 219, 220, 271, 272, 274-278, 308-315, 317, 318, 320, 321, 328, 332, 335

Marasmus (*Abnemme*)   33, 40, 85, 119, 237, 239, 240

Mark, the Evangelist   21, 79, 88, 106, 112, 113, 143, 144, 161, 168, 286, 311, 312, 314, 316, 318

marriage   67, 107, 141, 203, 220, 220, 260, 261, 275

Mary, the Virgin   59-63, 69, 70, 72, 76, 81, 86, 88, 90, 139, 153, 198, 199, 207, 240, 241, 266, 272, 278, 281, 294, 296, 301, 306

Matilda, St.   60, 144, 149, 150, 310

Matthew, the Evangelist   34, 79, 106, 110, 120, 125, 145, 168, 240, 271, 286, 304, 308, 314, 315, 323

Maundy Thursday (See Green Thursday)

May   91, 158, 174, 177, 260, 272

men   34, 67, 68, 193, 195, 216, 274-276

Mennig, Rev. Georg P.   39, 65, 98, 115, 116, 118, 119, 156, 308, 314

Mennonites   18, 29, 199, 267, 313, 316, 333

menopause   277, 278

menstruation   60, 115, 123, 143, 269, 277, 310, 315, 326

mice   158, 267

midwifery   135-138, 140, 212, 315

milk   63, 65, 86, 145, 175-177, 183, 184, 186, 198, 206, 207, 217, 219, 220, 222, 246, 260, 267, 268, 271, 277, 300, 304

Montgomery County   18, 39, 105, 159, 183, 213, 216, 217, 327, 335

moon   13, 15, 23-26, 37, 42, 45, 47, 102, 103, 105, 106, 114, 120, 135, 153, 154, 156, 157, 158, 166, 191, 201, 202, 209, 210, 211, 218, 219, 222, 227, 234, 252, 259, 260, 265, 266, 268, 270, 272, 274, 278, 290, 303, 306, 313

Moses   111, 116, 127, 217, 229

Moses, Sixth and Seventh Books (see *Sixth and Seventh Books of Moses*)

Mountain Bummy   (see Bumbaugh, Lamar)

Mountain Mary   54-57, 197, 309

Moravian (denomination)   29, 162, 275, 276, 329, 335

Moyer, Lilly A.   136, 137

murmele   82

Murray, Rufus   47, 245

Northampton County   93, 95, 96, 106-108, 130, 131, 136, 144, 147, 157, 158, 160, 162, 174, 179, 209, 225, 251, 266, 312-316, 321

Northumberland County   141-143, 164, 168, 284, 313, 318, 319

Oley   25, 37, 38, 39, 54, 56, 57, 147, 197, 208, 240, 245, 308, 319, 320, 322, 323, 335

onion   26, 103, 203, 224, 267, 299

Ontario   24, 146, 203, 307, 310, 311, 313, 327, 336

oral tradition   14, 16, 17, 23, 25, 26, 28, 29, 49, 81, 83, 91, 100, 116, 122, 127, 129, 130, 131, 151, 179, 257, 271, 307, 314

Ossman & Steel's Guide to Health   160, 163-167, 318, 320, 328, 329

Ossman, Ann   164

outhouse   107, 259, 271

Ozarks   24, 209, 321

parsley   199, 259, 272

patriarchs   59, 60, 149

Paul, St., the Apostle   101, 112, 143-146, 192, 199, 229, 274, 294, 297, 300, 303, 304, 323

payment   27, 34, 35, 71, 124, 125,

pelican   59, 140

Pennsylvania Dutch language   13, 17, 18, 20, 21, 47, 130, 175, 225, 255, 258, 326

penny   26, 108, 125, 263

peony   359

pig   33, 99, 108, 156, 261, 271, 278

pin   185, 209

placebo   109

plantain, broadleaf   47, 201, 205, 206

planting   24, 124, 149, 258, 265-267, 269, 277, 281

plug   104, 204, 205,

plugging, tree   158, 209-212, 228, 321

potato   13, 15, 23-26, 33, 42, 43, 47, 99, 104, 106, 202, 215, 244, 246, 265-267, 271, 278, 327

protection   15, 18, 21, 23, 35, 46, 47, 54, 61, 62, 66, 69, 71, 74-77, 79-81, 85, 92, 97, 100, 105, 110, 122, 129, 130, 135, 141, 145-147, 150, 153, 160, 161, 166, 171, 178, 182, 195, 205, 212, 217, 219, 222-228, 232, 236, 251, 258, 263, 270, 272, 274, 276, 277, 281, 283, 284, 305, 311, 320

rabbit   187, 275

Raber, Conrad   102, 103, 202, 269, 270, 313, 327, 332

Raber, Rev. William B.   40, 41, 308, 335

ramp (wild leek)   177, 204, 277

Reading, PA   35, 40, 42, 43, 49, 50, 51, 69, 77, 79, 134-136, 146-152, 155, 157, 160, 162, 163, 180, 191, 203, 204, 222, 231, 232, 234-238, 240, 242, 245, 251, 254, 271, 273, 274, 307-311, 316-320, 322-327, 329, 331-335

reciprocity   27, 43, 124, 190, 208

red string   115-118, 259, 268, 311, 320, 283

Reformed (denomination)   18, 20, 29, 39, 40, 60, 65, 94, 112, 113, 119, 141, 192, 232M, 268, 308, 324, 333, 335

Rehmeyer, Nelson D.   47, 169, 230, 231, 240, 244-251, 253, 319, 325

Reppert, William   28, 33-35, 124, 308

Rex, Dennis   9, 241-244, 315, 324, 325, 329

Rhine River   29, 91, 129, 130, 328

Ritter, Johann   134, 147, 315, 333

ritual   19, 23, 24, 29, 30, 31, 33, 99-125, 175, 215, 257-281

Ritual Arts (*Kunst-Stücke*)   133-135, 141, 147, 315

Roman Catholicism   19, 29, 31, 37, 39, 40, 60, 61, 63-65, 70-72, 75, 77, 80, 87, 88, 90, 91, 129, 130, 138, 146-148, 163, 168, 173, 181, 224, 225, 264, 266, 268, 311

Romanus-Büchlein   80, 81, 83, 85, 86, 97, 127, 138, 139, 145, 150, 151, 162, 173, 192, 208, 221, 307, 310, 311, 317, 318, 321, 331, 336

Ruhkbrief (Letter of Rest)   191, 192, 320

Ruhkschtee (Stone of Rest)   225-227, 323

Russian Germans (see Volga-Deitsch)

Ruth, Book of   260

Sage, Heinrich B.   147, 150,151, 155, 200, 308, 315, 317

saint   16, 20, 26, 31, 50-52, 54, 57, 59, 60, 62, 63, 66, 69, 70, 71, 72, 76, 77, 79, 80, 81, 86, 98, 100, 106, 108, 130, 138, 139, 145, 146, 149, 150, 157, 163, 198, 199, 205, 207, 224, 225, 237, 260, 264-267, 269, 272, 281, 283, 286, 308-310, 321, 324, 327

salt   13, 64, 70, 103, 105, 108, 191, 204, 205, 207, 224, 238, 265, 275, 292, 295, 300

saltpeter   166, 213

sator square palindrome   37, 38, 95-97, 133, 135, 139, 152, 155, 259, 312

Sauer, Christopher   197, 205, 206, 321

Saylor, Peter   107, 144, 209, 312, 321

Schuylkill County   13, 18, 20, 38-40, 51, 52, 117, 120, 143, 159, 164, 168, 188, 191, 217, 128, 224, 251, 252, 263, 266, 309, 314, 319, 321, 322

Secrets of Sympathy   21, 84, 127, 141-143, 146, 161, 164, 167, 224, 284-306, 313, 315, 316, 319SEED   125, 132, 149, 197, 202, 220, 258, 267, 301

serpent (snake)   5, 49, 65, 87, 90, 94, 110-112, 116, 132, 159, 165, 194, 216-219, 228, 234, 252, 268, 272, 273, 292, 293, 314, 322, 328, 336

snakeroot   199, 201

Seven Seals (*Sieben Schloss*)   76, 77

sewing   166, 262, 268, 278, 326

Shamokin, PA   141, 143, 167, 168, 316, 318, 319

Shaner, Richard   9, 228, 229, 311, 323

Shively, John   130, 131, 315

Shoemaker, Dr. Alfred L.   168, 177, 178, 307, 315, 319, 321, 328

shooter's blessing   195, 273, 274

Sixth and Seventh Books of Moses (*Moses, Sixth and Seventh Books*)   47, 161, 171-173, 209, 245, 252, 253, 307, 308, 315, 319, 326

skull   171, 173, 195, 208, 246, 319

Slatedale, PA   105, 241, 242, 244

smoke   103, 108, 116, 117, 207, 274

snake (see serpent)

Soli Deo Gloria (see *Secrets of Sympathy*)

sorcery   19, 29, 62, 65, 66, 69, 71, 77, 79, 80, 82, 84, 90, 125, 138, 139, 162, 173, 175, 183, 186, 189, 192-194, 203, 204, 240, 271, 300, 301, 304, 310

Spangenberg, Johannes Ernst   93-97, 273, 308, 328

Spiritual Shield (*Geistliche Schild*)   35, 77, 79, 80, 81, 83, 84, 150, 163, 171-173, 236, 237, 253, 311, 315, 317

Springer, Marty   45-48, 308

Stecher, Johannes   94-96, 312, 328

Steel, Isaac D.   164-167, 275, 318, 320, 328, 329

stone   7, 23, 26, 49, 65, 76, 86, 88, 100, 102-105, 113, 130, 140, 143, 144, 156, 166, 182, 208, 215, 225-227, 244, 268, 271, 273, 281, 293, 302, 316, 317

string   45, 72, 98, 103, 104, 115, 116, 117, 118, 119, 211, 215, 259, 268, 274, 275, 277, 280, 311, 329

sun   23, 33, 45, 65, 90, 102, 103, 105, 108, 114, 120, 122, 124, 129, 135, 139, 144, 154, 159, 167, 177, 184, 188, 191, 194, 201, 205, 206, 208, 209, 210, 211, 218, 220, 227, 234, 260, 265, 268, 272, 277, 281, 292, 296, 301, 303, 328

sweeny   26, 85, 130, 104, 156, 209, 269, 292, 303, 321

Switzerland   29, 80, 135, 225, 253, 254, 267

Swope, Harry Edward   43, 44, 45, 308

table   15, 27, 34, 36, 63, 65, 100, 104, 120, 124, 141, 150, 154, 259, 268, 269, 328

baptismal certificate (*Taufschein*)   93, 94, 146, 157, 279, 317, 329

Teacle, Joseph Littleton   46

teething   105, 188, 259

thief-blessing (*Dieb-Segen*)   66, 224, 225, 271, 272, 299, 310

Three Cross Knife (*Drei Kreitzer Messer*)   129, 219, 220, 221, 222, 223, 322

Three Kings (Magi)   60, 61, 64, 65, 70, 76, 90, 102, 106, 143, 221, 222, 259, 269, 327

Three Lillies Blessing   280, 281

Three Roses Blessing   129, 153, 280, 281

Three Things Ritual   105, 264, 265, 270, 313

tombstone   39, 120, 279-281, 312, 320, 325

toothache   62, 85, 92, 156, 158, 209, 281, 321

tree   46, 49, 67, 90, 130, 144, 149, 158, 160, 166, 197, 198, 199, 208, 209, 210, 211, 212, 218, 228, 259, 265, 270, 274, 275, 278, 292

Trinity   23, 59, 60, 81, 90, 100, 105, 106, 110, 116, 120, 141, 145, 146, 160, 168, 169, 211, 217, 219, 224, 229, 239, 268, 278, 286, 292, 294, 297, 299, 301, 302, 305, 319

trough, pig   33, 99, 261

Tulpehocken, Berks County   102, 116, 137, 202, 313

tumors   35, 45, 65, 104, 278, 280, 281, 329

urine   85, 166, 191, 211, 300, 318

veterinary medicine   109, 112, 127, 145, 146, 226, 328

Victorialis (*Allermansharnisch*)   203, 204, 319

Volga-Deitsch (Russian Germans)   125

votive   85, 223, 225, 264

wagon   45, 99, 155, 158, 241, 242, 244, 266

warts   23, 24, 25, 26, 33, 35, 37, 38, 42, 43, 47, 105, 108, 109, 124, 141, 148, 153, 155, 157, 158, 166, 202, 211, 248, 253, 264, 281, 292, 315, 318, 329

water   13, 49, 60, 64, 65, 66, 75, 77, 80, 86, 97, 104, 105, 108, 114-116, 118, 120, 121, 129, 135, 139, 143, 144, 152, 158, 177, 178, 190-192, 194, 198, 205, 206, 211, 226, 228, 229, 241, 244, 247, 253, 259, 260, 265, 268-272, 274-278, 292, 296, 300, 303, 306, 310, 311, 327

Weaver, William Woys   9, 20, 97, 214, 320, 321, 322, 328

whooping cough (*Blohe Huschde*)   35, 45, 46

wildfire (see erysipelas)

Wilhelm, Jacob   93, 94, 95, 96, 107, 312, 328

Wilhelm, John Henry   105, 313, 321

wine   19, 59, 85, 87, 101, 108, 109, 143, 149, 215, 216, 258, 259, 275, 278, 288, 294, 297, 318

witch bottle   145, 190-192, 316

witch trials   66-70, 176, 191

witchcraft   19, 27, 47, 66- 71, 82, 83, 107, 108, 139, 141, 145, 152, 175- 177, 179, 183, 185, 186, 188- 192, 194, 203, 206, 218-221, 228, 240, 241, 248- 250, 254, 255, 261, 262, 308, 310, 314, 319- 325, 326

Wittgenstein   82, 310

wolf-blessing (*Wolf-Segen*)   272

women   18, 28, 29, 51, 60, 65, 66, 66, 67, 68, 72, 84, 90, 123, 135, 136, 138, 143, 144, 149, 150, 169, 176, 189, 194, 195, 198, 203, 213, 221, 234, 237, 238, 241, 242, 251, 253, 254, 267, 269, 270, 276, 277, 293, 310, 315

worm-blessing (*Würm-Segen*)   66, 92, 144, 153, 281

wound-wood   154, 158

Yoder, Don   5, 20, 21, 32, 42, 52, 61, 69, 82, 98, 117, 118, 120, 123, 174, 216, 228, 283, 307, 308, 309, 310, 311, 312, 313, 314, 315, 316, 317, 318, 319, 320, 321, 323, 324, 326, 328, 329

York County   13, 38, 47, 56, 101, 135, 155, 169, 185, 199, 203, 225, 230, 231, 240, 244, 245, 246, 248, 249, 250, 253, 254, 273, 309, 312, 315, 320, 325, 326, 328

Zigeuner-Buch   81, 151, 317, 321

zodiac   102, 265, 266

Zwalley, Isaac W.   35, 308

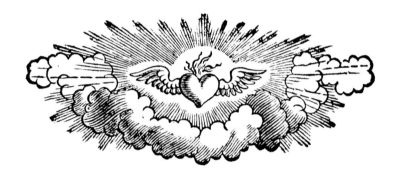